INTERPRETATION OF BREAST BIOPSIES

Fourth Edition

Biopsy Interpretation Series

BIOPSY INTERPRETATION SERIES

Series Editor: Jonathan I. Epstein, M.D.

Prostate Biopsy Interpretation, Third Edition
Jonathan I. Epstein and Ximing J. Yang, 2002, 320 Pages

Interpretation of Breast Biopsies, Fourth Edition
Darryl Carter, 2002, 440 Pages

INTERPRETATION OF BREAST BIOPSIES

Fourth Edition

Biopsy Interpretation Series

Darryl Carter, M.D.

Professor
Department of Pathology
Yale University School of Medicine;
Attending Pathologist
Yale-New Haven Hospital
New Haven, Connecticut

LIPPINCOTT WILLIAMS & WILKINS
A **Wolters Kluwer** Company
Philadelphia • Baltimore • New York • London
Buenos Aires • Hong Kong • Sydney • Tokyo

Acquisitions Editor: Ruth W. Weinberg
Developmental Editor: Lisa Consoli
Production Editor: Emmeline A. Parker
Manufacturing Manager: Timothy Reynolds
Cover Designer: Karen Quigley
Compositor: Lippincott Williams & Wilkins Desktop Division
Printer: Maple Press

530 Walnut Street
Philadelphia, PA 19106 USA
LWW.com

Printed in the USA

Library of Congress Cataloging-in-Publication Data
Carter, Darryl.
Interpretation of breast biopsies / Darryl Carter.—4th ed.
p.; cm.—(Biopsy interpretation series)
Includes bibliographical references and index.
ISBN 0-7817-3320-0
1. Breast—Cancer—Diagnosis. 2. Breast—Biopsy. I. Title. II. Series.
[DNLM: 1. Breast Diseases—pathology. 2. Biopsy—methods. 3. Breast Neoplasms—pathology. WP 815 C323i 2003]
RC280.B8 C39 2003
616.99′449075—dc21

2002072998

Care has been taken to confirm the accuracy of the information presented and to describe generally accepted practices. However, the author and publisher are not responsible for errors or omissions or for any consequences from application of the information in this book and make no warranty, expressed or implied, with respect to the currency, completeness, or accuracy of the contents of the publication. Application of this information in a particular situation remains the professional responsibility of the practitioner.

The author and publisher have exerted every effort to ensure that drug selection and dosage set forth in this text are in accordance with current recommendations and practice at the time of publication. However, in view of ongoing research, changes in government regulations, and the constant flow of information relating to drug therapy and drug reactions, the reader is urged to check the package insert for each drug for any change in indications and dosage and for added warnings and precautions. This is particularly important when the recommended agent is a new or infrequently employed drug.

Some drugs and medical devices presented in this publication have Food and Drug Administration (FDA) clearance for limited use in restricted research settings. It is the responsibility of the health care provider to ascertain the FDA status of each drug or device planned for use in their clinical practice.

10 9 8 7 6 5 4 3 2 1

To William Miles Shelley, M.D., (1928–1974) who provided the initial stimulus for my interest in the pathology of the breast.

Contents

Preface

Like its predecessors, the Fourth Edition of *Interpretation of Breast Biopsies* is fundamentally a guide to the principles of the surgical pathology of the breast. The focus is on the interpretation of breast histology and its correlation with clinical events. Wherever possible, I have pointed out the borderlines in pathology that have clinical implications, and those that do not, so that one may cross these borders knowing the effect on the patient. The book verbally describes, as well as illustrates in black and white figures and a color insert, the basic histopathology of the breast.

The exciting part of creating the Fourth Edition has been the ability to add over 600 color figures on an accompanying CD, which are noted in the text as (efigs.). This has given me the opportunity to expand the illustrative material so that I could show not only classic histologic features, but also a range of changes acceptable within a given diagnosis. The illustrations in the book and on the CD overlap each other so that one can look at either with some continuity but, obviously, the CD illustrates much more than could be shown in a book of this size. I hope the reader and viewer can use the CD as a reference for comparison with a problem case.

Chapter 1 describes the anatomy and physiology of the breast. Chapter 2 has been extensively rewritten to reflect new information concerning environmental factors, epidemiology, and genetic factors, which have impact on the epidemiology and pathogenesis of breast cancer. Chapter 3 describes biopsy and local treatment of breast cancer ranging from fine needle aspiration to extended mastectomy. Mammography and mammographic-pathologic correlations are described and the increasing role of core needle biopsy is discussed extensively. Frozen sections are done less frequently now but still have a place and they are discussed here. Finally, there is a discussion of the problem of examining margins, their reliability and their value in determining additional treatment.

Chapter 4 describes the intraductal lesions of the breast. As in the previous editions, the features of intraductal carcinoma are described and illustrated in detail so that the student may have a starting point from which to judge the nonmalignant intraductal proliferations. The subclassification of intraductal carcinoma is described and illustrated with an emphasis on the lower grade intraductal carcinomas, primarily the micropapillary type. The distinction between atypical ductal hyperplasia, which is also abundantly illustrated on the CD, and micropapillary DCIS is perhaps our most important problem at present. I have again separated the diffuse intraductal lesions from the localized papillomas and intracystic papillary carcinoma. New information has confirmed that this distinction is important clinically. In Chapter 5, the lobular lesions of the breast are described and illustrated and the problem of distinguishing large areas of lobular carcinoma in situ from bland types of intraductal carcinoma is abundantly illustrated and the clinical implications are described.

Chapter 6 describes the pseudoinfiltrative lesions, including sclerosing adenosis, microglandular adenosis and radial scar. All of these lesions are seen more often as mammography is used with increasing frequency. Chapter 7 describes the adnexal or salivary gland-like tumors that rarely occur in the breast. These include adenomyoepithelioma, pleomorphic adenoma, eccrine spiradenoma, adenoid cystic carcinoma, and collagenous spherulosis.

Chapter 8 is devoted to the description and illustration of the different types of invasive carcinoma of the breast. Chapter 9 is a description of grading and staging and the use of prognostic factors to determine outcome and clinical management of invasive carcinomas. Emphasis is placed on the sentinel lymph node biopsy and its place in determining prognosis. Chapter 9 concludes with the staging criteria currently in use.

Chapter 10 describes the stromal/ glandular and stromal lesions of the breast with emphasis on the problem of distinguishing cellular fibroadenoma from cystosarcoma phyllodes and the intermediate variants. These are illustrated abundantly, particularly on the CD. Vascular tumors of the breast are also illustrated abundantly. Distinction between the relatively few benign vascular tumors and the more frequently observed angiosarcoma, particularly as it occurs in the post-treatment breast, are abundantly illustrated. Metastatic carcinoma to the breast, lymphoma, and the reaction to silicone implants are also described here.

I find myself drawn to the preface of the First Edition, published in 1984, which suggested that the pathologist had become increasingly important as the diagnosis of cancer of the breast moved to earlier stages. Certainly that trend has continued and the pathologist is the pivotal diagnostician for radiologists, surgeons, radiotherapists, and oncologists. Because of that position, it is critical for us as pathologists to understand enough of the principles of treatment to provide meaningful guidance to our clinical colleagues. However, we must recognize that some of the distinctions made histologically can only be done by pathology but have enormous implication in the life of the patient. Better criteria and better support from molecular biology are likely to help us in the near future, but at present, most interpretations of clinical significance must be made with the light microscope. Therefore, the emphasis in this book is on the histology of the breast.

As always, I have been guided by questions asked by residents in Pathology and answers given by the clinical staff at Yale-New Haven Hospital. I hope this Fourth Edition is useful to all of those individuals.

Darryl Carter, M.D.
New Haven, Connecticut

Acknowledgments

I gratefully acknowledge the patience and help of Catherine Haynes in preparing the manuscript for this Fourth Edition and of my wife, Alice, for reading through the manuscript several times and pointing out the many errors which I had made. The book is much better because of her input. Photomicrographs from Drs. Paul Peter Rosen, Maria Merino, and Samuel Orr have been used in all editions and I gratefully acknowledge their use. Staging criteria are published intact with the permission of the American Joint Committee on Cancer (AJCC), Chicago, Illinois. The original source of this material is the *AJCC Cancer Staging Manual*, 5th Edition (1997), published by Lippincott–Raven Publishers, Philadelphia and the *AJCC Cancer Staging Manual,* 6th Edition (2002), Springer, New York.

INTERPRETATION OF BREAST BIOPSIES

Fourth Edition

Biopsy Interpretation Series

1

Anatomy

The breasts, located on the anterior chest wall between the second and seventh ribs, are normally paired organs. The nipples are centrally placed in the midclavicular lines, along which supernumerary nipples may occur. The breast is attached to the dermis by fibrous bands called suspensory (Cooper's) ligaments anteriorly, and the posterior surface is the pectoral fascia. Topographically, the mammary tissue is divided into upper inner, upper outer, lower inner, and lower outer quadrants, the subareolar area, and the axillary tail (of Spence) of the upper outer quadrant, which has as its posterior surface the axillary and serratus anterior fascia. The arterial blood supply is derived from axillary, intercostal, and internal mammary arteries, and venous drainage is into the axillary and internal mammary veins. Lymphatic drainage is to axillary, subclavicular, and internal mammary lymph node groups. From the upper outer quadrant, drainage is predominantly to axillary nodes. From the inner quadrants, drainage is greater to the internal mammary chain of nodes. A high degree of lymphatic overlap allows drainage to multiple lymph node areas. The nerves are branches of the thoracic segmentals.

MICROSCOPIC ANATOMY

The nipple is the focal point of the breast. Characteristically, the skin of the nipple projects 1 to 2 cm out over the skin of the breast to form the areola. Numerous sebaceous glands (the glands of Montgomery) are present within the areolar dermis. Paget's disease occurs in the epidermis of the nipple in association with 1% to 2% of breast cancers and may also involve the lactiferous ductal epithelium (Chapter 4). The nipple dermis and subcutaneous tissue contain circular and radiating smooth muscle bundles that serve to identify the nipple histologically.

Lactiferous ducts course through the nipple dermis and open onto the epidermis. On cross-sections of the nipple, 14 to 24 ducts may be seen (efig. 1.1). They connect the surface of the skin to underlying lactiferous sinuses that are formed by the confluence or dilatation of 14 to 24 collecting ductular units. These units radiate out into the mammary parenchyma and connect the lobules to the nipple (Fig. 1.1). The nipple, superficial to the lactiferous sinus, is rarely the site of neo-

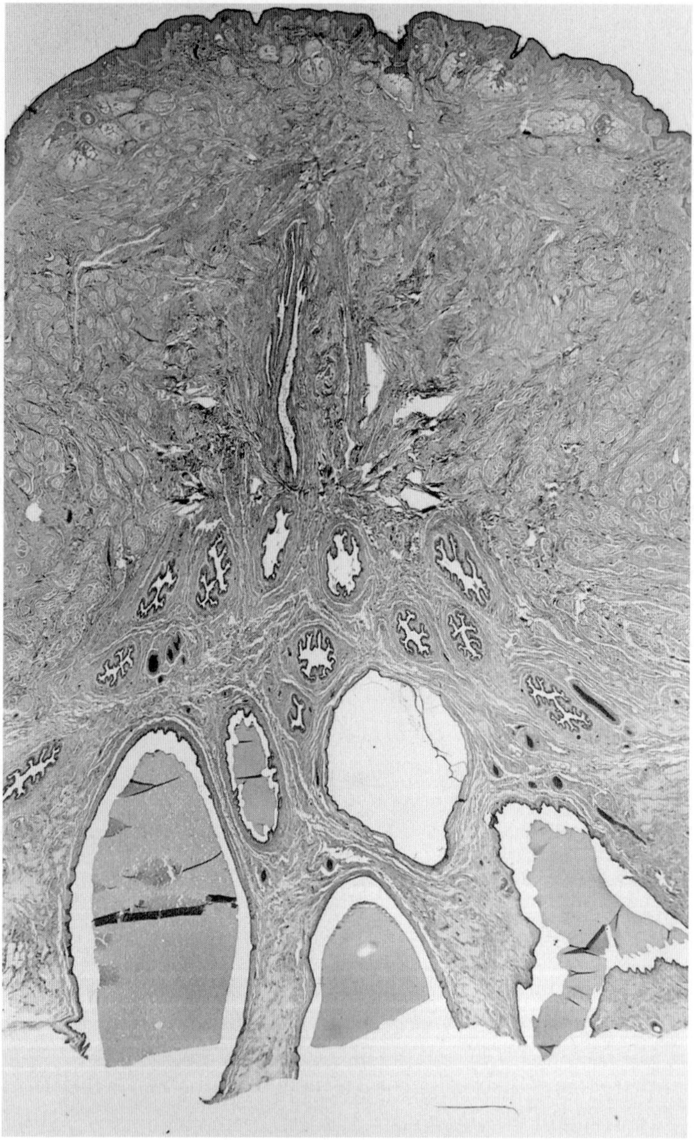

FIG. 1.1. Nipple, in sagittal section, has the deeply located dilated lactiferous sinuses that are connected to the surface by thinner lactiferous ducts. The specialized dermis contains numerous bundles of smooth muscle and prominent sebaceous glands.

plasms similar to adnexal tumors found elsewhere in the skin (e.g., syringomas or nipple adenomas) (Chapter 4). Invasive breast carcinoma infrequently involves the nipple; however, when it does, it is usually late in its course.

Each collecting ductular unit is made up of a large or main duct that progressively branches to form ever smaller branches throughout the interlobular stroma. These ductular units intertwine to make dissection of a single unit difficult, except when the most anterior segment is distended (e.g., in the presence of a papilloma). There is debate over whether the units anastomose normally or when harboring benign or especially malignant proliferations.

Lobules are composed of terminal ducts and acini and their specialized supporting stroma. Although their number has not been established, they are numerous and vary with age, physiologic state, and individual. The terminal duct–lobular unit was described by Wellings et al. (1,2) as the area in which secretion occurs and in which most carcinomas arise. The terminal ducts are either extralobular or intralobular—depending on their location relative to the specialized lobular stroma, which sharply defines the extent of the lobule—often limit inflammation, and participate in cyclic and reactive changes independent of the interlobular stroma (Fig. 1.2, efigs. 1.2 to 1.5). A desmoplasia-like reaction of the lobular stroma often is seen when intraductal carcinoma involves the lobule, making it difficult to distinguish *in-situ* from early invasive carcinoma. A striking fibroblastic reaction also may accompany benign proliferations and atrophy.

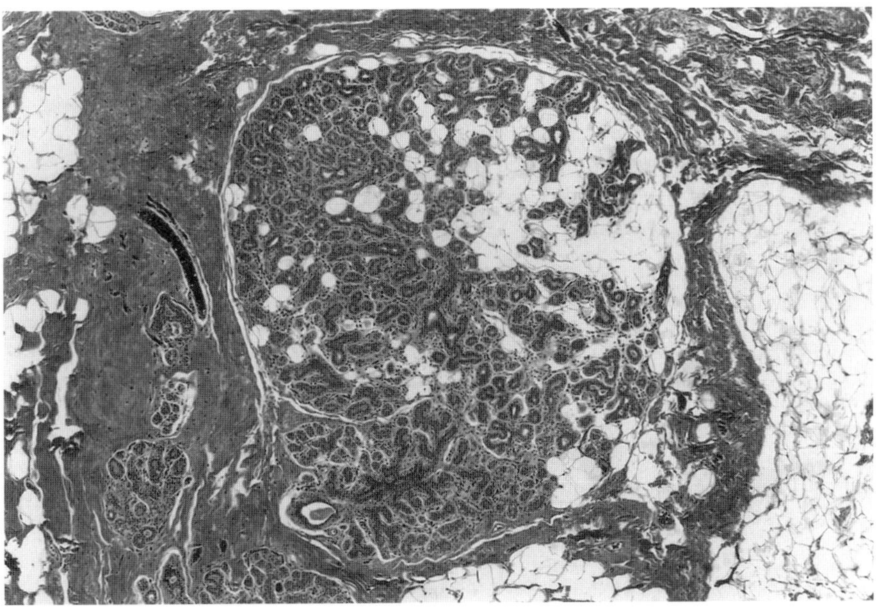

FIG. 1.2. Lobular stroma is distinct and participates in cyclical and reactive changes separate from the interlobular stroma. In this lobule, the stroma is half fatty and half fibrous.

Pseudoinvasive lesions (e.g., sclerosing adenosis) include proliferations of intralobular stroma. The most terminal part of the duct system is the site of secretion and may be referred to as the acinus, although some authors use that term only when lactational changes are present.

Lakhani et al. (3) studied reduction mammoplasty tissue and found loss of heterozygosity in one third of cases and benign areas from mastectomy done for cancer that showed loss of heterozygosity in half of the cases. Identification of loss of heterozygosity in normal lobular units suggested that they might be clonal in origin. Tsai et al. (4), using X-inactivation studies to study both reduction mammoplasty tissue and benign ducts from a mastectomy, found entire lobules and large ducts with the same X chromosome inactivated, suggesting that they were derived from a single progenitor cell. If confirmed, these findings might help to explain the focal nature of lobular changes in the breast and make the definition of neoplastic progression dependent on information other than the demonstration of clonality.

The epithelial elements of the breast are directly supported by specialized periductal and lobular stroma that is distinct from, and bound together by, interlobular stroma that is composed of varying amounts of adipose and fibrous tissue. Before puberty, there is little stroma, and adipose tissue is dominant. During adolescence, there is a marked increase in the amount of stroma with a predominantly fibrous component that becomes more cellular as the lobules develop within it. Virginal hypertrophy is an abundance of fibrous stroma with a dearth of lobular development, histologically similar to gynecomastia. During the postmenopausal period, there is usually a decrease in the cellularity of the stroma, with replacement of dense fibrous stroma with an adipose component, and a corresponding decrease in the number and size of lobules. Decrease in the frequency of lobular units is a better guide to age, but it is also quite variable. Irradiated breasts usually have a marked diminution in the number of lobules.

Mammary epithelium is ectodermally derived and similar in many ways to that of sweat glands. As such, it is composed of an inner epithelial cell layer and an outer myoepithelial layer that separates the epithelial cells from the basement membrane (Fig. 1.3) (5,6). In the resting breast, ductal morphology is similar from the collecting ducts to the lobules (Figs. 1.4 to 1.7) (7,8). The terminal ducts are arranged in two cell layers—a centrally placed layer of columnar cells that line the lumen and a continuous layer of myoepithelial cells between the columnar cells and basement membrane. Ultrastructurally, the columnar cells contain microvilli on their luminal surface and are joined to adjacent columnar cells by desmosomes located along their lateral borders (Fig. 1.4). Their cytoplasm may contain secretory granules, mitochondria, and rough endoplasmic reticulum. An "intracellular lumen"—a lumen surrounded by cytoplasm into which microvilli project—may be seen in the apical cytoplasm and might represent an invagination of the surface. Intracellular lumens may become markedly distended to form a signet-ring configuration of the nucleus, especially in lobu-

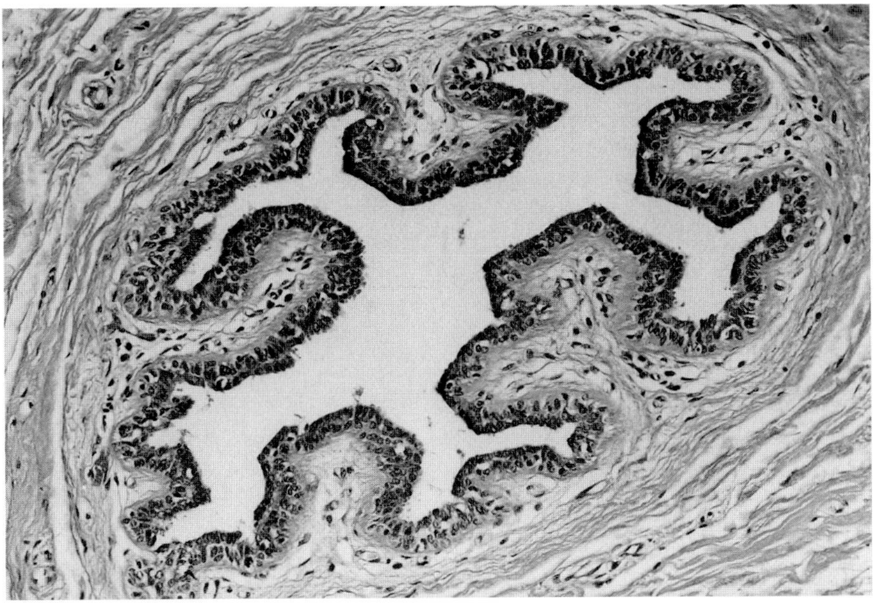

FIG. 1.3. Large collecting duct. This collapsed duct has a layer of epithelial cells bordering the central lumen and a layer of clear or myoepithelial cells adjacent to the basement membrane. It is invested with a distinct layer of fibrous stroma.

lar neoplasia and invasive lobular carcinoma (Fig. 1.5) (9). Myoepithelial cells are rounded or elongated cells attached to the basement membrane by hemidesmosomes with cytoplasm filled with intermediate filaments, shown immunohistochemically to be smooth muscle (Figs. 1.5 and 1.6). Immunohistochemical demonstration of the myoepithelium with antibodies to smooth muscle indicates integrity of the basement membrane and therefore absence of invasion.

Rudland (10) described subtle immunohistochemical differences between the epithelial cells of large ducts, lobular ducts, and acini. Ferguson (11) found mitotic activity of the nonlactating breast limited to the epithelial cells of the lobule. Russo and Russo (12) found the highest growth fraction in cells in the intralobular terminal duct.

When immunohistochemistry is employed, epithelial cells are usually well decorated when antibody to epithelial membrane antigen (EMA)—an antibody raised against a membrane component of a breast cancer cell line—is used, whereas myoepithelial cells are decorated when antibodies to smooth muscle actin or calponin are used. S-100 protein may be localized to the epithelial cells and/or myoepithelial cells, and different molecular weight keratins are variably distributed between the two cell types. Keratin 7 can reliably be found in both benign and malignant duct cells. Cells with apocrine metaplasia characteristically show intense granular cytoplasmic staining with many anti-

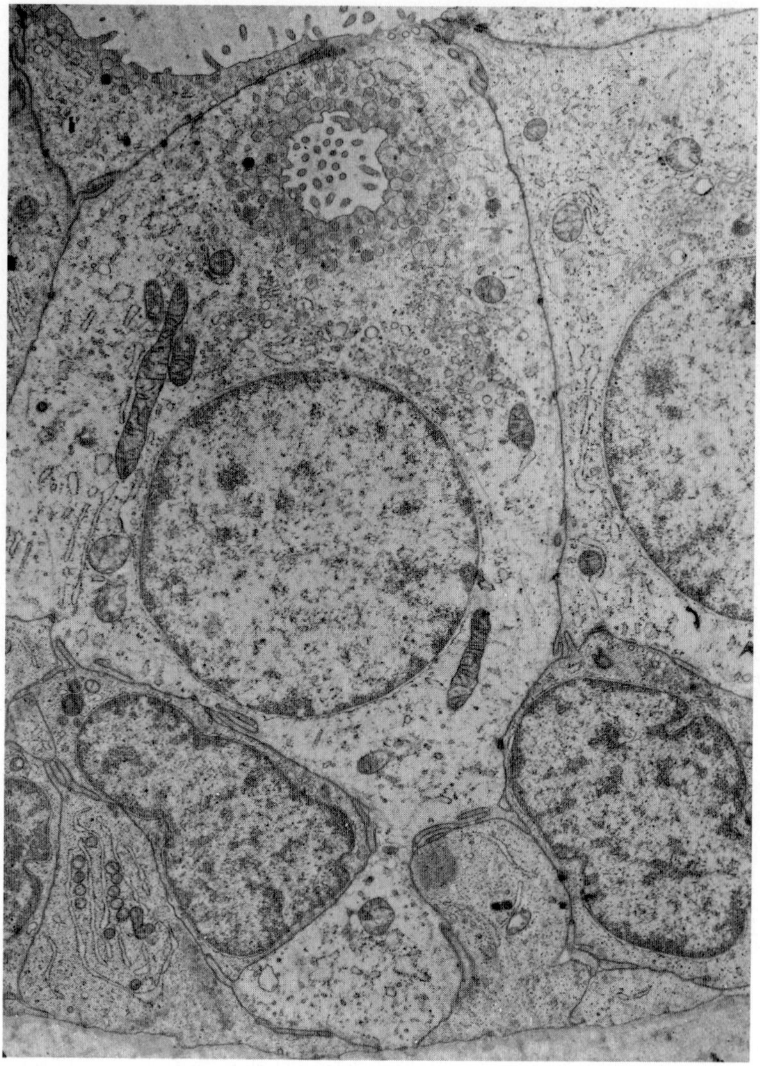

FIG. 1.4. Ultrastructure of normal terminal duct. The two cell layers are evident in this low-magnification electron micrograph. The columnar cell (**upper part**) is differentiated toward the luminal surface, with short microvilli projecting into the extracellular lumen. A vacuole-like intracellular lumen, into which microvilli project, is in the apical cytoplasm. The columnar cells are joined by desmosomal attachments in the long lateral cell border. A layer of more rounded myoepithelial cells (**lower part**) lies between the columnar cells and the basement membrane.

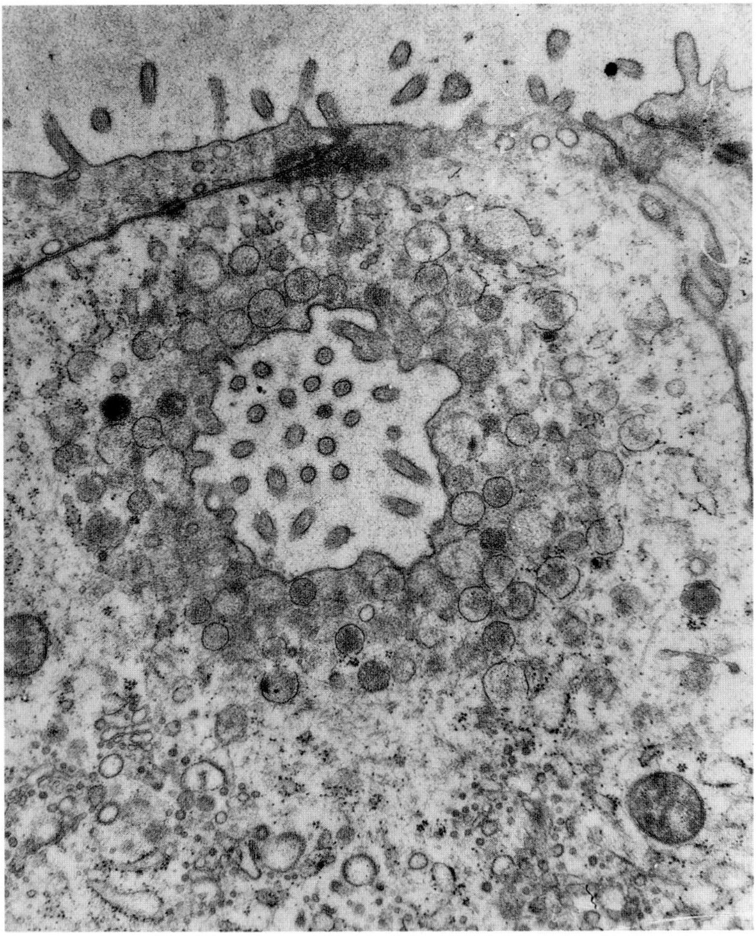

FIG. 1.5. Higher magnification of the epithelial cell shows the "intracellular lumen" in the apical cytoplasm, near the central extracellular lumen. Short stubby microvilli project into it, and the cytoplasm around it contains numerous membrane-bound vacuoles, which are probably secretory in nature. Although not demonstrated, it is possible that this apparently intracellular space connects with the extracellular space in another plane of section. Desmosomal attachments are prominent.

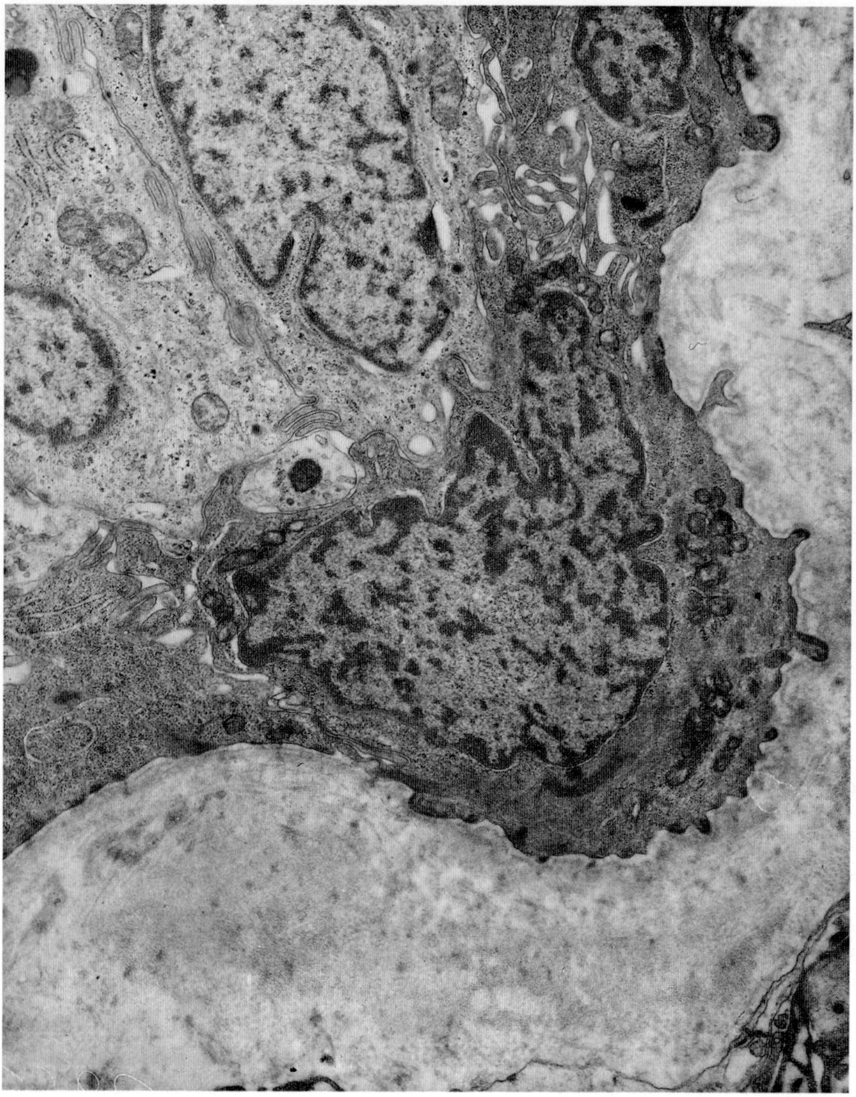

FIG. 1.6. Normal myoepithelial cell with an irregular elongated cell border attached to the basement membrane by hemidesmosomes. The cytoplasm is packed with intermediate filaments.

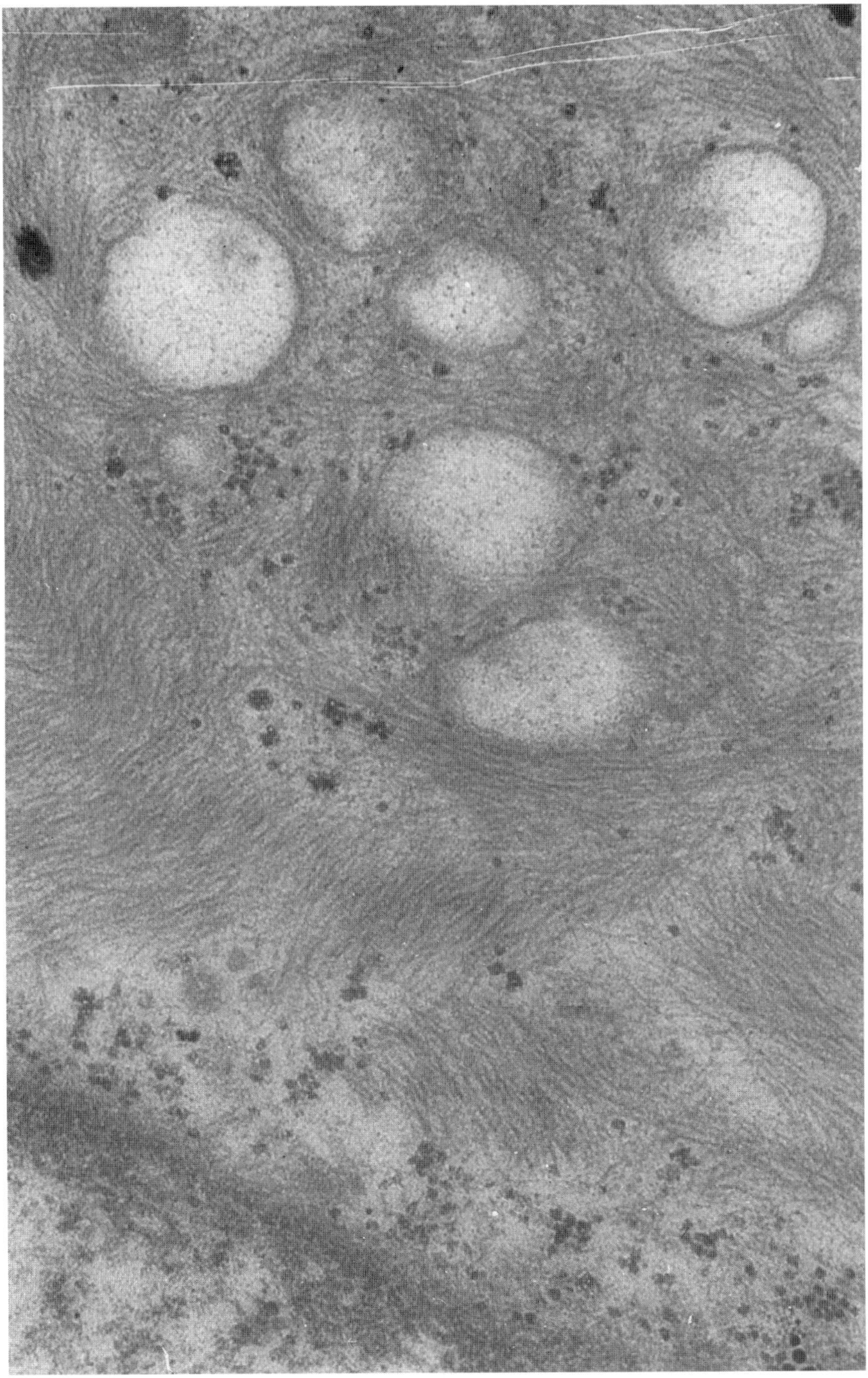

FIG. 1.7. Myoepithelial cell intermediate filaments. At high magnification, the cytoplasm contains numerous bundled intermediate filaments that are immunohistochemically stainable with antibody to smooth muscle.

bodies. Gross cystic disease fluid protein-15 (GCDFP-15) localizes to ductal and lobular epithelium, especially in areas with apocrine metaplasia. Antibodies to lactalbumin localize to terminal ducts, especially during lactation. Columnar cells variably express estrogen and progesterone receptors, but the myoepithelium usually does not.

PHYSIOLOGIC CHANGES

The breast is under the influence of several growth, differentiation, and control factors. In addition to estrogen, progesterone, and prolactin, it is also responsive to testosterone, glucocorticoids, insulin, insulin-like growth factor, growth hormone, and thyroid hormone (13,14). Fanger and Ree (15) and Longacre and Bartow (16) described increasing size of the lobules and their ter-

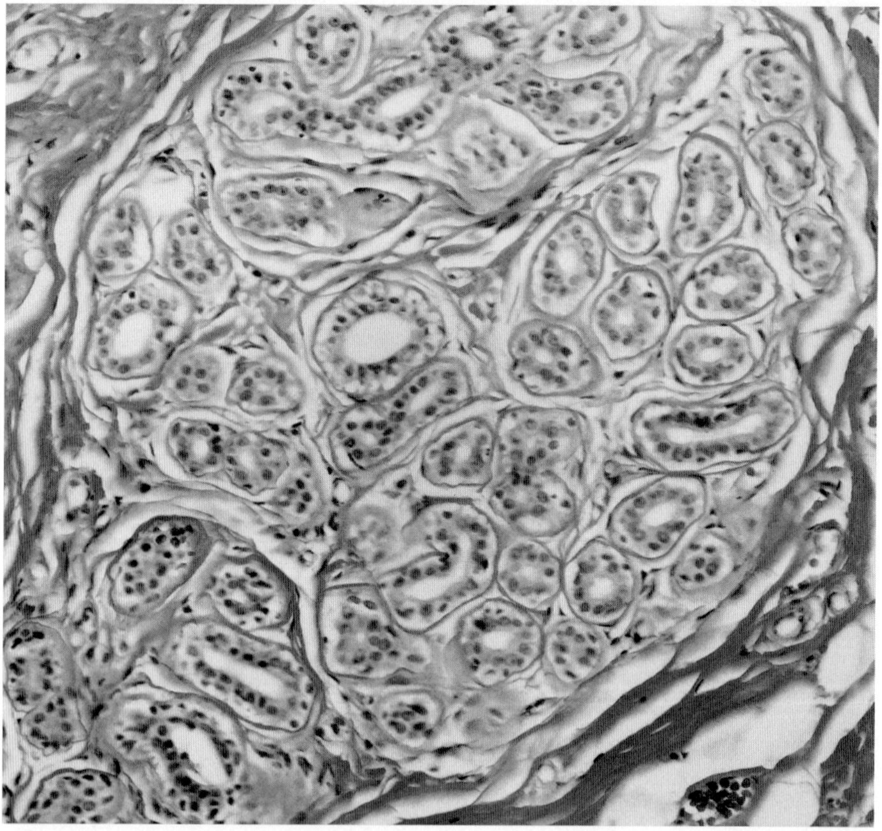

FIG. 1.8. In the early follicular phase, the lobule has dense stroma and a simple epithelium in which only a layer of columnar cells appears inside the basement membrane.

minal ducts with basal vacuolization of the epithelial cells during the secretory phase of the normal menstrual cycle. Stroma and epithelium of the lobule undergo extensive remodeling during the menstrual cycle. In the early follicular phase, the stroma is dense and collagenized and the epithelium is columnar, with only one type of cell apparent (Fig. 1.8). The later follicular phase, described as the "resting breast," is characterized by distinct epithelial and myoepithelial cell types and a dense fibrous lobular stroma. In the luteal phase, the lobular stroma is looser and more myxoid, both epithelial and myoepithelial cell layers are evident, and the acinar lumens are progressively distended with eosinophilic secretion (Fig. 1.9). These changes may not be observed synchronously in all lobules.

The terminal ducts (acini) of the lobular unit contain hormonally responsive cells that undergo secretory change for lactation. The luminal cells undergo marked hyperplasia, with enlargement of nuclei and distension of cytoplasm by one or several large secretory vacuoles, as they differentiate into lactating cells, whereas the myoepithelial component is difficult to find by light microscopy and the stroma becomes markedly attenuated (Figs. 1.10 and 1.11). The nuclei enlarge and, with nucleoli, become extremely prominent so that they have been mistaken for atypical ductal or lobular hyperplasia or even malignancy. With

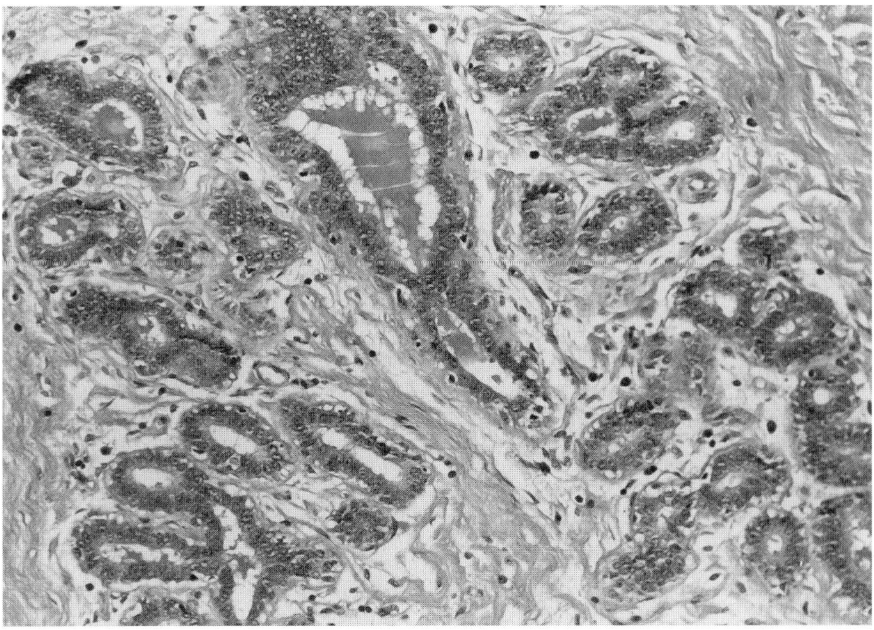

FIG. 1.9. In the late luteal phase, the lobule has a looser (more cellular) stroma and terminal ducts with two cell layers. The extracellular lumina contain eosinophilic secretion.

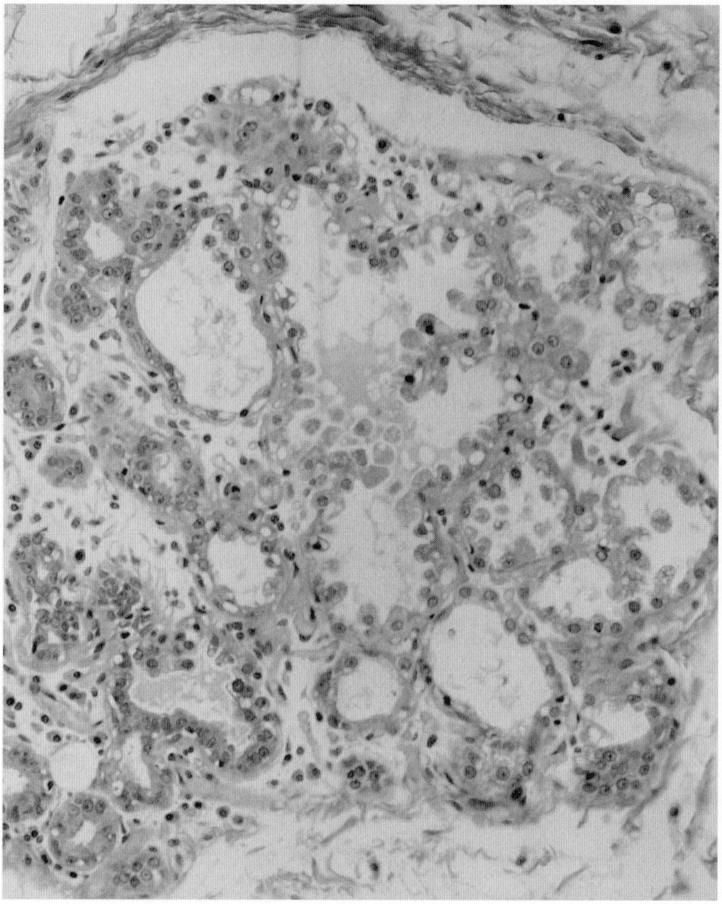

FIG. 1.10. The lactating lobule has been extensively remodeled and is characterized by distended acini that are lined by a single layer of large columnar cells with cytoplasm distended by secretory vacuoles. The myoepithelial layer is not apparent, and the stroma has become so attenuated that the only residual is an occasional capillary.

return to the follicular phase, the secretory cells are shed, the epithelial and myoepithelial layers are rebuilt, and the lobular stroma grows to become densely populated with fibroblasts and collagen. With this extensive variation in form, it is not surprising that minor variations may produce a variety of misshapen lobules with features resembling stromal invasion.

Tavassoli and Yeh (17) described the frequent, but very focal, occurrence of lactational changes in one or several lobules of women who were neither pregnant nor lactating.

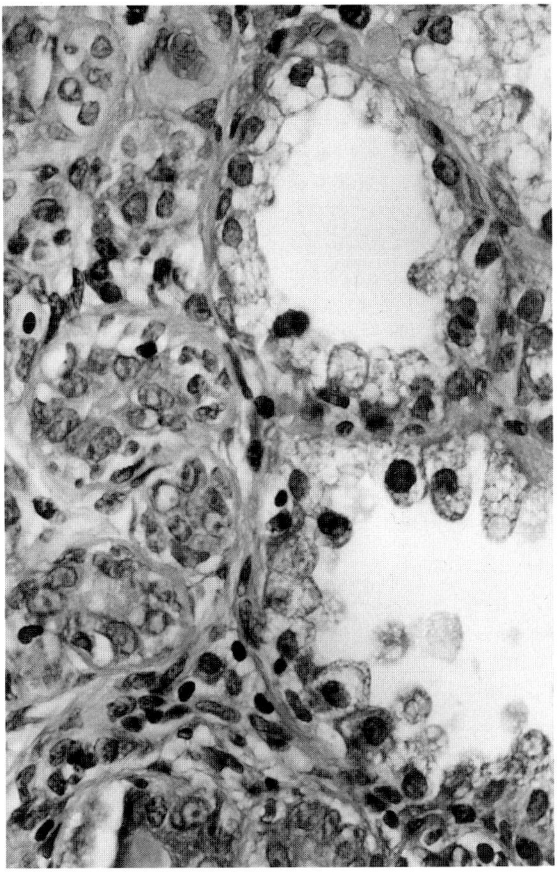

FIG. 1.11. Lactating lobule. At higher magnification, these lactating acini are composed of single layers of markedly vacuolated cells with large nuclei, some with prominent nucleoli. Mitotic figures may be present. The nuclei display a size and shape that might be mistaken for those of atypia, were it not for the vacuolated cytoplasm.

LACTATING ADENOMA

Localized collections of lobules are sometimes delineated from the rest of the breast during pregnancy or lactation, and nodules of lactating lobules may involute less rapidly than the rest of the breast to produce a lactating adenoma (Figs. 1.12 and 1.13). These do not appear to be neoplastic, but they are variations in an otherwise normal physiologic state. O'Hara and Page (18) described formation of lactating adenomas from lactational change within preexisting benign lesions. Fine needle aspirates of these potentially misleading lesions have been described by Grenko et al. (19).

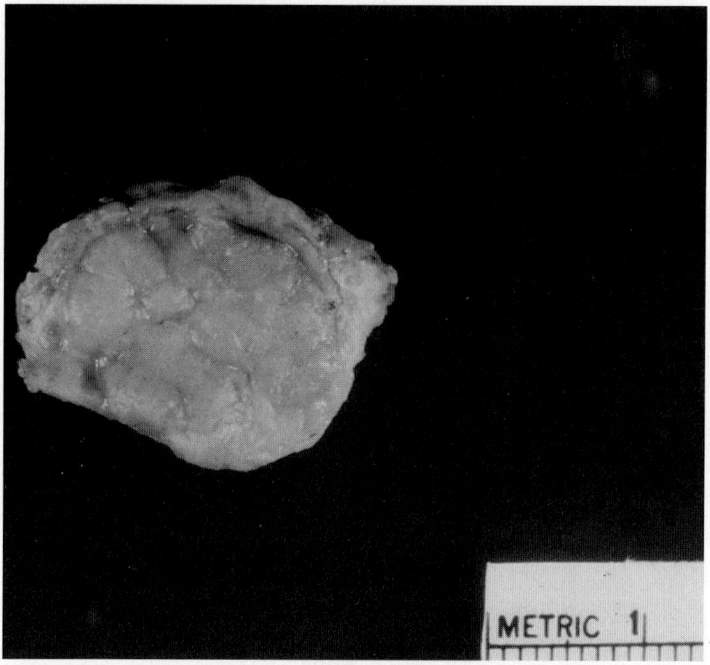

FIG. 1.12. Lactating adenoma. This circumscribed multilobulated nodule was removed from the breast of a lactating woman. Grossly, it was soft and pale and exuded milk when cut.

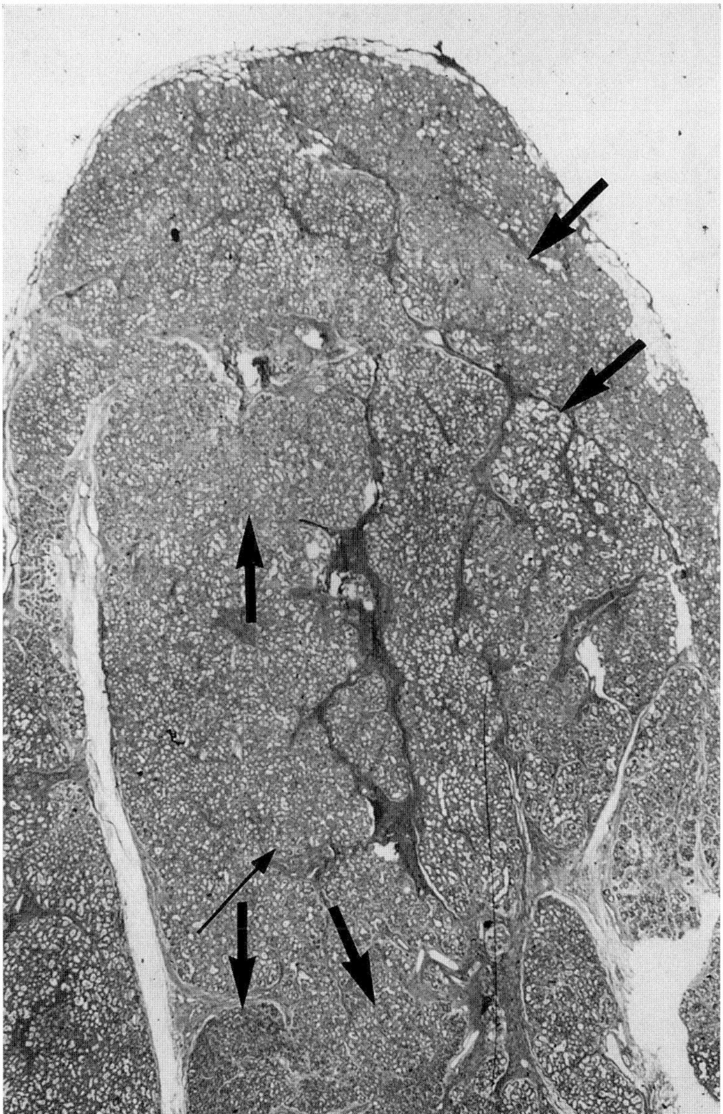

FIG. 1.13. Lactating adenoma. At low magnification, the lobular architecture is evident. The histological appearance is that of a lactating breast, as shown in Fig. 1.10.

REFERENCES

1. Wellings SR, Jensen HM, Marcum RG. An atlas of subgross pathology of the human breast with special reference to possible precancerous lesions. *J Natl Cancer Inst* 1971;55:231–273.
2. Wellings SR. Development of human breast cancer. *Adv Cancer Res* 1980;31:287–314.
3. Lakhani SR, Chaggar R, Davies S, et al. Genetic alterations in 'normal' luminal and myoepithelial cells of the breast. *J Pathol* 1999;189:496–503.
4. Tsai YC, Lu Y, Nichols PW, et al. Contiguous patches of normal human mammary epithelium derived from a single stem cell: implications for breast carcinogenesis. *Cancer Res* 1996;56:402–404.
5. Anderson RB. Embryonic and fetal development of the mammary apparatus. In: Larsen BL, ed. *Lactation: a comprehensive treatise*. New York: Academic Press, 1974:3–37.
6. Russo J, Calaf G, Russo, IH. Influence of age and gland topography on cell kinetics of normal human breast tissue. *J Natl Cancer Inst* 1987;78:413–418.
7. Tannenbaum M, Weiss M, Mark AJ. Fine structure of the human adult female breast. *Cancer* 1969; 23:958.
8. Wough D, Van der Hoeven E. Fine structure of the human adult female breast. *Lab Invest* 1962;2: 220–228.
9. Carter D, Yardley JH, Shelley WM. Lobular carcinoma of the breast: an ultrastructural comparison with certain duct carcinomas and benign lesions. *Johns Hopkins Med J* 1969;125:25–43.
10. Rudland PS. Epithelial stem cells and their possible role in the development of the normal and diseased human breast. *Histol Histopathol* 1993;8:385–404.
11. Ferguson D. Ultrastructural characterisation of the proliferative (stem?) cells within the parenchyma of the normal "resting" breast. *Virchows Arch* 1985;407:379–385.
12. Russo J, Russo I. Development of the human mammary gland. In: Neville ED, ed. *The mammary gland, development, regulation and function*. New York: Plenum Publishing, 1987.
13. McCarty KS. Proliferative stimuli in the normal breast estrogens or progestins? *Hum Pathol* 1989;20: 1137–1138.
14. McCarty K, Tucker J. Breast. In: Sternberg S, ed. *Histology for pathologists*. Raven Press: New York, 1992:893–902.
15. Fanger H, Ree HJ. Cyclic changes of human mammary gland epithelium in relation to the menstrual cycle—an ultrastructural study. *Cancer* 1974;34:574–585.
16. Longacre TA, Bartow SA. A correlative morphologic study of human breast and endometrium in the menstrual cycle. *Am J Surg Pathol* 1986;10:382.
17. Tavassoli FA, Yeh IT. Lactational and clear cell changes of the breast in nonlactating, nonpregnant women. *Am J Clin Pathol* 1987;87:23–29.
18. O'Hara MF, Page DL. Adenomas of the breast and ectopic breast under lactational influences. *Hum Pathol* 1985;16:707–712.
19. Grenko RT, Lee KP, Lee KR. Fine needle aspiration cytology of lactating adenoma of the breast. A comparative light microscopic and morphometric study. *Acta Cytol* 1990;34:21–26.

2

Risk Factors for Breast Cancer and Its Appearance in Girls, Young Women, and Men

RISK OF DEVELOPING BREAST CANCER

The breast is the leading site of cancer in women. There are 192,200 new cases per year, accounting for 31% of all female cancer cases. In 2001, the American Cancer Society estimated that one in eight American women would develop some form of breast cancer during her lifetime (1). With 40,200 deaths, breast cancer is third in female cancer deaths, behind pulmonary and digestive tract malignancies.

Henderson (2) stated that gender is the single most important risk factor, with 92% of breast cancers occurring in females. Age is the second most important risk factor, with a 14-fold increase from age 30 years (1 in 5,900) to age 60 years (1 in 420). Greenlee et al. (1) showed a 1 in 225 incidence of breast cancer in women under 39 years of age, 1 in 24 between 40 and 59 years, and 1 in 14 for ages 60 to 79 years. Carcinomas in younger women have a poorer prognosis, primarily attributable to the higher stage at the time of diagnosis (87,114). DeWaard et al. (3) described a bimodal age distribution of patients with mammary carcinoma, observing peaks at age 40 years and again at 65 years, which suggests that two types of human breast cancer may exist. A steep rise in the incidence of breast cancer is noted during the perimenopausal period (ages 45 to 49 years).

Because the fundamental cause of breast cancer remains unknown, there is intense speculation on how mammary cancer arises and what factors are critical in its development. In epidemiologic studies, subsets of women at higher risk for breast cancer have been identified through determination of germline genetics, effects of steroid hormones inferred from menstrual and childbearing status and administration of exogenous hormones, environmental exposures, and evaluation of benign breast biopsies. These factors suggest that environmental factors might interact with hereditary and growth factor activated changes. The Study of Tamoxifen and Raloxifene (STAR) prevention trial (4) seeks to determine if risk can be diminished with the use of antiestrogens. In benign biopsies, pathologists have recognized histologic features which, alone or in association with other factors, indicate a higher risk for development of carcinoma. However, the great majority of breast cancers are sporadic and unexpected, with none of the risk associations noted above.

Heritable Genetic Alterations

BRCA1, localized to chromosome 17 Q21 (5,6), is associated with an inherited predisposition to breast and ovarian cancer. Mutations within this gene have been identified in families in which linkage between breast and ovarian cancer is prominent (7), and it has been estimated that BRCA1 may be involved in up to one-half of site-specific breast cancers (8,9). Loss of function frameshift mutations with cancer-causing mutations occur in 66% (10). BRCA1 and BRCA2 interact with recombination DNA repair proteins in pathways that participate in preserving intact chromosome structure and act as tumor suppressor genes (11). BRCA1 may function as a scaffold in the assembly of a multiprotein complex that plays a role in gene transcription, DNA damage repair, and transcription coupled DNA damage repair (12). Expression has been identified in sporadic carcinoma cells.

The tumor suppressor gene, p53, is mutated in 25% to 40% of sporadic breast cancers and has also been associated with the Li–Fraumeni syndrome in which there is increased incidence of breast cancer, sarcomas, and other neoplasms in children and young adults (13).

A smaller group of women with heritable breast cancer, but not ovarian cancer—especially those women who developed breast cancer at an early age—have been associated with BRCA2 mutations that are localized to chromosome 13 Q12-13.

Claus et al. (14,15) derived estimates for risk of breast cancer with regard to family history. The lifetime risk of developing breast cancer for women with one first-degree relative affected with ovarian cancer was estimated at 13%; for two first-degree relatives with ovarian cancer, the risk rose to 31%. A woman with one first-degree relative affected with ovarian cancer and one first-degree relative affected with breast cancer had an estimated 40% risk of developing breast cancer by the age of 79 years. Henderson (2) provided a cumulative relative risk of 5.5 for bilateral breast cancer in a sister of a woman who developed breast cancer before the age of 50 years. Claus et al. (15) also described models for predicting risk according to the age of onset of breast cancer in the affected family member, with progression of breast cancer at an earlier age in succeeding generations noted. Lobular carcinoma *in situ* was found to be the only lesion associated with a family history of breast cancer when stratified according to histology (14).

Malone et al. (16) examined 203 women diagnosed with breast cancer before age 35 years and 225 women with a first-degree family history of breast carcinoma diagnosed before age 45 years. Of the women diagnosed before age 35 years, 9.4% carried germ line mutations (5.9% for BRCA1 and 3.4% for BRCA2). Of the women diagnosed before age 45 years who had a first-degree family history of breast cancer, 12% carried germ line mutations (7.1% with BRCA1 and 4.9% with BRCA2). Data such as these suggest an interrelationship between age of diagnosis and heritable breast cancer.

Are the breast cancers associated with BRCA1 and BRCA2 mutations recognizably different to the pathologist? Khurana et al. (17) examined a small group of patients with heritable cancer and found a 15% incidence of simultaneous occult malignant neoplasms in the contralateral breasts when prophylactic bilateral mastectomies were performed. Lakhani et al. (18) characterized the pathology of 82 breast cancers from BRCA1 or BRCA2 families and found a higher grade with more mitotic figures, more nuclear pleomorphism, and more lymphocytic infiltration of the tumors, which were more often necrotic. Foulkes et al. (19) compared a historical cohort with breast cancers in 118 Askhenazi Jewish women, in whom the BRCA1 mutation is more commonly found, with axillary lymph node negative breast cancer. The authors found the presence of BRCA1 mutation to be an independently poor prognostic factor in the node negative situation. Stoppa-Lyonnet et al. (20) reported a worse outcome for breast cancers related to BRCA1 mutations. The BRCA1 positive tumors were larger, had a higher histologic grade, and a higher incidence of negative estrogen and progesterone receptors. Overall prognosis for carriers of the gene was 80% versus 91% for a control group. Numerous epigenetic mutations, which are not directly associated with germ line changes, have been described in the breast cancer tumor cells themselves.

Ethnic considerations also have been considered as epidemiologic factors in assessing risk of breast cancer. Japanese women have long been known to have a lower incidence of breast cancer compared to citizens of the United States (21, 22). Environmental factors are likely to play a role in this discrepancy because of the increased incidence of breast cancer among Japanese women who move to the United States. The high incidence of BRCA1 mutations among Askhenazi Jewish women was noted above. African-American women appear to have larger and more advanced breast cancers at a younger age than a comparable population of white women (23). These data suggest that earlier screening may be appropriate for women who are at elevated risk.

Cowden's disease also has been associated with breast cancer (24).

Risk Factors Related to Steroid Hormones

The association of breast cancer with female gender has, naturally, led investigators to the view that steroid hormones play a pivotal role in breast carcinogenesis. Some breast cancer cells remain responsive to hormonal stimulation after they have become fully malignant, invasive, or even metastatic (25). Studies (26) have documented that nulliparous women have twice the risk of developing breast cancer as women who have borne children. Women who have borne children before 19 years of age have one-half the risk of breast cancer, compared to those who have borne their first child in the fourth decade. Women who reached menarche before the age of 13 years and had a late menopause have twice the incidence of carcinoma, compared to women with menarche after the age of 13 years and an early menopause. These features suggest that humoral or hormonal factors exert their influence over decades. Hahn and Moolgavkar (27) followed cohorts in Connecticut from 1855 to 1945. The authors found that nulliparity and advanced decades of first childbearing were associated with elevated risks of developing breast cancer, but also that the overall incidence of breast cancer had increased over the extended period, which suggests an environmental effect. Steroid hormone receptor evaluation of carcinoma of the breast is described in detail in Chapter 9.

Exogenous steroid hormones, especially birth control pills, have been studied intensively over the past three decades. Hulka and Lininger (28) summarized numerous epidemiologic studies as showing no clear-cut evidence that contraceptive medications either add to or detract from the incidence of breast cancer. Grabrick et al. (29) examined a subset of women with first-degree relatives with breast cancer who had used oral contraceptives prior to 1975. The authors reported an elevated risk of breast cancer associated with those contraceptives, many of which are no longer in clinical usage.

Metaanalysis of the use of postmenopausal estrogen replacement (28) and Colditz and Rosner (30) show a slight increase in the risk of developing breast cancer, but, if it does, and this issue is still debated, the decreased survival from breast cancer is apparently counterbalanced by increased survival from cardiovascular disease. Jacobs (31) reported that any associated increase in risk was comparable to the delay of menopause for a similar period of time.

Estrogen replacement therapy in patients with breast cancer is also a hotly debated issue, but it appears that it does not cause a discernible decrease in survival from breast cancer.

Risk Factors Related to the Environment

The association of gender, hormonal stimulation, and familial propensity are all features of the mouse mammary tumor virus model. Adult female mice of strains in which there is maternal history of a high incidence of breast cancer are at very high risk for the development of mammary tumors that are due to a transmissible viral agent. Although similar viral bodies have been found in human milk (32), there is no evidence to indicate that human breast cancer is virally induced. Women whose breasts have been exposed to radiation (33) are at elevated risk, as are women treated with reserpine for hypertension (34). Boyd et al. (35) presented a metaanalysis of studies of dietary fat and breast cancer risk. The authors reported a relative risk in the neighborhood of 1.1 to 1.2 for a high fat diet. They also found European studies to be more likely than studies done in other countries to show an increased relative risk associated with dietary fat and breast cancer (36–39).

Environmental toxins, especially chlorinated chemicals, including dichlorodiphenyl-trichloroethane (DDT) and its congeners, have been suspected of causing breast cancer; however, extensive epidemiologic studies [Zheng et al. (40–44) and Stellman et al. (45)] have failed to confirm this suspicion. Other environmental factors are under investigation, but no likely cause has been identified at this time.

Histologic Changes in the Breast

The majority of breast biopsies that are performed for the suspicion of cancer are found to be free of malignancy, but pathologists have identified histologic changes and determined emperically what, if any, association they have with cancer.

Fibrocystic changes are found so often in every tissue study of the breast that some consider them ubiquitous. Their ability to mimic or obscure cancer causes problems for the clinician, radiologist, and pathologist. The most noticeable change is dilatation of medium and large ducts, but it is the chronic inflammation and scarring around the dilated ducts that produces densities on palpation or appearances on mammogram that may mimic cancer. Apocrine metaplasia usually accompanies fibrocystic changes and is considered a component of cystic disease by many. It is tempting to suggest that fibrocystic changes result from a foreign body type reaction to ductal contents. Within the dilated ducts, foamy macrophages that contain lipid granules are often observed cytologically and in sections (Fig. 2.1). These macrophages, accompanied by a variable population of

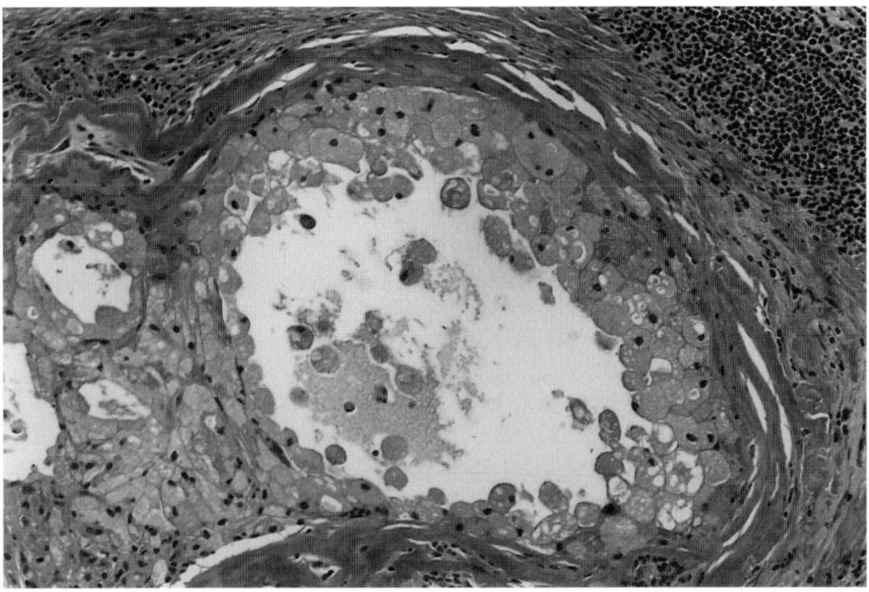

FIG. 2.1. Fibrocystic changes. Dilated duct is filled with foamy macrophages and epithelium is absent, presumed to have been destroyed by inflammatory reaction.

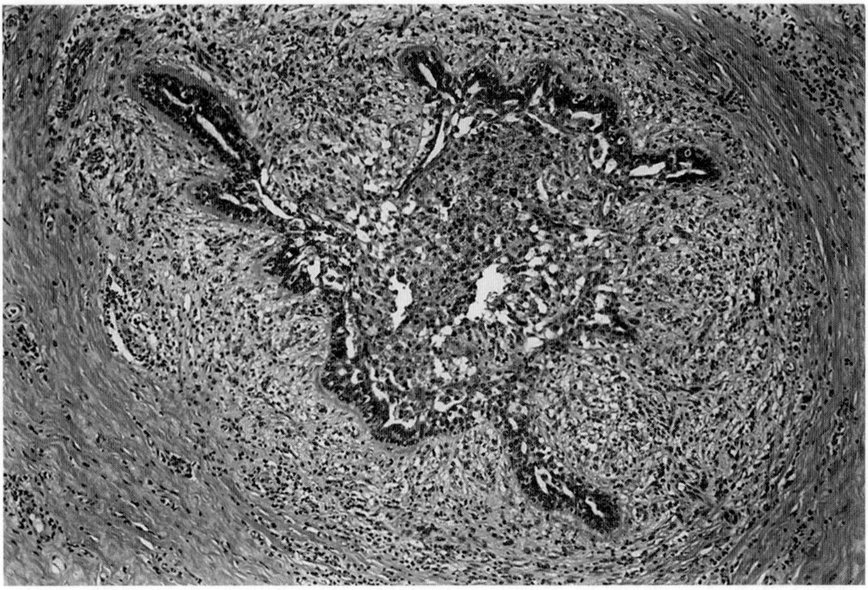

FIG. 2.2. Fibrocystic changes. Duct with intense inflammation in lumen and periductal stroma.

lymphocytes, plasma cells, and occasionally eosinophils, fill the periductal stroma, cross the basement membrane, damage or destroy the epithelium, and fill the lumens of ducts (Figs. 2.2 and 2.3). The periductal stroma undergoes fibrosis and angiogenesis to produce duct ectasia (Fig. 2.4, efigs. 2.1 to 2.9).

What role, if any, fibrocystic changes play as precursors or markers of elevated cancer risk is still debated. The risk of nonproliferative fibrocystic change alone is probably quite low, but distortions caused by associated scarring and reepithelialization of ducts denuded by inflammation may be factors in the initiation of proliferation, which is thought to indicate an elevated risk. Although the decision-making process of histopathologists is highly interpretive and has resulted in differences of opinion among serious students of this subject (46–51), it remains an important tool in the assignment of breast cancer risk clinically and is a significant point of departure for microdissected tissues for molecular analysis of early phases of breast carcinogenesis.

Hutter et al. (52), offered a consensus statement on the implications of each of the commonly observed benign lesions and gave numerical relative risk factors, but the database for these calculations was not described. The consensus group considered fibrocystic changes alone to be without increased risk. They also considered sclerosing or florid adenosis, apocrine metaplasia, cysts, duct ectasia, fibroadenoma, fibrosis, mild hyperplasia, mastitis, and squamous metaplasia to be without increased risk, but they assigned a slightly increased risk to

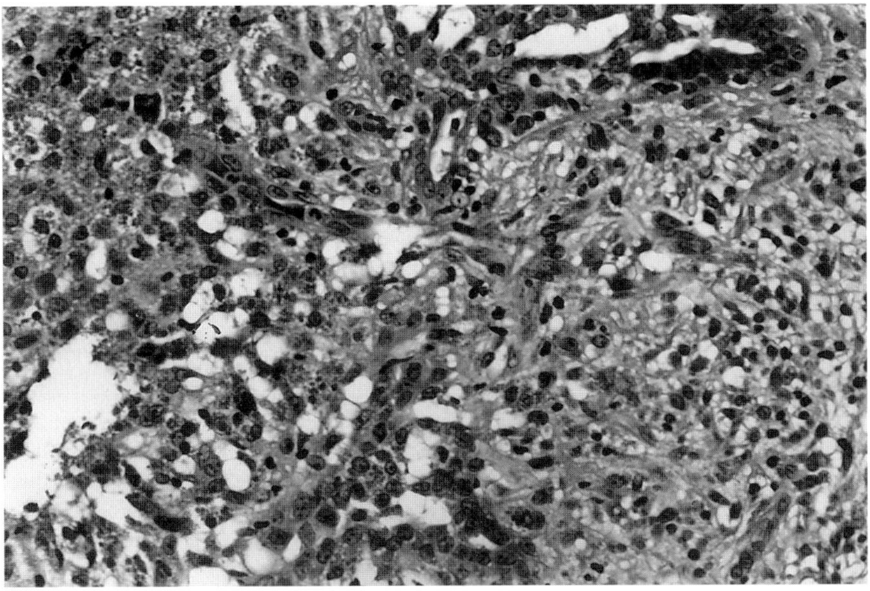

FIG. 2.3. Fibrocystic changes. Higher magnification of duct from Fig. 2.2 at the 3 o'clock position. Basement membrane is destroyed by macrophages, lymphocytes, and neutrophils.

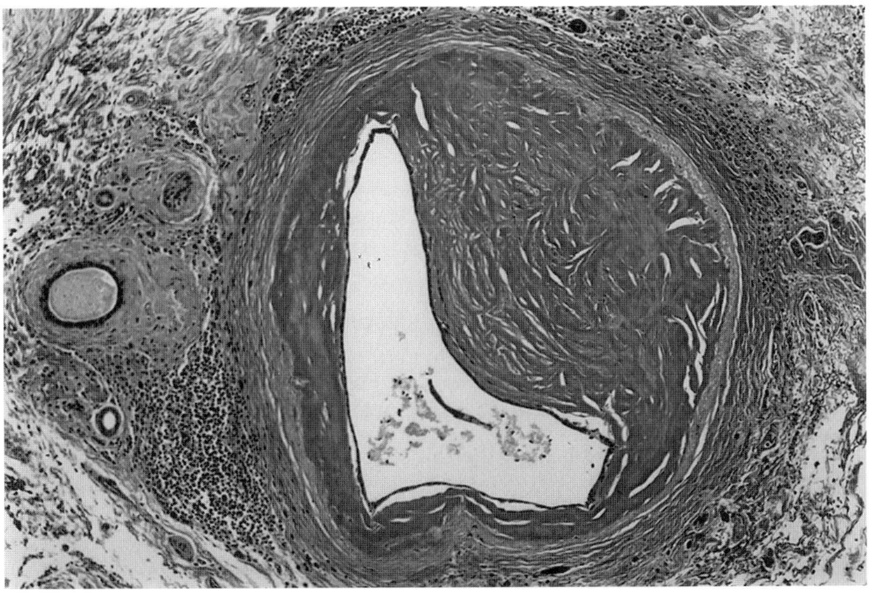

FIG. 2.4. Duct ectasia. End result of the inflammatory process (shown in Figs. 2.1 to 2.3) is this scarred ecstatic cystic duct that is lined by a minimal epithelial component.

TABLE 2.1. *Spectrum of intraepithelial breast lesions and their relationship to risk of ipsilateral or contralateral invasive cancer*

Risk of invasive cancer from:	
Baseline	Normal histology
Little or no risk (< 2 times)	Fibrocystic changes
	Fibroadenoma, fibroadenosis
Slight risk (2 times)	Sclerosing adenosis, Radial scar
	Papilloma, papillomatosis
	Ductal or lobular hyperplasia
Intermediate risk (3–8 times)	Atypical ductal or lobular hyperplasia
	Multiple papillomas
Highest risk (10 times or more)	Lobular carcinoma *in situ*
	Ductal carcinoma *in situ*

moderate, florid, solid, or papillary hyperplasia and to papilloma with a fibrovascular core. A moderately increased risk was assigned to ductal and lobular hyperplasia. The significance and diagnostic criteria for these and similar lesions are described in detail in Chapters 4, 5, and 6 and distinguished from the malignancies that they most closely resemble (see table 2.1).

Carter et al. (53) reviewed the relationship between benign changes in the breast seen at biopsy and the subsequent development of cancer of the breast in almost 17,000 women. The authors found relative risks of 1.5 for women with nonproliferative fibrocystic changes, 1.9 for women with ductal or lobular proliferation without atypia, and 3.0 for women displaying atypical hyperplasia—either ductal or lobular, when compared with "normal subjects" who were defined as those without clinical breast disease. The highest risk group (relative risk of 5.7) was found in women under the age of 46 years who displayed atypical ductal or lobular hyperplasia. Women with fibroadenomas and no other breast lesion had a relative risk of 1.7. Histologically, observed changes may interact with the family history (Chapters 4 and 5) to elevate the risk of developing breast cancer.

BREAST CANCER IN GIRLS AND YOUNG WOMEN AND IN PREGNANCY

Juvenile or Secretory Carcinoma

McDivitt and Stewart (54) described a rare carcinoma of the breast that occurs predominantly in children and is therefore designated juvenile carcinoma. In the original description, none of the patients (all of whom were children) had metastases from the tumor. Subsequently, however, metastases have been reported from secretory carcinoma in children and it has been seen in adults. In 1980, Tavassoli and Norris (55) reported on 19 patients with secretory carcinoma of the breast. Five of the patients were from 9 to 17 years of age, but eight of the patients were in their twenties, and six were in their thirties or older. The tumors ranged in size from 1 to 12 cm in diameter, had a rounded margin in most cases, and frequently resembled a fibroadenoma in gross appearance. Tumor cells were of two types: those with a granular cytoplasm and those with abundant secretory material within individual tumor cells and in extracellular lumina (Figs. 2.5 to 2.9 and efigs. 2.10 to 2.16). The secretory material was PAS-positive and diastase-resistant. Alcian blue stain was positive and resisted digestion with hyaluronidase. Staining with mucicarmine varied. Ultrastructurally, there were numerous intracellular lumens with microvilli extending into them. Extracellular lumina were also prominent. Mitochondria were numerous, and lipid droplets were occasionally present. Lamovec and Bracko (56) described five cases of secretory carcinoma of the breast. The most prominent histologic feature was the presence of intracellular and extracellular secretion. Immunohistochemically, all tumors showed strong positive reaction for lactalbumin and S-100 protein. Stains for CEA and GEFIGFP-15 were variable. Flow cytometry showed three of four cases to be diploid and all had a low S-phase.

Mitoses, anaplasia, and pleomorphism are minimal, but the tumors do display an invasive character. Four of the patients in the Tavassoli and Norris series (55) had axillary lymph node metastases and one patient died with disseminated carcinoma. The youngest patient with lymph node metastases was 24 years old. Oberman (57) reported six cases of secretory carcinoma of the breast in adults. Metastases were not observed in these patients, although associated intraductal carcinoma was noted occasionally. Karl et al. (58) reported positive lymph nodes in 5 of 18 childhood cases of secretory breast carcinoma, but metastases beyond the axilla were unusual.

In 1983, Akhtar et al. (59) reported on three adult cases of secretory carcinomas that were studied by both light and electron microscopy. Lymph node metastases were present in one case. Electron microscopy revealed numerous intracellular lumina and large numbers of membrane-bound intracytoplasmic secretory vacuoles. Guerry et al. (60) described a predominantly intraductal form of hypersecretory carcinoma that had an overall excellent prognosis.

In combined series, Oberman (57), Tavassoli and Norris (55), and Rosen and Cranor (61), with an aggregate of 40 cases, the age ranged from 9 to 87, 7 recurred (18%), 6 had node metastases (15%) and 2 died of disease (5%) at 10 months and 20 years, respectively.

Secretory carcinoma is the most common breast carcinoma of children and, in this age group, it is a relatively slowly growing neoplasm that is unlikely to metastasize. The reader is urged to read carefully the articles by Byrne et al. (62), Oberman and Stephens (63), and Oberman (64) whenever carcinoma is seen in the breast of a girl or adolescent, since ordinary invasive ductal carcinomas are quite rare in this age group. Secretory carcinoma also occurs in adults—women who are 20 years of age or older—in whom it has a greater propensity to metastasize, at least to axillary lymph nodes. It also has been described in boys (65) and men (66,67). Other more aggressive types of carcinoma (invasive ductal or lobular carcinoma) have rarely been observed in girls

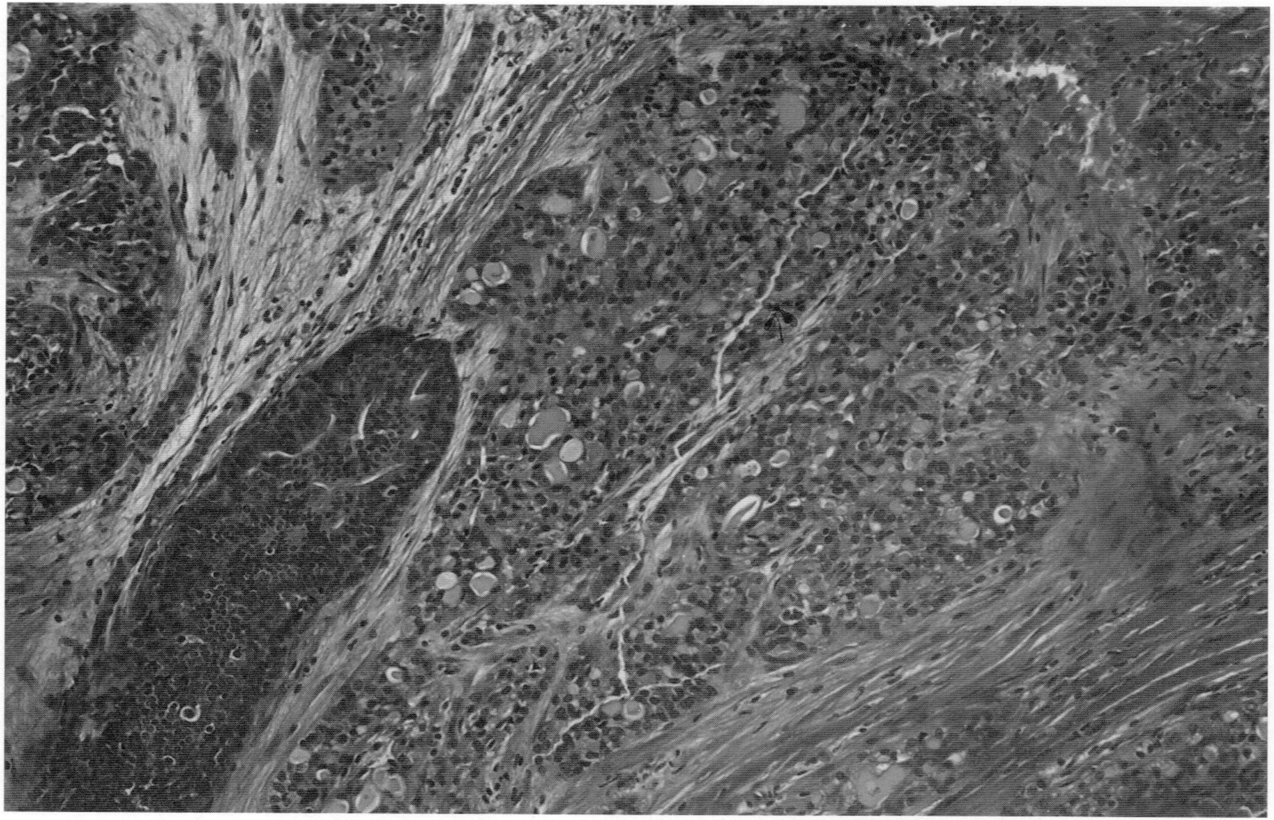

FIG. 2.5. Secretory carcinoma. Low magnification view shows an intraductal component and a nodular invasive component with a pushing border.

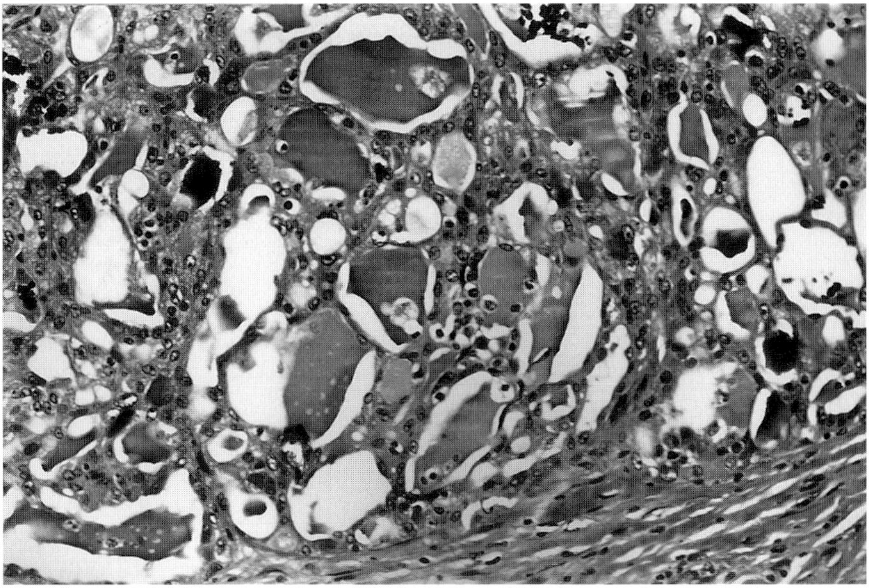

FIG. 2.6. Secretory carcinoma. Ducts are prominent, filled with secretion and lined by large and atypical cells.

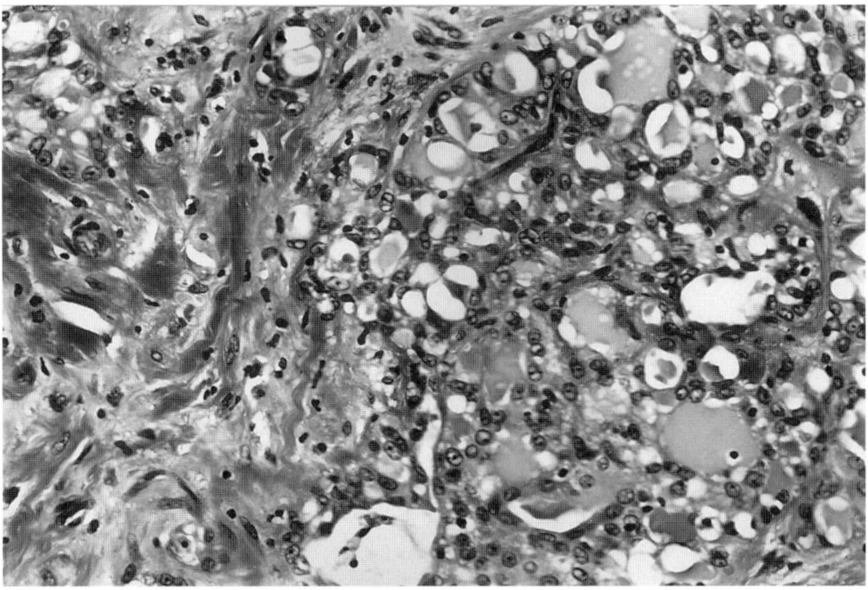

FIG. 2.7. Secretory carcinoma. Rounded lobular configuration of invasive secretory carcinoma with ducts distended by secretion and lined by abnormal cells. Compare this with the secretory lobule seen in Fig. 1.10.

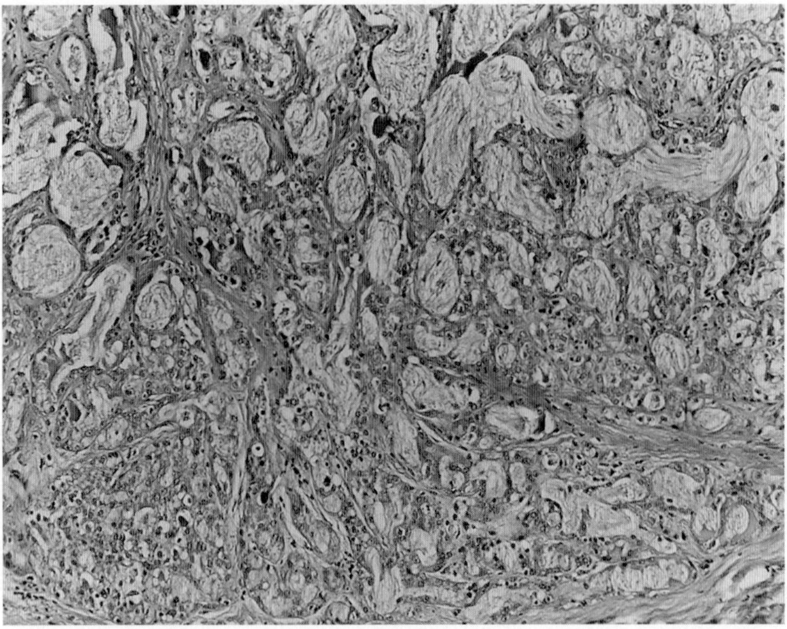

FIG. 2.8. Secretory carcinoma. In this carcinoma from a 23-year-old woman who had a breast mass for some time, the carcinoma infiltrating the stroma in large masses is evident. The age of the patient suggests the classification. The malignant cells are characterized by clear cytoplasm with abundant secretory material. (Case and photograph from P. Rosen, Memorial Sloan-Kettering Cancer Center, New York, NY, with permission.)

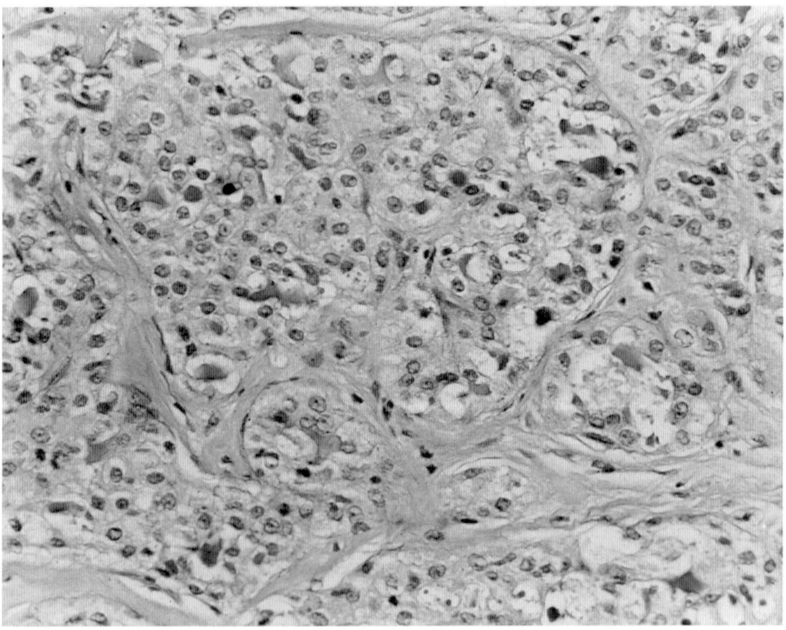

and adolescents and they may not share the good prognosis of secretory carcinoma [Ashikari et al. (68)].

Cancer in Young Women

Noyes et al. (69) reported on 125 women under the age of 30 years who were treated for breast cancer. In comparison to a matched group of over 3,000 women over the age of 30, the younger women had poorer survival in node negative cases and in those with primaries up to 5 cm in diameter. Among 125 cases, only 10 were found between the ages of 10 and 20 years, 26 were found between the ages of 21 and 25 years, and the remaining 96 were diagnosed in patients between 26 and 30 years of age. The great majority of cases were infiltrating ductal carcinoma. Fifty-one of 77 patients with axillary node dissections had lymph node metastases. Five-year survival was 41% in women who were less than 30 years of age; 10-year survival was 40%. Feldman and Welsh (70) recently reaffirmed the poor prognosis of breast cancer in women under the age of 30 years, with 22 of 29 dying from metastatic disease.

Cancer during Pregnancy and Lactation

Breast cancer is the most frequently seen cancer in pregnancy and lactation, but the incidence is low. Hoover (71) reported breast cancer in approximately 0.03% of pregnancies and stated that only 1% to 2% of breast cancer overall is diagnosed during pregnancy or during lactation the year after delivery. Kuerer et al. (72) reported an increased incidence of breast cancer concurrent with pregnancy, due to the increasing number of women electing to postpone pregnancy until their late thirties and forties, at which time breast cancer is more prevalent. Gemignani et al. (73) reviewed the literature on breast cancer and pregnancy and found an overall worse prognosis compared with nonpregnancy-associated breast cancers. This was due to the higher proportion of pregnant patients diagnosed at advanced disease stages. Hoover (71) reported that 70% to 89% of pregnant patients with operable primary breast carcinomas had axillary lymph node metastases.

Stage for stage, survival from pregnancy-associated breast cancer is not decreased. Ezzat et al. (74) reported a case control study of 28 women with breast cancer in pregnancy, where age and stage were matched with nonpregnant breast cancer controls. No statistically significant difference in relapse-free or overall survival was shown between the two groups. Reasons for the advanced

FIG. 2.9. Secretory carcinoma. At higher magnification, the granular and clear cell nature of the cytoplasm is evident. The nuclear contours are rounded and there is minimal pleomorphism. Mitotic figures are rare. (Case and photograph from P. Rosen, Memorial Sloan-Kettering Cancer Center, New York, NY, with permission.)

stage at time of diagnosis are probably multiple. Pregnancy does impede detection of cancer because of enlargement and increased density of the breast, and patient and physician delay may contribute to the advanced stage at the time of detection.

BREAST DEVELOPMENT IN THE MALE

Nipple development is normal in the male, and approximately 25% of adolescent males have some form of transitory development of breast tissue. In about 20% of those cases, there is persistence of breast tissue for a sufficient period of time so that removal for cosmetic purposes may be considered.

The development of breast tissue in adolescent males is limited to an increase in the amount of dense fibrous stroma, a proliferation of ducts, and a striking periductal stromal proliferation with a variable proliferation of the epithelial contents of the ducts to form a peculiar hyperplasia unlike that seen in hyperplasia or atypical ductal hyperplasia of the female breast. Acinar and lobular formation does not occur (Figs. 2.10 to 2.12 and efigs. 2.17 to 2.22).

Orchidectomy alone does not cause changes in the breast.

In men treated with nonprogestational antiandrogens for prostate cancer, there may be a slight to moderate amount of formation of acini or lobules. Kanhai et

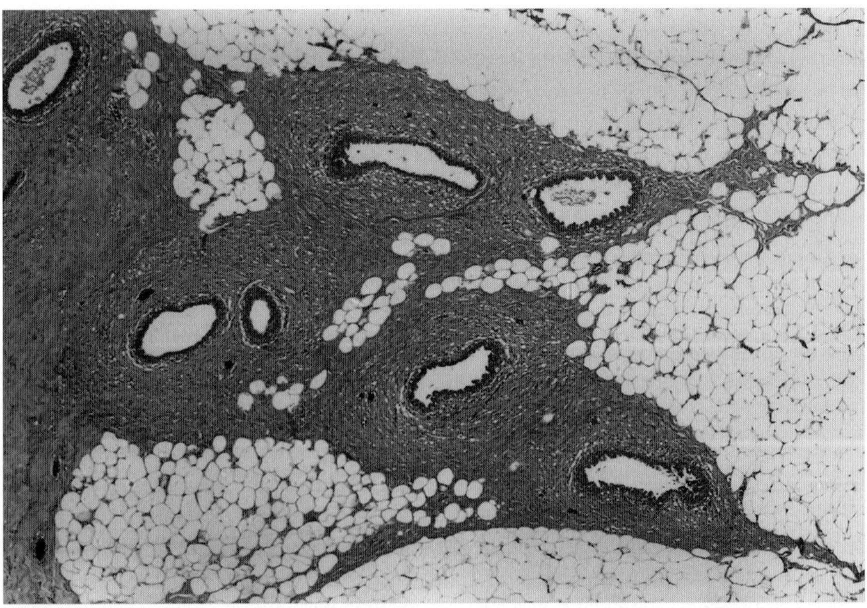

FIG. 2.10. Gynecomastia. Ducts with a dense and proliferative stroma are present, but lobules are not seen.

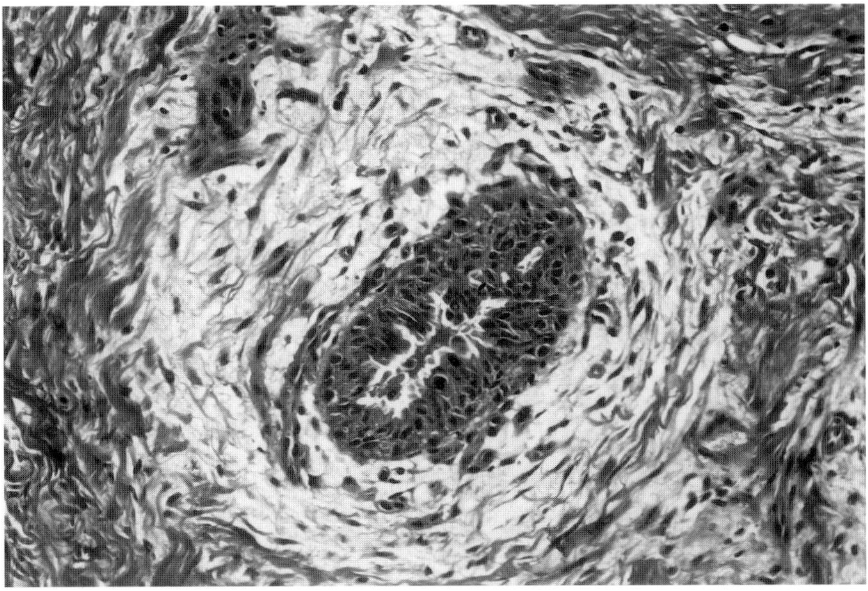

FIG. 2.11. Gynecomastia. The stroma is myxoid and filled with numerous proliferating fibroblasts. The exuberant proliferation of epithelium accompanies it.

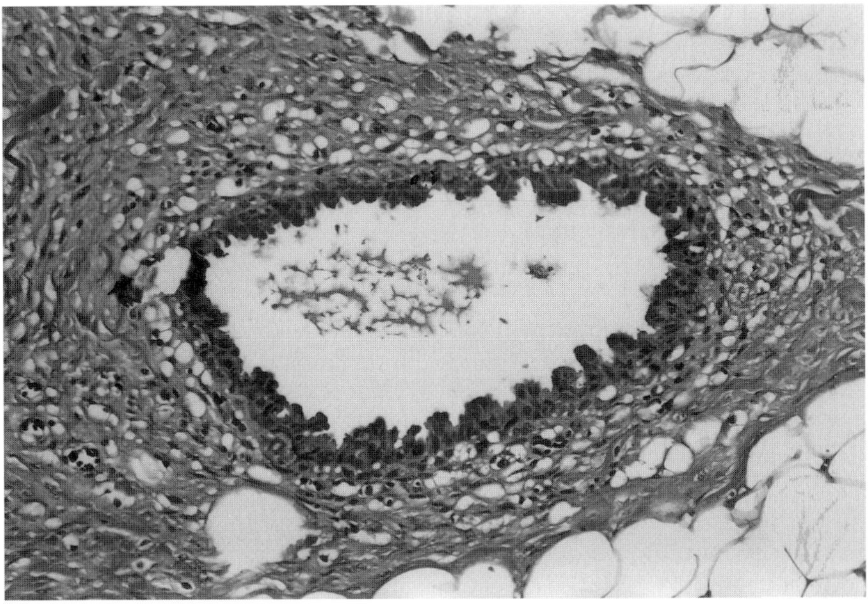

FIG. 2.12. Gynecomastia. Periductal stroma is dense and cellular, but less myxoid. Epithelium has a peculiar micropapillary appearance.

al. (75) described the histologic changes induced in the mammary glands of 14 male to female transsexuals in whom progestational chemical castration was combined with feminizing estrogen therapy to produce full development of acini or lobules with hormonally stimulated nuclei and pseudolactational changes. Apocrine metaplasia was also seen. Apotosis was observed in lobules when estrogen therapy was withdrawn.

As noted earlier, breast cancer is rare in the male, but, when it does occur, it is found in conjunction with gynecomastia. Volpe et al. (76) reviewed the records of 35 male patients who underwent subcutaneous mastectomy for a suspicious unilateral breast mass. Gynecomastia was diagnosed in 30 patients, lipoma in 4 patients, and invasive breast cancer in 1 patient. Of the 30 patients with gynecomastia, 60% gave a history of a medical condition and use of medications known to cause gynecomastia.

MALE BREAST CANCER

When cancer does occur in the male breast, it may be either pure intraductal carcinoma or intraductal carcinoma associated with invasive carcinoma. Hittmair et al. (77) reported 84 cases of pure intraductal carcinoma in men (median age 65 years) who presented with a typical nodular retroareolar partially cystic mass frequently associated with nipple discharge for a median duration of 2 months. Histologically, papillary carcinoma, often with a superimposed cribriform pattern was found in 74% of the cases. Intraductal extension beyond the main papillary lesion was commonly found. All cases of pure intraductal carcinoma were of low or intermediate grade. In 30 cases of invasive carcinoma, almost entirely of the ductal type, there was overall higher nuclear grade and associated necrosis.

Norris and Taylor (78) noted that only 2.4% of 4,810 breast cancers were found in men, and this was a series from the Armed Forces Institute of Pathology. Demeter et al. (79) described the familial association of breast cancer in males and showed a different pattern of inheritance. Hill et al. (80) found history of a first-degree relative with breast cancer among 15 of 142 men with breast cancer. Haraldsson et al. (81) found BRCA2 mutations in 21% of 34 men with breast cancer and Kwiatkowska et al. (82) reported BCA2 mutations in 7 of 37 men with four frameshift mutations and three missense variants.

Some older series suggest that survival from breast cancer in men is less than in women, but the series by Borgen et al. (83), Crichlow (84), Crichlow et al. (85), Visfeldt and Sheike (86), and Panettiere (87) all indicated that the prognosis is approximately the same in men and women, the most significant prognostic factors being the size of the primary tumor, axillary lymph node status, and fixation to skin or pectoral muscle. Hill et al. (80) reported 86% and 64% for 5- and 10- year survival, respectively.

Guinee et al. (88) described the course of breast cancer in 335 men with a mean follow-up of 65 months. Staging and prognostic indicators included fixation to the skin or chest wall and axillary lymph node metastases. Patients with fixation to either the chest wall or the skin did not have decreased survival, but, if ulceration of the skin was present, a marked decrease in the survival curve was observed. Men with a tumor 10 mm or less in diameter had a 94% 5-year survival, whereas those with tumor diameters between 11 and 40 mm had an 80% 5-year survival. Those with larger tumors had a 40% 5-year survival. Survival curves with regard to the clinical lymph node status of men and women were the same. The 10-year survival rate was 45% for men with clinically positive axillary nodes and 60% for those with negative nodes. Men with four or more positive nodes had a marked decrease in survival, starting 3 years after diagnosis, when compared with patients with one to three positive nodes. Eighty-four percent of men with histologically negative nodes were alive at 10 years, whereas only 14% of men with four or more histologically positive nodes were alive at this time. Men with one to three positive nodes fell in between these groups, with 44% survival at 10 years. In a study of 1,429 men, Adami et al. (89) found that the risk of dying from breast cancer was three times higher in men who developed breast cancer before the age of 40 years than it was in those who developed breast cancer after the age of 80 years. These studies confirm the previous impression that the course of cancer of the breast is essentially the same in men and women. The pathology and the principles of diagnosis and prognosis are also similar. The type of breast cancer that develops most commonly in men (and women) is infiltrating duct carcinoma. All other types, especially invasive lobular carcinoma, are less commonly found in men. Anelli et al. (90), Dawson et al. (91), and Yap and Tashima (92) described similarities in male and female breast cancer behavior and p53. Ansah-Boateng and Tavassoli (93) described cystosarcoma in men.

Older men with prostate cancer, for which they have been treated with estrogen, may develop gynecomastia. When carcinomas arise in this setting, the differential diagnosis of primary breast cancer or metastasis of prostate cancer (94) may be difficult to answer without the use of immunoperoxidase stains for prostate-specific antigen. Rosen (95) showed that carcinomas in the male breast often express steroid hormone receptors.

Munoz Toro et al. (96) reported 61% and 72% positivity for estrogen and progesterone receptors, respectively. Rayson et al. (97) studied 77 male breast cancers immunohistochemically and reported positive staining as follows: estrogen receptor, 91%; progesterone receptor, 96%; androgen receptor, 96%; bcl-2, 94%; cyclin D-1, 58%; MIB-1, 38%; HER2/neu, 29%; and p53, 21%. MIB-1 positivity and cyclin D-1 negativity predicted for poor prognosis.

REFERENCES

1. Greenlee R, Hill-Harmon M, Taylor M, et al. Cancer statistics. *Cancer* 2001;51:15–37.
2. Henderson CI. Risk factors for breast cancer development. *Cancer* 1993;71:2127–2140.
3. DeWaard F, Boanders-van Haleiujin EA, Huzinga J. The bimodal age distribution of patients with mammary carcinoma—evidence for the existence of two types of human breast cancer. *Cancer* 1964; 17:141–151.
4. Rhodes DJ, Hartmann LC, Perez EA. Breast cancer prevention trials. *Curr Oncol Rep* 2000;2:558–565.
5. Narod SA. Hereditary breast carcinoma syndromes. *Cancer* 1997;80[Suppl]:537–542.

6. Hall JM, Lee MK, Newman B. Linkage of early-onset familial breast cancer to chromosome 17q21. *Science* 1990;250:1684–1689.
7. Easton DF, Bishop DT, Ford D. Genetic linkage analysis in familial breast and ovarian cancer: results from 214 families. *Am J Hum Genet* 1993;52.
8. Colditz G, Rosner B. Cumulative risk to age 70 years according to risk factor status: data from the Nurses' Health Study. *Am J Epidemiol* 2000;152:950–964.
9. Lynch BJ, Holden JA, Buys SS, et al. Pathobiologic characteristics of hereditary breast cancer. *Hum Pathol* 1998;29:1140–1144.
10. Shen D, Vadgama JV. BRCA1 and BRCA2 gene mutation analysis: visit to the Breast Cancer Information Core (BIC). *Oncol Res* 1999;11:63–69.
11. Scully R, Livingston DM. In search of the tumour-suppressor functions of BRCA1 and BRCA2. *Nature* 2000;408:429–432.
12. Wang Q, Zhang H, Fishel R, et al. BRCA1 and cell signaling. *Oncogene* 2000;19:6152–6158.
13. Garber JEG, Kantor AF, Dreyfus MG, et al. Follow-up study of twenty-four families with Li–Fraumeni syndrome. *Cancer Res* 1991;51:6094–6097.
14. Claus EB, Risch N, Thompson DW, et al. Relationship between breast histopathology and family history of breast cancer. *Cancer* 1993;71:147–153.
15. Claus EB, Risch N, Thompson WD. Autosomal dominant inheritance of early-onset breast cancer: implications for risk prediction. *Cancer* 1994;73:643–651.
16. Malone KE, Daling JR, Neal C, et al. Frequency of BRCA1/BRCA2 mutations in a population-based sample of young breast carcinoma cases. *Cancer* 2000;88:1393–1402.
17. Khurana KK, Loosmann A, Numann PJ, et al. Prophylactic mastectomy: pathologic findings in high-risk patients. *Arch Pathol Lab Med* 2000;124:378–381.
18. Lakhani SR, Gusterson BA, Jacquemier J, et al. The pathology of familial breast cancer: histological features of cancers in families not attributable to mutations in BRCA1 or BRCA2. *Clin Cancer Res* 2000;6:782–789.
19. Foulkes WD, Chappuis PO, Wong N, et al. Primary node negative breast cancer in BRCA1 mutation carriers has a poor outcome. *Ann Oncol* 2000;11:307–313.
20. Stoppa-Lyonnet D, Ansquer Y, Dreyfus H, et al. Familial invasive breast cancers: worse outcome related to BRCA1 mutations. *J Clin Oncol* 2000;18:4053–4059.
21. Hoare T. Breast screening and ethnic minorities. *Br J Cancer* 1996;29[Suppl]:S38–S41.
22. Meng L, Maskarinec G, Wilkens L. Ethnic differences and factors related to breast cancer survival in Hawaii. *Int J Epidemiol* 1997;26:1151–1158.
23. Elmore JG, Moceri VM, Carter D, et al. Breast carcinoma tumor characteristics in black and white women. *Cancer* 1998;83:2509–2515.
24. Fackenthal JD, Marsh DJ, Richardson AL, et al. Male breast cancer in Cowden syndrome patients with germline PTEN mutations. *J Med Genet* 2001;38:159–164.
25. McClelland RA, Berger V, Miller LS. Immunocytochemical assay for estrogen receptor: relationship to outcome of therapy in patients with advanced breast cancer. *Cancer Res* 1986;46:4241s.
26. Cole P. Major aspects of epidemiology of breast cancer. *Cancer* 1980;46:865–867.
27. Hahn RA, Moolgavkar SH. Nulliparity, decade of first birth, and breast cancer in Connecticut cohorts, 1855 to 1945: an ecological study. *Am J Public Health* 1989;79:1503–1507.
28. Hulka BSL, Lininger RA. Steroid hormones and risk of breast cancer. *Cancer* 1994;74:1111–1124.
29. Grabrick DM, Hartmann LC, Cerhan JR, et al. Risk of breast cancer with oral contraceptive use in women with a family history of breast cancer. *JAMA* 2000;284:1791–1798.
30. Colditz GA, Rosner B. Cumulative risk of breast cancer to age 70 years according to risk factor status: data from the Nurses' Health Study. *Am J Epidemiol* 2000;152:950–964.
31. Jacobs HS. Postmenopausal hormone replacement therapy and breast cancer. *Medscape Women's Health* 2000;5:E2.
32. Seman G, Dmochowski L. Electron microscopic observation of virus-like particles in comedocarcinoma of the human breast. *Cancer* 1973;32:822.
33. Little MP, Boice JD. Comparison of breast cancer incidence in the Massachusetts tuberculosis fluoroscopy cohort and in the Japanese atomic bomb survivors. *Radiat Res* 1999;151:218–224.
34. Dankward K, McCarthy N. Reserpine and breast cancer. *Cancer* 1978;41:761–768.
35. Boyd NF, Martin LJ, Noffel M, et al. A meta-analysis of studies of dietary fat and breast cancer risk. *Br J Cancer* 1993;68:627–636.
36. Howe GR. Dietary fat and breast cancer risks: an epidemiologic perspective. *Cancer* 1994;74: 1078–1084.

37. Messina M, Barnes S. The role of soy products in reducing risk of cancer. *J Natl Cancer Inst* 1991; 83:541–547.
38. Schapira DV, Kumar NB, Lyman GH. Obesity, body fat distribution, and sex hormones in breast cancer patients. *Cancer* 1991;67:2215–2218.
39. Schapira DV, Kumar NB, Lyman GH. Estimate of breast cancer risk reduction with weight loss. *Cancer* 1991;67:2622–2625.
40. Zheng T, Holford TR, Mayne ST, et al. DDE and DDT in breast adipose tissue and risk of female breast cancer. *Am J Epidemiol* 1999;150:453–458.
41. Zheng T, Holford TR, Mayne ST, et al. Environmental exposure to hexachlorobenzene (HCB) and risk of female breast cancer in Connecticut. *Cancer Epidemiol Biomarkers Prev* 1999;8:407–411.
42. Zheng T, Holford TR, Mayne ST, et al. Beta-benzene hexachloride in breast adipose tissue and risk of breast carcinoma. *Cancer* 1999;85:2212–2218.
43. Zheng T, Holford TR, Mayne ST, et al. Risk of female breast cancer associated with serum polychlorinated biphenyls and 1,1-dichloro-2,2'-bis(p-chlorophenyl)ethylene. *Cancer Epidemiol Biomarkers Prev* 2000;9:167–174.
44. Zheng T, Holford TR, Mayne ST, et al. Exposure to electromagnetic fields from use of electric blankets and other in-home electrical appliances and breast cancer risk. *Am J Epidemiol* 2000;151:1103–1111.
45. Stellman SD, Djordjevic MV, Britton JA, et al. Breast cancer risk in relation to adipose concentrations of organochlorine pesticides and polychlorinated biphenyls in Long Island, New York. *Cancer Epidemiol Biomarkers Prev* 2000;9:1241–1249.
46. Devitt JE. Fibrocystic disease of the breast is not premalignant. *Surg Gynecol Obstet* 1972;134:803.
47. Haagensen DEJ. Is cystic disease related to breast cancer? *Am J Surg Pathol* 1991;15:687–694.
48. McDivitt RW, Stevens JA, Lee NC, et al. Histologic types of benign breast disease and the risk for breast cancer. *Cancer* 1992;69:1408–1414.
49. Noguchi S, Motomura K, Motomura, et al. Breast cancer risk associated with proliferative breast disease and atypical hyperplasia. *Cancer* 1993;71:1266–1272.
50. Page DL, Zwaag RV, Rogers L, et al. Relation between component parts of fibrocystic disease complex and breast cancer. *J Natl Cancer Inst* 1978;61:1055–1063.
51. Page DL, Jensen RA, Simpson JF. Premalignant and malignant disease of the breast: the roles of the pathologist. *Mod Pathol* 1998;11:120–128.
52. Hutter RVP, Albores-Saavedra J, Anderson E. Is fibrocystic disease of the breast precancerous? *Arch Pathol Lab Med* 1986;110:171–173.
53. Carter CL, Corle DK, Micozzi MS, et al. A prospective study of the development of breast cancer in 16,692 women with benign breast disease. *Am J Epidemiol* 1988;128:467–477.
54. McDivitt RW, Stewart FW. Breast carcinoma in children. *JAMA* 1966;195:388–390.
55. Tavassoli FA, Norris HJ. Secretory carcinoma of the breast. *Cancer* 1980;45:2404–2413.
56. Lamovec J, Bracko M. Secretory carcinoma of the breast: light microscopical, immunohistochemical and flow cytometric study. *Mod Pathol* 1994;7:475–479.
57. Oberman HA. Secretory carcinoma of the breast in adults. *Am J Surg Pathol* 1980;4:465–471.
58. Karl S, Ballantine T, Zaino R. Juvenile secretory carcinoma of the breast. *J Pediatr Surg* 1985;20: 368–371.
59. Akhtar M, Robinson C, Ali MA, et al. Secretory carcinoma of the breast in adults: light and electron microscopy study of three cases with review of the literature. *Cancer* 1983;51:2245–2254.
60. Guerry P, Erlandson RA, Rosen PP. Cystic hypersecretory hyperplasia and cystic hypersecretory duct carcinoma of the breast: pathology, therapy, and follow-up of 39 patients. *Cancer* 1988;61:1611–1620.
61. Rosen P, Cranor M. Secretory carcinoma of the breast. *Arch Pathol Lab Med* 1991;115:141–144.
62. Byrne MP, Fahey MM, Gooselaw JG. Breast cancer with axillary metastases in an 8½ year old girl. *Cancer* 1973;31:726.
63. Oberman HA, Stephens PJ. Carcinoma of the breast in childhood. *Cancer* 1972;30:470–474.
64. Oberman HA. Breast lesions in the adolescent female. *Pathol Ann* 1979;14(Pt. 1):175–201.
65. Bhagwandeen BS, Fenton L. Secretory carcinoma of the breast in a nine-year-old boy. *Pathology* 1999;31:166–168.
66. Roth JA, Discafani C, O'Malley M. Secretory breast carcinoma in a man. *Am J Surg Pathol* 1988;12: 150–154.
67. Kuwabara H, Yamane M, Okada S. Secretory breast carcinoma in a 66-year-old man. *J Clin Pathol* 1998;51:545–547.
68. Ashikari H, Jun MY, Farrow JH, et al. Breast carcinoma in children and adolescents. *Clin Bull* 1977; 7:55–62.

69. Noyes RD, Spanos WJ Jr, Montague ED. Breast cancer in women aged 30 and under. *Cancer* 1982; 49:1302–1307.
70. Feldman AL, Welch JP. Long-term outcome in women less than 30 years of age with breast cancer. *J Surg Oncol* 1998;68:193–198.
71. Hoover HC Jr. Breast cancer during pregnancy and lactation. *Surg Clin North Am* 1990;70:1151–1163.
72. Kuerer HM, Cunningham JD, Brower ST, et al. Breast carcinoma associated with pregnancy and lactation. *Surg Oncol* 1997;6:93–98.
73. Gemignani ML, Petrek JA, Borgen PI. Breast cancer and pregnancy. *Surg Clin North Am* 1999;79: 1157–1169.
74. Ezzat A, Raja MA, Berry J, et al. Impact of pregnancy on non-metastatic breast cancer: a case control study. *Clin Oncol* 1996;8:367–370.
75. Kanhai RC, Hage JJ, van Diest PJ, et al. Short-term and long-term histologic effects of castration and estrogen treatment on breast tissue of 14 male-to-female transsexuals in comparison with two chemically castrated men. *Am J Surg Pathol* 2000;24:74–80.
76. Volpe CM, Raffetto JD, Collure DW, et al. Unilateral male breast masses: cancer risk and their evaluation and management. *Am Surg* 1999;65:250–253.
77. Hittmair AP, Lininger RA, Tavassoli FA. Ductal carcinoma *in situ* (DCIS) in the male breast: a morphologic study of 84 cases of pure DCIS and 30 cases of DCIS associated with invasive carcinoma—a preliminary report. *Cancer* 1998;83:2139–2149.
78. Norris HJ, Taylor HB. Carcinoma of the male breast. *Cancer* 1969;23:1428–1435.
79. Demeter JG, Waterman NG, Verdi GD. Familial male breast carcinoma. *Cancer* 1990;65:2342–2343.
80. Hill A, Yagmur Y, Tran KN, et al. Localized male breast carcinoma and family history. An analysis of 142 patients. *Cancer* 1999;86:821–825.
81. Haraldsson K, Loman N, Zhang QX, et al. BRCA2 germ-line mutations are frequent in male breast cancer patients without a family history of the disease. *Cancer Res* 1998;58:1367–1371.
82. Kwiatkowska E, Teresiak M, Lamperska KM, et al. BRCA2 germline mutations in male breast cancer patients in the polish population. *Hum Mutat* 2001;17:73.
83. Borgen PI, Senie RT, McKinnon WM, et al. Carcinoma of the male breast: analysis of prognosis compared with matched female patients. *Ann Surg Oncol* 1997;4:385–388.
84. Crichlow RW. Carcinoma of the male breast. *Surg Gynecol Obstet* 1972;134:1011–1019.
85. Crichlow RW, Kaplan EL, Kearney WH. Male mammary cancer: an analysis of 32 cases. *Ann Surg* 1972;175:489.
86. Visfeldt J, Sheike O. Male breast cancer. I. Histologic typing and grading of 187 Danish cases. *Cancer* 1973;32:985–990.
87. Panettiere FJ. Cancer in the male breast. *Cancer* 1974;34:1324–1327.
88. Guinee VF, Olsson H, Moller T, et al. The prognosis of breast cancer in males: a report of 335 cases. *Cancer* 1993;71:154–161.
89. Adami HO, Hakulinen T, Ewertz M, et al. The survival pattern in male breast cancer: an analysis of 1429 patients from the Nordic Countries. *Cancer* 1989;64:1177–1182.
90. Anelli A, Anelli TFM, Youngson B, et al. Mutations of the p53 gene in male breast cancer. *Cancer* 1995;75:2233–2238.
91. Dawson PJ, Schroer KR, Wolman SR. Ras and p53 genes in male breast cancer. *Mod Pathol* 1996;9:367–370.
92. Yap HY, Tashima CK. Male breast cancer: a natural history study. *Cancer* 1979;44:748–754.
93. Ansah-Boateng Y, Tavassoli FA. Fibroadenoma and cytosarcoma phyllodes of the male breast. *Mod Pathol* 1992;5:114–116.
94. Salyer WR, Salyer DC. Metastases of prostatic carcinoma to the breast. *J Urol* 1973;109:671–675.
95. Rosen PP. Estrogen receptor proteins in lesions of the male breast: a preliminary report. *Cancer* 1976; 37:1866–1868.
96. Munoz de Toro MM, Maffini MV, Kass L, et al. Proliferative activity and steroid hormone receptor status in male breast carcinoma. *J Steroid Biochem Mol Biol* 1998;67:333–339.
97. Rayson D, Erlichman C, Suman VJ, et al. Molecular markers in male breast carcinoma. *Cancer* 1998; 83:1947–1955.

3

Biopsy and Local Treatment

With the survival of 150,000 of the 192,000 American women who are diagnosed with breast cancer, it is obvious that the disease is potentially curable in most cases. Early detection is the primary weapon in the battle to decrease the mortality rate from breast cancer, and the pathologist is the only physician who can diagnose breast cancer in its early stages. Much of the early detection effort is made by patients themselves with self examination, physicians with periodic physical examination, and radiologists with mammography screening who identify, obtain, and deliver specimens from suspiciously altered breast tissue, most of which does not harbor malignancy. Good communication among those involved in obtaining diagnostic specimens and among those who use the results of the diagnosis is required to maximize management of breast disease. The pathologist needs to know the history of both the patient and the lesion, the anatomic location and characteristics of the lesion, and whether the lesion was detected by mammography, with or without calcifications, as a result of nipple discharge, or from palpation of the mass by the patient herself or her surgeon. It is important to know how the biopsy was taken, how it is oriented, when it was collected, and the plans for therapy based upon the biopsy report. In turn, the pathologist must communicate his or her continuing evaluation to the surgeon, radiologist, radiotherapist, plastic surgeon, and oncologist, in order to obtain the necessary tissue for optimum diagnosis and staging, as well as to advise on management.

Biopsy takes one of several forms, each of which carries it's own special circumstances, requirements, and limitations. Biopsies include cytologic preparations, core needle biopsies, and open biopsies. Frozen sections are discussed, followed by a consideration of the current status of margins, the data on multifocality/multicentricity of breast cancer and, finally, features that predict for local recurrence.

BREAST CYTOLOGY

Material for cytologic examination may be gathered from nipple secretions, aspirates of cysts, aspirates of mammographically detected abnormalities, and aspirates of solid lesions.

Nipple Secretions

Papanicolaou et al. (1) described the exfoliative cytology of the breast from nipple secretions. Because these secretions are obtained without an invasive procedure, they are an important source of diagnostic material, even though the false negativity rate is high and it is easy to suggest a high rate of suspicious, but nondiagnostic findings. Nipple secretions are associated with proliferative changes within the ducts and most of these are benign. Fischermann et al. (2) reported on a series of patients in which none of the patients with a nonbloody discharge and no palpable mass had carcinoma on nipple secretion cytology, but 13% of patients with a bloody discharge without a mass had cancer, and 37% of patients with a bloody discharge and a mass in the underlying breast were found to have a carcinoma. Nipple discharge was associated with papillomatosis in 72% of the cases, and many of these patients had a bloody discharge. Takeda et al. (3) found a high likelihood of carcinoma in nipple secretions that were bloody and contained groups of 30 or more cells. Johnson and Kini (4) studied nipple secretions in 225 patients and diagnosed carcinoma in 3 of 216 (1.5%) women and 2 of 9 (22%) in men. Dunn et al. (5) diagnosed 16 of 29 breast cancers in women with nipple discharge from cytologic findings in nipple secretions. Nine of the 16 cases were in women with nonpalpable tumors. Shen et al. (6) performed ductoscopy with cytologic washings correlated with histology in 259 women with nipple discharge. None of the patients had cancer, 68 patients had single papillomas, 21 patients had multiple papillomas, and 3 patients had papillomatosis.

Aspiration of Cysts

Aspiration of presumptive breast cysts has long been practiced as both a diagnostic and therapeutic maneuver. Aspiration of clear fluid, in large volume, with disappearance of the palpated lesion is evidence of a benign cyst, and a few series have reported on its cytologic value. Takeda, et al. (7) studied 57 patients in which 10 of 17 cases subsequently shown to contain carcinoma were first discovered through cytologic examination of cyst fluid. No false positive results were found in this series. Bell et al. (8) reported comparable figures.

Aspiration of Solid Masses

Kline et al. (9–10), Oertel (12), Daum et al. (13), Giard and Hermans (14), and Gupta et al. (15) have described the value and problems associated with fine needle aspiration (FNA) of breast lesions. A range of abnormal cells and cell groupings may be obtained from benign proliferative changes found in the breast. Perhaps the most difficult pitfall is the appearance of proliferative epithelium from the elongated ducts of a fibroadenomas, which, of course, also presents as a mass lesion. These problems were described by Benoit et al. (16) and Dejmek and Lindholm (17). Rao et al. (18) described the malignant spindle cells of a phyllodes tumor. Bhagat and Kline (19) and Martin-Bates et al. (20) described changes in the male breast and problems in the diagnosis of gynecomastia. Grenko et al. (21) and Gupta et al. (22) described the appearance of secretory cells aspirated from a lactating adenoma. The distinction of carcinoma from any of these changes may be difficult, as is evident from false positive diagnoses which appear in several large series, as reviewed and described by Zarbo et al. (23).

In general, aspiration of a carcinoma provides abundant cellular material in groups and as single cells and this should be considered a baseline for interpretation of the specimen as diagnostic for malignancy. The individual cells display the characteristic features of cancer, primarily because of their large nuclei with irregular membranes and chromatin. The mere presence of nucleoli is not evidence of malignancy. Another major pitfall is the overinterpretation of poorly preserved material. The cytopathologist should insist upon those cytologic changes that are clearly characteristic of malignancy. Sneige (24) reported on 1,995 cases of FNA of palpable masses with biopsy follow-up. Sixty percent of cases were positive and 30% were benign. Eleven aspirations were suspicious and included three fibroadenomas, three ductal hyperplasias, two adenosis tumors, two mucoceles, and one nipple adenoma. Two false positive results included an apocrine cyst with atypia and a radial scar. de la Torre et al. (25) reported that aspirations of radial scars were relatively hypocellular, contained myoepithelial cells, and lacked prominent nucleoli; however, the aspirations did contain angular tubular structures similar to those of tubular carcinoma.

Malberger et al. (26) described the appearance of aspirates of scar formed in the breast following biopsy, Yeoh et al. (27) described mucoceles, and Dodd et al. (28) described the appearance of silicone in cells aspirated from the vicinity of an implant. Tanaka et al. (29) analyzed 14 factors associated with false negative results and found low nuclear grade, cellular distribution of cancer cells, and benign ultrasound appearance to be most significant. Increasingly, a diagnosis of suspicious for, or diagnostic of, carcinoma is followed by an excisional biopsy rather than mastectomy, which protects the pathologist and the patient somewhat from the consequences of false positive results. Good communication with the clinical staff about the implications of the diagnosis should be well established.

Distinctions between ductal hyperplasia, atypia, and ductal carcinoma *in situ* (DCIS) may be extremely difficult on fine needle aspirate smears. This problem has been discussed by Abendroth et al. (30), Markovic-Glamocak et al. (31), Stanley et al. (32), Venegas et al. (33), and Wang et al. (34). Chapter 4 presents problems relating to the histologic distinctions among these entities.

The use of FNA directed by radiographic technique (x-ray or ultrasound) has been discussed by Helvie et al. (35), Layfield et al. (36), Masood et al. (37), Rogers and Lee (38), and Sneige et al. (39,40). Thomas et al. (41) favorably compared the value of FNA to that of frozen section. Pisano et al. (42) reported on the Radiologic Diagnostic Oncology Group (RDOG) study of 377 cases in which core needle biopsy was found to be superior to fine needle aspirate, primarily because insufficient samples were obtained by FNA in 128 (34%) of the cases. Calcifications alone were associated with a significantly higher rate of insufficient sampling than were masses. Another shortcoming of FNA is the inability to definitively diagnose benign lesions and correlate them with mammography. The prospective RDOG study was prematurely terminated because of these deficiencies in the FNA material. Lee et al. (43) described the histologic changes that occur in the breast as a result of multiple passes with the fine needle for aspiration.

Salhany and Page (44) described FNA of lobular carcinoma *in situ* (LCIS) and atypical lobular hyperplasia (ALH) as loosely cohesive groups of uniform cells with eccentric nuclei, minimal atypia, and occasional intracytoplasmic lumina. Infiltrating lobular carcinomas had a higher proportion of noncohesive cells with more nuclear atypia and pleomorphism. Intracytoplasmic lumina were consistently found in invasive and noninvasive lobular lesions and were considered the single most useful cytologic clue for their recognition.

Sneige et al. (45) described FNA metastases to the breast from oat cell carcinoma, melanoma, serous ovarian carcinoma, lung cancer, lymphoma, carcinoid, myeloma, rhabdomyosarcoma, and bladder carcinoma. In most cases, the cytologic appearance gave the diagnosis of metastasis, but adenocarcinoma of the lung mimicked breast carcinoma. The authors recommended knowing the complete history, suspecting metastasis when the pattern was unusual, and employing immunohistochemistry.

Corkill et al. (46) described FNA of intracystic papillary carcinoma as cellular smears with papillary or cribriform clusters and numerous single cuboidal or columnar cells with minimal atypia. Seven of eight cases had diploid nuclei.

Fischler et al. (47) described the FNA of tubular carcinoma as cellular smears made up of angular tubular structures with single epithelial cells. Staining for smooth muscle actin was negative on the fragments. Gupta et al. (22,48) described the FNA of secretory carcinoma as cellular smears of cells with prominent cytoplasmic vacuoles and secretion in malignant cells with occasional signet ring forms.

The following photomicrographs in the text and on the CD display the spectrum of changes seen in breast cytopathology. Apocrine metaplasia is a common finding of cells seen in any type of material (Color Plate 1). The normal appearance of a terminal duct is seen only in aspirated material (Color Plate 2). The foam cells of fibrocystic change are in efig.3.1. Stromal fibroblasts are a common component of aspirates (Color Plate 3). Lactating cells are shown in efigs. 3.2 and 3.3. Some of the problems associated with the interpretation of material from fibroadenomas are shown in Color Plates 4 and 5 and efigs. 3.4 and 3.5. The extreme cellularity and the high level of activity within the individual cells make these lesions quite worrisome. Gynecomastia reveals cells and groups similar to those seen in fibroadenomas (Color Plate 6). Ductal hyperplasia is seen in both nipple secretions and aspirates. In hyperplasias, the number of groups is usually small and stratification of the cells with evident columnar cells forming a distinct luminal border is a helpful indicator of benignancy (Color Plates 7 and 8 and efigs. 3.6 to 3.8). Papillary carcinoma or intraductal carcinoma may shed cells in nipple secretion. These may present as papillary groups with clearly malignant cells (Color Plates 9 and 10). Aspiration of a group of malignant cells from a solid mass may present the difficult diagnostic dilemma of *in situ* versus invasive carcinoma. Color Plates 11 and 12 and efig. 3.9 show the solid variant of intraductal carcinoma. Efig. 3.10 shows micropapillary DCIS. The regularity of the cells and the central location of their nuclei, as well as the lack of regularity of the nuclear borders, chromatin, and nucleoli, indicate malignancy.

Efig.3.11 shows a low magnification of a smear aspirate from an invasive carcinoma. Color Plate 13 shows a large number of cells with extremely high nuclear/cytoplasmic ratios and angular irregular nuclei that denote malignancy. The formation of a small duct is indicative of a well-differentiated carcinoma. Color Plate 14 and efigs. 3.12 to 3.14 show malignant cells with extremely anaplastic nuclei and a small amount of cytoplasm. No architectural features are evident. This is indicative of a carcinoma with a high nuclear and histologic grade. Efigs.3.15 and 3.16 show an aspirate from a micropapillary invasive carcinoma. In Color Plate 15 and efigs. 3.17 and 3.18, the aspirate shows relatively few cells, but the nuclei clearly indicate malignancy and some cells have the signet ring appearance that is characteristic of a variant of invasive lobular carcinoma. Efig. 3.19 shows necrotic debris aspirated from a cancer. Color Plate 16 is an aspiration of a chest wall mass in a patient previously treated for carcinoma. The presence of the malignant cells in the fibroadipose stroma is diagnostic of recurrence of the carcinoma in the scar.

Mammographic Patterns

Radiologists interpreting mammograms now detect more breast cancers at an earlier stage than patients practicing self-detection or physicians palpating the breasts during physical examination. Wolfe et al. (49) described several patterns in mammograms: N1, normal; P1, prominent duct pattern; P2, more than 25% of the breast involved by prominent ducts where dense linear structures involve all of the parenchyma; DY, a markedly dense appearance to the entire breast; and QDY, markedly dense appearance to the entire breast (i.e., DY) with small islands of fat present in the breast of women under the age of 40 years. P2 and DY have been associated with an elevated risk of the development of breast cancer. Wolfe et al. (49) reported a 3.3 relative risk for P2 and DY compared to N1 plus P1. This was confirmed by Carlile et al. (50), Warner et al. (51), and Boyd et al. (52).

Calcifications

Mammographic abnormalities include architectural distortions, masses, and new, large, or clustered calcifications. Berend et al. (53) followed 91 women with indeterminate calcifications for 6 to 30 months and reported that five of them developed carcinoma. Thomas et al. (54) found a relative risk of 1.68 for the development of breast cancer in women with calcifications, 2.14 for bilateral calcifications, 2.09 for multiple ring or linear calcifications, and 3.64 when clustered calcifications were present. Ciatto et al. (55) reported on 1,182 consecutive cases detected by mammography of which 548 were malignant. The presence of isolated calcifications or irregular or stellate opacities were the most predictive of cancer.

Hall et al. (56) found calcified masses and abnormal calcifications equally predictive of cancer. Newstead et al. (57) noted masses or architectural distortion in all detected cancer cases. Calcifications were present in 47% of those with invasive ductal carcinoma, but in none of the patients with invasive lobular carcinoma.

Radial scars, which mimic cancer mammographically, grossly, and microscopically, have been reported as usually free of calcium, but Orel et al. (58) described four cases of radial scar with microcalcifications. The significance of radial scars remains somewhat controversial, with the radiology literature viewing them with greater alarm than the pathology literature (Chapter 6).

Localization of nonpalpable lesions requires preoperative needle localization (59). The excised area is then reexamined by specimen mammography to ascertain that the localizing wire was removed, as well as the entire lesion (Figs. 3.1 and 3.2 and efigs. 3.20 and 3.21). After that, the specimen is seen in surgical pathology and a determination is made as to whether frozen sections should be done (see frozen section discussion) (60). Blocks are then submitted to encompass the mammographically detected lesion. Owings et al. (61) described a study

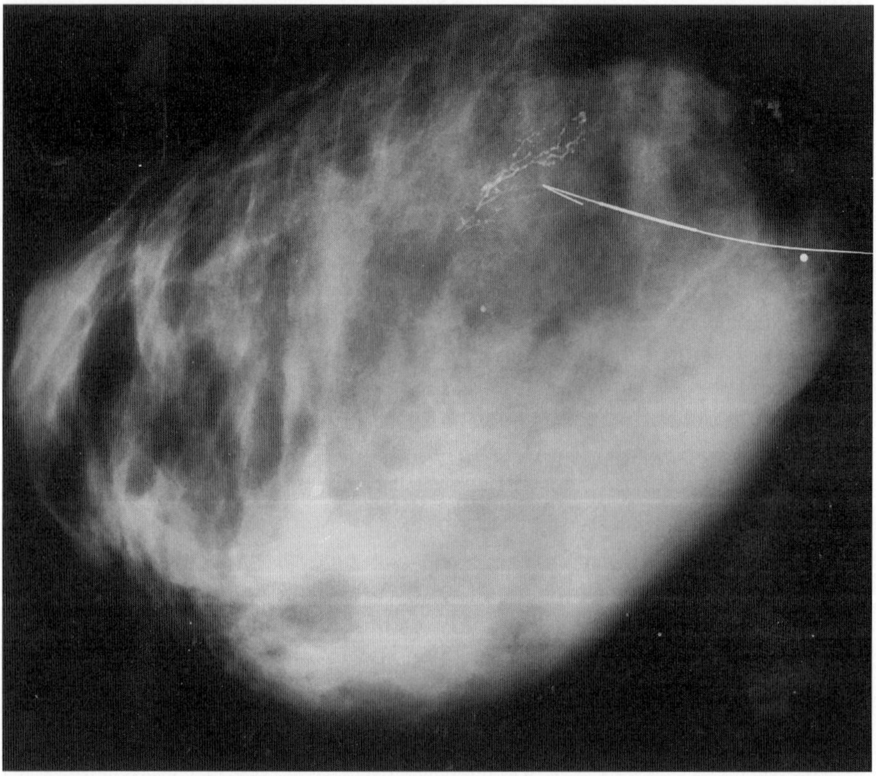

FIG. 3.1. Specimen radiograph. Clustered linear calcifications localized by an intact wire and a narrow rim of normal (uncalcified) tissue are documented.

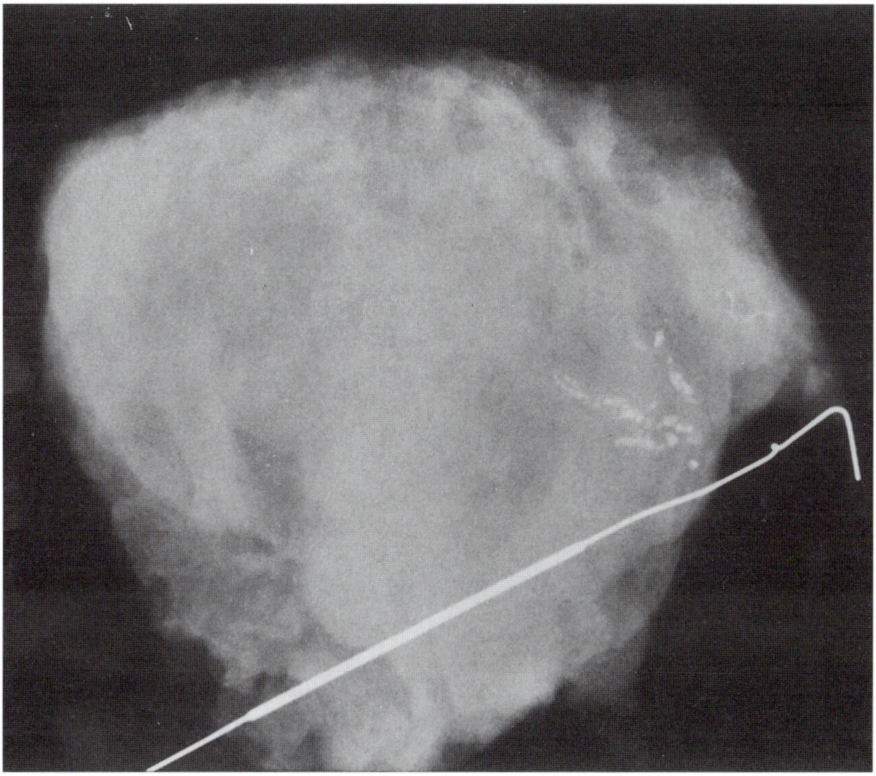

FIG. 3.2. Specimen radiograph. The intact (although displaced) localizing wire, the coarse linear calcifications suggestive of comedocarcinoma, and the absence of a margin of normal (uncalcified) tissue at the margin of the specimen are documented.

of 157 biopsies completely submitted to determine the best and most efficient way to sample these specimens. The authors recommended that blocks from the abnormal density and any area of calcification be submitted along with all the fibrous tissue, but not with the fat in the biopsy. Calcification was found in association with cancer in 94% of the cases, but atypical ductal hyperplasia (ADH) was not calcium associated in 5 of 19 cases.

Pathologists spend much time and effort trying to find the calcification for which biopsy was performed. If calcium cannot be found on the original sections, we recommend that all blocks be x-rayed. Those that are found to contain calcium should be resectioned. Calcium phosphate can be identified on carefully evaluated H&E sections by basophilia and sharp intensely basophilic borders; it may also be lamellar. Calcium phosphate is the most common form of calcification. It may be found in ducts that are proliferative or nonproliferative, benign or malignant, in the adjacent stroma or in the stroma of carcinomas or benign lesions, and especially in collagenized fibroadenomas where it may present as large, coarse, and linear structures like those seen in comedocarcinoma (Figs. 3.3 to 3.6, efigs. 3.22 to 3.24, and Table 3.1).

Poggi et al. (62) studied sections of breast tissue by scanning electron microscopy and backscattered electron microscopy energy and wavelength chemical analyses. The authors found mineral deposits of less than 1 to 50 μ in size to mostly contain calcium phosphate as single or compound aggregates of spherules of 1 to 4 μ in size. Differing ratios of calcium to phosphate were observed, depending on the site of deposition, with lower ratios in stromal calcifications in fibroadenomas than in the calcifications found in intraductal lesions, both benign and malignant. Calcifications found in fibroadenoma stroma had a bimodal size distribution of calcium phosphate spherules. Calcium oxalate crystallites were found in benign ducts and they were birefringent and ranged in size from 1 to 60 μ.

Stein and Karlan (63) described 277 cases in which biopsy was done solely for the presence of microcalcification. Calcium phosphate was found in 93% of the cases. In 2 of the 12 other cases, calcium oxalate was present. Calcium was also reported in 8% of cases in which the mammographer had reported no calcium. This points out the several order of magnitude difference in resolution between mammography and optical microscopy. Calcifications seen by the pathologist are from 10 μm to 1 mm in diameter and only 5 μ (the thickness of the section) deep, whereas those seen by the radiologist are 3-dimensional and may be about 1 mm in diameter, but are limited in depth only by the thickness of the mammary tissue. Radiologists and pathologists should keep in mind that each is accurately determining the presence of microcalcifications, but the cal-

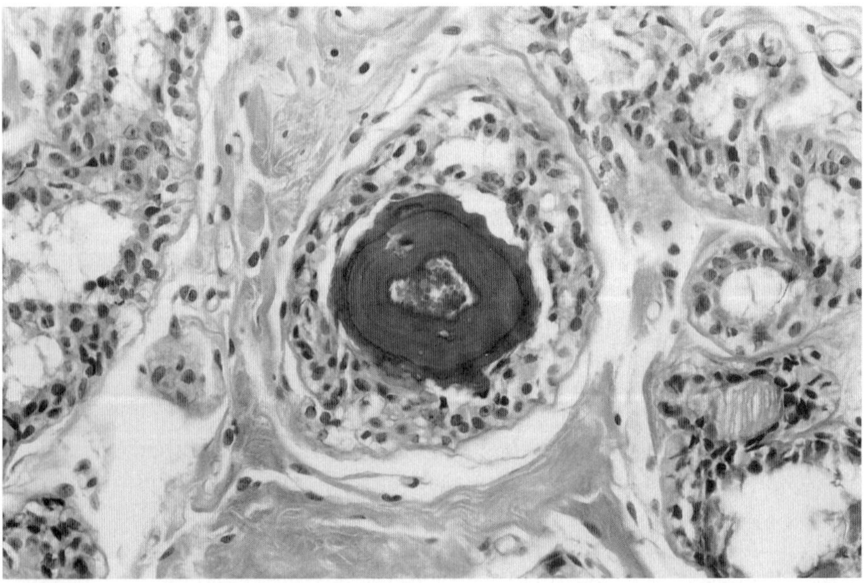

FIG. 3.3. Microcalcification. The characteristic features of calcium phosphate calculi-marked basophilia, a sharp blue border, and lamellar configuration are present in a benign, slightly hyperplastic, terminal duct.

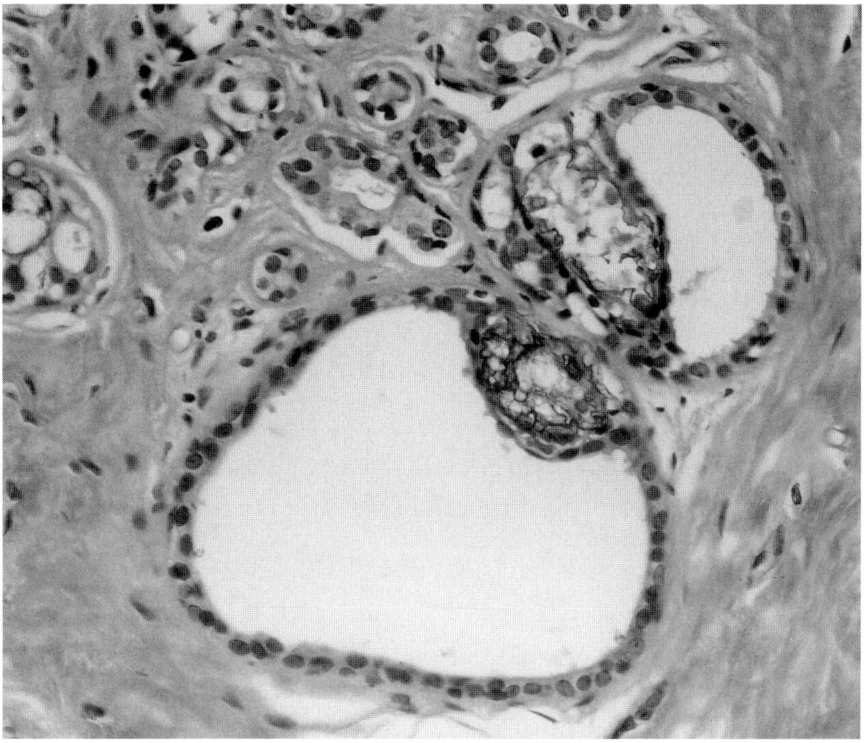

FIG. 3.4. Microcalcification (calcium phosphate) in the stroma adjacent to a dilated terminal duct of blunt ductal adenosis. The calcium deposit is an aggregate of numerous small basophilic calcifications with sharply circumscribed basophilic edges, but they are not lamellar.

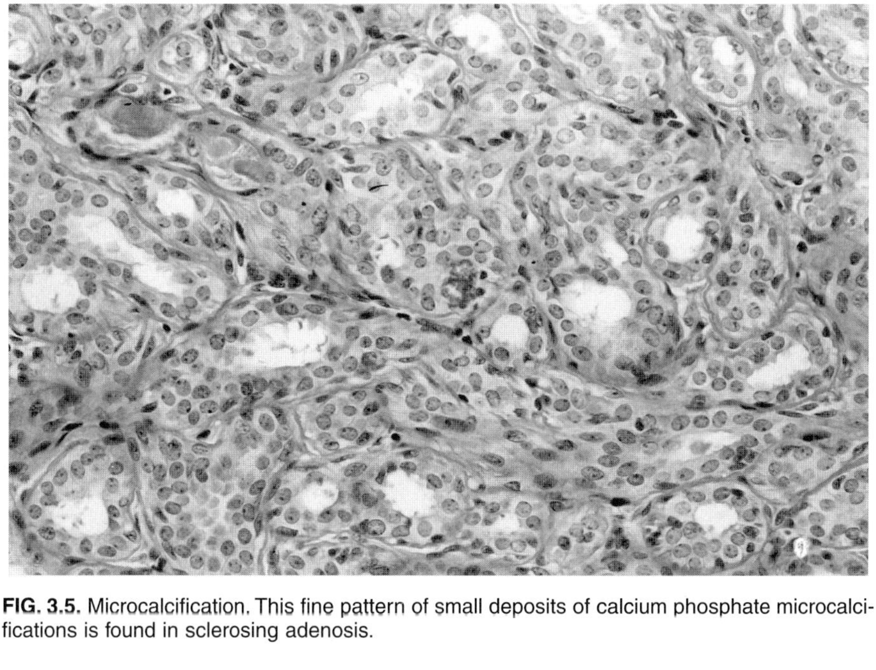

FIG. 3.5. Microcalcification. This fine pattern of small deposits of calcium phosphate microcalcifications is found in sclerosing adenosis.

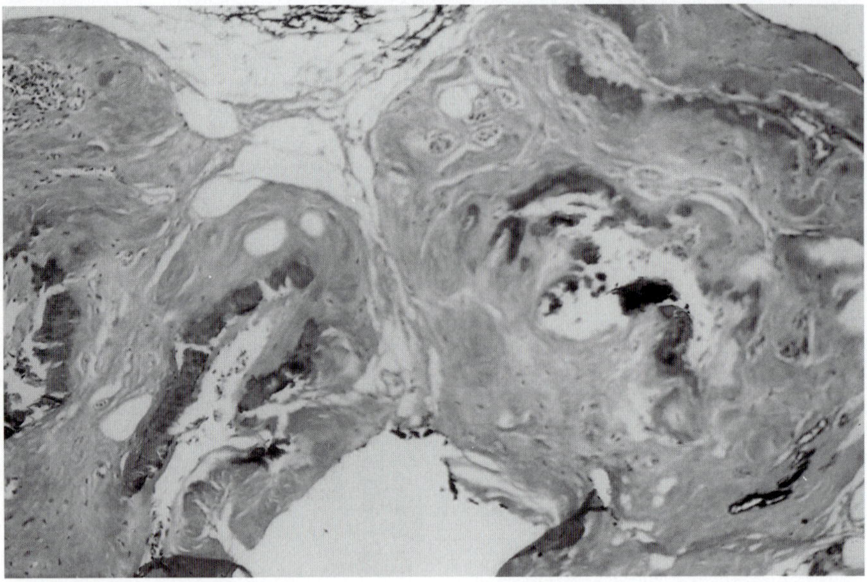

FIG. 3.6. Stromal microcalcification. These coarse deposits are characteristic of calcium phosphate laid down on some collagenized fibroadenomas. Their size and linearity produce a mammographic appearance that is suggestive of comedocarcinoma.

cifications described may be entirely different. The pathologist is finding calcifications that are not necessarily evident radiographically, and calcium is often not the most serious lesion in the biopsy! This last point deserves special emphasis. When microcalcifications are found in carcinoma, they are almost always found in the intraductal component and not in the invasive carcinoma.

Lee et al. (64) reported on 59 cases of intraductal carcinoma that were diagnosed on core needle biopsies done for microcalcifications and followed by open biopsy. Calcification was limited to DCIS in 49% of cases and to DCIS and benign areas in another 42%. Calcification was seen in both the DCIS and invasive carcinoma in 3% (two cases) and in benign tissue in only two other cases. In 17 of the 49 cases (29%), invasive carcinoma was found on open biopsy. Follow-up for calcifications may therefore overlook invasive carcinoma.

D'Orsi et al. (65) described the absence of calcification in 26% of blocks taken from tissue that was shown to contain calcification on specimen mammography.

TABLE 3.1. *Microcalcifications in the breast*

Calcium	Phosphate	Oxalate
White light	Yes	No
Polarized	No	Yes
Benign	Yes	Yes
Malignant	Yes	?No
Ducts	Yes	Yes
Stroma	Yes	No

Of those blocks found to be without calcium on the first section, 95.4% were found to contain calcium on x-ray of the blocks. Microcalcifications were found on 49% of new sections from these blocks. The blocks in which sections were still negative for calcification were x-rayed a second time, which demonstrated calcification in 45%, of which 64% were confirmed as having microcalcification on section. Of those still negative, another round of x-rays revealed calcification in 40%, and half of these produced microcalcification-bearing slides. If calcification is not found on the original section, but is seen on x-rays of the blocks, we recommend that those blocks be step-sectioned. It is rare that calcification is not detected in this manner. Symonds et al. (66) reported the value of von Kossa stains for the identification of microcalcifications in the 10% of cases in which microcalcification on the original H&E sections was not found.

Symonds et al. (66) reviewed 503 consecutive biopsies with specimen mammograms and found that 48% contained calcifications. Carcinoma was found in 17% of those with calcification, compared to 10% in the noncalcified group; however, the calcification was in DCIS and not the invasive carcinoma in 60% of the positive cases. Holland et al. (67) reviewed cases of DCIS detected by screening mammography, virtually all of which were unicentric, and found linear branching calcification or coarse granular calcification in high grade DCIS. Histologically, this calcium was amorphous. Multiple clusters of finely granular calcifications were mammographically detected in lower grades of DCIS. These were usually laminated histologically. Evans et al. (68) found diffuse calcification in 10 of 77 palpable cases of DCIS, but in none of 54 cases detected as part of a screening procedure. These symptomatic cases were larger and calcification was present in 48 of the 77 cases, but calcification was less likely to be in DCIS than in the cases detected in the screening group. The comedocarcinoma variant of DCIS was seen in 26% of the screened group and 45% of palpable group. Stomper et al. (69) found 78% of linear calcifications in comedocarcinomas and 53% of granular calcifications in noncomedo calcifications. LCIS may be calcified (70). Sonnenfeld et al. (71) reviewed 41 cases of LCIS in which biopsy followed the findings of a mammographic abnormality. Clustered calcifications were seen in 31 of the 41 cases (76%), but the calcifications were found in benign ducts in 24 of the 31 cases. The authors considered LCIS to be coincidentally found and not related to the presence of the calcifications. Kopans et al. (72) found 10 cases of apocrine intraductal carcinoma to be associated with a profuse deposition of heterogeneous forms of calcifications. Holland et al. described radiologic–pathologic correlations of small occult (67) and interval (73) carcinomas.

CALCIUM OXALATE

Going et al. (74), Tornos et al. (75), and Frouge et al. (76) described the presence of calcium oxalate (weddelite) in the luminal spaces of benign ducts with cystic change. Calcium oxalate may be inapparent in white light, but it is evident on polarized light (Figs. 3.7 to 3.10 and efigs. 3.25 to 3.26) (calcium phosphate is not birefringent). Winston et al. (77) reviewed cases in which the biopsies

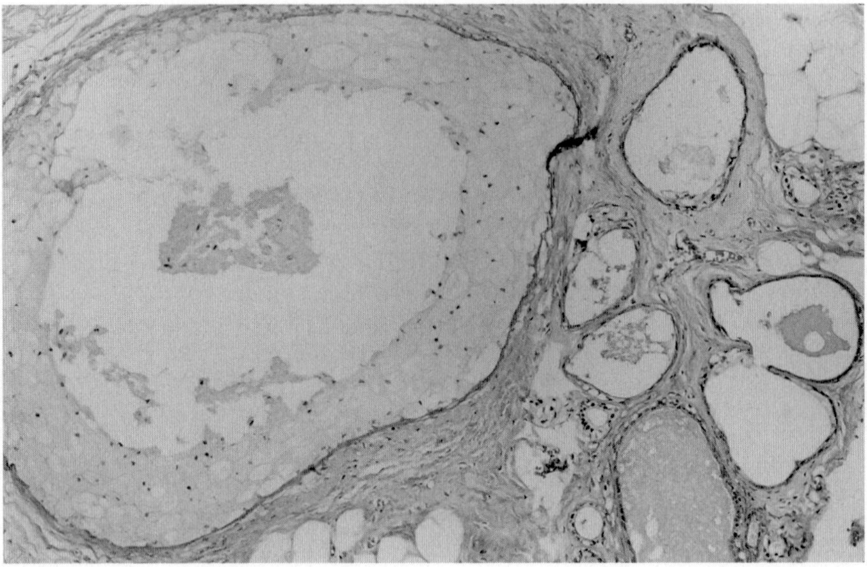

FIG. 3.7. Fibrocystic changes. This large duct is distended and filled with foamy macrophages. Several smaller ducts are also distended. No calcification is evident in this photomicrograph taken in white light, but this histologic appearance is often the site of calcium oxalate deposits.

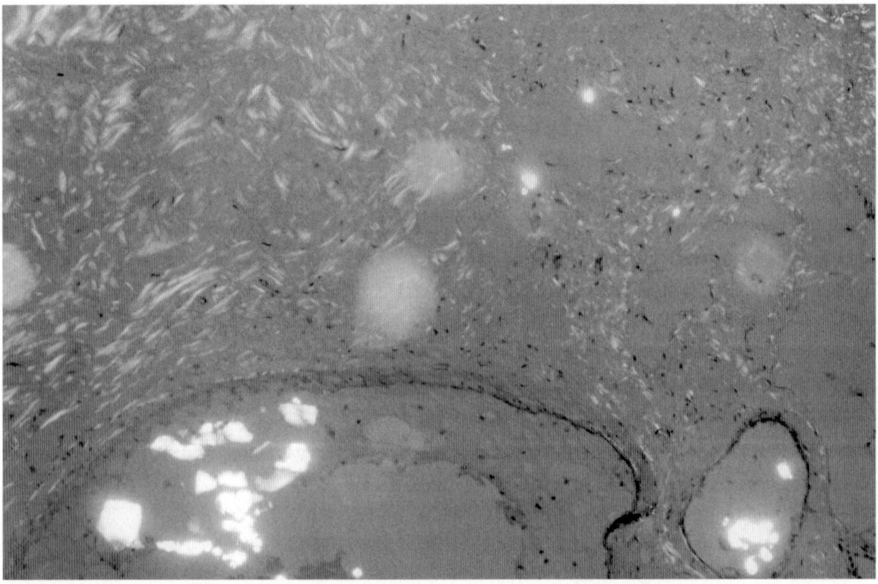

FIG. 3.8. Calcium oxalate in cystic duct. Field from Fig. 3.7 photographed in polarized light displays the birefringent crystals of calcium oxalate in the apparently empty zone of the larger duct and in one of the six smaller ducts.

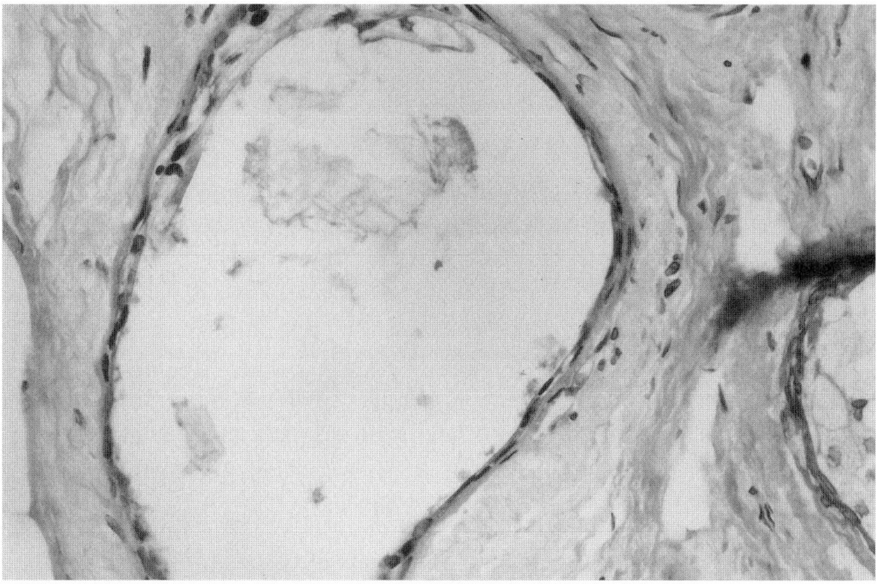

FIG. 3.9. Cystically dilated duct. At higher magnification, the smaller duct at the 1 o'clock position in Fig. 3.7 contains some apparently amorphous material with a negative image defined by sharp edges. In white light, it is easy to pass over the oxalate crystals.

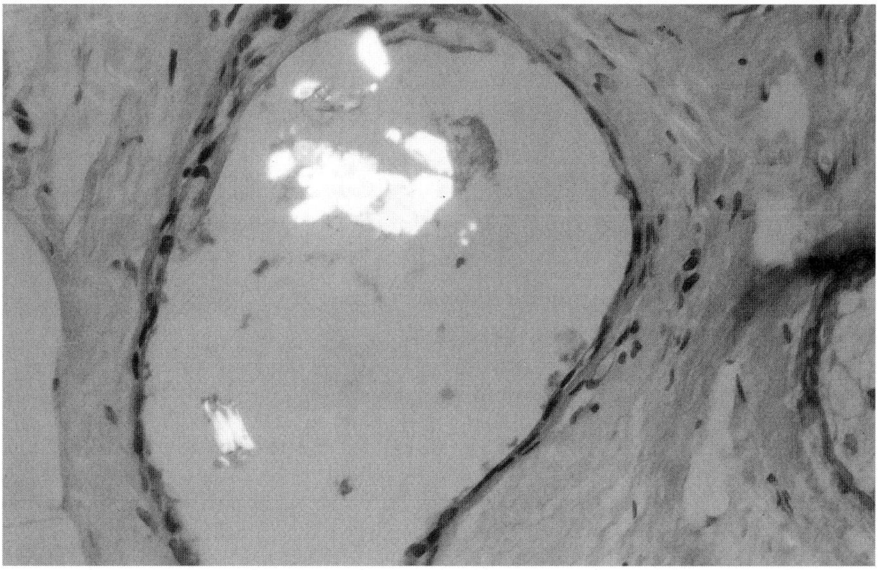

FIG. 3.10. Calcium oxalate in dilated duct. In polarized light, the duct from Fig. 3.9 contains birefringent crystals of calcium oxalate. A microscope that can provide polarized light is essential for finding this inapparent calcium and documenting that the abnormality that precipitated needle localized biopsy has been microscopically identified.

revealed calcium oxalate and found them to be associated with a low density and a scattered pattern on mammogram. Cystically dilated ducts with foamy macrophages and a flattened lining of apocrine epithelium is the best place to look for calcium oxalate, with its refractile appearance in white light confirmed by its birefringent appearance in polarized light.

Needle Biopsy

Stereotactically directed core needle biopsies (SCNB) have come into increased usage with the availability of improved imaging equipment and the use of larger (11-gauge) needles.

The primary purpose of SCNB is the precise diagnosis of a benign lesion that correlates with the suspicious radiographic abnormality. A diagnosis of fibroadenoma, especially when associated with stromal calcification, sclerosing adenosis, and of clustered calcifications when completely excised, may be sufficient to reassure the radiologist that the suspicious area is a benign lesion and that the patient may be safely followed radiographically. The finding of benign breast tissue, without these diagnoses and a lack of correlation between pathology and the radiographic appearance, indicates either another stereotactic biopsy or an open biopsy to resolve the suspicion. Intermediate diagnoses raise the suspicion for the mammographically detected lesion and consensus dictates that they should be followed by an open biopsy. These diagnoses primarily include ADH and an abnormality of suspicious histologic appearance that cannot be resolved by the pathologist. Incomplete removal of the suspicious areas of calcification should be followed up with additional diagnostic material. Consensus has not developed on the management of stereotactic core needle biopsy diagnosis of ALH, LCIS, or radial scar.

The diagnosis of malignancy on SCNB is normally followed by an open excisional biopsy. Distinction between intraductal carcinoma and invasive carcinoma on SCNB may be difficult and is discussed below. The finding of invasive carcinoma allows planning for a wider excision for margins and for addressing the issue of lymph node status at a single operation. In advanced cases of carcinoma or in those where neoadjuvant therapy is planned, it is possible to determine the steroid hormone receptor status, HER2/neu status, and proliferative level from the core needle biopsy. In these instances, the size of the mass on x-ray is probably the most accurate for staging purposes.

Accuracy of localization is high for both mass lesions and microcalcification. The value of this technique is its relatively low morbidity for lesions of moderate suspicion, which might otherwise go to open biopsy. SCNB diagnosis of fibroadenoma, sclerosing adenosis, or possibly benign ductal hyperplasia in a completely removed cluster of microcalcifications will often allow the patient to be followed mammographically without open biopsy. Needle biopsies presented to the pathologist pose special challenges, especially when pseudoinvasive lesions (e.g., sclerosing adenosis, radial scar, and atypical apocrine sclerosing

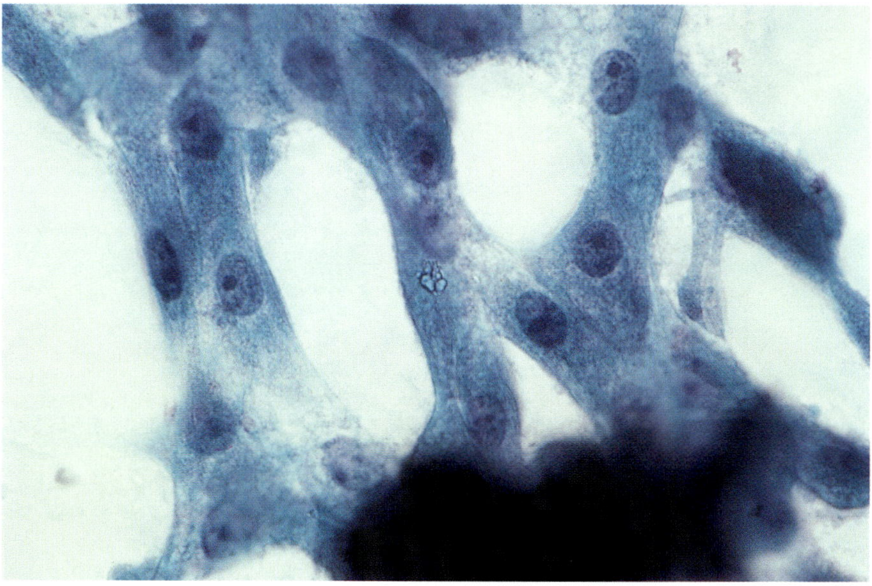

PLATE 1. Apocrine metaplasia. This fine needle aspiration of a cyst yielded numerous large cells with abundant granular cytoplasm. The nuclei are relatively small and rounded, but have large and prominent nucleoli. Papanicolaou's stain.

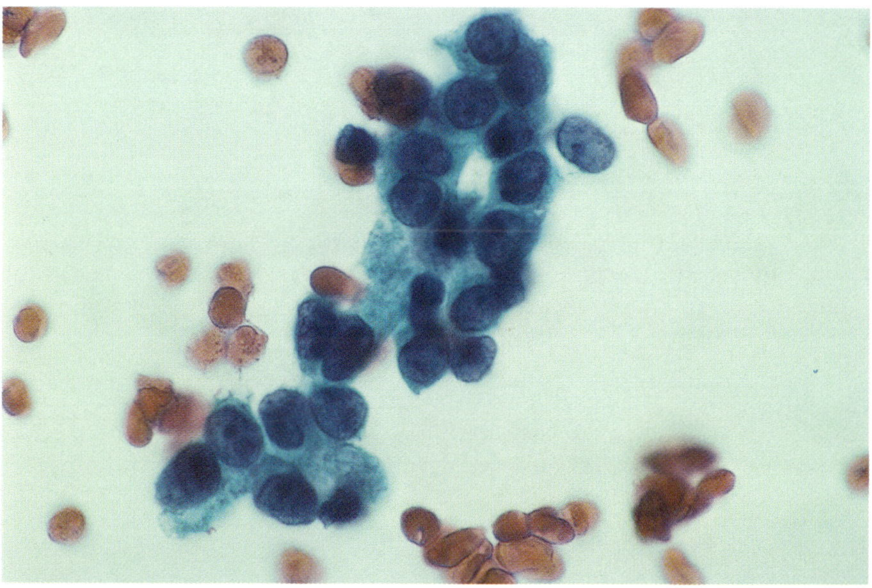

PLATE 2. Normal terminal duct. These aspirated cells form a small group with a central lumen. The cells are relatively small, some show a columnar configuration, and their nuclei are hyperchromatic, but regular in size and shape. The configuration of the group and appearance of the individual cells is that of a resting terminal duct. Papanicolaou's stain.

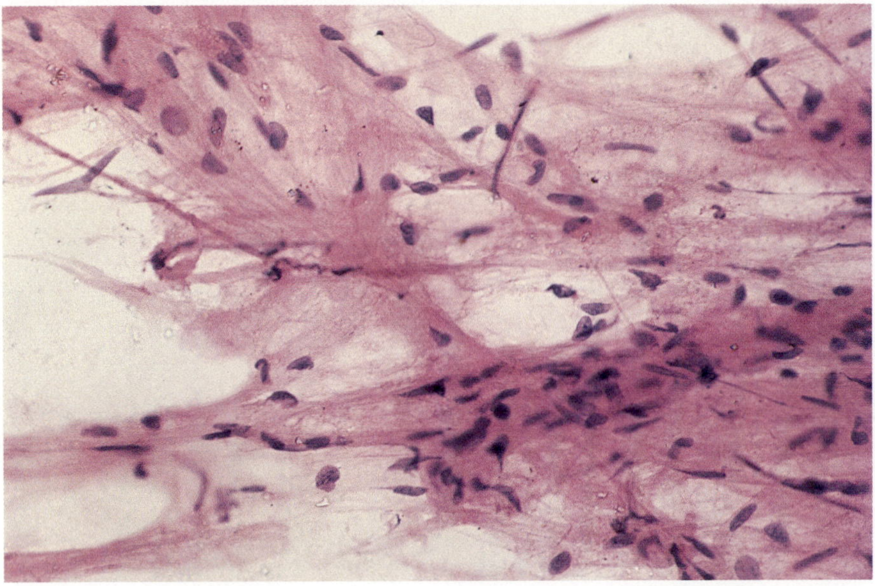

PLATE 3. Stromal fibroblasts and adipose tissue. The spindle-shaped fibroblasts are numerous and interwoven through the adipose tissue. The fibroblastic nuclei are small and regular. H&E stain.

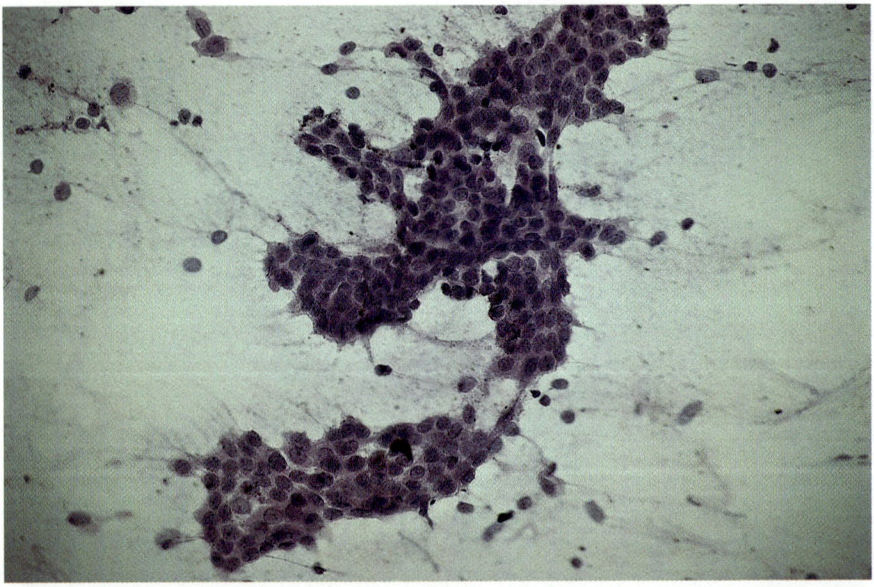

PLATE 4. Fibroadenoma. In this medium power view of a needle aspirate of a fibroadenoma, stroma is not evident and groups of epithelial cells are abundant, raising concern about malignancy; however, the staghorn configuration of the groupings is characteristic of fibroadenoma. H&E stain.

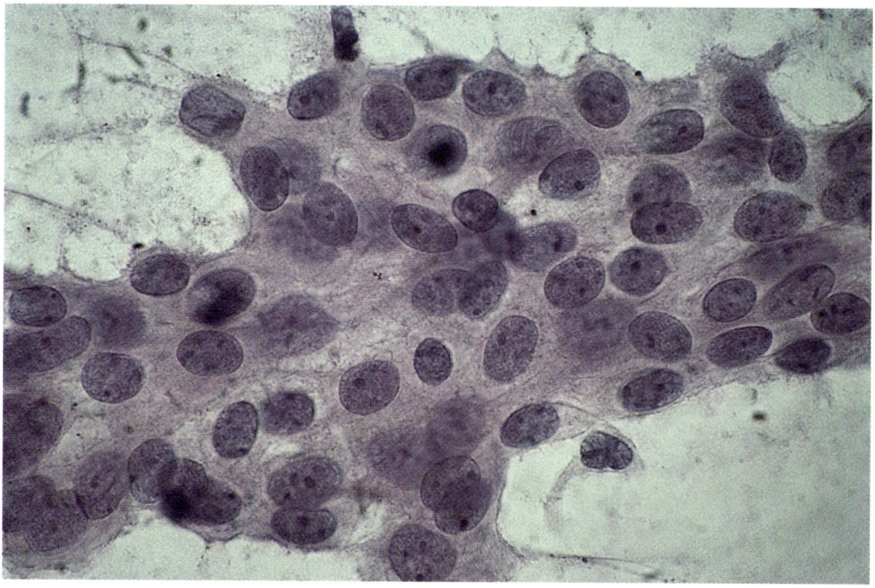

PLATE 5. Fibroadenoma. Same case as in Color Plate 4. At higher magnification, the epithelial cells are large with high nuclear/cytoplasmic ratios, moderate pleomorphism, and prominent nucleoli. The abundance of cell groups and the activity in their nuclei are reasons for difficulty in the cytologic interpretation of fibroadenomas. H&E stain.

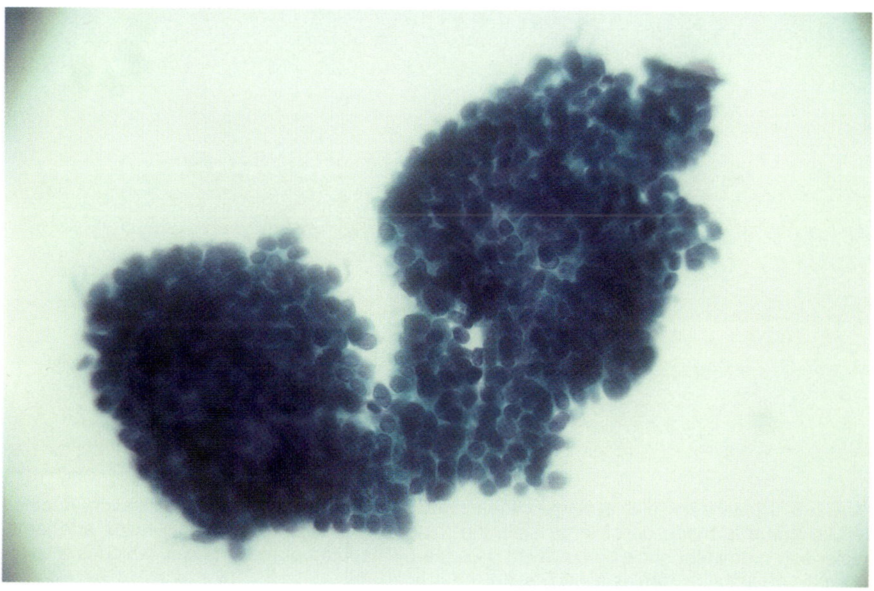

PLATE 6. Gynecomastia. Aspirate from an older man with a mass in his breast. A group of epithelial cells displays a level of cellularity, pleomorphism, and activity similar to that seen in the fibroadenoma in Fig. 3.5. Papanicolaou's stain.

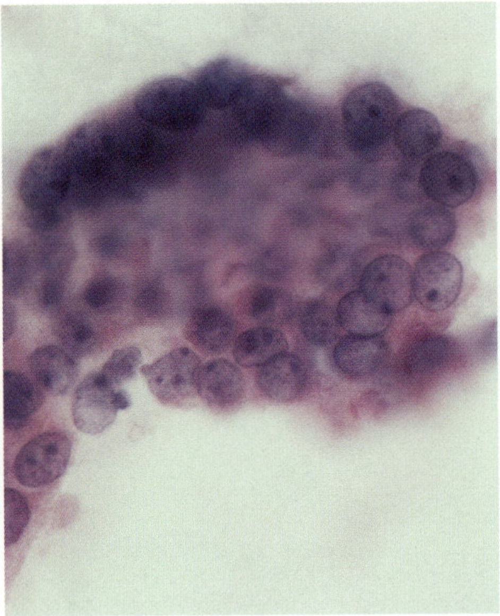

PLATE 7. Ductal hyperplasia. An aspirated specimen from a cystic lesion contains several clumps of cells, seen here at medium magnification. The stratification of the cells along the upper border is indicative of columnar differentiation and is useful in determining that the regular monomorphous pattern of ductal carcinoma *in situ* is not present. H&E stain.

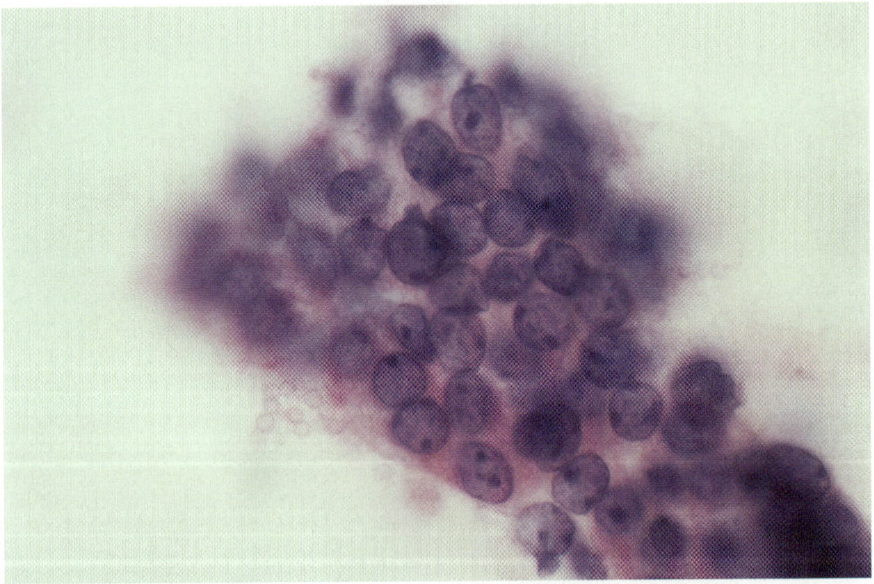

PLATE 8. Ductal hyperplasia. Same case as in Color Plate 7, at higher magnification. Another cellular group is made up of large cells that have high nuclear/cytoplasmic ratios and large nuclei with prominent nucleoli; however, note the overlapping at these nuclei, which is a characteristic of ductal hyperplasia. H&E stain.

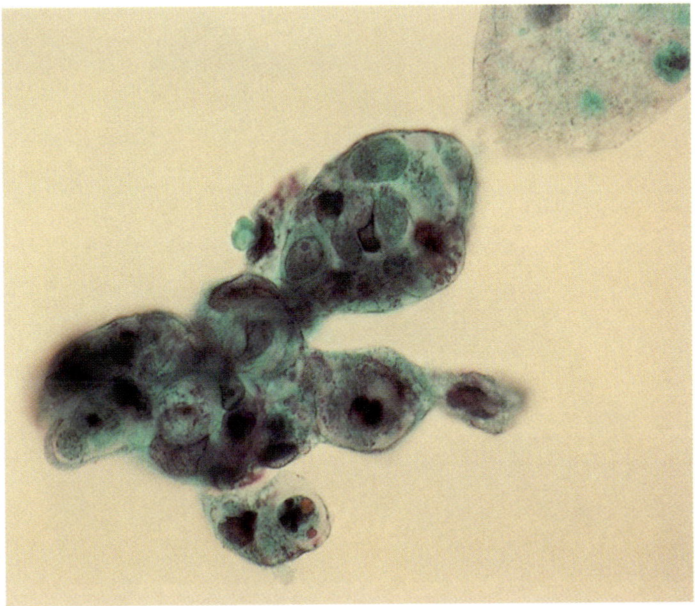

PLATE 9. Intraductal carcinoma. In this nipple discharge, a micropapillary group of large cells with large, hyperchromatic, and irregular nuclei is indicative of a micropapillary variant of ductal carcinoma *in situ*. Papanicolaou's stain.

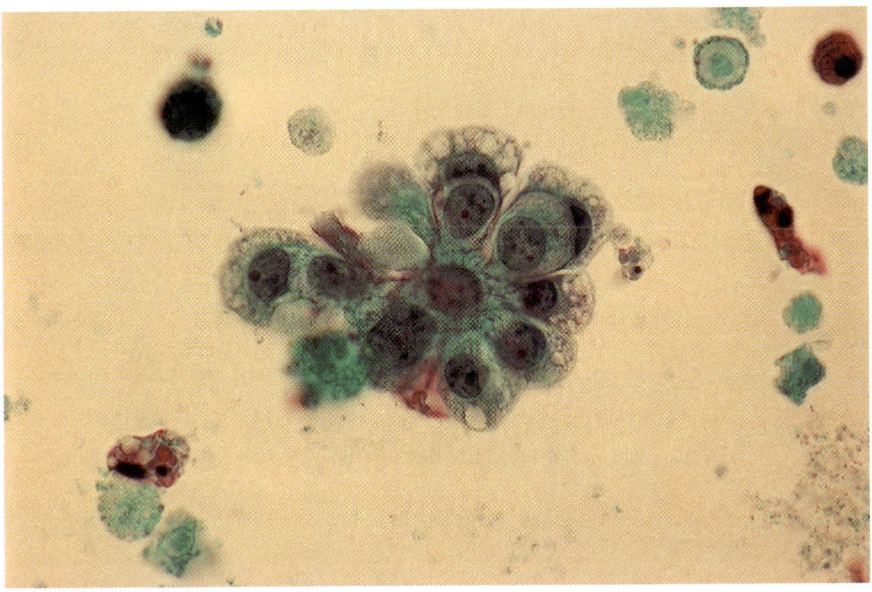

PLATE 10. Intraductal carcinoma. Nipple discharge with a micropapillary clump made up of large cells without overlapping of the large and irregular nuclei. No fibrovascular core is present. Papanicolaou's stain.

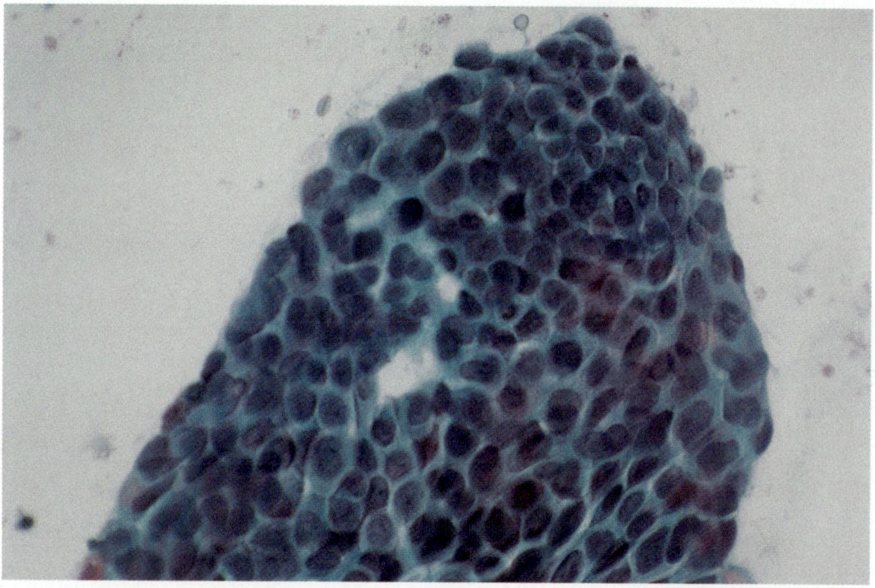

PLATE 11. Intraductal carcinoma. Aspiration of a firm area in the breast yielded large smooth-surfaced groups of a homogenous population of cells with centrally placed, irregular, hyperchromatic nuclei that are indicative of a solid variant of ductal carcinoma *in situ*. Papanicolaou's stain.

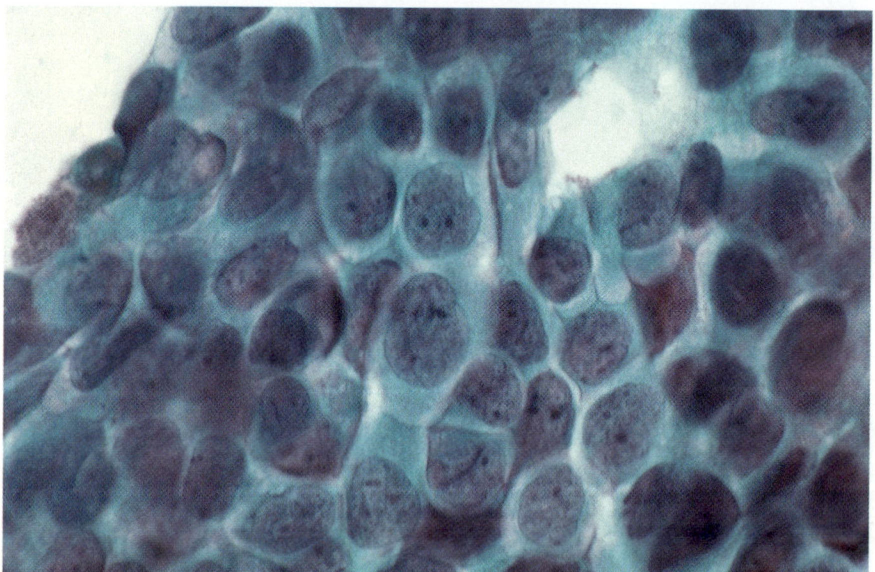

PLATE 12. Intraductal carcinoma. At higher magnification, a group from the same case (shown in Fig. 3.11) is composed of large cells with well-defined cytoplasmic membranes and large centrally placed nuclei with irregular nuclear borders, chromatin, and nucleoli. The nuclei do not overlap. The central location of the nuclei and the crispness of the cell borders lend an appearance of "rigidity" to this group of cells and is diagnostic of the solid variant of ductal carcinoma *in situ*. Papanicolaou's stain.

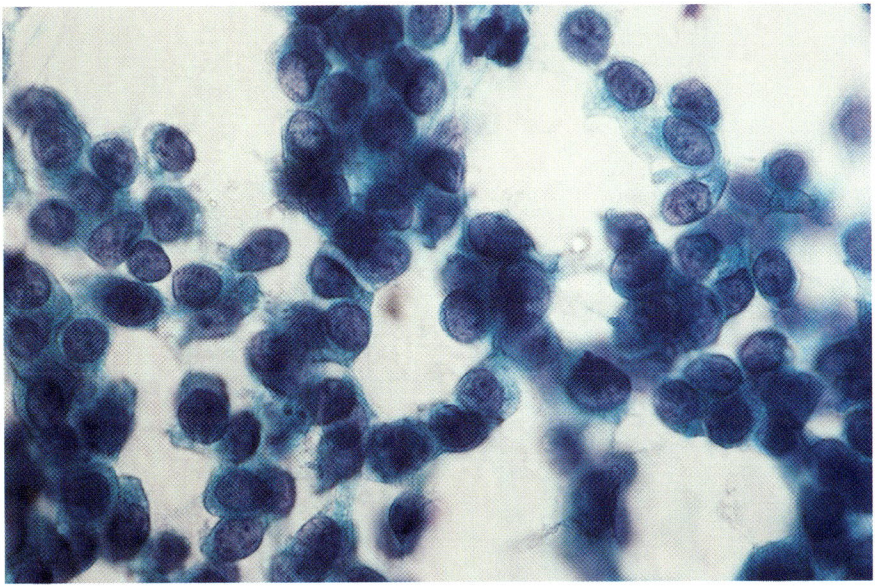

PLATE 13. Invasive ductal carcinoma of low nuclear and histologic grade. Aspirate of a breast mass reveals large cells with extremely high nuclear/cytoplasmic ratios and irregular hyperchromatic nuclei that form a small duct-like structure in the center of the photograph. Papanicolaou's stain.

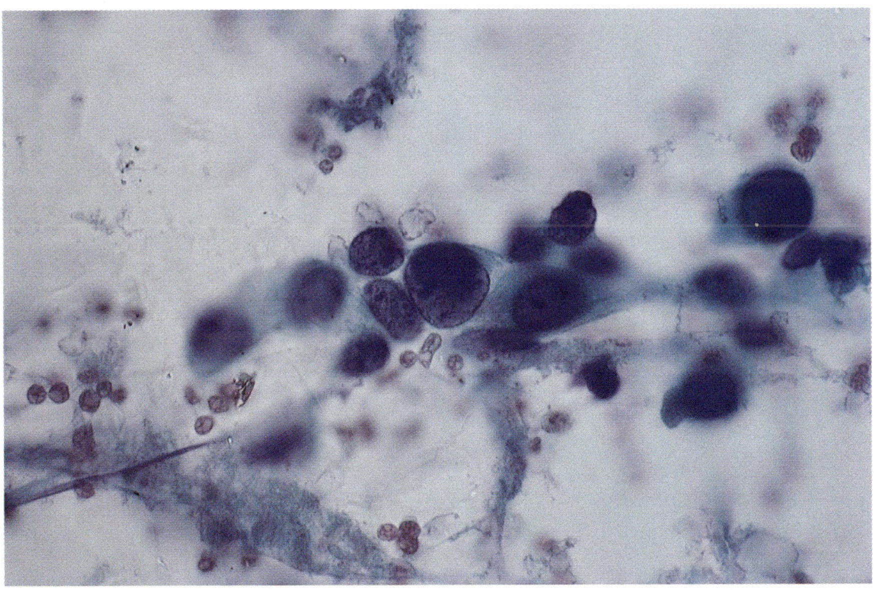

PLATE 14. Invasive ductal carcinoma of high nuclear and histologic grade. A breast aspirate yielded these extremely anaplastic individual malignant cells without architectural features. Papanicolaou's stain.

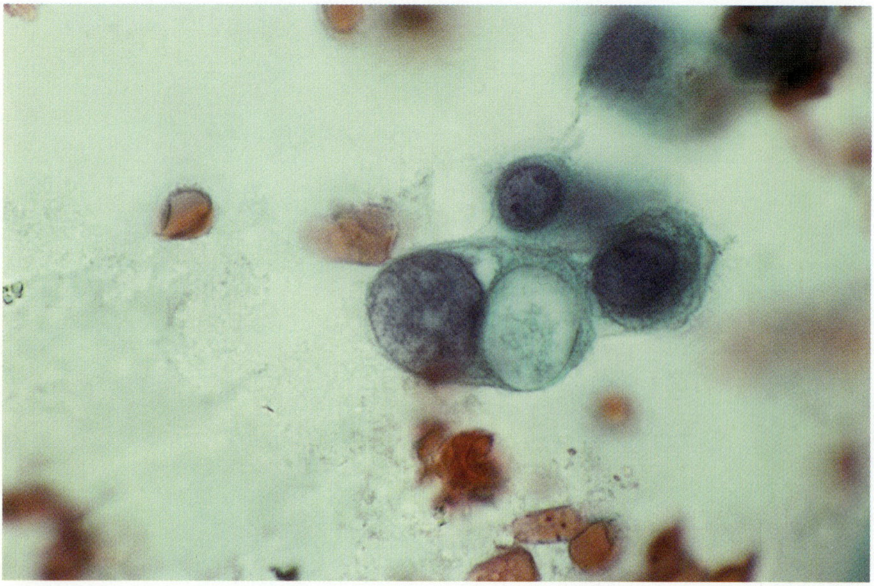

PLATE 15. Invasive lobular carcinoma, signet ring variant. This aspirate from a breast mass yielded relatively few cells, but the nuclei are large, hyperchromatic, and irregular. One large cell has a signet ring appearance, which is seen in some invasive lobular carcinomas. Papanicolaou's stain.

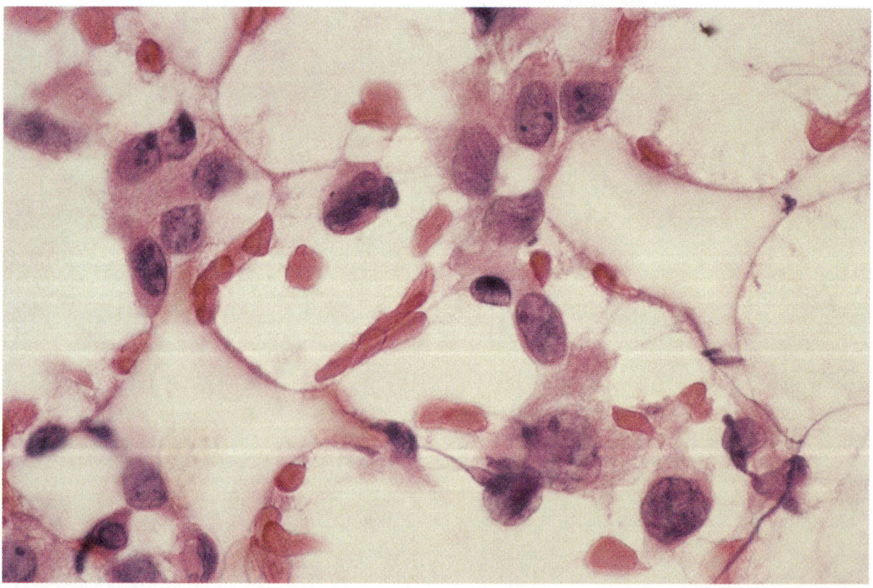

PLATE 16. Recurrent invasive ductal carcinoma. Aspiration of a chest wall mass revealed these anaplastic malignant epithelial cells in the fibroadipose stroma. H&E.

lesions) are biopsied (Chapter 6). Liberman et al. (78) described specimen radiographs of these SCNB biopsies. Calcification was found on 40% of cores and detected microscopically in 78% of cases. A specific diagnosis was made in 118 of 146 cases (81%). In those cases in which no calcification was found on x-ray of the core biopsy, histologic detection of calcification occurred in 13% and a specific diagnosis was made in only 38% of cases.

Ductal proliferative changes in core samples present special problems in distinguishing ductal hyperplasia from ADH and DCIS. The study reported by Liberman et al. (79) documented the difficulty. In 264 consecutive SCNB biopsies, the authors diagnosed 25 biopsies as ADH and received an open biopsy follow-up in 21 cases. Ductal hyperplasia without atypia was found in 4 of 21 (19%) biopsies, ADH was found in 6 (21%) biopsies, and DCIS was found in 8 (40%) biopsies. Invasive carcinoma was present in 3 of 21 (15%) biopsies. The authors recommended open biopsy for a diagnosis of ADH made on core biopsy. Philpotts et al. (80) reported on 26 cases diagnosed as ADH on SCNB and followed by open biopsy (efigs.3.27 and 3.28). In 6 of the 26 cases, cancer was found in open biopsy; 5 of the 6 cases were DCIS; and 1 case was invasive carcinoma. The other 20 cases were confirmed as ADH. Cases imaged as calcifications only were more often underestimated than those with masses. An issue especially pertinent to core biopsy is the finding of a single duct, which has many features of low grade DCIS. The size convention would suggest that this be termed ADH, but I include a note stating that a single duct with the features of DCIS is present and expect an open biopsy to clarify the severity and extent of the lesion. Open biopsy is recommended for a SCNB diagnosis of ADH.

ALH and LCIS also may be diagnosed on core needle biopsy. Liberman et al. (81) reported on 13 women with LCIS on CNB followed by open biopsy. The authors found 38% of the patients with synchronous or metachronous invasive carcinoma; open biopsy for LCIS was recommended. Philpotts et al. (80) found DCIS in 1 of 5 patients with LCIS on CNB.

Lee and Carter (82) reported on 59 cases diagnosed as DCIS on SCNB and followed by open biopsy. In 17 cases (29%), invasive carcinoma was detected surgically. The incidence of upstaging to invasive carcinoma was lower with 11-gauge than with 14-gauge needle biopsies. No difference between the confirmed DCIS cases and the upstaged cases was evident in retrospective review of mammographic features (size of lesion, number of cores, distribution, or morphology of calcifications or associated mass) and histologic features (type or nuclear grade of DCIS, necrosis, periductal fibrosis, or inflammation).

Complete removal of cancer on SCNB is also a potential problem. Gajdos et al. (83), Brenner (84), and Liberman et al. (85) reported on complete 11-gauge needle biopsy removal of an accurately diagnosed carcinoma, with no residual carcinoma found on open excision in 17% to 29% of cases. Completely removed carcinomas tended to be smaller and the number of cores tended to be higher than in those with residual carcinoma. Gajdos (83) found that 9 of 52 cases diagnosed on needle biopsy had no residual carcinoma on open biopsy; all 9 cases were DCIS, which presented as microcalcification without a mass. Liberman et al. (86) stressed that complete removal of the radiographically evident lesion does not imply complete removal of the carcinoma, but complete removal was accomplished in 4 of 12 cases of DCIS that presented as calcification without a mass. When reexcision fails to reveal residual carcinoma, the following steps should be taken. Evidence of the scar or needle track from the previous biopsy should be identified. A specimen mammogram may be useful for identification of calcification or, optimally, a clip placed at the time of biopsy. The surgeon and radiologist should be consulted for orientation and localization of the biopsy site and, of course, the sections from which the cancer diagnosis was established should be reviewed. DNA fingerprinting of the specimens is rarely required.

Youngston et al. (87) described histologic changes in 29 breast biopsies after SCNB, fine needle aspiration, needle localization, suture placement, or injection of local anesthesia in which benign and malignant epithelial cells were displaced in such a way as to simulate stromal or vascular invasion (efigs. 3.29 to 3.32). Benign epithelium was, of course, considered displaced. The authors determined that benign epithelial cells may be found in stroma or vessels and may be recognized for what they are—displaced benign lesions. When malignant cells are found in stroma, they may or may not have invaded, depending on stromal reaction, but the finding of malignant cells in vessels was considered indicative of invasion. The question of needle tract recurrence has often been raised, but rarely observed. In general, colloid carcinoma is most likely to be found along the needle tract. For this reason, colloid carcinoma is noted by type on needle biopsy to alert the surgeon to consider excision of the needle tract in the excisional biopsy (Figs. 3.11 and 3.12 and efigs. 3.33 and 3.34).

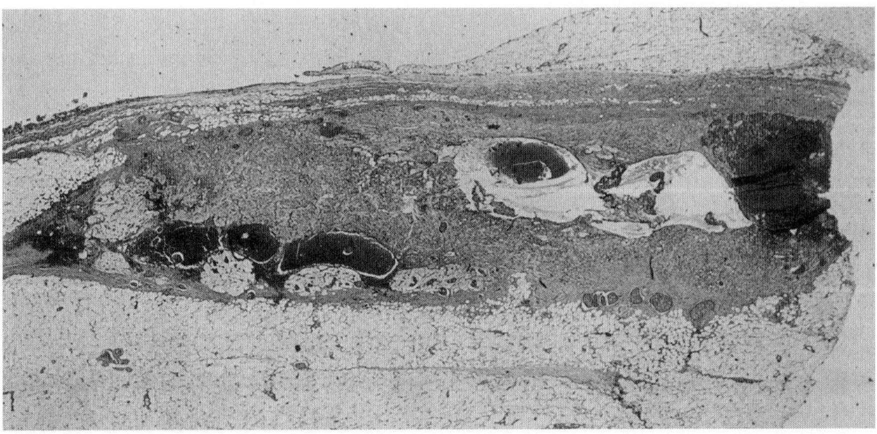

FIG. 3.11. Tract of needle biopsy. Excision of a breast lesion 2 weeks after a stereotactically directed needle biopsy revealed this stiletto-shaped scar in which pools of mucoid material can be seen.

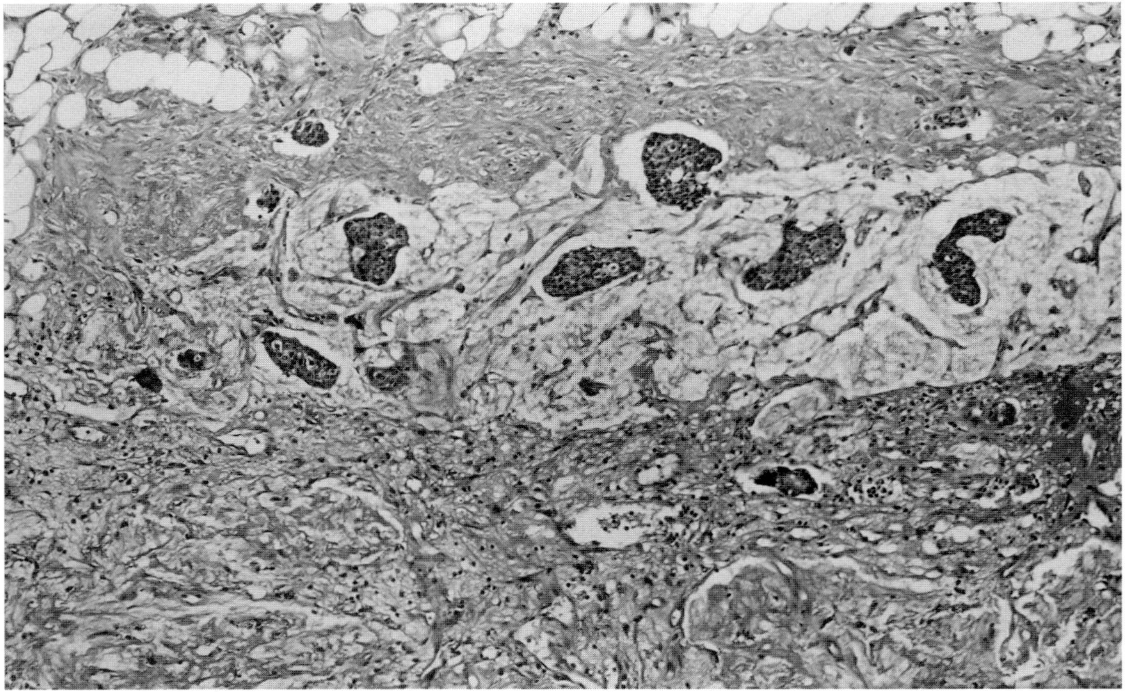

FIG. 3.12. Tract of needle biopsy. At higher magnification, it is evident that a mucinous or colloid carcinoma has seeded the granulation tissue that has formed along the tract of needle penetration. The entire tract should be excised in the open biopsy, especially after a diagnosis of mucinous carcinoma.

OPEN BIOPSY

Frozen Section

The first intraoperative frozen section was done by William Welch on a breast tumor excised by William Halsted, Professor of Surgery at Johns Hopkins Hospital, in 1895 (88). In that case, the frozen section diagnosis arrived after the operation was over and it was years before Halsted requested another. However, frozen sections on breast tumors were done with increasing frequency starting in the early 1930s and soon became a defining component of surgical pathology. In most institutions, they are done with a high degree of accuracy (89–91). Oberman (92) suggested (and the Association of Directors of Anatomic Pathology recommended) that frozen section not be performed on lesions smaller than 1 cm in diameter (60). The reasons given for this recommendation include lack of medical urgency of the diagnosis, the high level of difficulty of diagnosis for small lesions, and the possible ill effects of freezing tissue that contains a small early carcinoma, especially a noninvasive one, which must have a final evaluation by paraffin sections. In most situations, excisional biopsy is the extent of the planned procedure, and mastectomy no longer immediately follows receipt of a frozen section diagnosis of carcinoma. Mammographically detected lesions have a higher likelihood of being carcinoma *in situ*, which is better diagnosed on permanent section, and the absence of invasion must be confirmed on paraffin sections. Finally, small pseudoinfiltrative lesions, such as radial scars, are more difficult to diagnose on frozen section. In favor of frozen section diagnosis is the immediate determination that cancer is present, which affords the surgeon an opportunity to enlarge the excision for adequate margins, notify the patient of her status, begin planning the next step in treatment, and allow the pathologist to preserve tissue for prognostic indicators. The net effect of these considerations has been to defer the diagnosis on breast lesions to paraffin sections in the great majority of cases, and accurate interpretation of breast frozen sections is on its way to becoming a lost art.

If gross examination reveals what appears to be an invasive carcinoma (1 cm or more in diameter), frozen section is usually done. It also may be done as confirmation of a suspicious cytology or SCNB report, prior to definitive excision or node dissection.

Lesions detected by the surgeon as palpable masses may be excised and sent promptly to the surgical laboratory. A variety of simple expedients may preserve the fresh state of the tissue during transportation and the initial specimen examination. Biopsies may be wrapped in aluminum foil and placed on ice during transportation and initial examination. If the specimen is found to contain carcinoma, a sample may be quick frozen and stored at –70. Alternatively, frozen sections may be cut from the blocks used for diagnosis and stored for immunohistochemical or RNA assay.

Gross examination of such a specimen usually results in the production of a frozen section, and the results of this frozen section report may be used to determine if additional surgery is to be carried out. The pathologist should know about this eventuality and proceed with appropriate caution. Gross examination is of critical importance in identifying the lesion selected for sectioning. The biopsy should be cut to expose its greatest surface area first and then cut into slices of approximately 2- to 3-mm thickness. Visual inspection for cysts, streaks, abnormal color, texture, and so on is useful, but frequently palpation is of even greater value. Variations in consistency are usually the best guide to the presence of carcinoma, since a desmoplastic reaction is such a common feature of breast cancer. Invasive ductal carcinomas, especially their cut surfaces, usually have the consistency of a raw potato. With experience, one can learn this feeling and use it to distinguish carcinoma from other fibrous and inflammatory lesions of the breast with a high level of certainty.

Pitfalls in the frozen section diagnosis of breast cancer include:

1. The epithelial cells of an invasive carcinoma are usually well supported, but this is often not true of intraductal lesions, either benign or malignant, and architectural features may be the factor which distinguishes benign or atypical proliferative hyperplasias from carcinoma *in situ* (Chapter 4). Papillary tumors are notoriously difficult on frozen section and routinely are deferred to permanent section, unless they are obviously benign. In addition, the gross features of noninvasive lesions are usually not sufficiently characteristic to confirm the microscopic impression.

   If the pathologist is in doubt, he or she should warn the surgeon of the suspicion and defer diagnosis to permanent section. In this circumstance, all of the material may be needed for diagnosis, and evaluation of margins may not have the highest priority.
2. The diagnosis of *in situ* lobular carcinoma is extremely difficult on frozen section because the cellularity and size of the ducts are crucial determinants in this diagnosis. Thickness of frozen sections is difficult to control, which is reflected in marked changes in apparent cellularity. I consider it safest to defer this diagnosis to permanent section, but warn the surgeon of the suspicion that LCIS may be present. Gross examination is not a guide to the presence of this lesion.
3. The diagnosis of infiltrating lobular carcinoma is also difficult and may be mimicked by chronic mastitis with plump plasma cells with poorly preserved nuclear detail. Inflammatory cells may align themselves in the same single files and target fashion around ducts as invasive lobular carcinoma cells. The gross appearance of the two lesions may be quite similar because invasive lobular carcinoma frequently insinuates itself into normal tissues without eliciting the desmoplastic reaction that is characteristic of infiltrating duct carcinoma.
4. Radial scars and small tubular carcinomas both present as stellate puckered firm lesions with chalky or yellow streaks. Both may be associated with ductal proliferations, which histologically range from usual hyperplasia to

carcinoma *in situ*, all of which are difficult to interpret on frozen section. The 1-cm rule is useful for avoiding this differential diagnosis.

5. Medullary carcinoma also lacks the desmoplastic reaction that is characteristic of most breast cancers and may present the gross appearance of a lymph node. Histologically, the characteristic inflammatory reaction of medullary carcinoma may be so striking as to cause confusion with the histiocytic reaction of a lymph node. Histiocytoid and lipid rich carcinomas present a similar problem.
6. Epithelial–stromal lesions present the dual problems of sampling and cellularity. Distinction between fibroadenoma and phyllodes tumor (Chapter 10), is based, in part, on the cellularity of the stromal component. Most frozen sections are thicker than permanent sections and therefore falsely suggest a more cellular lesion. In addition, the cellularity of a phyllodes tumor may vary enormously, with some areas presenting an appearance that is indistinguishable from that of an ordinary fibroadenoma. As a result, the pathologist is at risk for both over- and underdiagnosis of stromal lesions.
7. In spindle cell tumors, the differential diagnosis of metaplastic carcinoma presents itself. Metaplastic carcinoma is statistically more likely than primary sarcoma of the breast, but sampling may not show the diagnostic epithelial component. This reservation should be communicated to the surgeon when dealing with what appears to be a primary sarcoma of the breast.

The frozen section report of carcinoma should be restricted to those cases in which both gross and microscopic appearances indicate carcinoma. A dichotomy in the two appearances should be a warning sign that the diagnosis should be deferred.

If no carcinoma is identified on frozen section, the biopsy should be liberally sampled with submission of blocks for paraffin sections, in an attempt to demonstrate the presence of inapparent *in situ* carcinoma (or even invasive carcinoma). The most suspicious areas, especially those that are firm to the touch, should, of course, be submitted. It is our practice to initially submit all tissue—up to eight randomly selected blocks in biopsies done for a mass and all fibrous tissue—when the lesion is detected by mammography alone to screen for inapparent lesions, even when there are no grossly evident abnormalities.

MARGINS

Pathologists are asked to determine the margins of resection of a carcinoma excised in a lumpectomy or partial mastectomy. It should be pointed out that the surgeon does a biopsy for diagnosis of breast cancer and this may require a great deal of skill and resourcefulness on the part of the pathologist. It is only after the pathologist's diagnosis of cancer has been established that the specimen ceases to be a biopsy and becomes an excision for removal of the carcinoma—a lumpectomy and the question of adequacy of margins becomes important. Diagnosis must take precedence. It is of limited value to know that the margins are negative if you don't know whether the diagnosis is cancer or whether the diagnosis is carcinoma *in situ* and invasive carcinoma cannot be ruled out. It is also as important to make certain that a mammographically detected lesion has been completely excised, as it is used to determine the margins at time of biopsy. Sometimes it is just not possible to get all of the needed information at the time of biopsy. However, in a reexcision lumpectomy or quadrectomy following a biopsy, the diagnosis has been established and the primary focus shifts to the adequacy of surgical margins.

Methods of Determining Margins

Margins are determined in a number of ways, none of which is entirely satisfactory.

Determination of surgical margins is traditionally done by inking the surface of the specimen with a dark marker, often India ink, and cutting sections from the central obvious tumor mass in a radial fashion to the margin at the periphery. If one assumes that the biopsy is roughly spherical, then the surface area of the biopsy is equal to pi times the diameter squared. A 4-cm biopsy has approximately a 50-cm^2 surface area. If the marginal sections are taken in a radial fashion, one has to consider the section used to look at the margin. The surface area of a cover slip, viewed in the way we are used to looking at it, is approximately 4×2 cm (or 8 cm^2) (Fig. 3.13), but traditionally taken marginal sections actually reveal only the end-on surface area (Fig. 3.14). This section is 5 μm thick and 2 cm long, revealing a surface area of only 0.001 cm^2. Review of even four marginal sections in this way can only document the gross impression of the pathologist that a margin is positive. A negative finding is of minimal value

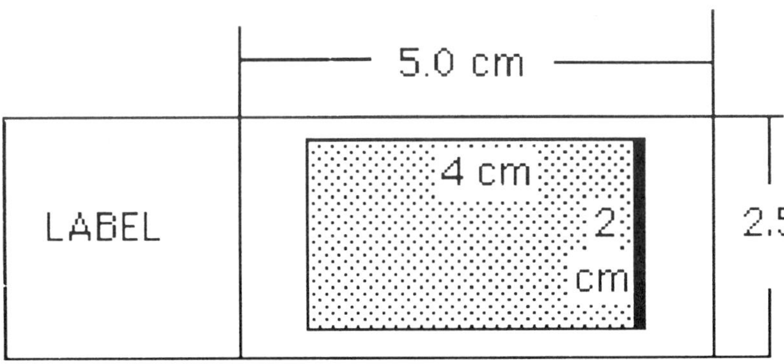

FIG. 3.13. Histologic sections have a maximum surface area of about 8 cm^2 (4×2 cm), which is the surface area of a coverslip. A section is 5 μm thick, however, and, if viewed on end, has a surface area of only 0.001 cm^2 (2 cm × 5 μm). The ratio of the end face to the end-on surface area is about 8000 to 1.

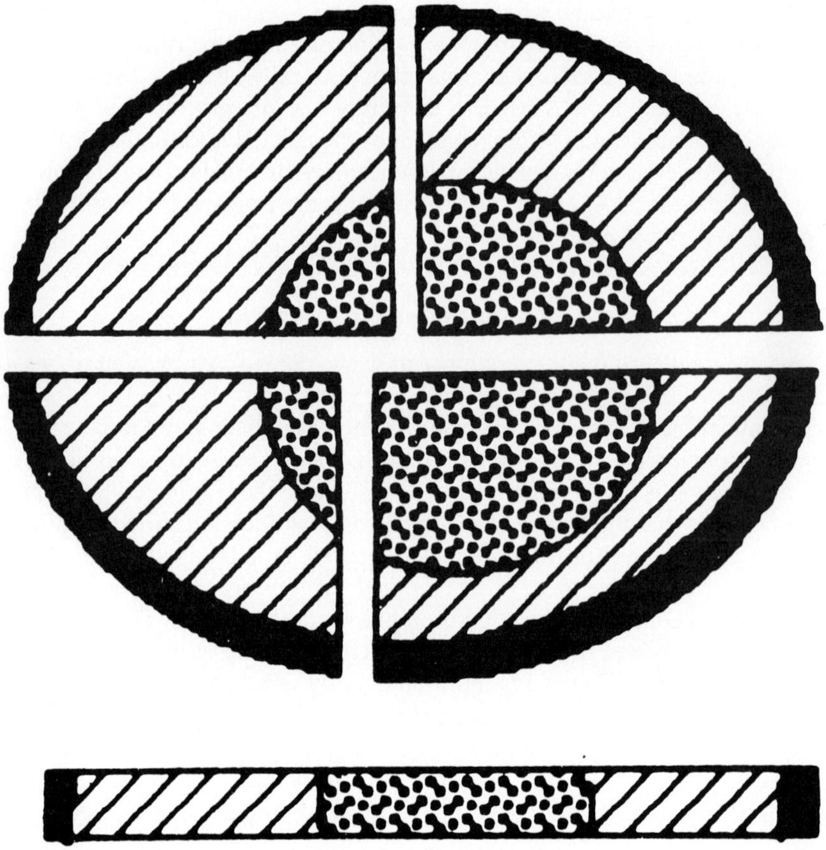

FIG. 3.14. Radial margins. Examination of a roughly spherical breast biopsy is usually done after the surface has been inked. Sections are taken radially from the apparent central tumor to the inked margin. The section displays the central tumor and its relationship to the margin, but the marginal surface area histologically examined is the end-on surface of only 0.001 cm^2.

because of the small sample size. Obviously, it is more efficient to view the margin with the open flat surface and the only way to do that is to take the margins en face. A technique for "orange-peeling" the biopsy was suggested by Carter (93) and is shown in Fig. 3.15. Using this technique for 100 consecutive lumpectomy specimens, microscopically positive margins were found in 36% of the specimens.

The "orange-peel" method requires inking of the surface of the specimen, removal of the peripheral tissue, embedding the peripheral tissue on the ink side down, and cutting sections parallel to the surface. The reason for sectioning in this plane is to use histologic sections to display the maximum surface area of the sphere-like reexcision. Approximately 20 sections, on average, were needed to display the margin of reexcision specimens. Although this number is high, it

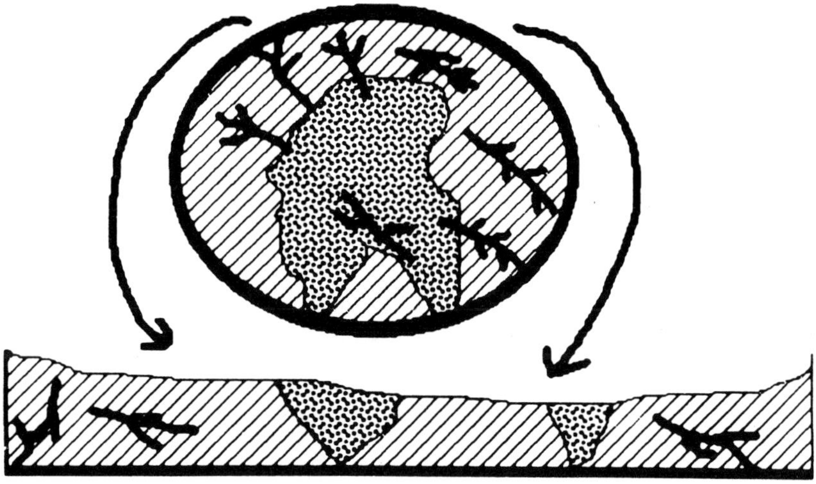

FIG. 3.15. "Orange-peeled" or shaved margin. If the surface area is inked, cut away, and embedded face down, the maximum surface area of the section can be utilized to histologically examine up to 8 cm^2 of the margin. Other sections, however, must be used to examine the central tumor.

is small in comparison to the number of sections required to display the margin of a resection specimen in the traditional method of cross sectioning, with slides taken perpendicular to the inked margin. In the radial method, less than 1% of the margin is histologically sampled, which could be predicted to lead to significant underestimation of grossly inapparent carcinoma, especially intraductal carcinoma. The van Nuys method (94) for margin sampling requires bookleafing, embedding, and cross sectioning the entire specimen to reveal all of the margins at right angles to the ink. The benefit of this technique is that it shows the entire specimen, although significantly less than 1% of the true margin. The drawback is that it still requires a large number of sections.

Noguchi et al. (95) studied 100 breast tumors embedded with this method. They found one-third of the excisions had positive or suspicious margins on frozen section analysis. Based on these findings, secondary excisions were performed in order to obtain negative margins; however, follow-up information was not given. Guidi et al. (96) described a study of shaved margins in 22 consecutive breast reexcision specimens. Ten of the specimens were intraductal carcinoma alone, six were infiltrating ductal carcinomas, and six were invasive lobular carcinoma. The surface area was inked and the periphery was reexcised with specimens embedded opposite to the inked surface. This would show the status of tissue approximately 3 mm from the true margin. All 22 excisions thus examined had a positive margin in at least one section. The authors then removed the tissue from the blocks, cut the tissue perpendicular to the inked margin, and reembedded the specimens. The authors found that only 55% of specimens reexamined in this way had positive margins. Their conclusion that many patients with positive shave margins do not have positive inked margins is not entirely appropriate. The shaved margins were not true margins, but were, in fact, 3 mm or more (the thickness of the block) from the true margin. In addition, the authors examined only about 1/1000 of the margin histologically in the reembedded specimens and did not offer clinical outcome based on the studies.

Another margin technique is to sample the margin of the reexcision specimen by traditional perpendicular margin sections and then to examine the cavity wall by shave margins. Beck et al. (97) found that margin analysis is a poor predictor of completeness of excision. Holland et al. (98) found that shavings of the cavity are not predictive of residual disease in a reexcision specimen.

Accuracy of Margins

In ten reported series in which margins were determined and subsequent excision provided follow-up to establish accuracy of the margin report, there were 169 true positive and 144 false positive results and 380 true negative and 190 false negative results. The aggregate calculated sensitivity of margins determination was 30%; specificity, 59%; positive predictive value, 56%; and negative predictive value, 33% (Table 3.2).

Campbell et al. (99) examined 37 reexcision specimens and found that 57% of the women had residual carcinoma. Sixty-four percent of those with a positive margin had residual disease and 42% of those with disease that was within 2 to 3 mm of the margin had residual disease. Seventy-two percent of patients with an extensive intraductal component (EIC) had residual disease, whereas only 17% of women with none or some *in situ* disease had residual carcinoma.

TABLE 3.2. *Residual disease, no followup*

Author	No. patients	+[a]	–[b]	Close[c]	?[d]	Comment
Solin (101)	185	60%	49%			
Kearney (104)	90	45%	42%		42%	
Beron (110)	87	29%	13%			N.S., extensive introductal component (EIC) and MAMM and MGN
Graham (114)	119	98%	32%			Mammography
Lee (82)	125	79%	44%			Mammography
Acosta (116)	93	22%	8%			
Campbell (99)	37	64%	0	42%	0	EIC +/– 72%, 17%
Frazier (106)	87	53%	26%	32		
Veronesi (119)	705	7%	2%			Lumpectomy vs. quadrant
Ghossein (120)	503	14%	7%			Lumpectomy vs. quadrant

N.S., not significant; EIC, extensive intraductal component; MAMM, mammographically detected; MGN, margin.

[a]+ is % residual disease when margin was reported as positive.

[b]– is % residual disease when margin was reported as negative.

[c]Close is % residual disease when margin was reported as close by several criteria.

[d]? is % residual disease when margin was reported as unknown.

Five of 16 women who had negative margins initially also were found to have residual disease in the resection specimen.

Morimoto et al. (100) found 23% of cases with residual carcinoma in 183 cases in which the carcinoma was less than 2 cm, and there was a 2-cm negative margin around the original excision. Solin et al. (101) found 63% of 251 reexcisions positive for residual carcinoma, with 85% revealing an invasive component. Fifteen percent revealed *in situ* carcinoma only. Fifty-one percent of patients with an apparently excisional biopsy had residual tumor in the reexcision specimen. When the pathologic margin of the initial biopsy was described as positive, 60% had residual tumor on reexcision, and 49% had residual carcinoma when the pathology margin was unknown. T1 carcinomas contained residual carcinoma in 45% and T2 lesions 63%. In those patients who had a post biopsy mammogram in which residual microcalcifications were present, 86% of them showed residual tumor in the reexcision specimen. The authors recommended reexcision when the initial margin was positive or unknown or if there were residual microcalcifications on post biopsy mammogram. When inked margins were negative, reexcision was not undertaken. McCormick et al. (102) found involved margins in 28% after initial resection and 15% after reexcision. Gwin et al. (103) reviewed 192 reexcisions. No residual carcinoma was found in 105 (55%) of the reexcisions, 24% had residual minimal microscopic disease, 12% had extensive microscopic disease, and 9% had gross residual carcinoma. The characteristics predicting for the quantity of residual disease included the original tumor stage and the margin status of the primary excision. Sixty-two percent of the cases with residual carcinoma had an invasive component. Kearney and Morrow (104) reviewed 239 cases in which the carcinoma was initially diagnosed by FNA and lumpectomy was performed in order to obtain negative margins. Reexcision was subsequently undertaken because of a positive margin in 42 cases and an unknown margin status in 48 cases. Only 19 of the reexcisions for positive margins and 20 of the reexcisions for unknown margins contained residual carcinoma. Jardines et al. (105) examined reexcisions after an initial excisional biopsy and found that the most significant factors associated with a positive reexcision were clinical tumor size, method of tumor detection, nodal status, and the presence of an invasive lobular component. Frazier et al. (106) examined 87 patients who underwent mastectomy or reexcision following a segmental resection. Forty-six percent of patients had involved margins, 32% of patients had close margins, and 22% of patients had clear margins. Residual carcinoma was found in 53% of those with positive margins, 32% of those with close margins, and 26% of those with negative margins. Of those with residual tumor, 31% had carcinoma in the same quadrant and 15% of 75 cases were found to have carcinoma in a different quadrant from the index tumor. The authors concluded that the methods used for assessment of microscopic margins may be misleading, since 30% of patients with clear or close margins subsequently had residual tumor and 48% of those with margins reported as positive were found to have no residual tumor. Schnitt et al. (107) found that 88% of patients with EIC had residual carcinoma, whereas only 48% of patients without EIC were found to have residual tumor in reexcision specimens. Wazer et al. (108) found the relative closeness of carcinoma to the specimen edge, and the extent of margin positivity was both predictive for residual tumor, as was the histopathology in the initial excision. DCIS was found in 60% of positive reexcision specimens with an initial histopathology of invasive carcinoma with EIC, compared to 26% in which there was only invasive carcinoma. Positive margins graded as focal, minimal, and extensive were associated with a positive reexcision in 26%, 58%, and 84% of cases, respectively. Tartter et al. (109) studied 674 excisional biopsy specimens after a FNA diagnosis of carcinoma. In the multivariate analysis, the authors found that only the diagnosis by FNA and small tumor size was associated with clear tumor margins.

None of the studies noted above have follow-up information regarding the number of failures associated with positive or negative margins, but all show that reexcision specimens have a considerable likelihood of demonstrating residual invasive tumor, depending upon factors that relate to the initial margin, as well as to the features of the carcinoma. False positive and false negative results occur with high frequency.

RADIOGRAPHIC–PATHOLOGIC CORRELATION OF MARGIN STATUS

Beron et al. (110) examined 87 patients with infiltrating ductal carcinoma who underwent excisional biopsy followed by reexcision of the tumor site. Reexcision specimens were evaluated for residual disease and correlated with initial mammographic and pathologic findings. The authors reported that initially positive margins did not predict residual disease at the reexcision significantly better than did initially negative margins (29% versus 13%). The authors found that patients with all three features (EIC, margin status, and mammography) negative had a 6% incidence of residual disease, whereas those patients in whom all three factors were positive had an 83% incidence of residual disease. Walls et al. (111) found that the presence of mammographic microcalcifications was associated with a 68% incidence of residual tumor in reexcision specimens, whereas only 36% of carcinomas without mammographic microcalcifications contained residual malignancy. Homer et al. (112) reported that microcalcifications that had prompted biopsy were confined to the tumor in 63% of 40 cases, within and contiguous to the tumor in 32% of cases, and within 13 mm of the tumor in 5% of cases. Oakley and Going (113) reported radiographic histologic correlation in 26 cancer excisions. Six invasive carcinomas, which were not detected by radiology, were found to reach a margin that was apparently radiologically clear. Six small invasive carcinoma satellites were not recognized. Adjacent DCIS was not detectable in 9 of 15 cases. Graham et al. (114) described single view radiographs of 119 consecutive surgical biopsy specimens of impalpable invasive or *in situ* carcinomas. Specimen radiographs showed carcinoma at the surgical margin in

63 cases, which was confirmed in 62 cases. Tumor free margins were shown radiographically in 56 cases, but only confirmed in 18 (32%) cases. The authors concluded that specimen mammogram margin positivity was predictive for residual disease, but negativity was not predictive for absence of residual disease.

Dixon et al. (115) studied 80 impalpable breast lesions that were excised by wide local excision. Clear histologic margins were obtained in 68% of 77 carcinomas. After inspection of the oriented specimen radiograph, additional tissue was excised from 22 patients, raising the rate of complete excision to 86%. Significantly more patients with invasive cancer had a complete excision than those with DCIS (91% versus 70%).

Lee and Carter (82) compared radiographs of tissue specimens obtained at initial biopsy of 125 impalpable breast cancers with the preoperative mammograms. The specimen mammogram was considered to show complete excision of the clinical mammographic lesion in 63% of the 125 cases. Tumor was found at mastectomy or reexcision in 35 of those cases, giving a false negative rate of 44% for a residual tumor. Incomplete excision was determined on 39 specimen radiographs. Eight of the radiographs had no residual tumor, giving a false positive rate of 21%. The sensitivity of the specimen radiograph for predicting the presence of residual tumor was 49% and specificity was 77%, with an overall accuracy rate of 62%. The overall accuracy of the pathologic examination of the margins was 58%. Specimen radiograph alone correctly identified 18 cases of residual tumor in the reexcision, where biopsy margins were either indeterminate or considered clear of tumor. The authors concluded that the specimen radiograph was of value only in those cases in which margins examined pathologically were indeterminate or considered negative, but the specimen radiograph showed incomplete excision of the mammographic lesion.

Acosta et al. (116) studied 96 patients with needle localization breast biopsy in which the margins were histologically determined. Forty-five patients were found to have positive margins and all of these patients underwent reexcision. Twenty-two percent of these patients were found to have residual carcinoma. Thirty-eight of 51 patients found initially to have negative margins underwent reexcision. In 8% of the cases, there was residual carcinoma. The authors concluded that reexcision was required for patients undergoing needle localization breast biopsy. Lind et al. (117) compared 69 patients with impalpable breast cancer who underwent biopsy by needle localization to 48 patients in whom impalpable lesions were first diagnosed by stereotactic core needle biopsy followed by excision. In the latter group, the volume of tissue was considerably larger than in the former group. Six percent of the patients who had SCNB had positive margins, whereas 55% of those undergoing a needle localization biopsy had positive margins. Kaufman et al. (118) reported that the use of SCNB was associated with breast excisions of larger volumes, more frequently negative margins and decreased need for reexcision.

Veronesi (119) reported a significantly higher incidence of local recurrence following lumpectomy than after quadrectomy. Ghossein et al. (120) reported that 41% of 323 patients in whom the tumor was excised with a minimal rim of tissue had involved margins. In 14% of 142 patients undergoing wide excision, the margin was positive, and in only 7% of 56 patients who underwent quadrectomy was the margin positive for carcinoma. Cosmetic results were not discussed. In T1 ductal carcinomas, only 4% of those with excisions greater than 5 cm had recurrences, but lesser excisions had a 20% rate of recurrence. The authors concluded that failure was inversely proportional to the amount of breast tissue resected.

MARGINS OF DUCTAL CARCINOMA *IN SITU*

Intraductal carcinoma, without associated invasive carcinoma, has been studied for margin status. Cheng et al. (121) reported that both the size and margin status of intraductal carcinoma were found to be independent predictors of residual disease. Ratanawichitrasin et al. (122) found residual disease in reexcision specimens of patients with intraductal carcinoma, without invasive cancer. It was found in 17% of patients with negative margins, 31% of patients with close margins (defined as being less than 2 mm from the margin), and 58% of patients with positive margins. One-half of 34 patients with margins of unknown status were also found to have residual disease in the reexcision specimen. Silverstein et al. (94) concluded that it was difficult to completely excise DCIS by using a wide local excision. Patients with comedocarcinoma had a greater tendency to positive initial histologic margins and residual DCIS. Histologically negative margins did not guarantee that residual DCIS had not been left behind.

LOCAL RECURRENCE BY MARGIN STATUS

The literature on margin analysis of cases in which both *in situ* and invasive carcinoma were present reveals that, in some reports, margin status is an independent predictor of local recurrence; however, in other reports, this was not found. Smitt et al. (123) studied 289 patients, examined margins in the traditional radial manner, and classified the margins as positive, close (less than 2 mm), negative, or indeterminate. The actuarial probability of local control at 10 years was 98% for those patients with negative surgical margins versus 82% for all others. The local control rate at 10 years was 97% for patients who underwent reexcision and 84% for those who did not. Anscher et al. (124) studied 259 patients with radially sectioned inked margins and considered the margins positive if tumor extended to the ink and negative if it did not. Twelve percent of patients had positive margins, 50% had negative margins, and 38% were indeterminate. There was 4% local failure overall—9% from the positive margin group, 2% from the negative margin group, and 6% from the indeterminate group. The difference between the positive and negative group was statistically significant, but the difference between the positive and indeterminate group was not. A total of 2 of 7 patients with positive margins after reexcision, who were subsequently irradiated, versus 1 of 56 patients, who had negative margins after local excision, had local recurrence. Heimann et al. (125) studied 852 patients who were treated with breast conservation surgery and radiation, including a boost to the tumor bed of

60 grays (Gy). In multivariate analysis, the only significant factor that affects local control is margin status. In patients who received a boost, the local control rate at 5 years was 98%, if the margins were negative, and 89%, if the margins were positive. The local control rate was dose dependent, with 91% local control with 60 Gy, compared to 76% for a dose less than 60 Gy.

Gage et al. (126) examined patients with stage I or stage II breast cancer who were treated by radiation and breast conserving surgery. The authors found that patients with negative margins of excision had a low rate of recurrence in the treated breast, whether the margin was 1 mm or greater and whether the carcinoma was EIC negative or EIC positive. Among patients with positive margins, those with focally positive margins had a considerably lower risk of local recurrence than those with more than focally positive margins. Focally positive was carcinoma, either invasive or *in situ*, at the margin in three or fewer low power fields. Schnitt et al. (127), following a similar group of cases, found local recurrence at or near the primary site in 12 of 181 patients. The local recurrence rate was zero in patients with negative margins, 4% in patients with close margins, 6% in those patients who were focally positive, and 21% in patients where margins were more than focally positive. In 127 patients with EIC negative carcinomas, the 5-year local recurrence rate was less than 10% in all margin groups. In 30 patients with EIC positive tumors, the 5-year rate of local recurrence was zero when margins were negative or close, but 50% when margins were more than focally positive.

DiBiase et al. (128) studied patients who were treated with conservative surgery, followed by radiation with either an electron boost or an iridium-192 implant to the tumor bed. Local control rates for patients with negative margins or one positive margin at 5 years and 10 years were 94% and 87%, respectively, compared with 86% and 69%, respectively, for those with two or more positive margins. There was no significant difference in local recurrence when those patients with one positive margin were compared to those with more than one positive margin. Spivack et al. (129) studied 272 patients who were treated with surgical resection, followed by radiotherapy. Local recurrence was observed in 18% of those with positive margins, 7% of those with unknown margins, and 4% of those with negative margins. The local recurrence rate was dose related, with 8% recurrence after radiation doses of 66 Gy, compared to 22% following lower doses. Kurtz et al. (130) studied 496 stage I and stage II breast cancer patients who were treated by conservative surgery and radiotherapy. Premenopausal patients had a low recurrence rate of 3% at 5 years, regardless of other factors. In postmenopausal patients, the risk of local recurrence was determined by the adequacy of resection margin and nuclear grade. Tafra et al. (131) compared patients who were treated by excisional biopsy and segmentectomy. The presence of carcinoma in the segmentectomy specimen was related to size of the primary tumor and presence of positive axillary lymph nodes. The overall recurrence rate was 7% and was related to tumor status of the segmentectomy margins. Lagios et al. (132) reported 43 segmental mastectomies without radiotherapy and found that detection of clinically unsuspected involvement of resection margins, by microscopic foci of carcinoma, was an important

TABLE 3.3. *Local recurrence correlated with margin status*

Author	No. patients	+[a]	–[b]	Close[c]	?[d]	Comment
Anscher (124)	259	9%	2%		6%	
Heimann (125)	852	11%	2%			
Gage (126)	340	16%	3%	2%		
Schnitt (127)	181	21%	0	4%		
DiBiase (128)	453	14%	6%			0 or 1 vs. 2 or more
Spivack (129)	272	18%	4%		7%	
Kurtz (130)	496	31%				Postmenopausal only
Tafra (131)	375	7%				
Lagios (132)	43	45%	9%			No radiation
Schmidt-Ullrich (137)	108	0	0	0		
Schmidt-Ullrich (138)	225	1%	1%			
Pittinger (139)	183	3%	3%			
Vicini (140)	0	0				
Solin (136)	697	NR	NR	NR	NR	N.S., but boost dose changed
Dalberg (142)	759	1.50%				Age, radiation, nodes
Sinn (143)	957					EIC, age, lobular type
Touboul (144)	528					EIC, age, bifocality

NR, not related.
[a]+ is % residual disease when margin was reported as positive.
[b]– is % residual disease when margin was reported as negative.
[c]Close is % residual disease when margin was reported as close by several criteria.
[d]? is % residual disease when margin was reported as unknown.

prognostic indicator of local recurrence. Five of 11 breast resections with this feature developed local recurrence, compared to 3 of 32 resections without margin involvement. Fisher et al. (133) studied 150 axillary node positive stage II and stage III breast cancer patients who did not receive radiation. The authors found that 22% of postmenopausal patients with positive resection margins and four or more axillary lymph node metastases developed local and regional recurrence and recommended radiation for this group (Tables 3.3 and 3.4).

TABLE 3.4. *Ductal carcinoma in situ: local recurrence correlated with margin status*

Author	No. patients	+[a]	–[b]	Close[c]	?[d]	Comment
Solin (101)	110	29%	7%		14%	10 institutions
Holland (98)	129		2%	36%		
Schwartz (150)	70	NR	NR			Comedocarcinoma
Solin (136)	172	NR	NR			Comedocarcinoma
Sneige (155)	49	NR	NR			Periductal fibrosis
Cataliotti (154)	183	NR	NR			N.S.
Fisher (156)	818	NR	NR			Radiation
Mariani (152)	705	NR	NR			Tumorectomy vs. quadrant

NR, not related.
[a]+ is % residual disease when margin was reported as positive.
[b]– is % residual disease when margin was reported as negative.
[c]Close is % residual disease when margin was reported as close by several criteria.
[d]? is % residual disease when margin was reported as unknown.

OTHER FACTORS PREDICTIVE OF LOCAL RECURRENCE

Other studies have not shown that margin status is the controlling factor in local recurrence. Harris et al. (134) reported that local recurrence was observed in 37% of patients with EIC—a prominent intraductal component in the "tumor mass," intraductal carcinoma in the grossly normal adjacent tissue, and a high nuclear grade. Vicini et al. (135) reported that EIC positive tumors with the largest resections had one-third the recurrence rate of those with narrow resections. In EIC negative cases, the rates were lower, but there was still substantially greater benefit in reduction of local recurrence by a wide resection margin. In 1994, Schnitt et al. (127) divided margins into the following categories: negative, close, focally positive, and more than focally positive. The recurrence rates in these four groups were 0%, 4%, 6%, and 21%, respectively. Distant failure also was observed more often in patients with positive margins.

Solin et al. (136) divided their cases into four groups: negative margin, positive margin, close margin, and indeterminate. The cases with a positive pathology margin were subdivided into those that were focally positive on microscopic examination and those with grossly positive or microscopically diffusely positive margins. The latter group was treated by mastectomy, but the focally microscopically positive group was treated with radiotherapy. No difference in local recurrence was observed among the four groups—negative, microscopically positive, close, or unknown.

Schmidt-Ullrich et al. (137) studied 115 stage I and stage II invasive mammary carcinomas that were treated with conservative surgery and radiation. Fifty-four percent of the patients had a positive resection margin, but none of the patients experienced a local recurrence at 60 months median follow-up. Schmidt-Ullrich et al. (138) reported on 225 patients that were treated with conservation surgery and dose-adjusted radiation to maximum doses of 70 Gy to the tumor bearing quadrant. The authors observed local control rates in the treated breast of 97.5% at 10 years, with only three local recurrences at a median follow-up of 4.5 years. Pittinger et al. (139) studied 211 patients with stage I and stage II breast cancers that were treated by breast conserving surgery. The patients were divided according to margin status as negative, close (3mm or less), positive, or unknown. Residual carcinoma was found in 0, 24%, 44%, and 48%, respectively. The local recurrence rate was equivalent in patients with negative and close final margins. Vicini et al. (140) reported on 50 early stage breast cancer cases with lumpectomy and interstitial brachytherapy. None of the patients experienced local, regional, or distant failure, regardless of tumor size, margin status, or axillary lymph node metastases. Wazer et al. (108) used the final margin status to guide the tumor bed dose of radiation in 509 cases of stage I and stage II breast cancer with a median follow-up of 72 months. Local control rates were excellent for patients who were older than 45 years, but, in those younger than 45 years, the local recurrence rate was proportional to the closeness of the final margin. Solin et al. (136) studied 697 patients with stage I or stage II invasive carcinoma who were treated with breast conserving surgery and definitive irradiation. Gross excision of the primary tumor was performed and axillary staging was determined. The patients were divided into four groups: 257 patients with a negative margin, 57 patients with a positive margin, 37 patients with a close margin (defined as within 2 mm of the resection margin), and 346 patients in whom the margin status was unknown. The patients with positive final pathology margins were focally positive on microscopic examination. There was no difference in the local recurrence rate at 5 years among these four groups. Patients with grossly positive margins or diffusely positive microscopic margins were treated by mastectomy. Fowble et al. (141) reported on 886 patients with stage I and stage II breast cancers who were treated by excisional biopsy, axillary dissection, and radiation. Final pathologic margin status was evaluated, in addition to other factors, and it was not found to predict for local recurrence. Dalberg et al. (142) reported on 759 patients with T1 and T2 carcinomas that were treated by breast conserving surgery. Eighty-eight percent also received postoperative radiotherapy. The yearly increase in ipsilateral breast tumor recurrence was between 1% and 1.5%. Univariate analysis showed that under the age of 50 years, tumor size, uncertain microscopic margins, axillary lymph node metastases, absence of postoperative tamoxifen treatment, premenopausal status, and no postoperative radiotherapy predicted for local recurrence, but multivariate analysis showed that only age less than 50 years, no postoperative radiation therapy, and positive lymph nodes independently predicted for ipsilateral local recurrence. Sinn et al. (143) reviewed 957 patients who were treated with breast conserving therapy. Again, the authors found in univariate analysis that EIC, histologic grade, angioinvasion, lobular tumor type, involved resection margin, and lymph node status predicted for local recurrence. In a multivariate logistical regression analysis, however, only EIC, angioinvasion, lobular tumor type, and age less than 40 years were independent predictors of local recurrence. Touboul et al. (144) reported on 528 patients with T1 or T2 carcinoma who were treated by local resection and radiotherapy. There were 44 local recurrences. Thirty-nine of the recurrences were pathologically evaluated as local recurrence and six of them were considered ipsilateral new primary carcinomas. Multivariate analysis showed the probability of local control was decreased by age less than 40 years, premenopausal status, bifocality of the tumor, and EIC, but not by margin status. Borger et al. (145) studied 1,026 patients with clinical stage I and stage II breast cancer that was treated with local excision, axillary dissection, and whole breast radiation. Only young age and vascular invasion were independent predictive factors of local recurrence. Ryoo et al. (146) reported on 393 patients with breast cancer (clinical stages T0-3, N0-2, and M0) that was treated by excisional biopsy and radiation. The three major factors that predicted for local treatment failure were age below 40 years, negative estrogen receptor assay, and failure to deliver a radiation boost (Table 3.4).

LOCAL RECURRENCE OF DUCTAL CARCINOMA *IN SITU*

In reports of cases with DCIS without invasive cancer, the effect of margin status are also mixed. McCormick et al. (147) reported on 54 patients with DCIS who were treated with breast conserving surgery and radiation. Eighteen percent of the patients had local recurrence. Close or involved margins were noted in 30% of the patients who locally recurred, despite the fact that 50% had a reexcision after the initial biopsy. Breasts with maintained local control had only 4% involved margins, and reexcision was performed in only 20% of cases. Vicini et al. (148) reported on 105 patients with DCIS who were only treated with breast conserving surgery and radiation. The authors found that margin status, as well as cancerization of the lobules near the surgical margin, appeared to be associated with local recurrence within or immediately adjacent to the lumpectomy cavity. Three of the recurrences were pure DCIS, but seven of the recurrences were invasive carcinomas. Solin et al. (149) reported on a multiinstitutional study of 110 patients with unilateral nonpalpable mammographically detected intraductal carcinoma who were treated by breast conserving surgery and definitive breast irradiation. The local recurrence rate was 7% when the final pathology margin of excision was negative and 29% when the margin was close or positive. In 51 patients in whom the margin was unknown, the local recurrence rate was 14%. The pathologic characteristics of the primary tumor did not appear to predict for local recurrence. Holland et al. (98) studied 129 women with DCIS who were treated with breast conserving surgery. Margins were evaluated by biopsy cavity shavings and by evaluation of the specimen margins. Ipsilateral recurrence was related to margin status. Only 2 of 101 patients with clear margins recurred, compared to 10 of 28 patients in whom margins were close. Cavity shavings were considered to be ineffective in ensuring complete excision. Those authors recommend a 10-mm margin of excision around all screen-detected DCIS lesions.

However, Schwartz et al. (150) reported on 70 patients with nonpalpable DCIS that was detected by mammography and treated by local excision. The authors related local recurrence to the comedo-type of DCIS, but not to margins. Fish et al. (151) reported on 106 patients with a diagnosis of DCIS that was treated by lumpectomy. Only 18 patients in the group received radiation. Lumpectomy alone patients experienced a 19% rate of DCIS recurrence in the ipsilateral breast. Predictors of local recurrence included the extent of involvement of the parenchyma and the initial presentation. Margins did not predict for local recurrence. Mariani et al. (152) reported on patients treated by quadrectomy, axillary dissection, and radiotherapy versus tumorectomy with axillary node dissection. Both groups also were treated by external radiotherapy and a localized boost with iridium-192 implantation. No second surgery was given to patients who had positive surgical margins. The ipsilateral breast recurrence rate was 4.7% and 7.4% at 5 and 10 years, respectively, in the group treated by quadrectomy and 12% and 19% at 5 and 10 years, respectively, in the group treated by local excision. The status of resection margins did not significantly influence the risk of local recurrence. Swensen et al. (153) reported on 121 patients in whom margins were not predictive of local recurrence. Cataliotti et al. (154) reported on 183 patients with DCIS who were treated by conservative surgery, with radiation added in 34 cases. Local recurrence, all infiltrating, occurred in the same breast after conservative surgery in eight cases, three of which had received postoperative radiotherapy. Local recurrence also occurred in three patients who were treated by mastectomy. No significant differences relating to mammographic pattern, size, histologic type, margin involvement, or radiotherapy were observed. Solin et al. (136) described the follow-up in 172 women with DCIS who underwent breast conserving surgery and definitive breast irradiation in multiple institutions in Europe and the United States. The only pathologic parameter that correlated with rate of local recurrence was the presence of the comedo subtype of intraductal carcinoma with nuclear grade 3. Sneige et al. (155) reported on 49 patients with DCIS who were treated by lumpectomy and radiation. The rate of local recurrence was 2% at 5 years and 6% at 10 years. Among the pathologic parameters studied, only periductal fibrosis showed a significant relationship with outcome. Fisher et al. (156), reporting on the National Surgical Adjuvant Breast and Bowel Project (NSABP) trial of 818 patients with localized DCIS (randomly assigned to lumpectomy or lumpectomy plus radiation), showed, through 8 years of follow-up, that lumpectomy plus radiation was more beneficial than lumpectomy alone for women with localized mammographically detected DCIS. The incidence of ipsilateral noninvasive breast cancer recurrence was reduced from 13% to 8%, and the incidence of invasive ipsilateral breast cancer was reduced from 13% to 4%, with the addition of radiation.

Silverstein et al. (157) proposed a prognostic index, including the size, type of intraductal carcinoma, and margin status in predicting for local recurrence, following local excision, without the addition of radiation. When the prognostic index is low, which necessitates the presence of negative margins by 1 cm, the local recurrence rate is low. Recently, Silverstein et al. suggested that a 1-cm margin of normal tissue all around the DCIS is sufficient treatment, regardless of other factors, for guaranteeing no recurrence.

Summary and Conclusion

In other organs, the pathologist's determination that margins are histologically free of cancer is a clear indication that residual primary malignant tumor does not remain in the patient. For technical and biological reasons, this is not true for locally excised breast cancer, and it is the residual carcinoma that remains in the breast that recurs locally. Because reported margin status fails to accurately predict the presence or absence of residual disease, the study of margins is frustrating and the results are disappointing to pathologists, surgeons, and radiotherapists. Assessment of margins by means of the standard radial method, although imperfect for detection of inapparent microscopic disease, is probably reliable for excluding gross or extensive disease and is therefore useful.

Comparison of specimen and clinical mammograms may help in some circumstances. Veronesi (119) recently described the uncertainty associated with assessment of margins by stating that the finding of "pathologic clear margins is not a reassuring factor and that it will not predict a low risk of recurrence."

MULTICENTRICITY/MULTIFOCALITY OR MULTIPLICITY OF BREAST CANCER

Multicentricity implies that two or more carcinomas have arisen independently and is recognized by the absence of genetic similarities, different histologies, or wide anatomic separation of the carcinomas. Most often it is used to describe anatomically separated carcinomas. The term "multifocal" implies that a single carcinoma has spread to separate foci. Intramammary metastases are multifocal, but these are rare. Most carcinomas described as multifocal are probably extremely stellate in shape and appear artifactually multiple, due to the 2-dimensional representation on sections. Because of the difficulty in determining the 3-dimensional structure of breast cancer, the terms "multifocality" and "multicentricity" often have been used interchangeably, and the suggestion has been made that the term multiplicity should replace both of them in most cases.

The breast is made up of 14 to 24 collecting duct systems (DS), each emptying into the nipple and arborizing toward the chest wall and branching into a large, but undetermined, number of terminal duct lobular units (TDLU). DCIS arises near the junction of collecting duct units and TDLU and spreads along the DS, perhaps spreading to other DS, and forming a complex 3-dimensional structure. When heavily calcified, the spread of DCIS, especially comedocarcinoma, may be evident and can be modeled radiographically, but, in most cases, all of the DCIS is not calcified, which renders radiographic demonstration incomplete. Invasive carcinoma that arises from DCIS probably follows the DS early, but, as invasion progresses, the carcinoma spreads aggressively to form a stellate 3-dimensional mass that does not relate to normal DS and is not calcified, thereby making radiographic or gross modeling even more difficult. Because biopsy is not done along anatomic structures, and because the advancing tips of carcinoma are not evident grossly or radiographically, the limits of the cancer are poorly defined. Lumpectomy describes the nonanatomic resection. In sampling the biopsy with 2-dimensional sections to visualize the advancing root-like tips of carcinoma, the impression of separate foci may be given, although the carcinoma is connected in other planes of the section. In the absence of genetic fingerprinting, differences in histology, and obvious intralymphatic metastases, the distinction between multicentric and multifocal is problematic. Most authors studying the problem have used wide anatomic separation as the definition of multicentricity, but even this feature is imperfect and is defined differently from study to study. One needs to read each published article to interpret the claim of multicentricity. Numerous published studies have reported that approximately one-third of carcinomas of the breast are multiple within the ipsilateral breast (Table 3.2). Although it may be difficult to confirm true multicentricity or multifocality, the apparent multiplicity of breast cancer must be considered in treatment planning.

Qualheim and Gall (158) found breast cancers to be multifocal in 54% of 157 mastectomies that were studied by a whole-mount technique. Multifocality was present in the same quadrant in 17% of cases and in other quadrants in 37% of cases.

Tellem et al. (159) took 2 to 5 sections from each quadrant of 64 mastectomy specimens and found multifocal breast cancer in quadrants other than in those from which the primary tumor had been excised in 27% of the cases. Gallagher and Martin (160) found multifocal breast cancer in other quadrants in 75% of 38 mastectomy specimens. Fisher et al. (161) reviewed the NSABP (B-04 cases), in which there were 904 mastectomies. Only one block was sampled per quadrant from these specimens, but even with this limited sampling technique, multifocal breast cancer was reported in other quadrants in 13% of the cases. Four percent were invasive and the other 9% of cases were carcinoma *in situ.*

Lagios (162) used a combination serial subgross sectioning and radiographic method to study 85 mastectomy specimens. With a definition of multicentric carcinoma as noncontiguous foci of cancer located at least 5 cm from the border of the residual tumor of the excisional biopsy cavity margin, the author found multicentricity in 21% of the cases with one-half of the second carcinomas invasive and the other half carcinoma *in situ* only. Those with multicentric breast carcinomas were more likely to have a positive family history of breast cancer or a tubular carcinoma. Patients with intraductal carcinoma that was less than 25 mm in diameter were unlikely to have occult invasive or significant *in situ* multicentricity, whereas larger intraductal carcinomas had a higher frequency of occult invasive carcinoma. Schwartz et al. (163) took four sections from each quadrant and the retroareolar area of 52 mastectomies that were done for nonpalpable mammographically detected carcinomas. Multicentricity was defined as the presence of invasive or noninvasive carcinoma in a quadrant other than that containing the index tumor, and 44% of the cases had multifocal carcinoma. The carcinoma was *in situ* in 37% of the cases and invasive in 7% of cases.

Egan (164) studied 161 mastectomy specimens by a combined radiographic and histopathologic whole-mount technique and found multifocality in 60% of the cases. Those women with multifocal carcinomas had a significantly worse mortality rate than those in whom carcinoma was unifocal. Noel et al. (165) used a topographic grid method for the study of node negative carcinomas that varied from 2 to 5 cm in diameter. Nine percent of patients had multifocal breast cancer and these patients had a significantly decreased survival rate. Cowen et al. (166) reported multifocality as a significant factor in determining local and distant recurrence when margins of resection were negative.

Shah et al. (167) examined 508 mastectomy specimens after an excisional biopsy and found carcinoma distant from the biopsy site in 59% of the cases. The second carcinoma was invasive in 33% of the cases and carcinoma *in situ* was invasive in 25% of cases. Rosen et al. (168) studied 203 mastectomy specimens by dissecting the quadrant from which the biopsy had been taken and submitting it separately from the rest of the breast. Thus examined, multicentricity was reported in other quadrants in 32% of the cases. Invasive cancer was present in 21% of cases and residual carcinoma *in situ* was present in the other 11% of cases. Sarnelli and Squartini (169) dissected mastectomy specimens and found less than 5-mm submacroscopic foci collateral to and independent of the clinical cancer in 36%, with *in situ* in 17% of cases, invasive in 12% of cases, and *in situ* and invasive in 7% of cases. The authors reported multicentricity as significantly associated with family history and advanced age.

Holland et al. (170) studied 282 mastectomies by specimen mammography, excluding all cases in which cancer extended to the chest wall or skin or was diffuse, clinically and radiographically inapparent, or greater than 5 cm in diameter. In 20% of the cases, multifocality was present within 2 cm of the site of excision; in 43% of cases, tumor was present at a distance of more than 2 cm from the "excisional biopsy." Of 264 invasive carcinomas that were 4 cm or less in diameter and which were removed with a 3- to 4-cm margin of apparently normal breast tissue, 7% to 9% of the patients had residual invasive carcinoma and 4% to 9% had foci of carcinoma *in situ*.

Faverly et al. (171,172) used a stereoscopic technique to study 60 mastectomy specimens for the growth pattern of DCIS. A multifocal distribution, defined as a gap of 4 cm or more between tumor foci, was found in only one case. Poorly differentiated DCIS showed a continuous growth pattern, in contrast to well-differentiated DCIS, which more frequently showed a multicentric pattern. Irrespective of histologic type, 8% of DCIS had a multifocal distribution with gaps greater than 1 cm. The earlier study by these authors showed that most minimal carcinomas arose in the terminal ductulo–lobular units and that DCIS may grow continuously by extending through the glandular tree, but it may also have a multifocal or stepwise progression in rare cases. Coombs et al. (173) studied 60 cases of DCIS that were treated by mastectomy. Eight percent of the lesions were multicentric and 45% of the lesions were multifocal. Lagios (174) found multicentricity of DCIS in 32% of cases. Multicentricity was observed in 13 of 24 cases of DCIS that were larger than 25 mm, but in only 4 of 29 cases of DCIS that were less than 25 mm. Alpers and Wellings (175) studied 292 breasts in a subgroup sampling technique with histologic confirmation. The authors found primary foci of DCIS that was unrelated to invasive breast cancer in 53% of cancer-containing breasts. DCIS was found in 48% of contralateral breasts and 6% of breasts from random autopsies. Simpson et al. (176) studied 36 patients who were treated for DCIS by mastectomy. The authors found multicentricity of DCIS in 78% of cases overall and in 88% of cases with comedocarcinoma, but in none of the cases with low-grade papillary DCIS. Schwartz et al. (177) found comedocarcinoma to be the most likely type of DCIS associated with multicentricity. Their solid and cribriform types of DCIS were rarely multicentric, but the micropapillary DCIS was often multicentric.

Luttges et al. (178) reported multicentricity in 76 of 166 patients who were treated by mastectomy. Nipple involvement was found in 38% of the cases and correlated with multicentricity of breast cancer as a disease of the whole organ.

CYTOGENETIC STUDIES

Confirmation of multicentricity with cytogenetic studies is not without difficulty. Heim et al. (179) described cytogenetically unrelated clones in one-half of all solitary breast cancers. The authors divided three primary carcinomas into 12 segments and found clonal chromosome aberrations in all 8 successfully analyzed samples. Between two and six cytogenetically unrelated clones were detected in each case and they were unevenly distributed among the tumor quadrants. It is not clear whether this indicated multicellular origin or progression of heterogeneity within a single tumor. Pandis et al. (180) described clonal heterogeneity in ten carcinomas of the breast. Teixeira et al. (181) studied 26 macroscopically distinct ipsilateral breast carcinomas from 12 patients. In 62% of the foci, the authors found clonal chromosome abnormalities. Two carcinoma foci were karyotypically abnormal in each of seven patients. Four of these cases had an evolutionarily related cytogenetically abnormal clone in the two lesions from the same breast and three cases had different clonal karyotypic aberrations in separate foci. These data were interpreted as showing that multiple synchronous breast carcinomas sometimes arise through intramammary spread from a single focus, but simultaneous emergence of pathogenetically independent carcinomas may also occur. Tsuda and Hirohashi (182) found both multicentricity and multifocality in 60 cases of multiple breast cancer studied by Southern blot analysis for loss of heterozygosity on chromosome 16q. In 5 of 11 cases of carcinomas identified as multicentric and also 5 of 11 synchronous bilateral breast cancers, loss of heterozygosity indicated independent occurrence and multicentric origin; however, in the other cases, there was genetic concordance consistent with monocentric origin and spread. In the carcinomas identified as multifocal or intramammary metastases, there was concordance and loss of heterozygosity.

Dawson et al. (183) reported an immunohistochemical study to distinguish between multifocal and multicentric synchronous tumors. Using markers B72.3, DF3, CERB2, SP1, CED and P53, evaluated by immunostaining, there was histologic and immunohistochemical identity in 10 cases, and, in 7 cases, the carcinomas were different both histologically and immunohistochemically. Five cases were histologically similar, but immunocytochemically different; two cases were histologically different, but immunocytochemically identical.

MULTIFOCALITY BY TYPE OF CARCINOMA

Few reports distinguish multicentricity of invasive carcinomas by histologic type. The study by Lagios et al. (184) showed that patients with tubular carcinomas were more likely to have multicentric invasive carcinomas. Green et al.

(185) reported multifocality of pure tubular carcinomas at 20%, with 33% of the multifocal cases and 7% of unifocal cases node positive, whereas tubulolobular carcinomas were multifocal in 29% of cases, with node positivity in 60% of multifocal cases and 33% of unifocal cases.

Crile (186) argued that the incidence of multifocality that is found histologically in mastectomy specimens does not necessarily relate to the likelihood of a clinical recurrent tumor, but Fisher et al. (187) reported a 28% incidence of local recurrence after segmental mastectomy without radiation compared to a 7.7% incidence of local recurrence after excisional biopsy and radiotherapy. The 28% incidence of local recurrence is essentially the same as the incidence of multifocality, as determined by a large number of studies, and it is a strong argument for additional treatment—surgery or radiation to the entire breast. Lobular carcinoma, both noninvasive and invasive, tubular carcinomas, and large intraductal carcinomas appear to have the highest likelihood of multifocality.

Bilateral Breast Cancer

Bilateral breast cancer is a special case for consideration of multicentricity or multifocality. In advanced cancer, metastasis to the contralateral breast is possible, but in follow-up of the great majority of local or regional breast cancer, the appearance of a contralateral carcinoma indicates a new primary cancer.

Bilateral breast cancer is associated with a family history of breast cancer, early onset breast cancer, and ovarian cancer through BRCA1 mutations (188,189). If BRCA1 status has not been determined, the presence of early onset breast cancer, a family history of breast cancer, or ovarian cancer, in association with breast cancer, should be a warning that bilateral breast cancer is likely to occur. Horn and Thompson (190) found a threefold risk in bilateral breast cancer when there was a family history of breast cancer in any first- or second-degree relative. Pandis et al. (191) studied 16 bilateral carcinomas cytogenetically. In two cases, the finding of identical clonal abnormalities was consistent with the interpretation that the contralateral carcinoma was a metastasis. In the other 14 cases, the absence of mutational similarities indicated independent bilateral origin. Deletions and translocations on chromosomes 1 and 3 were studied. Shibata et al. (192) studied 12 cases of bilateral breast cancer for trinucleotide repeat polymorphism in exon 1 of the androgen receptor gene on the X chromosome and for p53 mutations in pairs of bilateral breast cancers. Three cases had distinct alleles, which indicated that they arose independently, and, in 13 cases, mutations in the p53 gene were found. The authors concluded that some bilateral breast cancers originate independently, but some others may be related through a common p53 abnormality. Ackerman et al. (193), however, could not find that p53 mutations played a major role in the pathogenesis of bilateral disease in most women. Lidereau and Soussi (194) screened lymphocyte DNA from 19 unrelated bilateral breast cancer patients and detected no germ line mutation in p53 exons 5, 6, 7, or 8.

Mose et al. (195) found no difference in survival between unilateral and bilateral breast cancer patients. The 10-year survival rate was 54% in patients with unilateral disease and 56% in patients with bilateral breast cancer. Fung et al. (196) reported 5- and 10-year actuarial relapse-free survival rates of 90%, and 75%, respectively, for patients treated by lumpectomy and radiotherapy for the first breast cancer and 83% and 72%, respectively, after similar treatment for the second carcinoma.

Coradini et al. (197) studied estrogen receptors and progesterone receptors in both primary and contralateral breast cancers and found that estrogen and progesterone receptor levels did not differ significantly between the two carcinomas. They significantly correlated within the same patient, with higher correlation for synchronous than metachronous carcinomas for ER only. Correlation between estrogen and progesterone receptor levels in the same tumor was stronger than the correlation of either receptor between primary and contralateral breast cancer. The authors interpreted these data to show that contralateral breast cancers are second primaries that arise in a common predisposing milieu.

Dawson et al. (198) reported that adjuvant tamoxifen and ovarian ablation significantly reduced contralateral breast cancer in reported studies.

Fisher (199) reported on 29 patients with carcinoma that was detected on biopsy of one breast who were treated by bilateral mastectomy and found ten unexpected carcinomas in the contralateral breast.

de la Rochefordiere and Scholl (200) described 149 patients with simultaneous bilateral breast carcinomas, defined as those diagnosed with cancer in both breasts within 6 months. Forty percent of the second tumors were T0 to T1 and 45% were T2 tumors. Eighty-three percent of the patients were clinically node negative. The positive correlations that existed between the two carcinomas included lobular carcinoma in both breasts, the same histologic grade, and similar estrogen receptor and progesterone receptor status. Five-year rates of survival were high at 86%, with 70% disease-free rates. Patients with bilateral breast cancer that was staged according to the higher stage carcinoma did not fare worse than the matched group of patients with unilateral breast cancer.

Urban (201) found a 16% incidence of bilateral cancer among 159 women with blind biopsy of the contralateral breast. In 13 of the 31 cases, the carcinoma was noninvasive. Moertel et al. (202) estimated the true incidence of bilaterality at 6% to 8%. The authors found 110 interval malignant lesions and 8 simultaneous carcinomas among 2,945 patients that were followed for breast cancer. Robbins and Berg (203) found an incidence of 7 cases of contralateral carcinoma per 1,000 patients per year. The risk was 5 times that of the female population in general, 10 times in women under 50 years, and 2 times in women over 50 years. Lobular carcinoma was the histologic type most often bilateral. The authors pointed out that a relatively low-grade or nonfatal initial carcinoma was needed for sufficient follow-up time to observe the occurrence of a second carcinoma. McCredie et al. (204) found an incidence of 1% per year, constant over 20 years, for contralateral carcinoma.

Ringberg et al. (205) summarized three series of patients. Fifty-two percent of 46 patients with unilateral breast cancer who underwent subcutaneous mastectomy of the contralateral breast for cosmesis had bilateral malignant lesions. There were 24 contralateral carcinomas; 4 were invasive and 20 were *in situ*. Among 52 other women with unilateral diagnosis of *in situ* carcinoma who underwent bilateral subcutaneous mastectomy for cosmesis, 48% had bilateral malignant lesions; 24 of 25 contralateral carcinomas were *in situ*. Twelve of the 20 cases of lobular carcinoma *in situ* were bilateral. In a series of 64 autopsies of women with unilateral mastectomy, 23% were found to have contralateral primary carcinoma; 4 were invasive and 11 were *in situ*. The authors also looked at multifocality of carcinoma in 47 subcutaneous mastectomy specimens after excisional biopsy for *in situ* carcinoma. Seventy-five percent of these patients had additional malignant lesions, despite normal mammography and clinical findings. Thirty-one of the 35 patients had *in situ* lesions and 4 patients had invasive carcinomas. The clinical development of a second primary carcinoma, however, was somewhat less frequently observed. Parker (206) obtained follow-up data 5 to 30 years after mastectomy on 1,630 women. The rate of development of nonsimultaneous contralateral breast carcinoma was 2.5 per 1,000 person years at risk. Beller et al. (207), however, found a five- to sevenfold risk of occurrence of breast cancer in the contralateral breast, with 15 frankly invasive carcinomas, 4 metastases, and 28 carcinomas *in situ* among 365 patients. Wanebo et al. (208) described a group of 62 patients who underwent elective contralateral biopsies after mastectomy for primary breast cancer. The biopsies were either mirror image (i.e., contralateral to the site at which the first breast cancer was found) or, more often, a biopsy of the upper outer quadrant. Thirteen of the 62 had simultaneous contralateral carcinomas, of which 11 were clinically occult. Occult carcinomas were more often noninvasive than the original clinically diagnosed carcinoma. In a series of 500 primary breast cancer patients, 37 (7.4%) patients developed second breast primaries and 33 of them were metachronous. Thirty-five of the 37 carcinomas were invasive. The authors concluded that elective contralateral biopsy may detect and treat carcinoma at an earlier stage. Brenner et al. (209) studied 250 patients with bilateral breast cancer and compared them to 9,585 patients with a first diagnosis of breast cancer. Women with bilateral breast cancer were younger on average, and women younger than age 50 years had a much less favorable stage distribution of second breast cancers. Survival rates after diagnosis of the second breast cancer were not as good as survival after a first breast cancer diagnosis. Boice (210) conducted a case control study in a cohort of 41,109 women who were diagnosed with breast cancer in Connecticut between 1935 and 1982. Among women who survived for at least 10 years after treatment, radiation was associated with a small, but marginally significant, elevation in the risk of a second breast primary. This risk was confined to women who were under 45 years of age when they were treated (relative risk of 1.59, compared to a relative risk of 1.01 among women older than 45 years when treated for their first breast primary).

In summary, it is clear that as breast cancer is detected and effectively treated at an earlier stage, the development of carcinoma in the contralateral breast will assume a more important role in the management of the woman with breast cancer. A rule of thumb for estimating this risk is about 1% per year of follow-up.

PRIMARY THERAPEUTIC OPTIONS

Surgery Alone

When mastectomy was the treatment of choice, study of the intact breast led to a well-defined list of predictors of therapeutic success. Type of carcinoma present, size, stage, status of axillary lymph nodes, presence or absence of fixation to the skin or to the underlying fascia, presence or absence of vascular invasion, tumor grade (as suggested by a number of schemes), and presence or absence of carcinoma *in situ* were all reported to predict for local failure.

Mastectomy has ceased to be the only treatment option for limited stage carcinoma of the breast; lumpectomy plus radiotherapy is an increasingly popular choice and consideration is now being given to limited surgery alone in selected cases. A number of factors have contributed to the change in thinking about the treatment of the primary tumor. Detection of carcinoma of the breast at an earlier stage has obviated the necessity for removal of skin and fascia, which are involved, by definition, late in the local spread of the disease. Perhaps more important has been an understanding that removal of all local and regionally metastatic disease has little impact on prevention of systemic metastases. The extent of local and regional spread is now viewed primarily as an important predictor of the presence of distant metastases, which are treated medically. However, local and regional recurrences are still significant problems, and the pathologist is called upon to predict the success of local treatment.

With the entire breast and regional nodes available for study, this was less of a challenge, but the pathologist must now make recommendations over a broader range of therapeutic options, from a biopsy of the primary tumor. We need to predict invasiveness, metastatic potential radiosensitivity, responsiveness to hormonal manipulation, or specific chemotherapy.

Local Recurrence after Mastectomy

The incidence of recurrence of carcinoma in the chest wall following radical, super radical or modified radical mastectomy has been well established. Controversy over the need for removal of large amounts of skin that require skin grafting to close the wound led to a more conservative trend, with a decrease in the use of skin grafting. Chest wall recurrences after removal of the entire breast varied from 3% to 22%, according to stage of disease and the operation. In the Haagensen (211) series, only 4% of stage A patients had chest wall recurrence within 10 years, whereas 14% of stage B, 16% of stage C, and 66% of stage D carcinomas experienced chest wall recurrence within that timeframe. Local recurrence of carcinoma after mastectomy is considered a harbinger of distant metastases. The cases in this series were of relatively good prognosis, but 30% of those with local recurrence were dead within one year and only 12% were alive 5 years after local recurrence.

Radiotherapy

Local Recurrence after Radiotherapy

Local recurrence in the breast after radiation is not necessarily as ominous as chest wall recurrence after mastectomy. Early recurrence indicates persistence of an aggressive carcinoma, unresponsiveness to radiotherapy, and/or multifocality. Later recurrence could be persistence of the primary carcinoma, but it might also be development of a new carcinoma or possibly a radiation-induced neoplasm.

Amalric et al. (212) reported on 1,440 women who were treated with conservative surgery and radiation. Patients with primaries smaller than 5 cm in diameter (generally treated by lumpectomy or wedge resection followed by radiation) had a 10-year survival rate of 77%. Those with larger primaries (generally treated primarily with radiation after less than excisional biopsy) had a 10-year survival rate of only 34%. Thirty-five percent of the patients required a second operation for what was presumed to be a local recurrence, but no tumor was found in 24% of those operative specimens. The authors noted that earlier reports with local failure rates of only 10% were based on follow-up of 5 years or less and most of their local recurrences were found between 5 and 10 years. In their study, local recurrence did not adversely affect survival. The authors analyzed only size and type of excision. Twenty percent of 122 patients with excisional biopsy recurred, whereas 40% of 192 patients without complete excision failed locally. Size did not predict local recurrence. The histology of these carcinomas was not reported.

Calle et al. (213) reported on 120 patients with breast primaries that were 3 cm or less in size and without palpable axillary lymph nodes who were treated by lumpectomy and radiation. These cases were compared to 394 patients with larger primaries or palpable axillary nodes who were treated by radiation without lumpectomy. In those patients who were treated by lumpectomy and radiation, 12% had local recurrence; the 5- and 10-year survivals, free of disease, were 85% and 75%, respectively. In the group treated by radiation without lumpectomy, the 5- and 10-year survivals were 68% and 43%, respectively; 55% had local recurrence, with 81% of these having locally persistent disease that required surgery within 4.5 months after completion of radiation. Fifty-five percent of the patients needing secondary surgery were alive at 5 years. No other predictors of local failure were analyzed.

Albert and Ghossein (214) found a local recurrence rate of 8% in 109 cases of breast cancer that were treated by tumorectomy and radiotherapy or by radiotherapy alone. In reviewing the factors associated with local failure, microscopic involvement of the surgical margin did not affect local control rate; an 8% local failure rate occurred in patients with both positive and negative margins. Follow-up time for this study averaged only 4 years, with a minimum of 2 years. Absolute survival, free of disease, was 65%. As mentioned above, local failure between 5 and 10 years has been observed by several groups. No data that relates to the histologic predictors of local recurrence were reported.

Bataini and Picco (215) reported local recurrence in 10 of 67 patients that were treated by lumpectomy and radiotherapy and followed for a total of 5 years. Eight patients had recurred by the fifth year. In 122 patients treated by radiotherapy without excisional biopsy, 57% had persistent disease or local recurrence within 5 years. Seventy-four percent of these patients had recurred within 6 months of the completion of radiotherapy. The authors studied the histology of the carcinomas and reported briefly that patients with grade III (high grade) cancers had a local control rate of only 26%, compared to 58% and 57% local control for carcinomas that were of grade I and grade II histology, respectively. The grading system used in the study is not noted. Fisher et al. (161) reported on a large series of patients who were treated by either segmental mastectomy alone or by segmental mastectomy in combination with radiotherapy. This series differs from the others, since all of the patients had dissection of axillary lymph nodes. The patients were compared to a group of patients who were treated by total mastectomy without radiation. At 5 years, 7.7% of patients with segmental resection plus radiation therapy had local recurrence in the breast, whereas 27.9% of those treated by segmental mastectomy without radiation had recurrence within the breast. The authors found that the stage of disease played an important role in the prediction of the likelihood of local recurrence. Only 2% of patients with negative lymph nodes who were irradiated had local recurrence, compared to 36% of those with positive nodes who did not undergo radiation. In patients with primary tumors of less than 2 cm in diameter, 6.5% had local recurrence following segmental mastectomy alone. In those patients with tumors between 2 and 4 cm in diameter, the figures were approximately the same—8% after segmental mastectomy with radiation and 23% without radiation. Size did not play a major role in determining the likelihood of failure, but it did play a role in predicting the likelihood of a positive surgical margin following segmental mastectomy. The incidence of a positive specimen margin was 13% in patients with tumors that varied from 2 to 4 cm in diameter and only 7% in those patients with tumors that were smaller than 2 cm in diameter. Patients with centrally located tumors were most likely to have a positive surgical margin. The authors did not report on the histologic predictors of local or distant recurrence following segmental mastectomy and radiation.

Schnitt et al. (107) studied 34 gross and histologic predictors of failure after radiotherapy in 231 cases of clinical stage I and stage II invasive breast cancer that was treated by biopsy and primary radiotherapy. The overall incidence of local recurrence was 7% at 44 months. Distribution of the types of invasive carcinomas in the 231 cases was approximately that of carcinoma of the breast in general. One hundred seventy-six cases were infiltrating duct carcinomas, 15 were infiltrating lobular carcinomas, 5 each were medullary and colloid carcinomas, 1 was a papillary carcinoma, and 1 was an adenoid cystic carcinoma. Fifteen of the duct carcinomas, one of the lobular carcinomas, and the adenoid cystic carcinoma failed locally. Eight percent of those in which the margins of resection were considered negative failed locally. All were infiltrating duct carcinomas. Thirty-six percent of the 19 cases in which the biopsy was less than excisional failed locally. Four of these cases were invasive ductal carcinomas, one was a lobular carcinoma, and the other was the adenoid cystic carcinoma. The largest group of carcinomas in this series, as in all others, was the invasive ductal carcinoma, and there were several predictors of the likelihood of local control within this group. Twenty-three percent of the 59 cases in which there was EIC, defined as DCIS both in the area of the invasive carcinoma and adjacent to it, failed locally. In the other 95 cases in which there was no intraductal carcinoma or the intraductal carcinoma was localized to either the area of the invasive carcinoma or to the area adjacent to it, but not both, only 1% failed locally. In addition, these carcinomas were graded according to Fisher's criteria (noted above). Fifteen percent of grade III carcinomas failed locally, whereas only 3% of those carcinomas considered grade I or grade II were not locally controlled by radiation. In patients in whom mitoses were absent or scanty, 3% failed locally; in those patients who had a moderate to marked number of mitotic figures, the local failure rate was 16%. In cases where there was both EIC and grade III histology, the local recurrence rate was 39%, compared to the rest of the cases, in which the local recurrence rate was only 4%. The other 34 descriptors, including the presence or absence of lymph node metastases and the size of the primary tumor, did not predict local failure in a statistically significant way.

Mate et al. (216) reported on a group of 180 women who had clinical stage I or stage II breast carcinoma, which was treated by local tumor excision followed by radiotherapy, with a median follow-up time of 6.9 years. The 5-year local recurrence-free survival rate was 92%. In this series, numerous histologic descriptors, similar in many ways to those reported by Schnitt et al. (107), were assessed. Descriptors that were found to be significant include the size of the carcinoma, the presence of necrosis within the tumor, and an infiltrating lobular carcinoma pattern. Histologic grade and the presence of an intraductal component had no impact on the outcome. The presence of less than excisional biopsy was not a frequent event. Clinical stage I carcinomas (i.e., carcinomas 2 cm or less in diameter) had a 20% recurrence rate, with 9% recurring in the breast. Clinical stage II carcinoma (i.e., carcinomas between 2 and 5 cm in diameter) had a 43% recurrence rate, with an 18% local failure rate. There were only 12 infiltrating lobular carcinomas, but they did so poorly, so as to suggest that they should be considered a poor prognostic indicator. Statistically, the difference between the invasive lobular type of carcinoma and other types of invasive carcinomas was significant, although with this small number of cases, further studies are needed to validate the observation. The multifocality and difficulty in establishing negative margins in lobular carcinoma may have been contributing factors. Poen et al. (217) reviewed 60 patients with stage I and stage II invasive lobular carcinoma who were treated with local excision and radiotherapy, with a mean follow-up of 5.5 years. The 5-year actuarial risk of local regional recurrence was 5%, with two of the failures in regional lymphatics. However, the 5-year actuarial disease-free survival and overall survival were comparable to those in other published series of invasive ductal carcinomas. Contralateral breast cancers occurred in 6 per 1,000 per year. White et al. (218) compared 30 patients with infiltrating lobular carcinomas with 346 patients with invasive ductal carcinomas and 26 cases with other types of invasive carcinomas. Median follow-up was 5 years. No significant difference in local recurrence rate was found between the invasive lobular and ductal carcinomas. The authors relied heavily on mammograms for determining the presence or absence of residual carcinoma following excision. Intraductal carcinoma was only evaluated for presence or absence and not for EIC. The presence of intraductal carcinoma alone was not found to be a reliable predictor of failure. One-third of the patients had invasive carcinoma in which tumor necrosis was evident; 37% of these patients died, 43% had a recurrence, and 20% had recurrence in the breast. In the other two-thirds of patients in which necrosis was not evident in the invasive carcinoma, 16% died, 21% had a recurrence, and 9% had a recurrence within the breast. The difference in these figures is statistically significant. Grading system did not segregate the behavior of the carcinomas, although the presence of necrosis was more likely in high-grade carcinomas in the large study by Fisher et al. (219). Those authors also found tumor necrosis to correlate with a marked intraductal component. Clark et al. (220) noted that the failure rate was higher in less well-differentiated carcinomas, using the Bloom grading system (221). The NSABP study by Fisher et al. (187), which showed that the results of treatment with lumpectomy and radiation were comparable to those achieved by mastectomy, created a consensus that breast conservation treatment with radiation was an appropriate method of primary therapy for the majority of women with stage I and stage II breast cancer. A subsequent study by Janjan et al. (222) that compared the results of 558 patients who were treated by mastectomy with the results in 201 patients who were treated by breast conserving surgery and radiation showed a better prognosis in node negative patients who underwent breast conservative surgery and radiation. Krishnan et al. (223) described 245 patients who were treated by lumpectomy, immediate boost interstitial radiation, and external beam radiation to the entire breast. EIC was found in 61 of the cases. The 10-year actuarial recurrence rate in patients with EIC was 9.1%. For those without EIC, the 10-year actuarial recurrence rate was 5.2%, but this difference was not statistically significantly.

Recht et al. (224) described 40 women with intraductal carcinoma of the breast who were treated satisfactorily by radiotherapy. Four patients had local recurrence, but all were satisfactorily salvaged by mastectomy. Solin et al. (149)

reported on 259 patients with intraductal carcinoma who were treated with lumpectomy and radiation in nine institutions in Europe and the United States with 10-year follow-up. The 10-year actuarial survival rate was 94% and the 10-year actuarial cause-specific survival rate was 97%. Ninety-six percent of patients were judged to be free of distant metastases, but a local failure rate of 16% was noted at 10 years, and one-half of those recurrences (14 of 28) showed invasive ductal carcinoma. Twenty-four of the 28 patients with local failure were salvaged, but 4 of the 28 patients who failed locally with invasive carcinoma subsequently developed distant metastases. Two patients without local failure also developed distant metastases, but one of these occurred after a contralateral breast carcinoma, which was invasive and node positive. The overall survival rate was high, but not 100%.

Kurtz et al. (225) described 61 patients (a subgroup of 586 unilateral stage I to stage II breast cancer patients) who were treated by conservative surgery and radiotherapy, in which two or more grossly evident cancers were present. After a median follow-up of 71 months, 25% of the patients with multiple tumors developed recurrence in the treated breast, compared to only 11% of patients with single carcinomas. Local failure occurred in 6 of 37 patients with two carcinomas and in 9 of 24 patients with three or more carcinomas. Failure in these patients tended to be located at a distance from the original tumors, multifocal or diffuse, and had a high incidence of skin involvement. Failure was more often seen when margins were positive. Reports by Baird et al. (226) and Fisher et al. (156,227)) have shown that DCIS can be treated successfully by lumpectomy and radiotherapy. In the series by Fisher et al. (227), radiotherapy reduced local recurrence from 39% to 13% over 8 years. Only comedocarcinoma predicted for local recurrence, 40% of which were invasive carcinomas. Mortality at 8 years, however, was 2%.

Surgery Alone for Ductal Carcinoma **In Situ**

Is there a subset of cases of DCIS that can be treated safely by local excision without radiotherapy? Silverstein et al. (157) proposed the Van Nuys Prognostic Index to give guidance on this question. The index was composed of three factors: tumor size, margin width, and pathologic classification. Scores of 1 (most favorable) to 3 (least favorable) were assigned to each of these features. The 8-year local recurrence-free survival was reported. It must be noted, however, that this was not a randomized study, but one in which some patients were treated with surgery alone and other patients received radiation. With that in mind, the findings show that a Van Nuys Prognostic Index score of 3 or 4 was associated with virtually 100% local recurrence-free survival, regardless of whether radiation was given or not. Radiation therapy did increase the local recurrence-free survival rate from 60% to 85% in those with scores of 5, 6, or 7. In patients with index scores of 8 or 9, local recurrence rates in excess of 60% were observed at 8 years, although this rate was reduced by addition of radiation therapy. The authors concluded that patients with intraductal carcinoma, with index scores of 3 or 4, could be considered for treatment with excision only. They went on to suggest that patients with DCIS, with intermediate scores of 5, 6, or 7, would benefit from the addition of radiotherapy, but that patients with DCIS with scores of 8 or 9 had such high local recurrence rates that they should be considered for mastectomy.

Three years later (228), the same group presented an updated analysis of their data on 469 patients with intraductal carcinoma who were treated with breast conserving surgery, with or without postoperative radiation therapy. They found a probability of recurrence of 0.04 at 8 years among 133 patients whose excised lesions had margin widths of 10 mm or more in every direction. These patients did not benefit from postoperative radiation therapy. Patients with margin widths between 1 and 10 mm also showed no benefit from postoperative radiation, but those with margin widths of less than 1 mm did show significant benefit from radiation. It appears then that the controlling factor in the Van Nuys Prognostic Index is the margin width. Tumor size and pathologic classification influence the size of the required excision, but not the final outcome, which was entirely margin related.

After reviewing these reports, it appears that the pathologist has several interrelated factors to report as predictors of local recurrence. No single feature of a carcinoma or its excision is likely to provide enough data for predicting local recurrence.

1. Margins of lumpectomy
   Although several authors have reported that positive margins correlate with local failure, other studies have found that they are not a contraindication to treatment with radiotherapy without reexcision. In DCIS cases, Silverstein et al. (228) found that margin status was the only important factor.
2. Size
   Data relating to the usefulness of size as a predictor of local recurrence are also mixed and probably are related to margin status.
3. Histologic type
   The study by Mate et al. (216) suggested that lobular carcinoma may be a predictor of local recurrence, although later reports failed to confirm this observation. Lobular histology also probably relates to margin status.
4. Grade
   Some authors reported that tumor grade correlates positively with local recurrence, but the grading schemes for these studies vary, and grade may correlate with size, which may correlate with margin status.
5. Tumor necrosis
   Tumor necrosis may be a useful predictor of response to radiotherapy, but it correlates with high tumor grade.
6. *In situ* carcinoma associated with invasive carcinoma
   EIC (intraductal carcinoma both within the invasive tumor and in the adjacent tissue) may be predictive of local failure in certain cases.

Although local recurrence occurs after radiotherapy, it is much more of a problem when radiation therapy is not given after lumpectomy for invasive carcinoma. Cajucom et al. (229) reported local recurrence in 25 of 128 stage I or stage II breast cancer patients who were treated by breast conservation surgery without radiation after a median disease-free interval of only 20 months. Mastectomy was carried out in these patients. After a median interval of 52 months, one-half of the patients had chest wall and/or distant recurrences. The 5-year actuarial disease-free and overall survival rates after salvage mastectomy were 51% and 65%, respectively. The authors noted that the size of the local recurrence and the number of pathologically positive axillary lymph nodes, at the time of the modified radical mastectomy, were prognostic indicators.

One infrequent, but serious, complication of radiotherapy is the appearance, in the irradiated tissues of sarcoma, especially angiosarcoma, often of high histologic grade and biological aggressiveness in a very short time after completion or radiotherapy. The incidence is low and the cases are mainly published as case reports (Chapter 10), but their number, localization to the irradiated area, and time course make it difficult to escape the conclusion that they are radiation-induced.

In summary, the rate of local recurrence after lumpectomy and radiotherapy is approximately 0.5% to 1% per year in the ipsilateral breast, which is approximately the incidence of the appearance of carcinoma in the contralateral breast. It appears that as more experience is gained with conservative surgery and radiotherapy as a primary modality of treatment, there are few absolute contraindications to its use, when this is the desire of the patient. It should be remembered, however, that this technique is employed primarily for an improvement in morbidity from treatment, rather than as an advance for limiting mortality from breast cancer.

Prognosis of Local Recurrence after Radiation.

Haffty et al. (230) described 50 local failures among 433 patients with clinical stage I and stage II breast cancer who were treated by conservative surgery and radiotherapy. Flow cytometric techniques were employed for a study of both the original carcinoma and the local recurrence. Sixty-three percent of the recurrent tumors were diploid and 37% were aneuploid. Both ploidy and S-phase fraction were statistically significant prognostic indicators for 5-year survival and disease-free survival after local recurrence. The 5-year survival rate of diploid recurrences was 64%, whereas it was only 15% for the aneuploid recurrences. Patients with recurrent tumors that showed an S-phase fraction that was lower than 12% had an 83% 5-year survival rate, compared with a 24% survival rate for those with a higher S-phase fraction. When combined, the favorable group of recurrences, which were diploid and low S-phase, experienced an 89% 5-year post recurrence survival rate. The poor prognostic group with aneuploid tumors with a high S-phase had only a 24% 5-year survival and a 32% disease-free survival rate. Flow cytometry correlated with other clinical parameters that were shown to be of prognostic significance in this patient population. A large recurrence shortly after treatment demonstrated poor survival, whereas patients with a small recurrence at 5 years or more after survival had a much superior survival post recurrence. It was speculated that the latter group might represent the emergence of a new carcinoma, rather than recurrence of the original carcinoma. Molecular biologic data is valuable in distinguishing recurrence from a new primary cancer.

Fisher et al. (231) described ipsilateral breast cancer recurrence in 42 of 488 patients, with a mean potential follow-up of 103 months. The recurrences were observed at or close to the same quadrant as the index cancers and their histologic types and nuclear grades were similar, if not identical, in 95% of the cases. The authors concluded that multicentricity was of little or no clinical significance in the treatment of breast cancer by conservative surgery and x-ray therapy. It was their conclusion that most, if not all, of the local recurrences represented residual cancer. Pathologic features of the index cancers were not found to predict for local recurrence; patients treated before age 35 years had a significantly elevated local recurrence rate. Kurtz et al. (232) analyzed 178 local recurrences among 1,593 patients with clinical stage I and stage II breast cancers who were treated by conservative surgery and radiotherapy. The 71 patients who were diagnosed with recurrence 5 years after treatment had a more favorable survival 5 years post recurrence (84%) than those with early recurrences (61%). Late recurrences were more often located at a distance from the primary tumor than were early recurrences. Most significantly, patients with late local recurrences had identical 15-year survivals to those who had never experienced local failure. The authors also found that local recurrence was more frequent in patients who were younger than the age of 40 years at initial treatment. Chauvet and Fetissof (233) identified the disappearance of carcinoma *in situ* in recurrence as predictive of systemic metastases after local relapse. In 17 patients with local recurrence, there was no shift in the presence or absence of an *in situ* component between the index cancer and the recurrence. Two of these 17 patients experienced systemic metastases. In contrast, 12 patients were shown to have a decrease in the proportion of noninvasive cancer and recurrence; 9 of these 12 patients developed systemic metastases. The authors concluded that early relapses had a poor prognosis and disappearance of the *in situ* component was also predictive of a poor prognosis.

Baird et al. (226) reported that comedo-type of intraductal carcinoma was the most commonly recurrent type after treatment by conservative surgery and radiotherapy. With a mean follow-up of 39 months, 4 of 30 patients with comedocarcinoma who were treated by local resection alone and 2 of 8 patients who were treated with local resection and radiotherapy recurred locally.

Girling et al. (234) illustrated radiotherapy-induced epithelial and stromal atypia, which are easily confused with recurrent malignancy, especially when a core needle biopsy is available for review. The use of antibodies to keratin may be useful in distinguishing atypia in stromal cells from single cell anaplastic carcinoma.

In 1998, Silverstein et al. (235) observed 74 local recurrences among 707 patients who were treated for DCIS between 1972 and 1997. Invasive carcinoma was present in 47% of the recurrences; 51% of the invasive carcinomas were in stage I cancers. The 8-year breast cancer specific mortality and distant disease probability for patients with local recurrence was 8.8% and 20.8%, respectively; however, for the 35 patients with invasive carcinoma in the recurrence, the rates were 14.4% and 27.1%, respectively.

REFERENCES

1. Papanicolaou GM, Holmquist DG, Bader GM, et al. Exfoliative cytology of the human mammary gland and its value in the diagnosis of cancer and other diseases of the breast. *Cancer* 1958;11: 377–409.
2. Fischermann K, Bech I, Foged P, et al. Nipple discharge: diagnosis and treatment. *Acta Chir Scand* 1969;135:403–406.
3. Takeda T, Suzuki M, Soto Y, et al. Cytologic studies of nipple discharges. *Acta Cytol* 1982;26:35–36.
4. Johnson TL, Kini SR. Cytologic and clinicopathologic features of abnormal nipple secretions: 225 cases. *Diagn Cytopathol* 1991;7:17–22.
5. Dunn JM, Lucarotti ME, Wood SJ, et al. Exfoliative cytology in the diagnosis of breast disease. *Br J Surg* 1995;82:789–791.
6. Shen KW, Wu J, Lu JS, et al. Fiberoptic ductoscopy for patients with nipple discharge. *Cancer* 2000;89:1512–1519.
7. Takeda T, Suzuki M, Soto Y, et al. Aspiration cytology of breast cysts. *Acta Cytol* 1982;26:37–38.
8. Bell DA, Hajdu SI, Urban JA, et al. Role of aspiration cytology in the diagnosis and management of mammary lesions in office practice. *Cancer* 1983;51:1182–1189.
9. Kline TS, Joshi LP, Neal HS. Fine-needle aspiration of the breast: diagnosis and pitfalls; a review of 3,545 cases. *Cancer* 1979;44:1458–1464.
10. Kline TS. Masquerades of malignancy: a review of 4,241 aspirates from the breast. *Acta Cytol* 1981;25:263–266.
11. Kline TS, Kannan V. Papillary carcinoma of the breast. A cytomorphologic analysis. *Arch Pathol Lab Med* 1986;110:189–191.
12. Oertel YC. *Fine needle aspiration of the breast*. Butterworth-Heineman: Boston, 1987.
13. Daum GS, Kline TS, Artymyshyn RL, et al. Aspiration biopsy cytology of occult breast lesions by use of the "scouting needle." A prospective study of 261 cases. *Cancer* 1991;67:2150–2152.
14. Giard RWM, Hermans J. The value of aspiration cytologic examination of the breast: a statistical review of the medical literature. *Cancer* 1992;69:2104–2110.
15. Gupta RK, Dowle CS, Simpson JS. The value of needle aspiration cytology of the breast, with an emphasis on the diagnosis of breast disease in young women below the age of 30. *Acta Cytol* 1990; 34:461–471.
16. Benoit JL, Kara R, McGregor SE, et al. Fibroadenoma of the breast: diagnostic pitfalls of fine-needle aspiration. *Diagn Cytopathol* 1992;8:647–648.
17. Dejmek A, Lindholm K. Frequency of cytologic features in fine needle aspirates from histologically and cytologically diagnosed fibroadenomas. *Acta Cytol* 1991;35:695–699.
18. Rao CR, Narasimhamurthy NK, Jaganathan K, et al. Cystosarcoma phyllodes. Diagnosis by fine needle aspiration cytology. *Acta Cytol* 1992;36:203–207.
19. Bhagat P, Kline TS. The male breast and malignant neoplasms: diagnosis by aspiration biopsy cytology. *Cancer* 1990;65:2338–2341.
20. Martin-Bates E, Krausz T, Phillips I. Evaluation of fine needle aspiration of the male breast for the diagnosis of gynaecomastia. *Cytopathology* 1990;1:79–85.
21. Grenko RT, Lee KP, Lee KR. Fine needle aspiration cytology of lactating adenoma of the breast. A comparative light microscopic and morphometric study. *Acta Cytol* 1990;34:21–26.
22. Gupta RK, McHutchison AG, Dowle CS, et al. Fine-needle aspiration cytodiagnosis of breast masses in pregnant and lactating women and its impact on management. *Diagn Cytopathol* 1993;9:156–159.

23. Zarbo RJ, Howanitz PJ, Bachner P. Interinstitutional comparison of performance in breast fine-needle aspiration cytology: a Q-probe quality indicator study. *Arch Pathol Lab Med* 1991;115:743–750.
24. Sneige N. Fine-needle aspiration of the breast: a review of 1,995 cases with emphasis on diagnostic pitfalls. *Diagn Cytopathol* 1993;9:106–112.
25. de la Torre M, Lindholm K, Lindgren A. Fine needle aspiration cytology of tubular breast carcinoma and radial scar. *Acta Cytol* 1994;38:884–890.
26. Malberger E, Yeouda E, Toledano O, et al. Fine-needle aspiration and cytologic findings of surgical scar lesions in women with breast cancer. *Cancer* 1992;69:148–152.
27. Yeoh GP, Cheung PS, Chan KW. Fine-needle aspiration cytology of mucocele-like tumors of the breast. *Am J Surg Pathol* 1999;23:552–559.
28. Dodd LG, Sneige N, Reece GP, et al. Fine-needle aspiration cytology of silicone granulomas in the augmented breast. *Diagn Cytopathol* 1993;9:498–502.
29. Tanaka K, Shoji T, Tominaga Y, et al. Statistical analysis of diagnostic failure of fine needle aspiration cytology (FNAC) in breast cancer. *J Surg Oncol* 2001;76:100–105.
30. Abendroth CS, Wang HH, Ducatman BS. Comparative features of carcinoma *in situ* and atypical ductal hyperplasia of the breast on fine-needle aspiration biopsy specimens. *Am J Clin Pathol* 1991; 96:654–659.
31. Markovic-Glamocak M, Boban D, Sucic M, et al. Significance of proliferative epithelial changes in breast fine-needle aspiration. *Cancer* 1992;70:781–783.
32. Stanley MW, Henry-Stanley MJ, Zera R. Atypia in breast fine-needle aspiration smears correlates poorly with the presence of a prognostically significant proliferative lesion of ductal epithelium. *Hum Pathol* 1993;24:630–635.
33. Venegas R, Rutgers JL, Cameron BL, et al. Fine needle aspiration cytology of breast ductal carcinoma *in situ*. *Acta Cytol* 1994;38:136–143.
34. Wang HH, Ducatman BS, Eick D. Comparative features of ductal carcinoma *in situ* and infiltrating ductal carcinoma of the breast on fine-needle aspiration biopsy. *Am J Clin Pathol* 1989;92:736–740.
35. Helvie MA, Baker DE, Adler DD, et al. Radiographically guided fine-needle aspiration of nonpalpable breast lesions. *Radiology* 1990;174:657–61.
36. Layfield LJ, Parkinson B, Wong J, et al. Mammographically guided fine-needle aspiration biopsy of nonpalpable breast lesions: Can it replace open biopsy? *Cancer* 1991;68:2007–2011.
37. Masood S, Frykberg ER, McLellan GL, et al. Prospective evaluation of radiologically directed fine-needle aspiration biopsy of nonpalpable breast lesions. *Cancer* 1990;66:1480–1487.
38. Rogers LA, Lee KR. Breast carcinoma simulating fibroadenoma or fibrocystic change by fine-needle aspiration: a study of 16 cases. *Am J Clin Pathol* 1992;98:155–160.
39. Sneige N. Fine-needle aspiration of the breast: a review of 1,995 cases with emphasis on diagnostic pitfalls. *Diagn Cytopathol* 1993;9:106–112.
40. Sneige N, Fornage BD, Saleh G. Ultrasound-guided fine-needle aspiration of nonpalpable breast lesions: cytologic and histologic findings. *Am J Clin Pathol* 1994;102:98–101.
41. Thomas PA, Vazquez MF, Waisman J. Comparison of fine-needle aspiration and frozen section of palpable mammary lesions. *Mod Pathol* 1990;3:570–574.
42. Pisano ED, Fajardo LL, Tsimikas J, et al. Rate of insufficient samples for fine-needle aspiration for nonpalpable breast lesions in a multicenter clinical trial: the Radiologic Diagnostic Oncology Group 5 study. *Cancer* 1998;82:679–688.
43. Lee KC, Chan JKC, Ho LC. Histologic changes in the breast after fine-needle aspiration. *Am J Surg Pathol* 1994;18:1039–1047.
44. Salhany KE, Page DL. Fine-needle aspiration of mammary lobular carcinoma *in situ* and atypical lobular hyperplasia. *Am J Clin Pathol* 1989;92:22–26.
45. Sneige N, Zachariah S, Fanning TV, et al. Fine-needle aspiration cytology of metastatic neoplasms in the breast. *Am J Clin Pathol* 1989;92:27–35.
46. Corkill ME, Sneige N, Fanning T, et al. Fine-needle aspiration cytology and flow cytometry of intracystic papillary carcinoma of breast. *Am J Clin Pathol* 1990;94:673–680.
47. Fischler DF, Sneige N, Ordonez NG, et al. Tubular carcinoma of the breast: cytologic features in fine-needle aspirations and application of monoclonal anti-alpha-smooth muscle actin in diagnosis. *Diagn Cytopathol* 1994;10:120–125.
48. Gupta RK, Kenwright D, Naran S, et al. Fine needle aspiration cytodiagnosis of secretory carcinoma of the breast. *Cytopathology* 2000;11:496–502.
49. Wolfe JN, Saftlas AF, Salane M. Mammographic parenchymal patterns and quantitative evaluation of mammographic densities: a case-control study. *Am J Roentgenol* 1987;148:1082–1092.

50. Carlile T, Kopecky KJ, Thompson DJ, et al. Breast cancer prediction and the Wolfe classification of mammograms. *JAMA* 1985;254:1050–1053.
51. Warner E, Lockwood G, Tritchler D, et al. The risk of breast cancer associated with mammographic parenchymal patterns: a meta-analysis of the published literature to examine the effect of method of classification. *Cancer Detect Prev* 1992;16:67–72.
52. Boyd NF, Jensen HM, Cooke G, et al. Relationship between mammographic and histological risk factors for breast cancer. *J Natl Cancer Inst* 1992;84:1170–1179.
53. Berend ME, Sullivan DC, Kornguth PJ, et al. The natural history of mammographic calcifications subjected to interval follow-up. *Arch Surg* 1992;127:1309–1313.
54. Thomas DB, Whitehead J, Dorse C, et al. Mammographic calcifications and risk of subsequent breast cancer. *J Natl Cancer Inst* 1993;85:230–235.
55. Ciatto S, Del Turco MR, Bonardi R, et al. Non-palpable lesions of the breast detected by mammography—review of 1182 consecutive histologically confirmed cases. *Eur J Cancer* 1994;30A:40–44.
56. Hall JA, Murphy DC, Hall BR, et al. Mammographic abnormalities and the detection of carcinoma of the breast. *Am J Obstet Gynecol* 1993;168:1677–1680.
57. Newstead GM, Baute PB, Toth HK. Invasive lobular and ductal carcinoma: mammographic findings and stage at diagnosis. *Radiology* 1992;184:623–627.
58. Orel SG, Evers K, Yeh IT, et al. Radial scar with microcalcifications: radiologic-pathologic correlation. *Radiology* 1992;183:479–482.
59. de Paredes ES, Abbitt PL, Tabbarah S, et al. Mammographic and histologic correlations of microcalcifications. *Radiographics* 1990;10:577–589.
60. Fechner R. Immediate management of mammographically detected breast lesions. *Am J Clin Pathol* 1993;100:92–93.
61. Owings DV, Hann L, Schnitt SJ. How thoroughly should needle localization breast biopsies be sampled for microscopic examination? A prospective mammographic/pathologic correlative study. *Am J Surg Pathol* 1990;14:578–583.
62. Poggi S, Skinner H, Ague J, et al. Using scanning electron microscopy to study mineral deposits in breast tissues. *Am Minerologist* 1998;83:1122–1126.
63. Stein MA, Karlan MS. Calcifications in breast biopsy specimens: discrepancies in radiologic-pathologic identification. *Radiology* 1991;179:111–114.
64. Lee CH, Carter D, Philpotts LE, et al. Ductal carcinoma *in situ* diagnosed with stereotactic core needle biopsy: can invasion be predicted? *Radiology* 2000;217:466–470.
65. D'Orsi CJ, Reale FR, Davis MA, et al. Breast specimen microcalcifications: radiographic validation and pathologic-radiologic correlation. *Radiology* 1991;180:397–401.
66. Symonds DA, Copeland BE, Drane A, et al. Pathologic correlation in mammographically directed breast biopsies. *Arch Pathol Lab Med* 1992;116:28–32.
67. Holland R, Hendriks JHCL, Mravunac M. Mammographically occult breast cancer: a pathologic and radiologic study. *Cancer* 1983;101:1810–1819.
68. Evans AJ, Pinder S, Ellis IO, et al. Screening-detected and symptomatic ductal carcinoma *in situ*: mammographic features with pathologic correlation. *Radiology* 1994;191:237–240.
69. Stomper PC, Connolly JL, Meyer JE. Clinically occult ductal carcinoma *in situ* detected with mammography: analysis of 100 cases with radiologic-pathologic correlation. *Radiology* 1989;172:235.
70. Beute BJ, Kalisher L, Hutter RVP. Lobular carcinoma *in situ* of the breast: clinical, pathologic and mammographic features. *Am J Roentgenol* 1991;157:257.
71. Sonnenfeld MR, Frenna TH, Weidner N, et al. Lobular carcinoma *in situ*: mammographic-pathologic correlation of results of needle-directed biopsy. *Radiology* 1991;181:363–367.
72. Kopans DB, Nguyen PL, Koerner FC, et al. Mixed form, diffusely scattered calcifications in breast cancer with apocrine features. *Radiology* 1990;177:807–811.
73. Holland R, Mravunac M, Hendriks JH, et al. So-called interval cancers of the breast. Pathologic and radiologic analysis of sixty-four cases. *Cancer* 1982;49:2527–2533.
74. Going JJ, Anderson TJ, Crocker PR, et al. Weddellite calcification in the breast: eighteen cases with implications for breast cancer screening. *Histopathology* 1990;16:119–124.
75. Tornos C, Silva E, El-Nagar A, et al. Calcium oxalate crystals in breast biopsies: the missing microcalcifications. *Am J Surg Pathol* 1990;14:961–968.
76. Frouge C, Meunier M, Guinebretiere JM, et al. Polyhedral microcalcifications at mammography: histologic correlation with calcium oxalate. *Radiology* 1993;186:681–684.
77. Winston JS, Yeh IT, Evers K, et al. Calcium oxalate is associated with benign breast tissue. Can we avoid biopsy? *Am J Clin Pathol* 1993;100:488–492.

78. Liberman L, Evans WPR, Dershaw DD, et al. Radiography of microcalcifications in stereotaxic mammary core biopsy specimens. *Radiology* 1994;190:223–225.
79. Liberman L, Cohen MA, Dershaw DD, et al. Atypical ductal hyperplasia diagnosed at stereotaxic core biopsy of breast lesions: an indication for surgical biopsy. *Am J Roentgenol* 1995;164:1111–1113.
80. Philpotts LE, Lee CH, Horvath LJ, et al. Underestimation of breast cancer with II-gauge vacuum suction biopsy. *Am J Roentgenol* 2000;175:1047–1050.
81. Liberman L, Sama M, Susnik B, et al. Lobular carcinoma *in situ* at percutaneous breast biopsy: surgical biopsy findings. *Am J Roentgenol* 1999;173:291–299.
82. Lee CH, Carter D. Detecting residual tumor after excisional biopsy of impalpable breast carcinoma: efficacy of comparing preoperative mammograms with radiographs of the biopsy specimen. *Am J Roentgenol* 1995;164:81–86.
83. Gajdos C, Levy M, Herman Z, et al. Complete removal of nonpalpable breast malignancies with a stereotactic percutaneous vacuum-assisted biopsy instrument. *J Am Coll Surg* 1999;189:237–240.
84. Brenner RJ. Lesions entirely removed during stereotactic biopsy: preoperative localization on the basis of mammographic landmarks and feasibility of freehand technique—initial experience. *Radiology* 2000;214:585–590.
85. Liberman L, Dershaw DD, Rosen PP, et al. Percutaneous removal of malignant mammographic lesions at stereotactic vacuum-assisted biopsy. *Radiology* 1998;206:711–715.
86. Liberman L, Zakowski MF, Avery S, et al. Complete percutaneous excision of infiltrating carcinoma at stereotactic breast biopsy: how can tumor size be assessed? *Am J Roentgenol* 1999;173:1315–1322.
87. Youngston BJ, Cranor M, Rosen PP. Epithelial displacement in surgical breast specimens following needling procedures. *Am J Surg Pathol* 1994;18:896–903.
88. Wright J. The development of frozen section technique, the evolution of surgical biopsy and the origins of surgical pathology. *Bull Hist Med* 1985;59:295–326.
89. Bianchi S, Palli D, Ciatto S, et al. Accuracy and reliability of frozen section diagnosis in a series of 672 nonpalpable breast lesions. *Am J Clin Pathol* 1995;103:199–205.
90. Howanitz PJ, Hoffman GG, Zarbo RJ. The accuracy of frozen-section diagnoses in 34 hospitals. *Arch Pathol Lab Med* 1990;114:355–359.
91. Speights VO Jr. Evaluation of frozen sections in grossly benign breast biopsies. *Mod Pathol* 1995;7: 762–765.
92. Oberman HA. A modest proposal. *Am J Surg Pathol* 1992;16:69–70.
93. Carter D. Margins of lumpectomy for breast cancer. *Hum Pathol* 1986;17:330–333.
94. Silverstein MJ, Gierson ED, Colburn WJ, et al. Can intraductal breast carcinoma be excised completely by local excision? Clinical and pathologic predictors. *Cancer* 1994;73:2985–2989.
95. Noguchi M, Minami M, Earashi M, et al. Intraoperative histologic assessment of surgical margins and lymph node metastases in breast-conserving therapy. *J Surg Oncol* 1995;60:185–190.
96. Guidi AJ, Connolly JL, Harris JR, et al. The relationship between shaved margin and inked margin status in breast excision specimens (see comments). *Cancer* 1997;79:1568–1573.
97. Beck NE, Bradburn MJ, Vincenti AC, et al. Detection of residual disease following breast-conserving surgery. *Br J Surg* 1998;85:1273–1276.
98. Holland PA, Gandhi A, Knox WF, et al. The importance of complete excision in the prevention of local recurrence of ductal carcinoma *in situ*. *Br J Cancer* 1998;77:110–114.
99. Campbell ID, Theaker JM, Royle GT, et al. Impact of an extensive *in situ* component on the presence of residual disease in screen detected breast cancer. *J R Soc Med* 1991;84:652–656.
100. Morimoto T, Okazaki K, Komaki K, et al. Cancerous residue in breast-conserving surgery. *J Surg Oncol* 1993;52:71–76.
101. Solin LJ, Fowble B, Martz K, et al. Results of re-excisional biopsy of the primary tumor in preparation for definitive irradiation of patients with early stage breast cancer. *Int J Radiat Oncol Biol Phys* 1986;12:721–725.
102. McCormick B, Kinne D, Petrek J, et al. Limited resection for breast cancer: a study of inked specimen margins before radiotherapy. *Int J Radiat Oncol Biol Phys* 1987;13:1667–1671.
103. Gwin JL, Eisenberg BL, Hoffman JP, et al. Incidence of gross and microscopic carcinoma in specimens from patients with breast cancer after re-excision lumpectomy. *Ann Surg* 1993;218:729–734.
104. Kearney TJ, Morrow M. Effect of reexcision on the success of breast-conserving surgery. *Ann Surg Oncol* 1995;2:303–207.
105. Jardines L, Fowble B, Schultz D, et al. Factors associated with a positive reexcision after excisional biopsy for invasive breast cancer. *Surgery* 1995;118:803–809.

106. Frazier TG, Wong RW, Rose D. Implications of accurate pathologic margins in the treatment of primary breast cancer. *Arch Surg* 1989;124:37–38.
107. Schnitt SJ, Connolly JL, Harris JR, et al. Pathologic predictors of early local recurrence in stage I and II breast cancer treated by primary radiation therapy. *Cancer* 1984;53:1049–1057.
108. Wazer DE, Schmidt-Ullrich RK, Schmid CH, et al. The value of breast lumpectomy margin assessment as a predictor of residual tumor burden. *Int J Radiat Oncol Biol Phys* 1997;38:291–299.
109. Tartter P, Bleiweiss I, Levchenko S. Factors associated with clear biopsy margins and clear reexcision margins in breast cancer specimens from candidates for breast conservation. *J Am Coll Surg* 1997;185:268–273.
110. Beron PJ, Horwitz EM, Martinez AA, et al. Pathologic and mammographic findings predicting the adequacy of tumor excision before breast-conserving therapy. *Am J Roentgenol* 1996;167: 1409–1414.
111. Walls J, Knox F, Baildam AD, et al. Can preoperative factors predict for residual malignancy after breast biopsy for invasive cancer? (Comment). *Ann R Coll Surg Engl* 1995;77:248–251.
112. Homer MJ, Safaii H, Smith TJ, et al. The relationship of mammographic microcalcification to histologic malignancy: radiologic-pathologic correlation. *Am J Roentgenol* 1989;153:1187–1189.
113. Oakley KL, Going JJ. Specimen slice radiography of cancer in breast conserving excisions. *J Clin Pathol* 1995;48:1028–1030.
114. Graham RA, Homer MJ, Sigler CJ, et al. The efficacy of specimen radiography in evaluating the surgical margins of impalpable breast carcinoma (Comment). *Am J Roentgenol* 1994;162:33–36.
115. Dixon JM, Ravi Sekar O, Walsh J, et al. Specimen-orientated radiography helps define excision margins of malignant lesions detected by breast screening (Comment). *Br J Surg* 1993;80:1001–1002.
116. Acosta JA, Greenlee JA, Gubler KD, et al. Surgical margins after needle-localization breast biopsy. *Am J Surg* 1995;170:643–645; discussion 645–646.
117. Lind DS, Minter R, Steinbach B, et al. Stereotactic core biopsy reduces the reexcision rate and the cost of mammographically detected cancer. *J Surg Res* 1998;78:23–26.
118. Kaufman CS, Delbecq R, Jacobson L. Excising the reexcision: stereotactic core-needle biopsy decreases need for reexcision of breast cancer. *World J Surg* 1998;22:1023–1027; discussion 1028.
119. Veronesi U. How important is the assessment of resection margins of conservative surgery for breast cancer? *Cancer* 1994;74:1660–1661.
120. Ghossein NA, Alpert S, Barba J, et al. Breast cancer. Importance of adequate surgical excision prior to radiotherapy in the local control of breast cancer in patients treated conservatively. *Arch Surg* 1992;127:411–415.
121. Cheng L, Al-Kaisi NK, Gordon NH, et al. Relationship between the size and margin status of ductal carcinoma *in situ* of the breast and residual disease (Comment). *J Natl Cancer Inst* 1997;89: 1356–1360.
122. Ratanawichitrasin A, Rybicki LA, Steiger E, et al. Predicting the likelihood of residual disease in women treated for ductal carcinoma *in situ*. *J Am Coll Surg* 1999;188:17–21.
123. Smitt MC, Nowels KW, Zdeblick MJ, et al. The importance of the lumpectomy surgical margin status in long-term results of breast conservation. *Cancer* 1995;76:259–267.
124. Anscher MS, Jones P, Prosnitz LR, et al. Local failure and margin status in early-stage breast carcinoma treated with conservation surgery and radiation therapy. *Ann Surg* 1993;218:22–28.
125. Heimann R, Powers C, Halpem HJ, et al. Breast preservation in stage I and II carcinoma of the breast. The University of Chicago experience. *Cancer* 1996;78:1722–1730.
126. Gage I, Schnitt SJ, Nixon AJ, et al. Pathologic margin involvement and the risk of recurrence in patients treated with breast-conserving therapy. *Cancer* 1996;78:1921–1928.
127. Schnitt SJ, Abner A, Gelman R, et al. The relationship between microscopic margins of resection and the risk of local recurrence in patients with breast cancer treated with breast-conserving surgery and radiation therapy (Comment). *Cancer* 1994;74:1746–1751.
128. DiBiase SJ, Komarnicky LT, Schwartz GF, et al. The number of positive margins influences the outcome of women treated with breast preservation for early stage breast carcinoma. *Cancer* 1998;82: 2212–2220.
129. Spivack B, Khanna MM, Tafra L, et al. Margin status and local recurrence after breast-conserving surgery. *Arch Surg* 1994;129:952–956; discussion 956–957.
130. Kurtz JM, Amalric R, Brandone H, et al. Results of wide excision for mammary recurrence after breast-conserving therapy. *Cancer* 1988;61:1969–1972.
131. Tafra L, Guenther JM, Giuliano AE. Planned segmentectomy. A necessity for breast carcinoma. *Arch Surg* 1993;128:1014–1018; discussion 1018–1020.

132. Lagios MD, Richards VE, Rose MR, et al. Segmental mastectomy without radiotherapy. Short-term follow-up. *Cancer* 1983;52:2173–2179.
133. Fisher B, Redmond C, Poisson R, et al. Eight-year results of a randomized clinical trial comparing total mastectomy and lumpectomy with or without irradiation in the treatment of breast cancer (published erratum appears in *N Engl J Med* 1994 May 19;330(20):1467) (Comment). *N Engl J Med* 1989;320:822–828.
134. Harris JR, Connolly JL, Schnitt SJ. The use of pathologic features in selecting the extent of surgical resection necessary for breast cancer patients treated by primary radiation therapy. *Ann Surg* 1985; 201:164–169.
135. Vicini FA, Eberlein TJ, Connolly JL, et al. The optimal extent of resection for patients with stages I or II breast cancer treated with conservative surgery and radiotherapy. *Ann Surg* 1991;214:200–204.
136. Solin LJ, Fowble BL, Schultz DJ, et al. The significance of the pathology margins of the tumor excision on the outcome of patients treated with definitive irradiation for early stage breast cancer (Comment). *Int J Radiat Oncol Biol Phys* 1991;21:279–287.
137. Schmidt-Ullrich R, Wazer DE, Tercilla O, et al. Tumor margin assessment as a guide to optimal conservation surgery and irradiation in early stage breast carcinoma. *Int J Radiat Oncol Biol Phys* 1989; 17:733–738.
138. Schmidt-Ullrich RK, Wazer DE, DiPetrillo T, et al. Breast conservation therapy for early stage breast carcinoma with outstanding 10-year locoregional control rates: a case for aggressive therapy to the tumor bearing quadrant (Comment). *Int J Radiat Oncol Biol Phys* 1993;27:545–552.
139. Pittinger TP, Maronian NC, Poulter CA, et al. Importance of margin status in outcome of breast-conserving surgery for carcinoma. *Surgery* 1994;116:605–608; discussion 608–609.
140. Vicini F, Kini VR, Chen P, et al. Irradiation of the tumor bed alone after lumpectomy in selected patients with early-stage breast cancer treated with breast conserving therapy. *J Surg Oncol* 1999;70: 33–40.
141. Fowble BL, et al. Ten-year results of conservative surgery and irradiation for stage I and II breast cancer. *Int J Radiat Oncol Biol Phys* 1991;21:269–277.
142. Dalberg K, Mattsson A, Rutqvist LE, et al. Breast conserving surgery for invasive breast cancer: risk actors for ipsilateral breast tumor recurrences. *Breast Cancer Res Treat* 1997;43:73–86.
143. Sinn HP, Anton HW, Magener A, et al. Extensive and predominant *in situ* component in breast carcinoma: their influence on treatment results after breast-conserving therapy. *Eur J Cancer* 1998;34: 646–653.
144. Touboul E, Buffat L, Belkacemi Y, et al. Local recurrences and distant metastases after breast-conserving surgery and radiation therapy for early breast cancer. *Int J Radiat Oncol Biol Phys* 1999;43: 25–38.
145. Borger J, Kemperman H, Hart A, et al. Risk factors in breast-conservation therapy (Comment). *J Clin Oncol* 1994;12:653–660.
146. Ryoo MC, Kagan AR, Wollin M, et al. Prognostic factors for recurrence and cosmesis in 393 patients after radiation therapy for early mammary carcinoma. *Radiology* 1989;172:555–559.
147. McCormick B, Rosen PP, Kinne D, et al. Duct carcinoma *in situ* of the breast: an analysis of local control after conservation surgery and radiotherapy. *Int J Radiat Oncol Biol Phys* 1991;21:289–292.
148. Vicini FA, Lacerna MD, Goldstein NS, et al. Ductal carcinoma *in situ* detected in the mammographic era: an analysis of clinical, pathologic, and treatment-related factors affecting outcome with breast-conserving therapy. *Int J Radiat Oncol Biol Phys* 1997;39:627–635.
149. Solin LJ, Recht A, Fourquet A, et al. Ten-year survival of breast-conserving surgery and definitive irradiation for intraductal carcinoma (ductal carcinoma *in situ*) of the breast. *Cancer* 1991;68: 2337–2344.
150. Schwartz GF, Finkel GC, Garcia JC, et al. Subclinical ductal carcinoma *in situ* of the breast: treatment by local excision and surveillance alone. *Cancer* 1992;70:2468–2474.
151. Fish EB, Chapman JA, Miller NA, et al. Assessment of treatment for patients with primary ductal carcinoma *in situ* in the breast. *Ann Surg Oncol* 1998;5:724–732.
152. Mariani L, Salvadori B, Marubini E, et al. Ten year results of a randomised trial comparing two conservative treatment strategies for small size breast cancer (Comment). *Eur J Cancer* 1998;34: 1156–1162.
153. Swenson KK, Decher L, Haselow R, et al. Prognostic factors after conservative surgery and radiation therapy for early stage breast cancer. *Am J Clin Oncol* 1998;21:111–116.
154. Cataliotti L, Distante V, Ciatto S, et al. Intraductal breast cancer: review of 183 consecutive cases. *Eur J Cancer* 1992:917–920.

155. Sneige N, McNeese MD, Atkinson EN, et al. Ductal carcinoma *in situ* treated with lumpectomy and irradiation: histopathological analysis of 49 specimens with emphasis on risk factors and long term results (Comment). *Hum Pathol* 1995;26:642–649.
156. Fisher ER, Costantino J, Fisher B, et al. Pathologic findings from the National Surgical Adjuvant Breast Project (NSABP) Protocol B-17: intraductal carcinoma (ductal carcinoma *in situ*). *Cancer* 1995;75:1310–1319.
157. Silverstein M, Lagios M, Craig P, et al. A prognostic index for ductal carcinoma *in situ* of the breast. *Cancer* 1996;77:2267–2279.
158. Qualheim RE, Gall EA, Breast carcinoma with multiple sites of origin. *Cancer* 1957;10:460–468.
159. Tellem M, Prive L, Meranze DR. Four quadrant study of breasts removed for carcinoma. *Cancer* 1962;15:10–17.
160. Gallagher HS, Martin JE. The study of mammary carcinoma by mammography and whole organ sectioning. *Cancer* 1969;23:855–873.
161. Fisher B, Wolmark N, Redmond C, et al. Findings from NSABP Protocol No. B-04: comparison of radical mastectomy with alternative treatments. II. The clinical and biologic significance of medial-central breast cancers. *Cancer* 1981;48:1863–1872.
162. Lagios MD. Multicentricity of breast carcinoma demonstrated by routine correlated serial subgross and radiographic examination. *Cancer* 1977;40:1726-1734.
163. Schwartz GF, Patchefsky AS, Feig SA, et al. Multicentricity of non-palpable breast cancer. *Cancer* 1980;45:2913–2916.
164. Egan RL. Multicentric breast carcinomas: clinical-radiographic-pathologic whole organ studies and 10-year survival. *Cancer* 1982;49:1123–1130.
165. Noel P, Chauvin F, Bailly C, et al. Prognostic value of the topographic grid method in women with T2 N-breast cancer. *Cancer* 1985;55:1987–1990.
166. Cowen D, Jacquemier J, Houvenaeghel G, et al. Local and distant recurrence after conservative management of "very low-risk" breast cancer are dependent events: a 10-year follow-up. *Int J Radiat Oncol Biol Phys* 1998;41:801–807.
167. Shah JP, Rosen PP, Robbins GF. Pitfalls of local excision in the treatment of carcinoma of the breast. *Surg Gynecol Obstet* 1973;136:721–725.
168. Rosen PP, Fracchia AA, Urban JA, et al. "Residual" mammary carcinoma following simulated partial mastectomy. *Cancer* 1975;35:739–747.
169. Sarnelli R, Squartini F. Multicentricity in breast cancer: a submacroscopic study. *Pathol Ann* 1986; 21:143–158.
170. Holland R, Veling SHJ, Mravunac M, et al. Histologic multifocality of T1's, T1-2 breast carcinomas. *Cancer* 1989;56:979–990.
171. Faverly D, Holland R, Burgers L. An original stereomicroscopic analysis of the mammary glandular tree. *Virchows Arch A Pathol Anal Histopathol* 1992;421:115–119.
172. Faverly DR, Burgers L, Bult P, et al. Three dimensional imaging of mammary ductal carcinoma *in situ*: clinical implications. *Semin Diagn Pathol* 1994;11:193–198.
173. Coombs JH, Hubbard E, Hudson K, et al. Ductal carcinoma *in situ* of the breast: correlation of pathologic and mammographic features with extent of disease. *Am Surg* 1997;63:1079–1083.
174. Lagios MD, Westdahl PR, Margolin FR, et al. Ductal carcinoma *in situ*. Relationship of extent of noninvasive disease to the frequency of occult invasion, multicentricity, lymph node metastases, and short-term treatment failures. *Cancer* 1982;50:1309–1314.
175. Alpers CE, Wellings SR. The prevalence of carcinoma *in situ* in normal and cancer-associated breasts. *Hum Pathol* 1985;16:796–807.
176. Simpson T, Thirlby RC, Dail DH. Surgical treatment of ductal carcinoma *in situ* of the breast—10- to 20- year follow-up. *Arch Surg* 1992;127:468–472.
177. Schwartz GF, Patchefsky AS, Finklestein SD, et al. Nonpalpable *in situ* ductal carcinoma of the breast. Predictors of multicentricity and microinvasion and implications for treatment. *Arch Surg* 1989;124:29–32.
178. Luttges J, Kalbfleisch H, Prinz P. Nipple involvement and multicentricity in breast cancer. A study on whole organ sections. *J Cancer Res Clin Oncol* 1987;113:481–487.
179. Heim S, Teixeira MR, Dietrich CU, et al. Cytogenetic polyclonality in tumors of the breast. *Cancer Genet Cytogenet* 1997;95:16–19.
180. Pandis N, Heim S, Bardi G, et al. Chromosome analysis of 20 breast carcinomas: cytogenetic multiclonality and karyotypic-pathologic correlations. *Genes Chromosomes Cancer* 1993;6:51–57.
181. Teixeira MR, Pandis N, Bardi G, et al. Cytogenetic analysis of multifocal breast carcinomas: detec-

tion of karyotypically unrelated clones as well as clonal similarities between tumour foci. *Br J Cancer* 1994;70:922–927.
182. Tsuda H, Hirohashi S. Identification of multiple breast cancers of multicentric origin by histological observations and distribution of allele loss on chromosome 16q. *Cancer Res* 1995;55:3395–3398.
183. Dawson PJ, Baekey PA, Clark RA. Mechanisms of multifocal breast cancer: an immunocytochemical study. *Hum Pathol* 1995;26:965–969.
184. Lagios MD, Rose MR, Margolin FR. Tubular carcinoma of the breast: association with multicentricity, bilaterality, and family history of mammary carcinoma. *Am J Clin Pathol* 1980;73:25–30.
185. Green I, McCormick B, Cranor M, et al. A comparative study of pure tubular and tubulolobular carcinoma of the breast. *Am J Surg Pathol* 1997;21:653–657.
186. Crile GJ. Multicentric breast cancer—the incidence of new cancers in the homolateral breast after partial mastectomy. *Cancer* 1975;35:475–477.
187. Fisher B, Bauer M, Margolese R, et al. Five-year results of a randomized clinical trial comparing total mastectomy and segmental mastectomy with or without radiation in the treatment of breast cancer. *N Engl J Med* 1985;312:665–673.
188. Panguluri RC, Brody LC, Modali R, et al. BRCA1 mutations in African Americans. *Hum Genet* 1999;105:28–31.
189. Vaittinen P, Hemminki K. Risk factors and age-incidence relationships for contralateral breast cancer. *Int J Cancer* 2000;88:998–1002.
190. Horn P, Thompson W. Risk of bilateral breast cancer: associations with factors related to initial breast cancer. *Am J Epidemiol* 1988;128:309–323.
191. Pandis N, Teixeira MR, Gerdes AM, et al. Chromosome abnormalities in bilateral breast carcinomas. Cytogenetic evaluation of the clonal origin of multiple primary tumors. *Cancer* 1995;76:250–258.
192. Shibata A, Tsai YC, Press MF, et al. Clonal analysis of bilateral breast cancer. *Clin Cancer Res* 1996;2:743–748.
193. Ackerman J, Baunoch DA, Gimotty P, et al. The role of p53 mutations in bilateral breast carcinoma. *Mod Pathol* 1995;8:244–248.
194. Lidereau R, Soussi T. Absence of p53 germ-line mutations in bilateral breast cancer patients. *Hum Genet* 1992;89:250–252.
195. Mose S, Adamietz IA, Thilmann C, et al. Bilateral breast carcinoma versus unilateral disease. Review of 498 patients. *Am J Clin Oncol* 1997;20:541–545.
196. Fung MC, Schultz DJ, Solin LJ. Early-stage bilateral breast cancer treated with breast-conserving surgery and definitive irradiation: the University of Pennsylvania experience. *Int J Radiat Oncol Biol Phys* 1997;38:959–967.
197. Coradini D, Oriana S, Mariani L, et al. Is steroid receptor profile in contralateral breast cancer a marker of independence of the corresponding primary tumour? *Eur J Cancer* 1998;34:825–830.
198. Dawson PJ, Maloney T, Gimotty P, et al. Bilateral breast cancer: one disease or two? *Breast Cancer Res Treat* 1991;19:233–244.
199. Fisher. The impact of pathology on the biologic, diagnostic, prognostic and therapeutic considerations in breast cancer. *Surg Clin North Am* 1984;64:1073–1093.
200. de la Rochefordiere A, Scholl S. Simultaneous bilateral breast cancer: a retrospective review of 149 cases. *Int J Radiat Oncol Biol Phys* 1994;30:35–41.
201. Urban JA. Bilaterality of cancer of the breast: biopsy of the opposite breast. *Cancer* 1967;20:1867.
202. Moertel CG, Dockerty MB, Bagenstoss AH. Multiple primary malignant neoplasms. III. Tumors of multicentric origin. *Cancer* 1961;14:238–247.
203. Robbins GF, Berg JW. Bilateral primary breast cancer: a prospective clinicopathological study. *Cancer* 1964;17.
204. McCredie JA, Inch WR, Aldersin M. Consecutive primary carcinomas of the breast. *Cancer* 1975;35:1472–1477.
205. Ringberg A, Palmer B, Linell F, et al. Bilateral and multifocal breast carcinoma. A clinical and autopsy study with special emphasis on carcinoma *in situ*. *Eur J Surg Oncol* 1991;17:20–29.
206. Parker R. Contralateral breast cancer following treatment for initial breast cancer. *Am J Clin Oncol* 1989;12:213–216.
207. Beller F, Nieder W, Holzgreve W. Bilateral breast cancer: the frequency of undiagnosed cancers. *Am J Obstet Gynecol* 1986;155:247–255.
208. Wanebo HJ, Senofsky GM, Fechner RE, et al. Bilateral breast cancer. Risk reduction by contralateral biopsy. *Ann Surg* 1985;201:667–677.

209. Brenner H, Engelsmann B, Stegmaier C, et al. Clinical epidemiology of bilateral breast cancer. *Cancer* 1993;72:3629–3635.
210. Boice JD. Cancer in the contralateral breast after radiotherapy for breast cancer. *N Engl J Med* 1992;326:781.
211. Haagensen CD. *Diseases of the breast.* Philadelphia: WB Saunders, 1971:710–711.
212. Amalric R, Santamaria F, Robert F, et al. Radiation therapy with or without primary limited surgery for operable breast cancer: a 20-year experience at the Marseilles Cancer Institute. *Cancer* 1982;49:30–34.
213. Calle R, Pilleron JP, Schleinger P, et al. Conservative management of operable breast cancer: Ten years experience at the Foundation Curie. *Cancer* 1978;42:2045–2053.
214. Albert S, Ghossein N. Primary management of operable breast cancer by minimal surgery and radiotherapy. *Cancer* 1979;42:2054–2058.
215. Bataini J, Picco C. Relation between time-dose and local control of preoperable breast cancer treated by tumorectomy and radiotherapy alone. *Cancer* 1978;42:2059–2065.
216. Mate TP, Carter D, Fisher DB, et al. A clinical and histopathologic analysis of the results of primary radiation therapy in stage I and II breast carcinoma. *Cancer* 1986;58:1995–2002.
217. Poen JC, Tran L, Juillard G, et al. Conservation therapy for invasive lobular carcinoma of the breast. *Cancer* 1992;69:2789–2795.
218. White JR, Gustafson GS, Wimbish K, et al. Conservative surgery and radiation therapy for infiltrating lobular carcinoma of the breast: the role of preoperative mammograms in guiding treatment. *Cancer* 1994;74:640–647.
219. Fisher ER, Gregario RM, Fisher B. The pathology of invasive breast cancer. *Cancer* 1975;36:1–85.
220. Clark RM, Wilkinson RH, Miceli PN, et al. Breast cancer: experiences with conservation therapy. *Am J Clin Oncol* 1987;10:461–468.
221. Bloom HJG. Prognosis in carcinoma of the breast. *Br J Cancer* 1950;4:259–288.
222. Janjan NA, Murray KJ, Conway P, et al. Prognosis for breast cancer surgery and radiation therapy compared with mastectomy alone: a retrospective analysis of 759 patients with stage I/II breast cancer. *Cancer* 1992;69:2842–2848.
223. Krishnan L, Jewell WR, Krishnan EC, et al. Breast cancer with extensive intraductal component: treatment with immediate interstitial boost irradiation. *Radiology* 1992;183:273–276.
224. Recht A, Danoff BS, Solin LJ. Intraductal carcinoma of the breast: results of treatment with excisional biopsy and irradiation. *J Clin Oncol* 1985;3:1339–1343.
225. Kurtz JM, Jacquemier J, Amalric R, et al. Risk factors for breast recurrence in premenopausal and postmenopausal patients with ductal cancers treated by conservation therapy. *Cancer* 1990;65:1867–1878.
226. Baird RM, Worth A, Hislop G. Recurrence after lumpectomy for comedo-type intraductal carcinoma of the breast. *Am J Surg* 1990;159:479–481.
227. Fisher B, Dignam J, Wolmark N, et al. Lumpectomy and radiation therapy for the treatment of intraductal breast cancer: findings from National Surgical Adjuvant Breast and Bowel Project B-17. *J Clin Oncol* 1998;16:441–452.
228. Silverstein M, Lagios M, Groshen S, et al. The influence of margin width on local control of ductal carcinoma *in situ* of the breast. *N Engl J Med* 1999;340:1455–1461.
229. Cajucom CC, Tsangaris TN, Nemoto T, et al. Results of salvage mastectomy for local recurrence after breast-conserving surgery without radiation therapy. *Cancer* 1993;71:1774–1779.
230. Haffty BG, Carter D, Flynn SD, et al. Local recurrence versus new primary: clinical analysis of 82 breast relapses and potential applications for genetic fingerprinting. *Int J Radiat Oncol Biol Phys* 1993;27:575–583.
231. Fisher E, Redmond C, Fisher B. Ipsilateral breast tumor recurrence and survival following lumpectomy and irradiation. *Semin Surg Oncol* 1992;8:161–166.
232. Kurtz JM, Spitalier JM, Amalric R. The prognostic significance of late local recurrence after breast-conserving therapy. *Int J Radiat Oncol Biol Phys* 1990;18:87–93.
233. Chauvet B, Fetissof F. Disappearance of the *in situ* component: a criterion predictive of metastasis in breast cancer after local recurrence. *Radiother Oncol* 1992;25:181–185.
234. Girling A, Hanby A, Millis R. Radiation and other pathological changes in breast tissue after conservation treatment for carcinoma. *J Clin Pathol* 1990;43:152–156.
235. Silverstein MJ, Lagios MD, Martino S, et al. Outcome after invasive local recurrence in patients with ductal carcinoma *in situ* of the breast. *J Clin Oncol* 1998;16:1367–1373.

4

Intraductal Lesions of the Breast

The most common and perhaps the most difficult histologic problem in breast pathology is the interpretation of proliferations of cells within the basement membranes of the ducts. These lesions fall into one of the following three groups: (a) ductal hyperplasia (DH), with little precancerous implication; (b) atypical ductal hyperplasia (ADH), which requires close follow-up; and (c) intraductal carcinoma, which is frequently accompanied by invasive cancer. How should one go about learning to distinguish one lesion from another? Rather than starting with benign proliferations and atypias, it is most expeditious to teach the types of intraductal carcinomas because they have relatively few patterns that can be recognized as *in situ* carcinoma. These are illustrated, along with guidelines for their recognition. One can readily enhance these illustrations by looking at the variants of intraductal carcinoma while examining multiple sections from a case with extensive full-blown intraductal carcinoma. It should be emphasized that intraductal carcinoma that is not associated with invasive cancer is an unusual lesion, and benign proliferations are much more common. Similarly, there are relatively few patterns of intraductal carcinoma, but there is an almost infinite variety of patterns of DH. As a first approximation, therefore, one can learn to recognize the great majority of intraductal carcinomas fairly quickly and assign those lesions that do not have this histologic appearance to a category that requires more study or consultation. It should be emphasized that this is only a first approximation. There are variations within the intraductal carcinomas that are extremely difficult to master, even though they are far fewer than the array of changes seen in DH.

Diffuse and localized forms of intraductal proliferations occur. The diffuse forms are DH, epitheliosis or papillomatosis, ADH, or intraductal carcinoma (DCIS). Localized forms are referred to as intraductal papilloma (IP) or intracystic papillary carcinoma (IPC). Localized and diffuse forms occur together or independently.

DIFFUSE INTRADUCTAL LESIONS

Intraductal Carcinomas

Intraductal carcinoma assumes one (or more) of the following patterns: comedocarcinoma, solid, cribriform, papillary, micropapillary, clinging, and hypersecretory. An apocrine variant also has been described. The cells that make up these patterns are all abnormal, but they may be graded according to their nuclear appearance. Comedocarcinomas are, by definition, of high nuclear grade with large bizarre mitotically active cells. Most papillary variants are of low nuclear grade with hyperchromatic round nuclei without mitotic figures, but intermediate grade comedocarcinoma and high-grade micropapillary carcinomas are recognized. The other patterns may be of high or low nuclear grade, or an intermediate grade that is characterized by large and prominent nucleoli.

Intraductal Carcinoma in General

Some rules of thumb about intraductal carcinoma (DCIS), in general, may be useful (Table 4.1).

1. DCIS is usually found and best recognized in medium-sized ducts, defined as larger than the ducts associated with lobules, but smaller than the ducts of the subareolar region. In size, they measure from 3 to 10 mm. In small ducts, everything tends to look more regular, and the irregularity inherent in benign hyperplasia does not manifest itself. DCIS may involve lobular ducts

TABLE 4.1. *Comparison of characteristics of benign and malignant intraductal lesions*

Parameter	Ductal hyperplasia/ papilloma	Ductal carcinoma *in situ*/ intracystic papillary carcinoma
Low power		
Lumina	Slit-like, distorted, angulated, irregularly spaced, varied in size and shape	More similar in size, shape and location, especially centrally
Stroma	Often prominent fibrovascular cores; irregularly spaced	Fibrovascular support often absent or minimal
Medium power		
Nuclear location	Irregular, overlapping, touching	Regular, central in cell, mosaic pattern
Cell types	Two or more: epithelial, myoepithelial, apocrine	Take over by single population
Necrosis	Rare	Common, often prominent
High power		
Chromatin pattern	Regular; may contain nucleoli	From regular to coarse nucleoli common
Mitoses	Rare, normal	Common, abnormal

(cancerization), but it is usually evident and more readily diagnosed from accompanying larger ducts.

2. In DCIS, there is a takeover of the duct by a monomorphic population of large cells with pale or granular cytoplasm, evident cell borders, and centrally placed nonoverlapping nuclei that extend from the lumen to the basement membrane. The addition of a second cell type—apocrine (spindle or small)—is a strong indication of benignancy. Myoepithelial cells are usually not large and proliferative in DCIS, but a rim of small myoepithelial cells with dark nuclei can usually be found in ducts otherwise involved by DCIS. A nonproliferative layer of myoepithelial cells is both an indication that the malignant cells are spreading along a duct and that the basement membrane is anatomically intact.
3. Patterns are helpful and usually reliable guides, and most examples of DCIS are recognized by the pattern of proliferation. The presence of angular, bizarre, clearly malignant cells with abnormal mitotic figures supersedes pattern, but to make a purely cytologic diagnosis of DCIS requires obvious cancer cells, and in many cases of DCIS, nuclear morphology is not the decisive feature. Nucleoli alone do not indicate cancer because they are prominent in benign proliferations, including normal lactation.
4. Necrosis is frequently seen in DCIS and its presence is a strong indicator of the diagnosis. Rarely, benign lesions also may be necrotic.
5. Finally, no single criterion—with the possible exception of clearly bizarre nuclei with abnormal mitotic figures—determines the diagnosis. All of the factors must be weighed and synthesized in a manner that can best be summarized by the following photomicrographs. The variants are described below by pattern.

Comedocarcinoma

Comedocarcinoma is usually found in larger ducts. It is composed of cells with higher nuclear grades, frequently contains mitotic figures, and forms a solid mass of tumor cells around the periphery of a centrally necrotic zone that occupies one-half or more of the diameter of the duct. Frequently, there is a dense or cellular fibrosis at the periphery of the comedocarcinoma, which raises the possibility of microinvasion. Cases with comedocarcinoma often display DCIS in the lobules where the pattern may not have central comedonecrosis. Microcalcification is frequently present in the centrally necrotic material, giving the mammographic appearance of elongated large tubular calcifications (Figs. 4.1 to 4.3 and efigs. 4.1 to 4.10).

Solid Intraductal Carcinoma

Solid intraductal carcinoma is composed of a monomorphic population of cells that extend from the basement membrane on one side of the duct to the

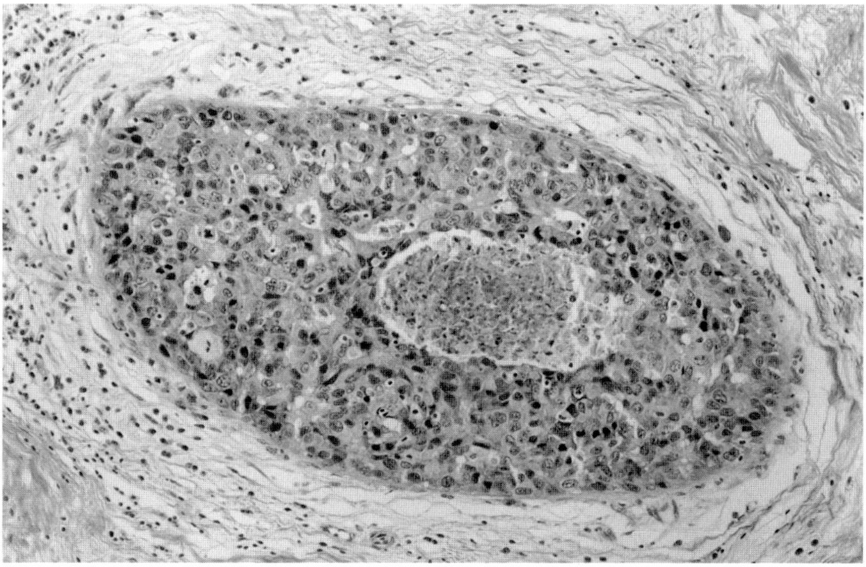

FIG. 4.1. Comedocarcinoma. This form of ductal carcinoma *in situ* is characterized by central massive necrosis, a solid proliferation of malignant cells of high nuclear grade, and periductal fibrosis. Microinvasion is frequently considered.

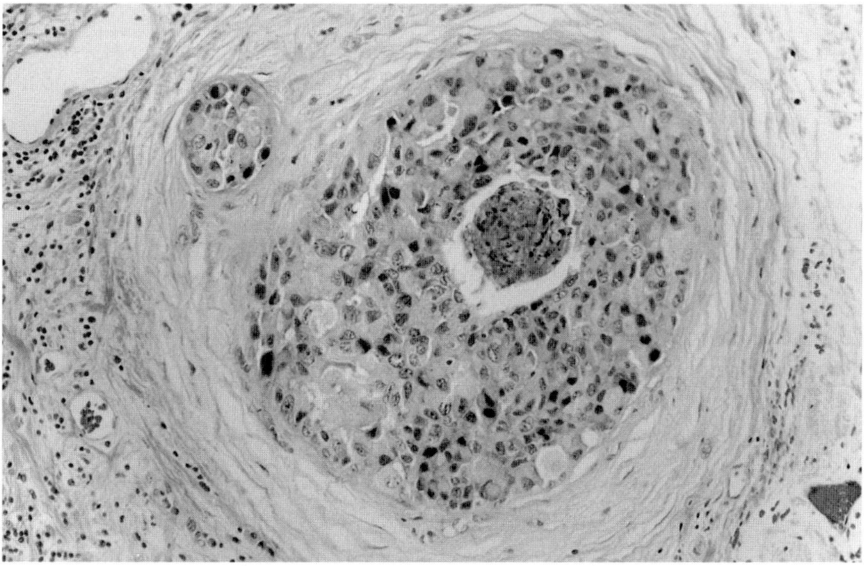

FIG. 4.2. Comedocarcinoma. This higher magnification photomicrograph depicts nuclear grade 3. The problem of microinvasion is presented (**upper left corner**). Does the small duct represent a branch involved by ductal carcinoma *in situ* or does it represent microinvasive carcinoma? The layer of myoepithelium is inapparent, but the basement membrane appears to be intact around the larger and smaller ducts, which indicates that invasion is not present.

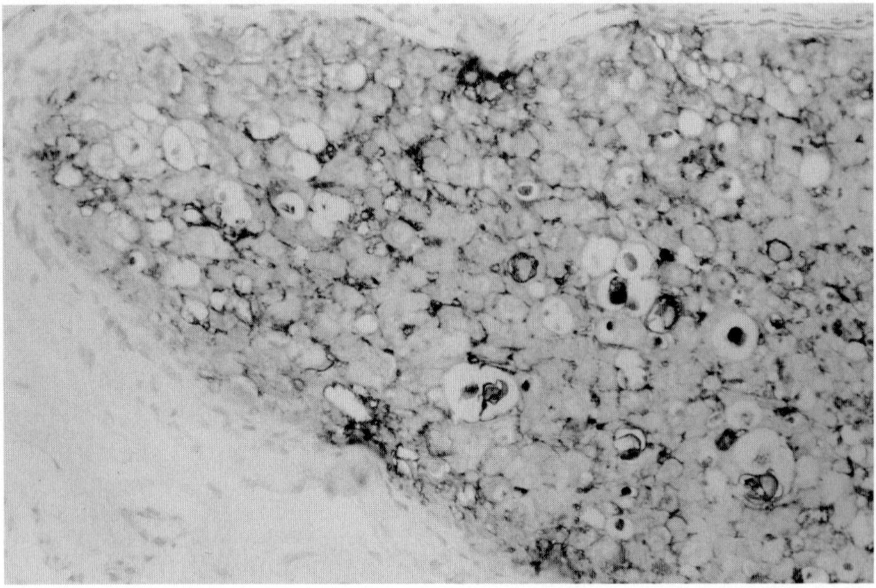

FIG. 4.3. Comedocarcinoma. Immunostain for HER2/neu reveals the membranous staining characteristic of this antigen, which is found in about one-half of comedocarcinomas.

other. The nuclear grade is frequently high, but it may be moderate or even low. When the nuclear grade is low, differential diagnosis from lobular carcinoma *in situ* (LCIS) is a problem (Chapter 5). Cellular necrosis may be present (Figs. 4.4 to 4.6 and efigs. 4.10 to 4.13).

Cribriform Intraductal Carcinoma

Cribriform intraductal carcinoma is a common variant of intraductal carcinoma. It has a regular or lace-like pattern that is composed of large cells with centrally placed nuclei that form regular rounded (not slit-like) intercellular lumina of approximately the same size, which are placed regularly across the lumen of the duct. Nuclear grade varies from high to low. Necrosis and calcification may be present (Figs. 4.7 to 4.12 and efigs. 4.14 to 4.21).

Papillary Intraductal Carcinoma

Papillary carcinoma is composed of a monomorphic population of cells that are usually of low to moderate nuclear grade, proliferating often as a monolayer of cells on a fibrovascular core or several fibrovascular cores that extend into the ductal lumen. Necrosis and calcification may be present but usually are not (Figs. 4.13 and 4.14)

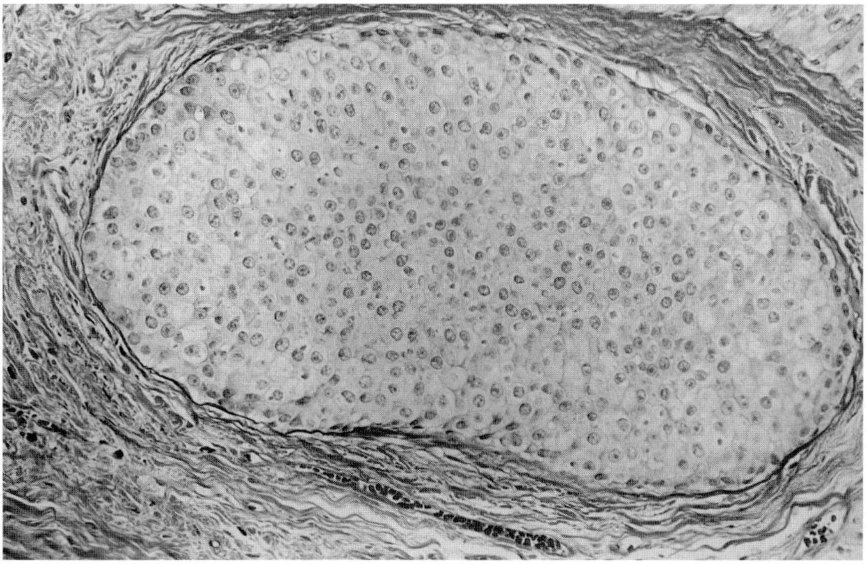

FIG. 4.4. Solid ductal carcinoma *in situ*. In this large duct, there is complete effacement by a solid proliferation of uniformly cuboidal cells with centrally placed, nonoverlapping, large nuclei of grade 2. The layer of myoepithelium is inapparent.

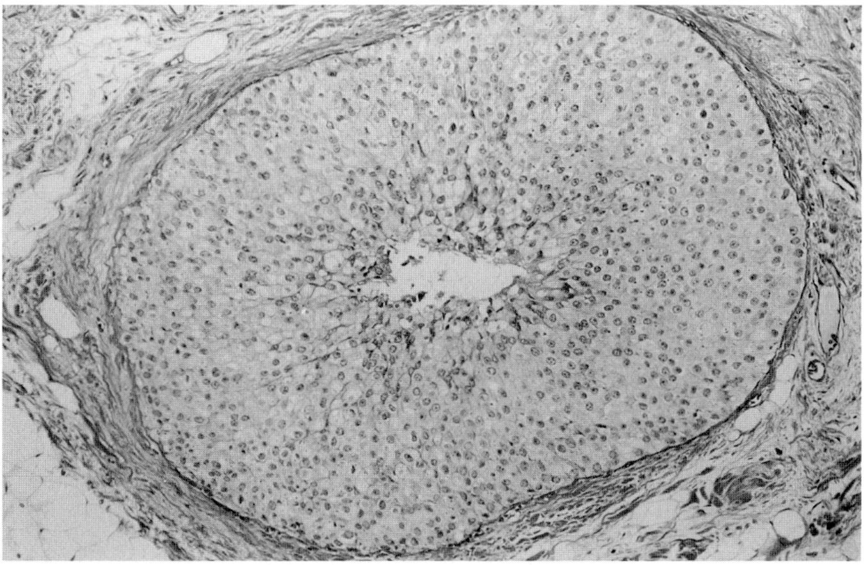

FIG. 4.5. Solid ductal carcinoma *in situ*. Central lumen with necrosis is seen in this duct with nuclear grade 2. Periductal fibrosis is not present.

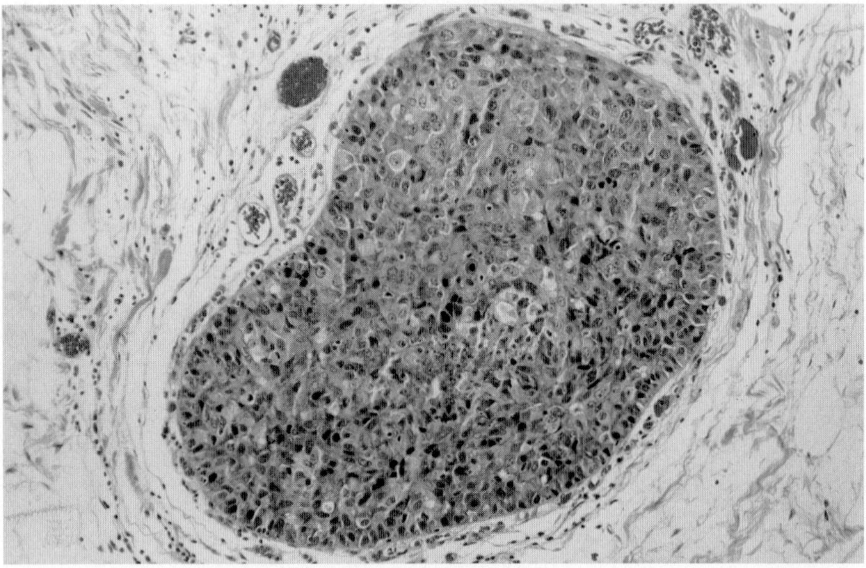

FIG. 4.6. Solid ductal carcinoma *in situ*. The individual cells are of nuclear grade 3. Note the striking increase in vascularity at the periphery of the involved duct. The layer of myoepithelium is inapparent.

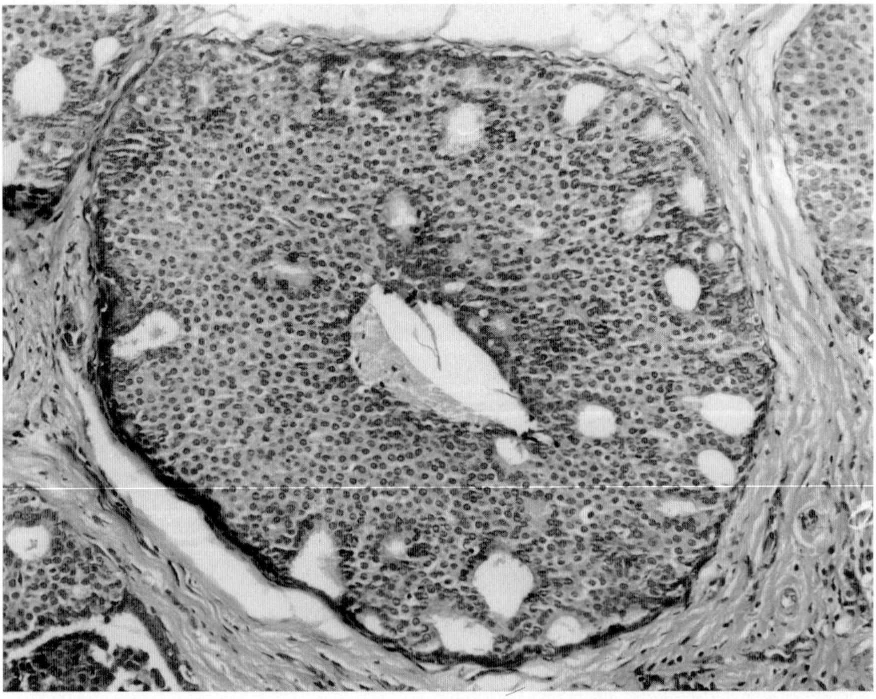

FIG 4.7. Cribriform ductal carcinoma *in situ*. A solid pattern of cells with grade 2 nuclei is focally interrupted by cells that form glands.

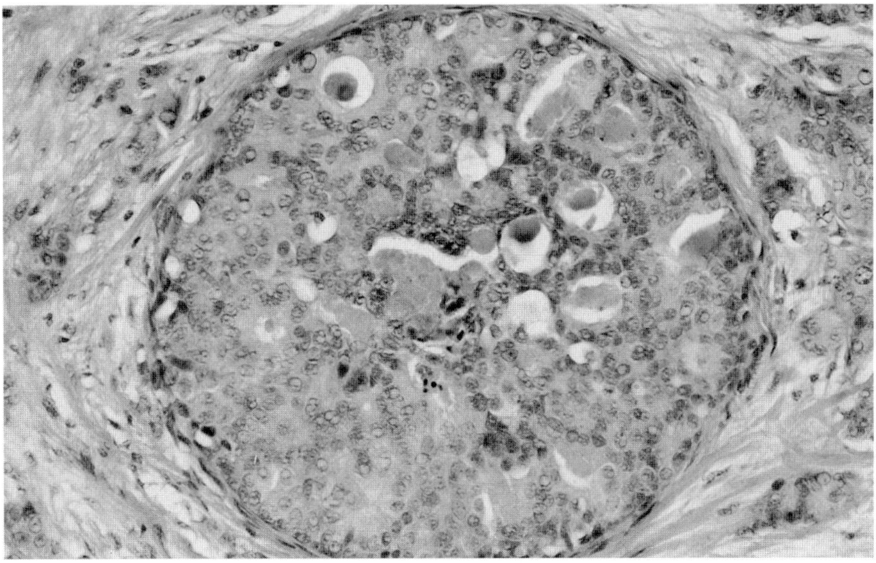

FIG. 4.8. Cribriform ductal carcinoma *in situ*. This type of intraductal carcinoma can be thought of as solid, but fenestrated by of a series of extracellular lumina and formed by the monomorphous cells with grade 2 nuclei. The extracellular lumina in this duct are regular, round, and surrounded by cuboidal cells. The central lumen has necrosis and microcalcification. Note the fibrous reaction at the periphery of this duct.

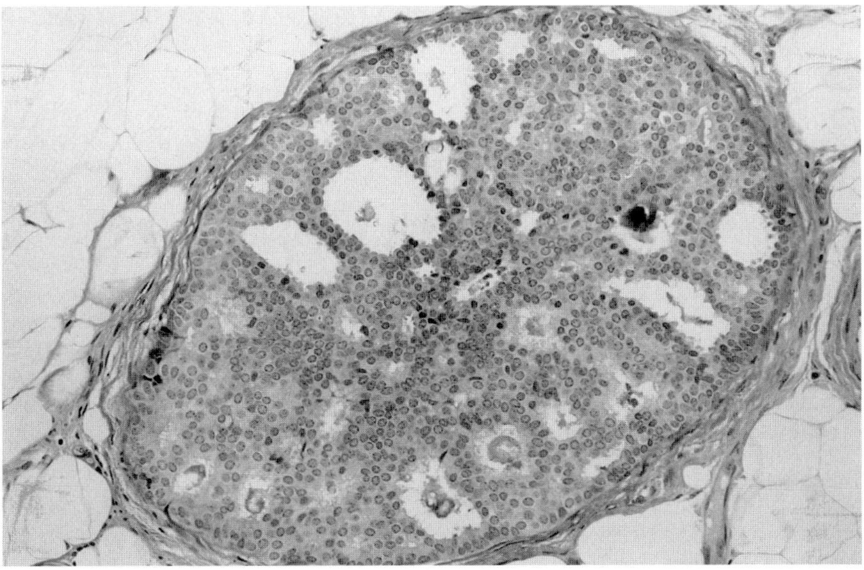

FIG. 4.9. Cribriform ductal carcinoma *in situ*. A series of extracellular lumens is formed by the monomorphous proliferation of cuboidal cells. Lamellar microcalcifications are present in several of these lumina (**lower half**). This is nuclear grade 2 and there is no necrosis. Note the absence of a fibrous reaction at the periphery of this duct.

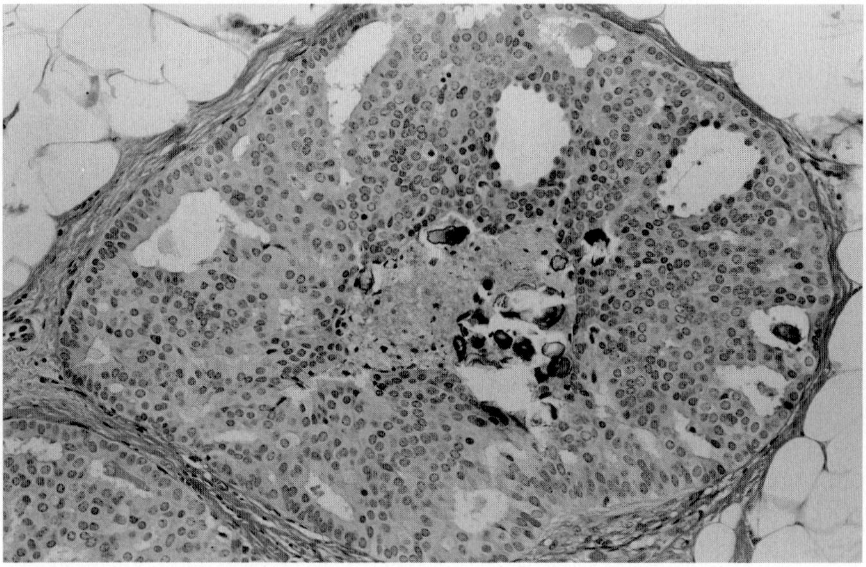

FIG. 4.10. Cribriform ductal carcinoma *in situ*, nuclear grade 2, with central necrosis and microcalcification.

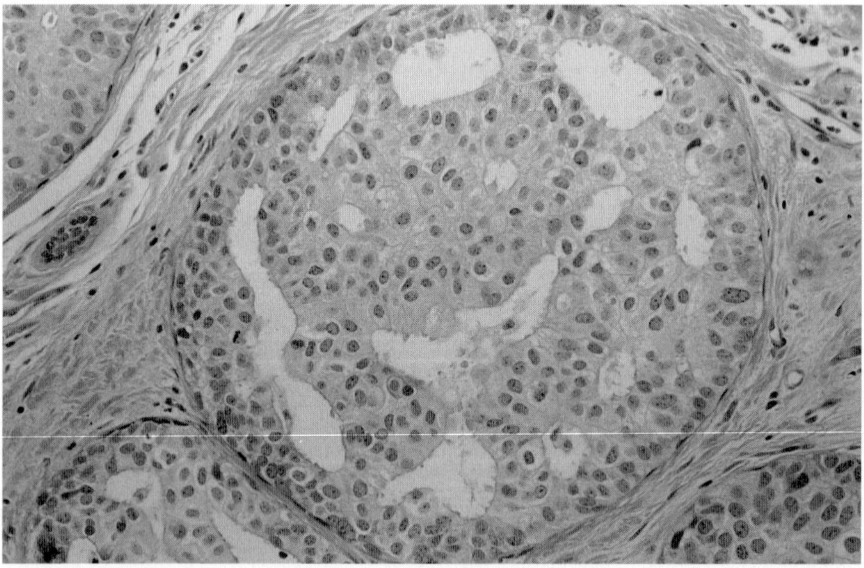

FIG. 411. Cribriform ductal carcinoma *in situ*. This medium duct is characterized by the presence of a monomorphous population of cuboidal cells with centrally placed, large, grade 1 nuclei that form regular, but not entirely rounded, extracellular lumens.

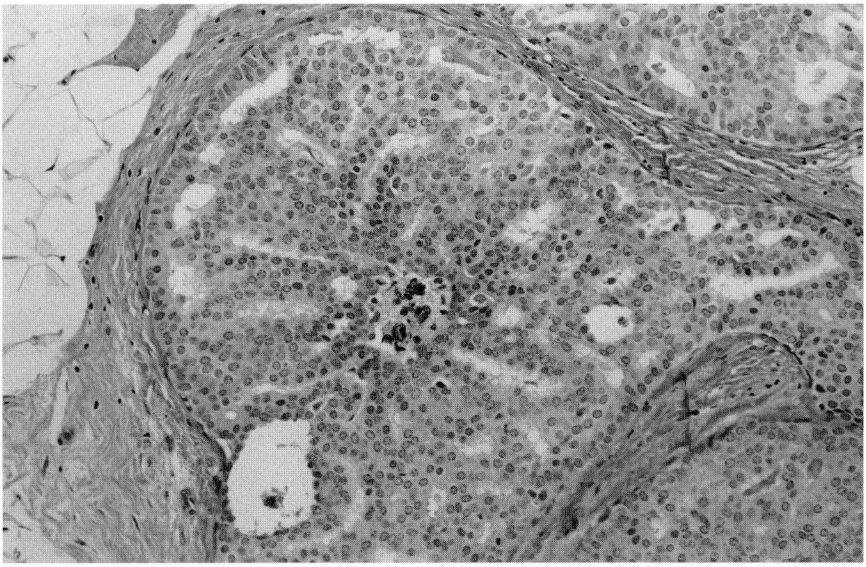

FIG. 4.12. Cribriform ductal carcinoma *in situ.* This medium- sized duct is filled with proliferating, mostly cuboidal, cells with grade 1 nuclei. Although extracellular lumens are present and regular, they are elongated, indicating that this pattern is basically micropapillary and arcuate. Central calcification is present.

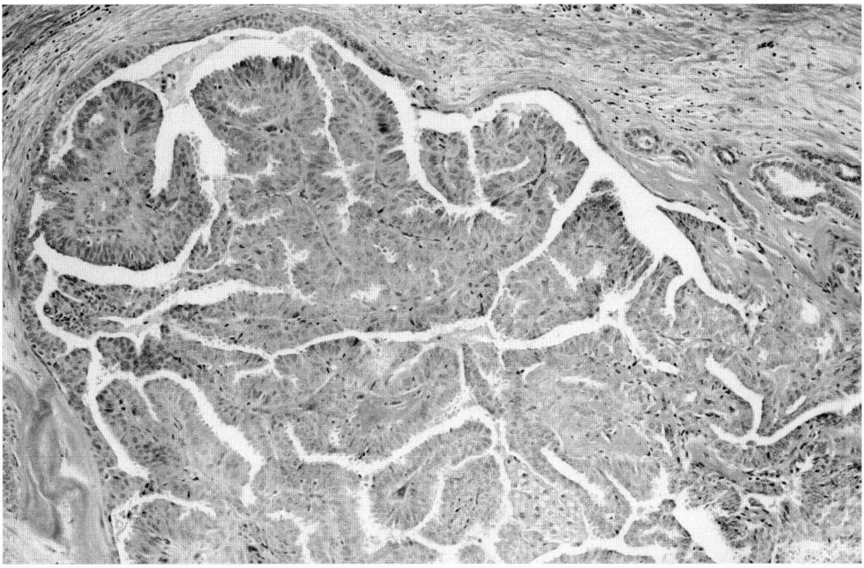

FIG. 4.13. Papillary ductal carcinoma *in situ* in which fibrovascular cores are prominent.

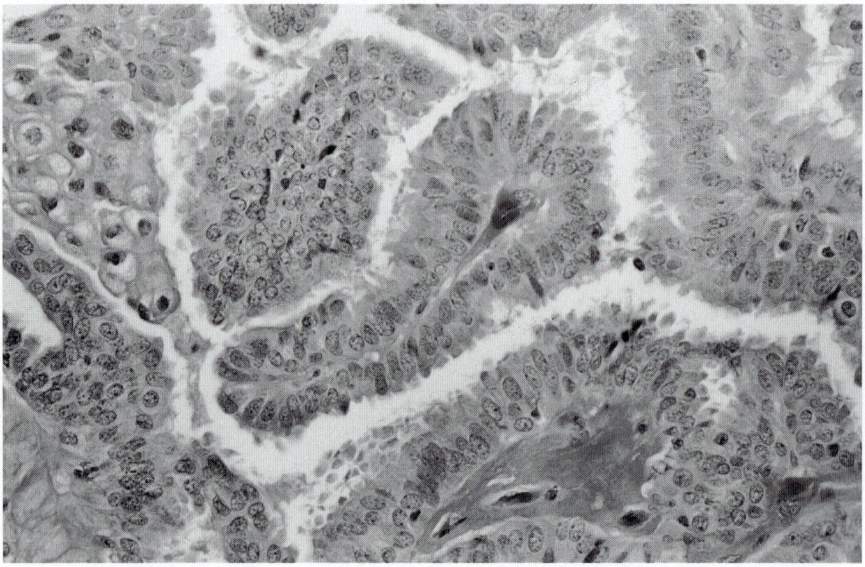

FIG. 4.14. Papillary ductal carcinoma *in situ*. In this higher power photomicrograph of the duct in Fig. 4.13, the fibrovascular cores are covered by a single layer of columnar cells with grade 2 nuclei. No myoepithelial layer is evident.

Micropapillary Intraductal Carcinoma

The micropapillary variant is a common form of DCIS and is probably the most difficult to diagnose because of its frequent low nuclear grade and lack of geometric regularity. Micropapillary DCIS has projections similar to papillary carcinoma, but they lack fibrovascular cores. The cells frequently present a knobby appearance as they project into the lumen of the duct and may join together centrally to form what Fisher et al.(1) called an arcuate pattern, forming the so-called Roman bridge (Figs. 4.15 and 4.16 and efigs. 4.22 to 4.44). Extracellular lumens in micropapillary DCIS are more slit-like and irregular than in cribriform DCIS. Necrosis, even comedonecrosis, may be present.

Apocrine Intraductal Carcinoma

A rare apocrine variant of DCIS has been described (2) in which the cells display apocrine metaplasia in a variety of patterns, usually micropapillary or cribriform. The nuclei, however, are usually of moderate to high grade, demonstrating the malignancy of the lesion. The DCIS patterns are made up of a monomorphic population of apocrine cells (Fig. 4.17 and efigs. 4.45 and 4.46). Because apocrine metaplasia usually is associated with benign changes, it is difficult to diagnose apocrine DCIS, unless both the nuclear abnormality and a recognizable DCIS pattern are abundantly present. Leal et al. (3) studied 35 cases

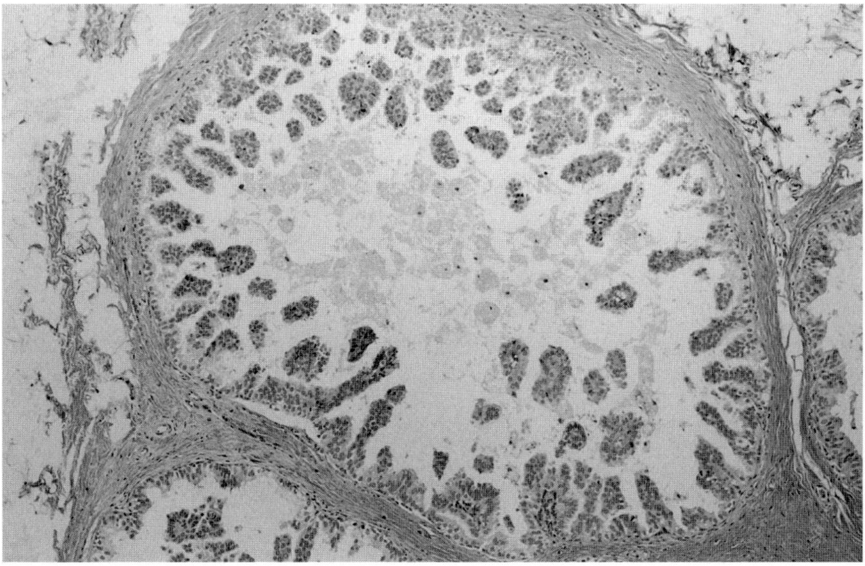

FIG. 4.15. Micropapillary ductal carcinoma *in situ.* A proliferation of micropapillae (without fibrovascular cores) extends into the lumen of a large duct.

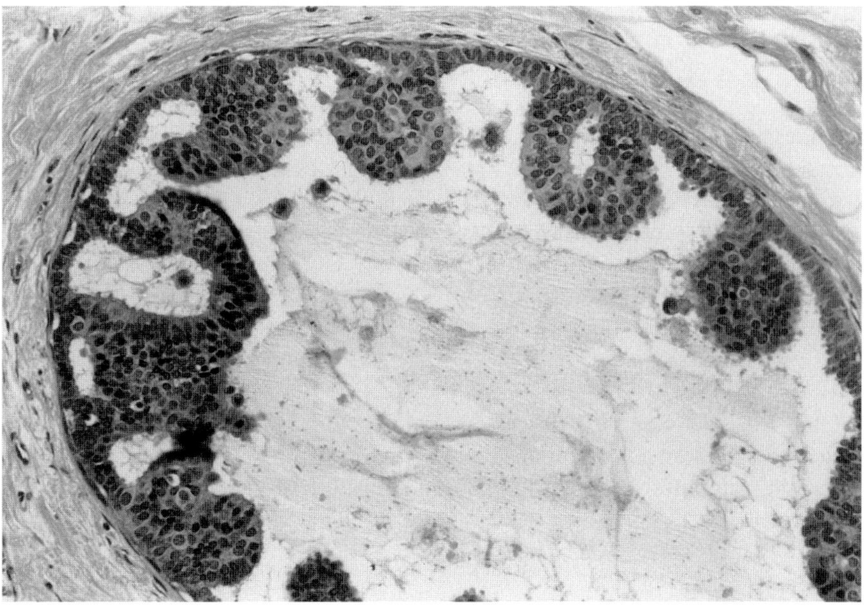

FIG. 4.16. Micropapillary ductal carcinoma *in situ* (DCIS). This form of DCIS has been likened to a Roman bridge. It also has been described as arcuate and may be conceived of as the joining of micropapillary segments composed of cuboidal cells with grade 1 nuclei.

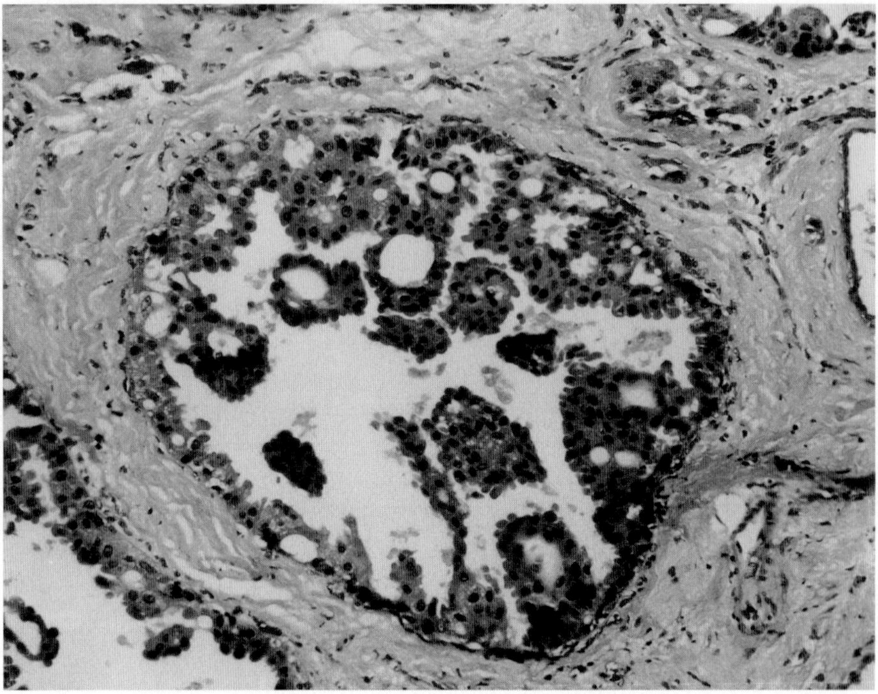

FIG. 4.17. Apocrine ductal carcinoma *in situ* (DCIS). The individual cells have apocrine cytoplasm and bland nuclei, but they form the micropapillary pattern of DCIS.

of apocrine DCIS, 22 of the cases without invasion and 13 cases with invasive carcinoma. The authors reported that 97% of the cases were androgen receptor positive. Ninety-four percent and 97% of the cases were estrogen and progesterone receptor negative, respectively. Fifteen cases were classified as high nuclear grade, ten cases were intermediate, and 10 cases low nuclear grade. Follow-up information is not available.

Clinging Carcinoma

Clinging carcinoma was described by Azzopardi (4) as a monolayer of cytologically malignant cells around a distended duct. No architectural pattern is present in this variant of DCIS (Fig. 4.18 and efigs. 4.47 and 4.48). See page 114.

Hypersecretory Carcinoma

Hypersecretory carcinoma was described by Guerry et al. (5) as being composed of malignant cells that secrete lactalbumin. The nuclear features are moderately anaplastic (nuclear grade 2), and there is a micropapillary pattern with

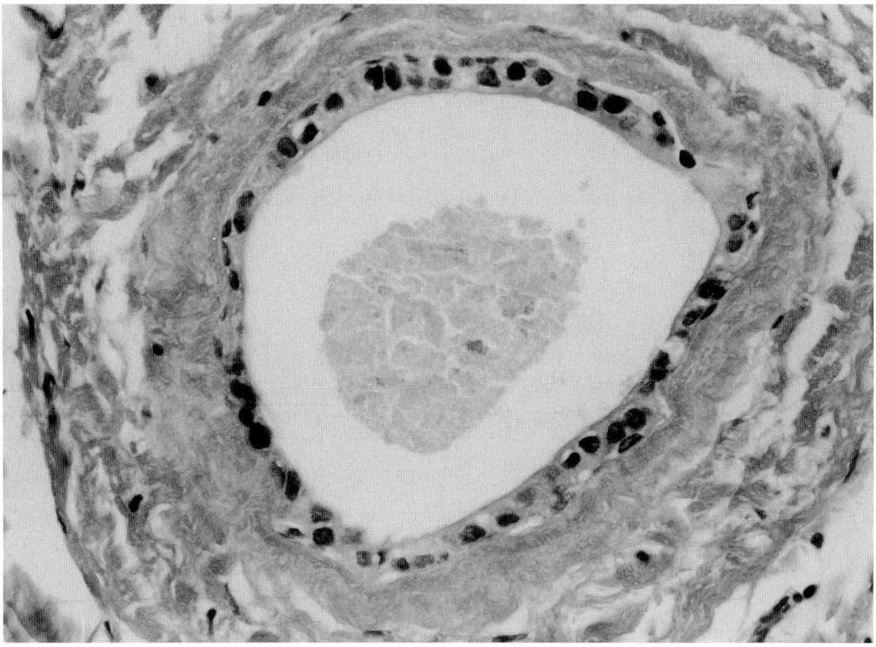

FIG. 4.18. Clinging carcinoma. There is a single layer of cytologically abnormal cells lining the duct. No myoepithelial layer is evident. The individual nuclei are so hyperchromatic and irregular that the diagnosis of malignancy is primarily made on the basis of their cytologic appearance. Note the dense fibrosis around this duct and the necrosis in the central lumen.

involved ducts with secretion (Figs. 4.19 and 4.20 and efigs. 4.49 to 4.54). (Compare with secretory DCIS in efigs. 4.55 and 4.56). See page 114.

Other Intraductal Carcinomas

Some cases of DCIS do not follow all the rules. Figure 4.21 is DCIS by nuclear grade alone. Immunostaining for HER2/neu and ER and demonstration of the neovascularity of DCIS are shown in efigs. 4.59 to 4.64. Tsang and Chan (6) described 14 cases of DCIS with neuroendocrine differentiation, frequently found in association with IPs (efigs. 4.57 and 4.58).

Significance of Ductal Carcinoma In Situ

Although there was considerable debate over the significance of LCIS, there has been less debate over the significance of intraductal carcinoma. It has long been considered a serious lesion, even though studies that document the relationships to infiltrating carcinoma are few in comparison to those documenting the follow-up of patients with LCIS. Patients with a diagnosis of intraductal carcinoma were usu-

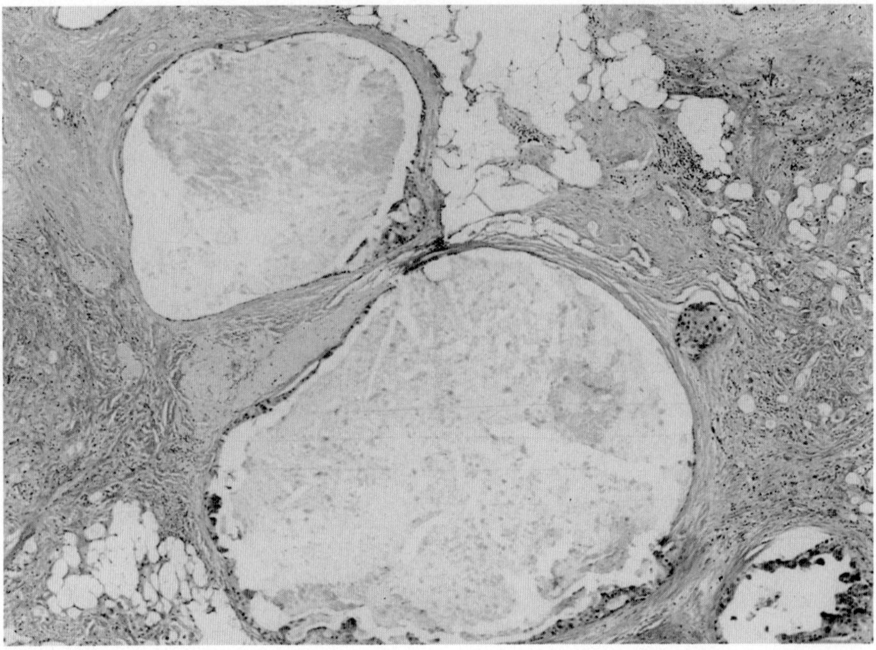

FIG. 4.19. Hypersecretory ductal carcinoma *in situ.* These distended ducts are filled with secretory material and lined very focally by a micropapillary proliferation. Note the elastosis at the periphery of the larger duct (**lower half**).

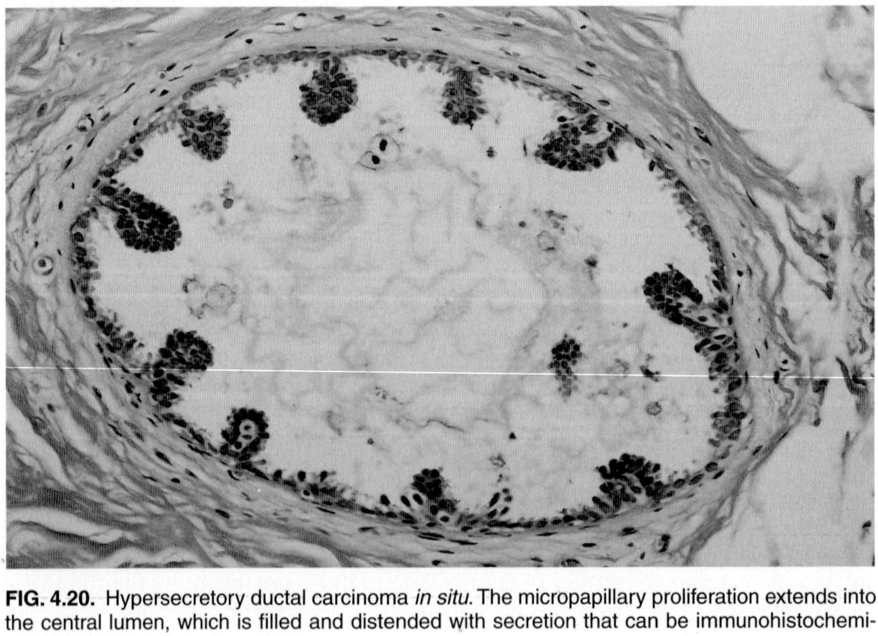

FIG. 4.20. Hypersecretory ductal carcinoma *in situ.* The micropapillary proliferation extends into the central lumen, which is filled and distended with secretion that can be immunohistochemically shown to contain lactalbumin.

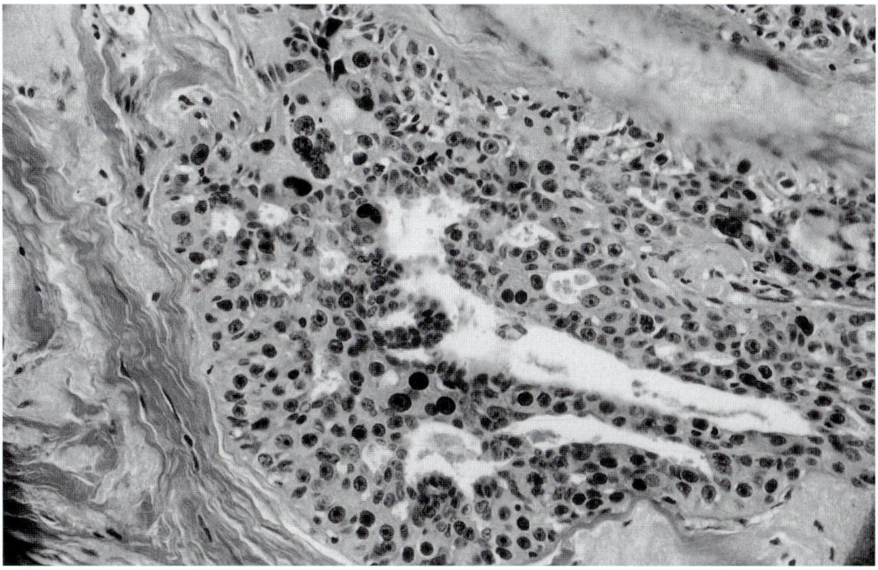

FIG. 4.21. Ductal carcinoma *in situ.* In this example of intraductal carcinoma, there is minimal regularity to the architectural features of the duct, but the nuclei are so large, hyperchromatic, irregular, and nonoverlapping that a cytologic diagnosis of carcinoma is unavoidable. Note the lack of a myoepithelial layer in this large duct.

ally treated with mastectomy, which produced excellent survival results. Several studies have documented that DCIS is often, but not invariably, followed by invasive cancer. Betsill et al. (7) reported on a group of 24 cases of DCIS that, for one reason or another, were not treated after biopsy. Thirty-four percent of those patients developed invasive cancer in the ipsilateral breast within a relatively short period of time after the DCIS diagnosis. Carter and Smith (8) studied a group of 38 patients who underwent mastectomy shortly after an open biopsy that was diagnostic of DCIS. In the mastectomy specimens, 7 of the 38 patients had either microinvasive or grossly invasive ductal carcinoma in the vicinity of the biopsy; 25 patients had residual intraductal carcinoma. Five patients had Paget's disease, and only six patients were found not to have residual cancer in the mastectomy specimen. Twenty-nine patients underwent lymphadenectomy in addition to the mastectomy. Three of these patients had axillary lymph node metastases. One patient, who was found to have intraductal carcinoma and no evidence of invasive cancer in either the biopsy or the mastectomy specimen, had axillary lymph node metastasis 16 months later. Another such patient, who had no axillary dissection, died of disseminated breast cancer. Shah et al. (9) found that 8 of 45 (18%) patients who were considered to have intraductal carcinoma in a biopsy specimen had invasive carcinoma in the mastectomy specimen. These data warn us that intraductal carcinoma may be associated with invasive carcinoma at the time DCIS is discovered, as well as during the follow-up period. The finding of metastases from a biopsy

TABLE 4.2. *Mastectomy status of 38 patients with ductal carcinoma in situ on biopsy*

Residual ductal carcinoma *in situ*	25 (66%)
Invasive carcinoma	7 (18%)
No residual cancer	6 (16%)
Positive nodes	4 (11%)
No invasion seen	1
Positive at 2 yr	1

From Carter D, Smith RR. Carcinoma *in situ* of the breast. *Cancer* 1977;40:1189–1193, with permission.

specimen that was diagnosed as intraductal carcinoma, without evident invasive carcinoma, is not unique to this series. Ashikari et al. (10) found one such patient in a series of 50 cases. Ozello and Sanpitak (11) observed that intraductal carcinoma is often associated with significant alterations at the epithelial stromal junction, when this area is observed by electron microscopy. A similar observation was made by Barsky et al. (12) using antibodies to type IV collagen and laminin. (In contrast, epithelial–stromal junction disruption has not been observed in LCIS). Invasive carcinoma that is found in association with DCIS is usually adjacent to the intraductal carcinoma. Carter and Smith (8) observed that 33 of 38 patients had residual intraductal or invasive cancer in the mastectomy specimen, which is consistent with figures in other series and a strong indication that some treatment is required for intraductal carcinoma. The interval between diagnosis and treatment should not be prolonged (Table 4.2).

Subclassification of Ductal Carcinoma In Situ

Several efforts have been made to subclassify intraductal carcinoma in order to better predict the distribution of the lesion, its likelihood of recurrence following treatment, and its relationship to invasive carcinoma. The number of types of DCIS ranges from three to seven and the number of nuclear grades ranges from two to four (Table 4.3).

Patchefsky et al. (13) separated 51 DCIS cases into six types—comedocarcinoma, solid, cribriform, papillary, micropapillary, and a mixed category. Comedocarcinoma was defined as any DCIS with central necrosis. The authors also used three nuclear grades and compared mammographically detected and incidentally found tumors. Microinvasion was most often found with comedocarcinoma and, second, with micropapillary carcinoma. Multicentricity was more often found with the micropapillary variant, but it was found overall in 44% of the 51 cases. A mixed category was found in 29% of the reported cases. Lagios et al. (14) described 79 cases of DCIS and classified them in three nuclear grades and four types—comedocarcinoma, cribriform carcinoma with necrosis, cribriform carcinoma with anaplasia, and micropapillary carcinoma; micropapillary carcinoma was the most common type. Comedocarcinoma was defined as DCIS with central necrosis, solid pattern, and high nuclear grade. The intraduc-

TABLE 4.3. *Reported classifications of ductal carcinoma in situ*

First author (reference)	No. cases	No. types	No. nuclear grades	Comedocarcinoma
Patchefsky (13)	51	6	3	Necrosis
Lagios (14)	79	4	3	Necrosis Solid HNG
Bellamy (15)	130	5	3	50% of necrosis Solid HNG
Poller (16)	76	3	3	Necrosis HNG High SPF
Holland (17)	—	3	3	—
Bobrow (19)	105	3	3	—
Lennington (19)	100	5	4	HNG Necrosis
Fisher (1)	573	7	2	—

HNG, high nuclear grade; SPF, S-phase fraction.

tal carcinomas were 25 mm or less in extent and the patients were treated by tylectomy alone, without irradiation. Eight patients had recurrence in the immediate vicinity of the biopsy site; four patients had invasive carcinoma and four patients had DCIS. DCIS with high nuclear grade and comedo-type necrosis was associated with a 19% local recurrence rate after 26 months, whereas only 1 of 43 patients with intermediate- or low-grade DCIS recurred.

Bellamy et al. (15) reported on 130 patients with DCIS, divided into three nuclear grades and five histologic types. Comedocarcinoma was described as those cases of DCIS with 50% central necrosis, a solid histologic pattern, and high nuclear grade. Thus defined, comedocarcinoma had an occult presentation more often than the other types. Micropapillary intraductal carcinoma was more likely to involve multiple quadrants, solid intraductal carcinoma was more often completely excised, and high-grade DCIS was more often incompletely excised. Of patients treated primarily by local excision alone, 16% had recurrence and, of these, 22% had invasive carcinoma, which followed only the high-grade DCIS, most often the comedo type. Poller et al. (16) described 76 DCIS cases, divided into three nuclear grades and three histologic types—pure comedocarcinoma, DCIS with necrosis, and DCIS without necrosis. A high S-phase was associated with the comedocarcinoma subtype.

In 1994, Holland et al. (17) proposed a classification of DCIS, with stratification according to 1 of 3 nuclear grades and also according to the degree of cellular polarization. The authors described DCIS as well—intermediately and poorly differentiated, based on these features. Using this classification, Bobrow et al. (18) described 105 cases of DCIS. Fifty-four percent of the cases were poorly differentiated, and necrosis was present in all of these cases. Forty-seven percent of those cases were classified as comedocarcinomas. Twenty-five percent of the cases were intermediately differentiated. Necrosis was present in all but three of those cases. Twenty-one percent were regarded as well-differentiated DCIS, and necrosis was present in 10 of the 22 cases. The poorly differentiated intraductal carcinomas were associated with a high proliferation rate, the expression of c-erbB-2 and p53 proteins, and the absence of progesterone receptors. The reverse was true for the well-differentiated intraductal carcinomas. Paget's disease was seen only in association with the poorly differentiated intraductal carcinomas.

Lennington et al. (19) analyzed 100 consecutive cases of intraductal carcinoma, using four nuclear grades (low, low moderate, high moderate, and high) to define five separate groups. Comedocarcinoma was diagnosed when necrosis and a high nuclear grade were present, but the histologic pattern was disregarded in making this designation. Forty-six percent of the cases were of mixed type. The authors reported that the highest grade of DCIS was present in the central part of the lesion, with progressively lower grade variants of intraductal carcinoma toward the periphery. ADH was associated with 17 of the DCIS cases, but none of the cases were comedocarcinoma.

Fisher et al. (1) reported 573 cases of intraductal carcinoma and used only two nuclear grades—high and low—to describe seven types of intraductal carcinoma. The authors reported that intraductal carcinoma generally could be successfully treated with lumpectomy and radiotherapy. Predictors of ipsilateral breast recurrence after lumpectomy were the presence of moderate to marked comedonecrosis and the presence of intraductal carcinoma at the margins of lumpectomy. The authors did not use the term "comedocarcinoma," but instead used descriptors to modify solid, cribriform, low papillary (micropapillary), high papillary (papillary), clinging, and arcuate types, as well as a mixed variety of intraductal carcinomas.

Eusebi et al. (20) reported on long-term follow-up of 80 cases of intraductal carcinoma, of which 41 cases were of the clinging type. The clinging type carcinomas were found among a group of 9,446 breast biopsy cases that were originally diagnosed as benign. Two of the patients with clinging carcinoma developed recurrent DCIS 3 years and 9 years after the breast biopsy. One of 28 cases of the flat type of clinging carcinoma and 1 of 13 cases of micropapillary variant of clinging carcinoma had recurrence. Invasive carcinoma was not found in the follow-up of any of the cases of clinging carcinoma. Because of these data that showed a low incidence of recurrence of this controversial entity and the absence of an association with invasive carcinoma, clinging carcinoma could be considered a type of ADH, mandating a thorough search for a definitive form of DCIS. Follow-up data on hypersecretory intraductal carcinoma did not show the development of invasive carcinoma (5).

Cataliotti et al. (21) reported on 183 cases of DCIS, of which 60% were multifocal and 22% were multicentric. Local recurrences, all of invasive carcinoma, occurred in the same breast after conservative surgery in eight cases. Three of these eight patients had received postoperative radiotherapy. Local recurrence was also noted in 3 of the 103 patients who were treated by mastectomy. Contralateral breast cancer was recorded in 12 cases—synchronously in 4 cases and metachronously in 8 cases—with invasive carcinoma recorded in 11 of the bilateral cases. Baird et al. (22) reported on 38 patients with comedo-type DCIS (not further defined) who were treated with less than total mastectomy. Thirteen of 35 patients for whom a family history was available had a family member with breast cancer, of which 11 were a first-degree relative. Four of 30 patients who were treated with local resection alone and 2 of 8 patients treated with local resection plus radiotherapy had recurrence during a mean follow-up period of 39 months.

O'Malley et al. (23) reported on 54 cases of proliferative intraductal apocrine lesions, of which 32 were classified as DCIS, based on size and nuclear abnormalities. Abati et al. (24) reported on 55 cases of intraductal apocrine carcinoma. Twenty of the 55 patients were treated by biopsy alone. Three of the patients recurred—one with axillary lymph node metastases and systemic spread. Tavassoli and Norris (2) reported on apocrine DCIS with behavior similar to that of micropapillary DCIS, without apocrine change.

Van de Vijver et al. (25) and Varley et al. (26) associated the comedo-type of intraductal carcinoma with the expression of c-erbB-2 oncogene. Liu et al. (27), Lodato et al. (28), and Somerville et al. (29) confirmed this observation. Lodato et al. (28) found that 55% of 33 cases of DCIS, but only 10% of 21 cases of ADH, expressed c-erbB-2. All 10 of the comedocarcinomas showed strong membrane staining, but micropapillary and cribriform variants did not. Paget's disease also was found to express the c-erb-2 frequently. Aasmundstad and Haugen (30) found aneuploidy in 55% of 29 comedocarcinomas, but only in 27% of 45 noncomedo DCIS cases. Ohuchi et al. (31) described 17 patients who presented initially with bloody nipple discharge and were treated by ductal–lobular segmentectomy, the linear removal of the area from which the blood could be expressed. The authors found intraductal spread of the DCIS in 8 of 16 segmentectomy specimens; 6 of the 8 patients had residual intraductal carcinoma in the subsequent mastectomy specimens. No residual DCIS was found in the mastectomy specimens from the other eight patients, in whom there was no intraductal spread of DCIS.

Guidi et al. (32) reported on the microvascular density and distribution in intraductal carcinoma. Comedocarcinoma was associated with marked stromal desmoplasia, which, in turn, was associated with a diffuse increase in stromal microvessels. Other histologic types were associated with a more sporadic microvascular cuffing of the involved spaces. Tsang and Chan (33) reported perineural invasion by a cribriform variant of intraductal carcinoma. Because perineural invasion has been observed with sclerosing adenosis, it is not surprising that, on extremely rare occasions, this might be seen with intraductal carcinoma as well.

Schwartz et al. (34,35) reported on 70 women who had intraductal carcinoma that was no larger than 25 mm. The patients were treated by local excision and surveillance, with a mean follow-up of 47 months. Recurrence was observed in

11 patients. Ten of these patients were recurrent comedocarcinomas, from among 21 cases of comedocarcinoma in the original series. One patient, who originally had a papillary DCIS, had recurrence as comedocarcinoma. In three patients, invasive carcinoma was recurrent, with positive axillary lymph nodes in one case. The comedocarcinomas were defined as had been described by Patchefsky et al. (13) as those DCIS cases with necrosis.

Badve et al. (36) analyzed a case control group of patients with DCIS that was histologically unequivocal, not associated with invasive carcinoma at first presentation, without relapse of ipsilateral invasive carcinoma within 6 months, and with surgery as the first line of therapy. Forty-three patients suffered recurrence (cases), whereas 81 patients did not have recurrence (controls). Cases and controls were blinded, and the cases were all analyzed according to the following architectural classification: the European Pathologists Working Group Classification, in which both nuclear grade and cellular polarization were utilized; the classification of the United Kingdom and European Commission Breast Screening Pathology Working Group, in which classification was made according to the highest nuclear grade; the Nottingham classification, in which cases of DCIS were divided into pure comedocarcinoma, other types of DCIS with necrosis, and DCIS without necrosis; and the Van Nuys classification, in which there was a high grade group with high nuclear grade with necrosis, a nonhigh grade group with necrosis, and a nonhigh grade group without necrosis. The follow-up period ranged from 7 to 125 months for the cases and 15 to 221 months for the controls. The best predictor of local recurrence was the nuclear grade, which achieved statistical significance. Histologic pattern was not useful in predicting recurrence. The Van Nuys classification, based on both nuclear grade and necrosis, also predicted for local recurrence. No factor predicted for the presence or absence of invasion when recurrence was observed or the time course to local recurrence.

A consensus conference (37) suggested that the following features should be recorded. For intraductal carcinoma, features included nuclear grade, the presence and type of necrosis, architectural pattern, margins, size, microcalcifications, and correlation of the tissue specimen with the specimen radiographic and mammographic findings. Nuclear grade was defined as low grade with nuclei 1.5 to 2 times the size of a normal red blood cell or ductal epithelial cell, with even chromatin and only occasional nucleoli and mitotic figures. High-grade nuclei were those that were highly pleomorphic, more than 2.5 times the size of a red blood cell or normal ductal epithelial cell, with prominent nucleoli, irregular chromatin, and conspicuous mitotic figures. Intermediate grade nuclei were those with features between those of low- and high-grade nuclei. Comedo necrosis was central zonal linear necrosis, whereas punctate necrosis was nonzonal and nonlinear. Cell polarization was described when the cytoplasm was oriented toward an intercellular lumen with the nuclei away from the lumen. The five architectural patterns recognized were comedo, cribriform, papillary, micropapillary, and solid. Recommendations were made for optimal tissue processing. A synoptic report including these features is shown as Table 4.4.

TABLE 4.4. *Synoptic ductal carcinoma in situ report*

SP No. ____________________________	
Name ____________________________	
Part No. _____ Left/right breast _____ Specimen _____	
Diagnosis: the carcinoma is intraductal	
Size	cm
Type	
Nuclear grade	
Necrosis	
Periductal fibrosis is present	
Microinvasion is possible, but not confirmed	
Orientation of cells	
Lobular involvement is present	
Extensive intraductal component is present	
Calcification is present in ductal carcinoma *in situ*	
Calcification is present in benign ducts	
Multifocal	
Multicentric	
Margins are positive/negative	
Distance to closest margin:	
(from designated margin)	cm

Microinvasion

The place of microinvasion as a stage of breast cancer has been unsettled since the acceptance of the concept of intraductal carcinoma as an entity. When rephrased in the context of measuring melanomas, the question is: What is the smallest invasive carcinoma that is capable of metastasis?

In 1997, the American Joint Commission on Cancer Staging (38) defined microinvasion as the extension of cancer cells beyond the basement membrane into adjacent tissues, with no focus more than 1 mm in greatest dimension. When multiple foci of microinvasion were present, the size of only the largest focus was used to classify the lesion as microinvasive. Thus defined, microinvasion was classified as T1mic, a subset of T1 invasive breast cancer. This definition did not include any restriction on the location of the apparently invasive component. Most observers agree that DCIS within the lobule may be so distorted that it is extremely difficult to reliably determine the presence or absence of invasion. The penetration of cells into the periductal stroma may present a similar challenge (Figs. 4.22 to 4.24 and efigs. 4.65 to 4.72). The consensus appears to be that microinvasion is found in the interlobular stroma. I have used the phrase "microinvasion is possible, but not demonstrated" when the area in question is confined to the periductal or lobular stroma and there is restricted unequivocal microinvasion to those areas that are clearly outside of the ductal and lobular stroma and measure no more than 1 mm in diameter. These T1mic lesions are predominantly intraductal carcinoma and usually of high nuclear grade with central zonal necrosis, thereby fulfilling most, if not all, of the criteria of comedocarcinoma (Fig. 4.25 and efigs. 4.73 to 4.79).

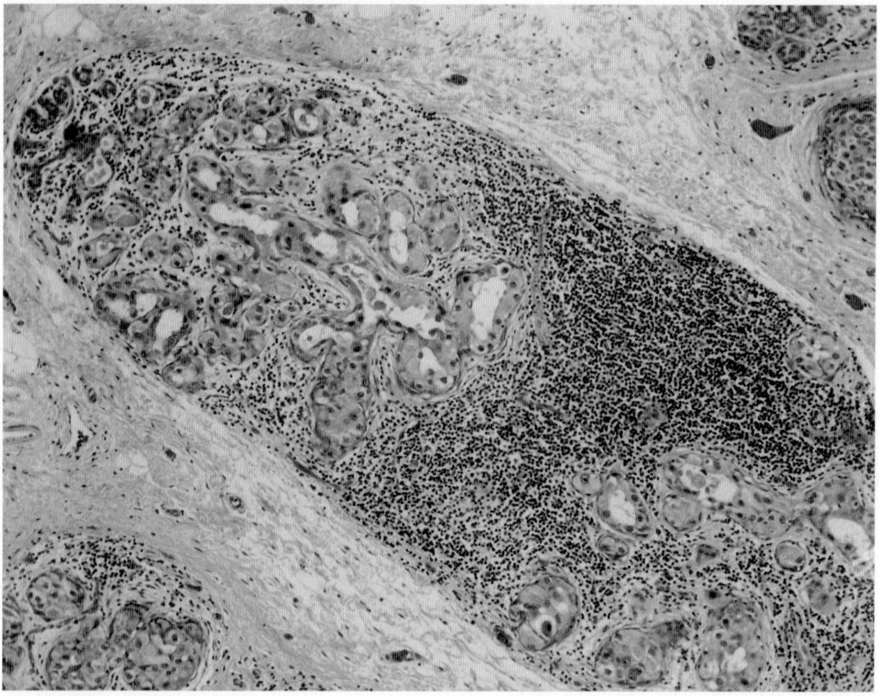

FIG. 4.22. Ductal carcinoma *in situ* (DCIS) with lobular involvement (cancerization of the lobule). The lobule has been involved by extension of DCIS into the terminal ducts, which is associated with an intense lymphocytic infiltrate (**right**).

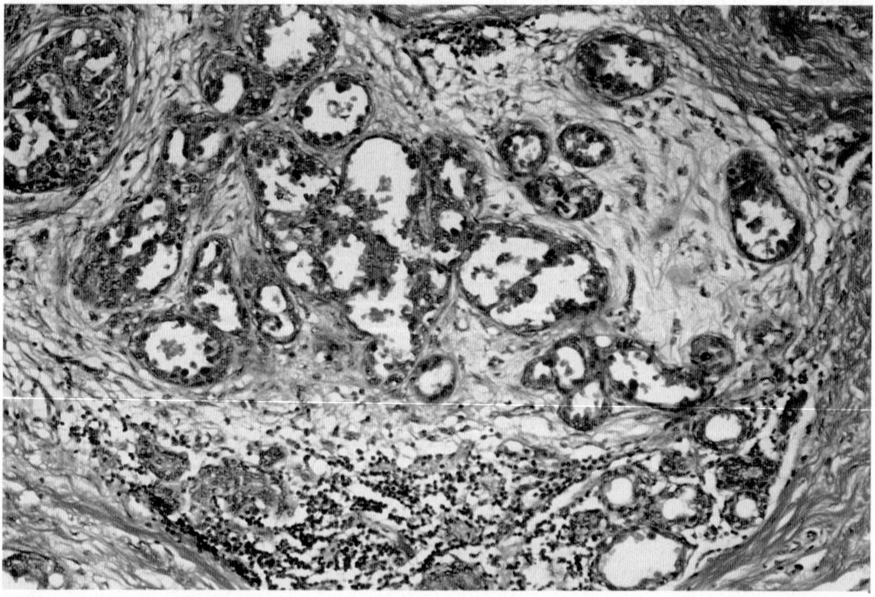

FIG. 4.23. Cancerization of the lobule. Micropapillary ductal carcinoma *in situ* has extended into the terminal ducts and caused dense fibrosis in the lobular stroma. Although the reaction appears to be desmoplastic, the basement membranes can be shown to be intact and this is not invasion or microinvasion.

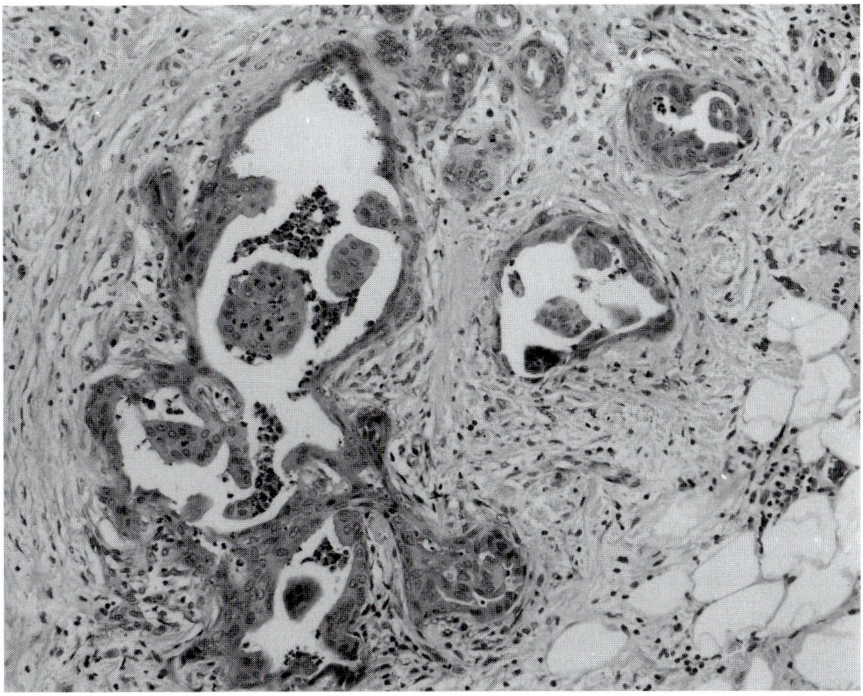

FIG. 4.24. Cancerization of the lobule with a question of microinvasion. Terminal ducts have been involved by a micropapillary variant of ductal carcinoma *in situ* with low nuclear grade. A question of microinvasion is raised by the extensive fibroblastic reaction, but identification of microinvasion is problematic. In cases like this, microinvasion may be present, but cannot be confirmed.

Unfortunately, the concept of microinvasion is not supported by very much reliable data, due to the relative rarity of breast cancer diagnosed in this stage, the variety of definitions used to define microinvasion, and the problems in making an accurate diagnosis. As a result, there is little in the literature that allows the pathologist to reliably indicate the likelihood of lymph node metastases from a T1mic carcinoma. The incidence is almost certainly quite low. Rosner et al. (39) found no positive nodes among 36 cases of intraductal carcinoma with microinvasion, but these cases were selected from amongst a group of node negative cases. Prasad et al. (40) reported on lymph node metastases in 2 of 15 T1mic cases. Zavotsky et al. (41) found that 2 of 14 T1mic cases had positive sentinel lymph nodes, but Wong et al. (42) found no lymph node metastases in 31 T1mic cases with axillary lymph node dissections. Silver and Tavassoli (43) found no lymph node metastases among 33 patients with microinvasion, and their definition of microinvasion was 1 focus (2 mm or less) or up to 3 foci, each of which was 1 mm or less. Patchefsky et al. (13) found 2 of 41 patients with microinvasion to have lymph node metastases, but their definition of microinvasion was no more than 10% of the entire area of DCIS. The authors found microinvasion in 1 of 15 papillary carcinomas *in situ*, 3 of 10 micropapillary carcinomas *in situ*, and 12 of 19 comedocarcinomas.

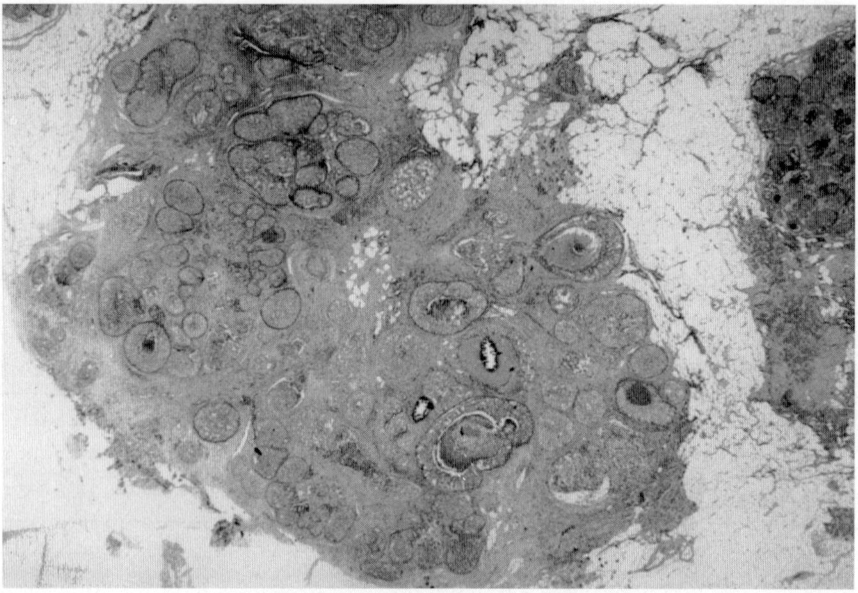

FIG. 4.25. Microinvasion. **A:** Area of extensive ductal carcinoma *in situ* (DCIS), predominantly comedo type with periductal fibrosis and lobular involvement. Attention is directed to the stellate area at the 1 o'clock position (**upper part**).

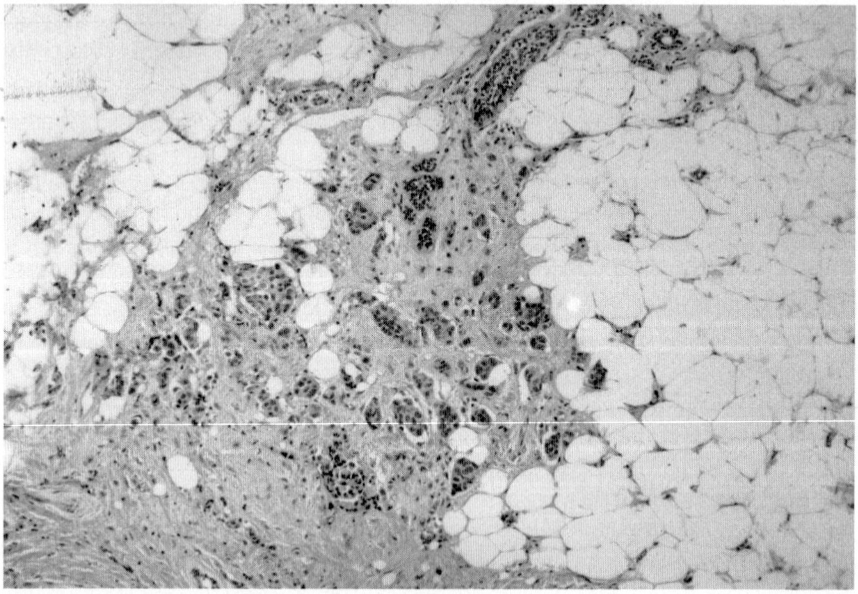

FIG. 4.25. B: Higher magnification of the area that is ordinary invasive ductal carcinoma with a desmoplastic reaction, but without a DCIS pattern. It is microinvasion because it is less than 1 mm in greatest dimension. See efig. 4.73 to 4.75.

The incidence of lymph node metastases from T1mic lesions must be considered in the same context as lymph node metastases from cases diagnosed as entirely intraductal carcinoma without microinvasion. Carter and Smith (8) described lymph node metastases that followed a diagnosis of intraductal carcinoma in 14% of cases. Kinne et al. (44) found 1 of 128 DCIS patients with positive axillary lymph nodes. Hardman et al. (45) reported on 62 cases diagnosed as comedocarcinoma, of which 14 showed evidence of clear-cut invasive carcinoma upon reexcision. Two of these patients had positive axillary lymph nodes. Lagios et al. (46) reported on 53 patients who underwent resection for a biopsy diagnosis of DCIS, in which the reexcision was studied with subgross and radiographic correlation. Among 4 lesions that were 2.5 cm or larger in extent, 11 of the lesions showed occult foci of invasive carcinoma, but there were no instances of occult invasive carcinoma found among 29 DCIS lesions that were smaller than 2.5 cm in diameter.

Schnitt (47) described the histologic problems presented by extensive intraductal carcinoma in which invasion may have started. Artifactual problems included crush and cautery effect and the artifactual displacement of intraductal carcinoma cells into the surrounding stroma by puncture wounds of needles or wires that were designed to obtain a biopsy or to localize a radiographic lesion. Intraductal carcinoma that involved a benign sclerosing process, such as sclerosing adenosis or extensive involvement of a lobule by DCIS (the so-called cancerization of the lobules), may also simulate invasive carcinoma. The branching of ducts, especially those distorted by periductal fibrosis, may also create difficulties in the accurate assessment of invasion. Entrapment of involved ducts or papillary structures is problematic, especially at the periphery of IPCs.

Microinvasion is associated with DCIS, but is virtually never found in association with LCIS. Distinction between these two entities may be difficult and is aided by staining for E-cadherin and HER2/neu (Chapter 5). Neovascularization occurs around the basement membranes of DCIS, especially those of high grade and those with periductal fibrosis; however, it is not an indicator of invasion, although it probably indicates signaling between stromal and epithelial components.

Immunohistochemistry may be useful in determining the integrity of the basement membrane and therefore ruling out the presence of invasion. Immunohistochemical stains for the basement membrane component, especially type IV collagen, are supplemented by immunohistochemical stains for calponin or smooth muscle actin, which demonstrate the presence of the myoepithelial cells known to be anchored in the basement membrane and therefore defining the absence of stromal invasion. The combination of these two stains is useful, and I insist that both show absence of basement membrane before invasion is considered. However, microscopic foci of putative microinvasion are, by definition, quite small and frequently not found on recuts that are made for immunohistochemical studies. In such cases, the diagnosis of invasive carcinoma rests upon the identification of malignant cells that are found in a stroma that is exhibiting a desmoplastic reaction to their presence.

In summary, pathologists spend considerable effort and anxiety determining if microinvasion has occurred in the setting of DCIS, but T1mic lesions are unlikely to be associated with lymph node metastases. A certain low incidence of metastases does occur, but it is nearly the same as that found after a diagnosis of DCIS without evident microinvasion. This seems to be an ideal setting for sentinel lymph node biopsy, but data are needed before a firm recommendation for that procedure can be made. Microinvasion and lesions that may be mistaken for it are illustrated abundantly, as noted above.

Atypical Ductal Hyperplasia

In 1985, Page et al. (48) defined ADH as a significant premalignant lesion, especially in women with a family history of breast cancer. The histologic appearance was defined as a ductal proliferation having some, but not all, features of DCIS. The authors described DCIS as composed of large round or polygonal cells with round, oval, monotonous, and hyperchromatic nuclei. Cell borders were distinct and the cells were evenly placed to form a rigid pattern, without swirls or streaming, and with smooth, round, and regular extracellular lumina. Micropapillae, frequently without a fibrovascular stalk, also were present. "ADH was present when some but not all of these criteria were fulfilled" (Figs. 4.26 to 4.31 and efigs. 4.80 to 92, 4.94 to 98, and 4.109). The risk of breast cancer in women with ADH was found to be 4.3 times greater than in women without it and 10 times greater in women with both ADH and a family history of breast cancer than in those with neither. Cancer developed in either breast over a long follow-up period. ADH, with these risks, was not a common lesion; it was found in only 150 cases among over 10,000 benign breast biopsy specimens (1.5%) and, among those 150 women, only 18 (12%) developed invasive cancer.

In the definition of Page et al. (48), at least two ducts were completely involved. Tavassoli and Norris (49) added an additional stipulation to the diagnosis of ADH, stating that it must be larger than 2 mm in aggregate cross-section of involved ducts.

O'Connell et al. (50) analyzed 399 cases of microdissected archival specimens by polymerase chain reaction (PCR) reaction for loss of heterozygosity at 15 polymorphic genetic loci that were known to exhibit high rates of loss in invasive breast cancer. In hyperplasias from noncancerous breasts, loss of heterozygosity at any given locus was rare, although 37% of usual DH and 42% of ADH lesions showed loss for at least one locus. In intraductal carcinoma, from breasts without invasive carcinoma, loss of heterozygosity was found in 70% of noncomedo DCIS and 79% of comedocarcinomas. In intraductal carcinoma, substantial rates of loss, up to 37%, were observed at loci on chromosome 16q, 17p, and 17q. Comparison of DCIS that was associated with invasive cancer with DCIS not associated with invasive cancer showed substantially more loss of heterozygosity on chromosomes 2p, 11p and 17q in the former group. From cancerous breasts, 36% of usual DH, 45% of atypical hyperplasia, 77% of noncomedo DCIS, and 80% of comedocarcinoma shared loss of heterozygosity with synchronous invasive carcinomas at one locus or more. The authors suggested

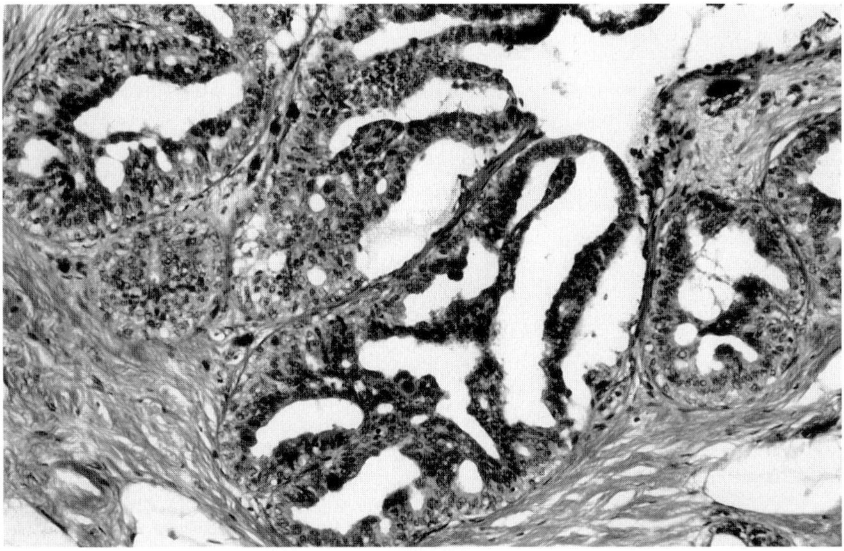

FIG. 4.26. Borderline or markedly atypical ductal hyperplasia. This borderline category contains intraductal proliferation with some of the features of ductal carcinoma *in situ*—a micropapillary projection of atypical cells into the lumen of a medium-sized duct. Against the diagnosis of carcinoma is the presence of a prominent myoepithelial layer and a lack of regularity of the pattern and cell type. The predominant cell type is cuboidal, but focally there are columnar cells. Different observers might place this lesion on either side of the borderline of intraductal carcinoma and atypical ductal hyperplasia. Lesions such as this are best dealt with according to their size and association with proliferations that are more definitively benign or malignant, as may be shown with recuts.

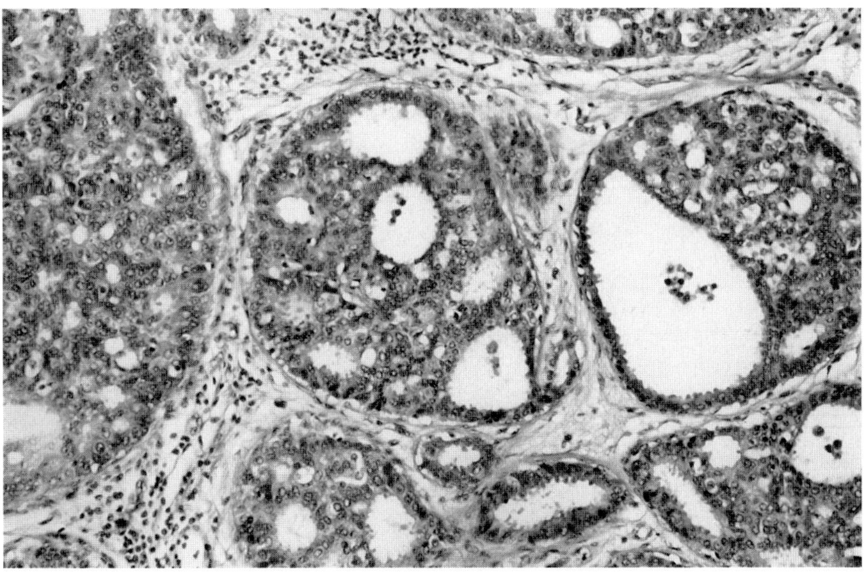

FIG. 4.27. Borderline or markedly atypical ductal hyperplasia. A micropapillary or cribriform proliferation of cells across the lumen forms a regular architecture without fibrovascular support, but there is a partial prominent myoepithelial layer, overlapping of the nuclei, and marked variation in the size and configuration of the extracellular lumina.

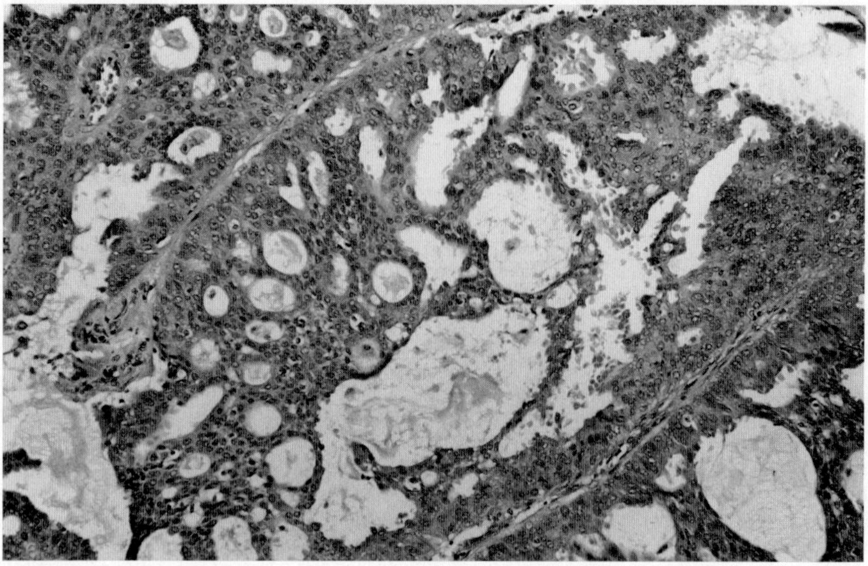

FIG. 4.28. Borderline or markedly atypical ductal hyperplasia. There is a cribriform or micropapillary pattern; however, there is a lack of regularity in the size of the lumens, a partial myoepithelial layer, focal overlapping of the nuclei, and variation from cuboidal to columnar cells with focal apocrine metaplasia.

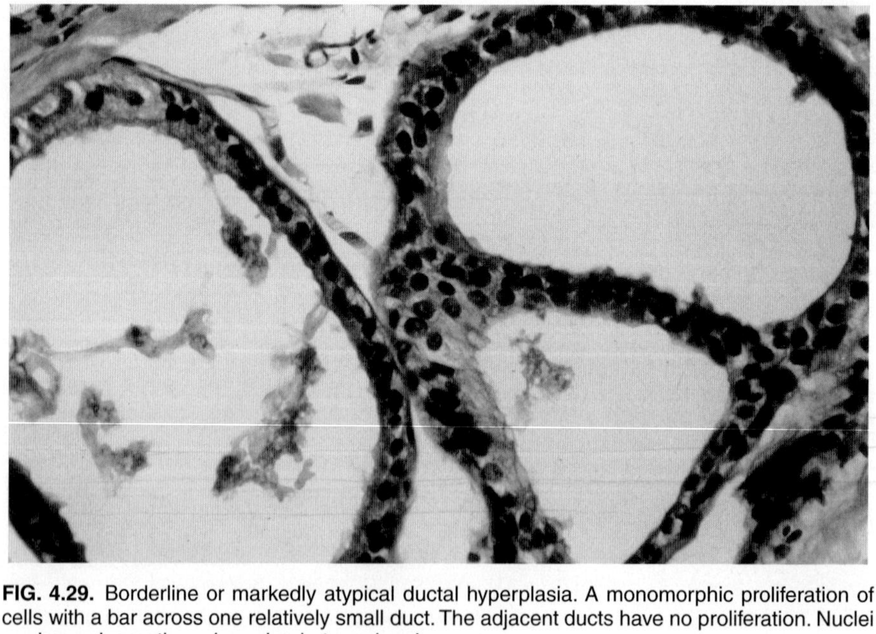

FIG. 4.29. Borderline or markedly atypical ductal hyperplasia. A monomorphic proliferation of cells with a bar across one relatively small duct. The adjacent ducts have no proliferation. Nuclei are hyperchromatic and regular, but overlapping.

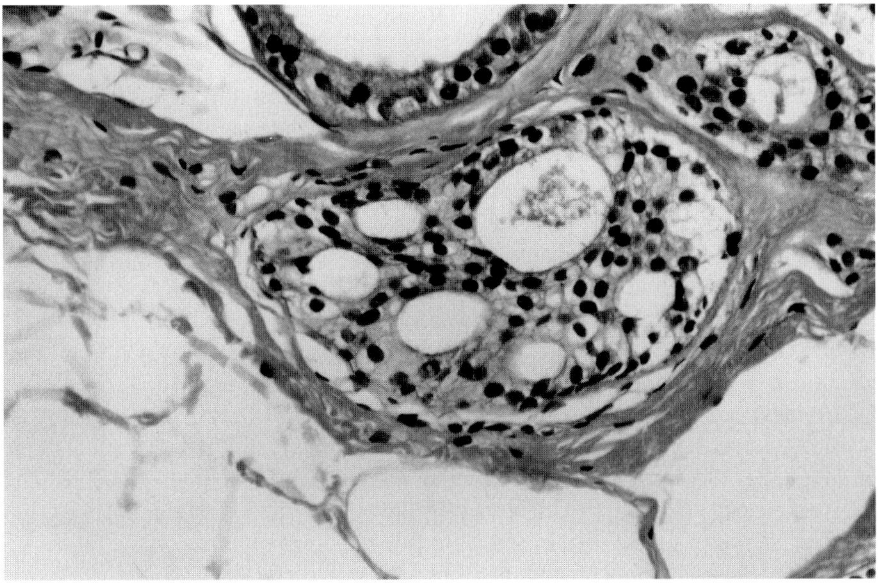

FIG. 4.30. Borderline or markedly atypical ductal hyperplasia. This small duct has a cribriform pattern and isolated nuclei, and the adjacent ducts show no similar change.

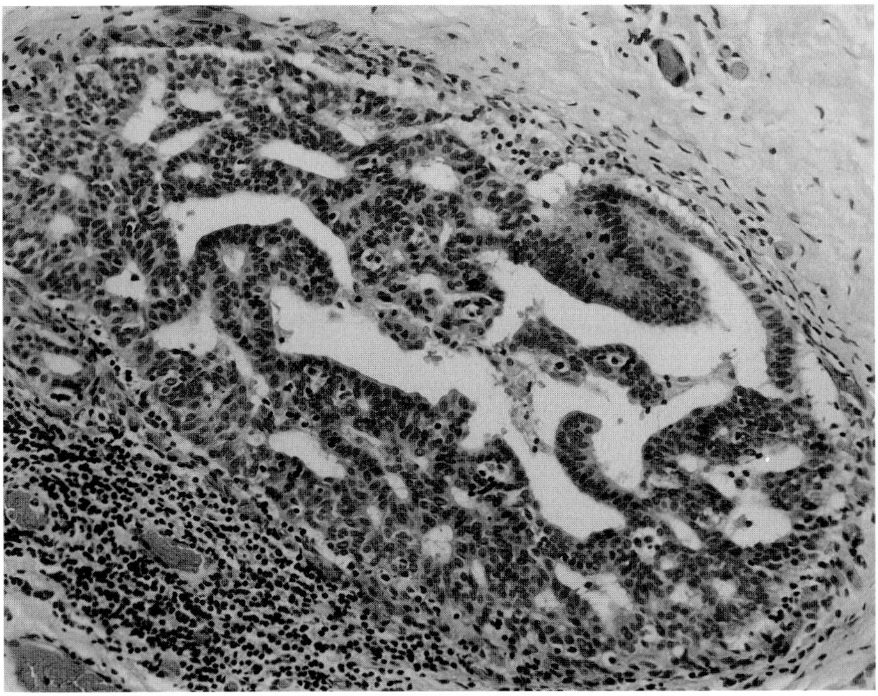

FIG. 4.31. Borderline or markedly atypical ductal hyperplasia. Duct with micropapillary pattern with small round touching nuclei.

progression from hyperplasia to atypia to DCIS and finally to invasive carcinoma, but the differences are relatively small and the overlap is too great for them to be applied in the clinical distinctions among usual DH, ADH, and DCIS.

The landmark study by Page et al. (48) has strong clinical implications and presents correspondingly serious diagnostic challenges. The report by Rosai (51) showed the difficulty of this diagnosis. The subsequent report by Schnitt et al. (52) showed that a different group of pathologists reviewing different cases and with agreed upon criteria could be more consistent in the diagnosis. Bodian et al. (53) reported on a series of reviewed breast biopsy specimens, some of which were rereviewed in a blinded study. There was good intraobserver agreement for DCIS, LCIS, papilloma, and adenosis, but poor agreement on levels of hyperplasia and atypia. As noted in Chapter 2, the consensus group divided DH into three grades, although they did not give definitions for any of them. ADH obviously falls into the most severe category. All investigators have not agreed on the criteria of ADH or on its precancerous implications. In 1993, Bodian et al. (53) reported on the follow-up of 1,799 patients who had undergone a breast biopsy (between 1930 and 1982) that was interpreted as a benign lesion. These biopsy specimens were reviewed and classified according to degree of hyperplasia and atypia present. The criteria set forth by Page et al. (48) were followed, except the criterion that only one duct involved by what appeared to be DCIS was still called ADH. Bodian et al. (53) classified cases with a single duct, which met all of the criteria for intraductal carcinoma, as DCIS. The authors found 1,521 patients with proliferative disease, compared with 278 cases in which there was no proliferative disease. The risk of subsequent carcinoma was equal to 2.2 times the population rate in the proliferative group. The authors found 272 patients with mildly atypical hyperplasia and 70 patients with moderately or severely atypical hyperplasia, with relative risks increasing to 2.3 for mild atypia and 3.0 for moderate to severe atypia; however, these differences in relative risk were not statistically significant. Curiously, the presence of adenosis had a relative risk that was approximately the same as that of moderate or severe atypia. Among the 272 patients with proliferative disease with mild atypia, 25 developed carcinoma. Among the 70 patients with moderate or severe atypia, 8 patients developed cancer. Linkage of family history with levels of proliferation was not established in this study or by Eliasen et al. (54) in nine young women.

Rosen (55) reviewed the subject of the precancerous implications of atypical hyperplasia and found that the reported percentage of patients who develop breast cancer following the observation of atypical hyperplasia ranges from 5% to 12%. It is clear that these patients represent a small, but important, subset of those who develop carcinoma of the breast and that the vast majority of patients are diagnosed with breast cancer on the first biopsy.

Distinction between ADH and ordinary DH also has serious clinical implications. One can easily fall into the habit of finding atypia in many DHs, but properly used, the term ADH should be reserved for the 2% of cases in which the most severe abnormalities are seen. Some of these changes are illustrated here, but the reader is also referred to the illustrations in reports by Page et al. (48) and Tavassoli and Norris (49).

Ductal Hyperplasia

There is a slight, but statistically significant, increase in the risk of invasive cancer associated with DH. The risk is not as great as family history, parity plus menstrual history, or presence of contralateral carcinoma and is therefore not considered to be the basis for action by the clinician, even though the distinction from malignant lesions may require considerable effort by the surgical pathologist. Careful follow-up is, of course, indicated.

A wide variety of proliferations that occur within the ducts of the breast are gathered together under this term. Paradoxically, these benign proliferations are less regular and predictable than malignancies. Fewer generalities can be stated for benign lesions than for DCIS, but a few are helpful. A prominent proliferative myoepithelial layer and the presence of more than one kind of cell (e.g., epithelial, myoepithelial, or apocrine) are benign features, as are dominant apocrine metaplasia (although apocrine carcinomas occur), irregularity, and lack of predictability. Lack of regularity is better seen in larger ducts. Although the nuclei of benign proliferations may be large, hyperchromatic, contain nucleoli, and rarely contain mitotic figures, they are not bizarre or angular and do not have abnormal mitoses (Table 4.1). Some of the variations are illustrated in Figs. 4.32 to 4.41 and efigs. 4.93 and 4.99 to 4.112.

What is the significance of DH in the breast? There is a consensus (53,56–63) that the risk of breast cancer in patients who have DH is slightly higher than in patients who have no breast abnormality, but lower than for patients who have

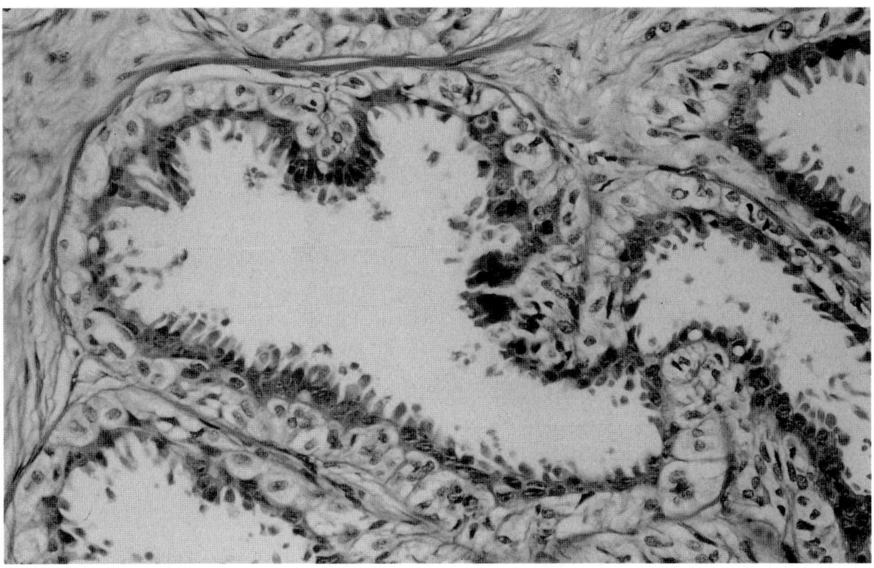

FIG. 4.32. Ductal hyperplasia with a striking proliferation of myoepithelial cells in the clear zone between the basement membrane and the columnar epithelium that lines the extracellular lumen. The columnar cells are oriented in a vertical fashion and display prominent apocrine snouts.

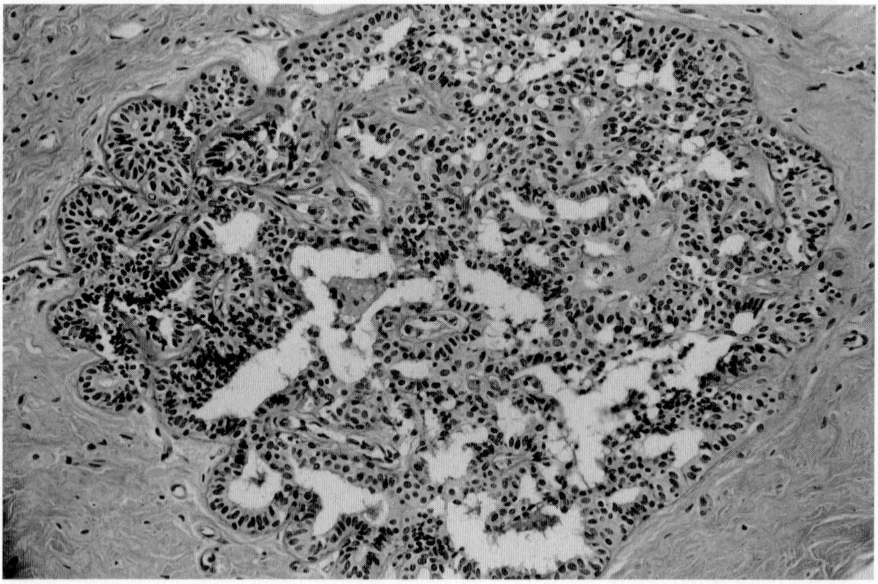

FIG. 4.33. Ductal hyperplasia. The proliferative lesion within a lobule is characterized by the presence of rounded, fairly regular extracellular lumens that vary in size and are round to elongated. There is also a two-cell population, which indicates that this a benign ductal hyperplasia.

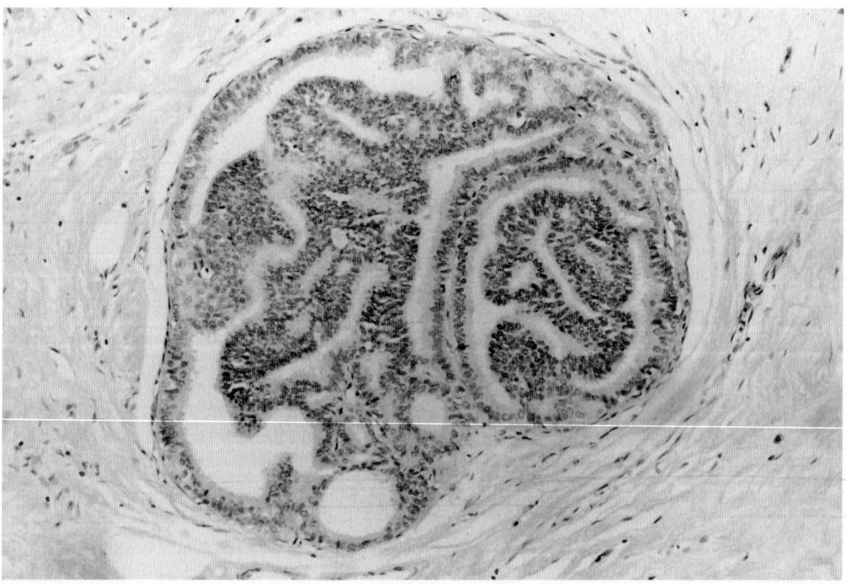

FIG. 4.34. Papillomatosis. Fibrovascular cores covered by layers of epithelium extending across the extracellular lumen in an irregular way. Nuclei are small and touching and there is a prominent myoepithelial layer.

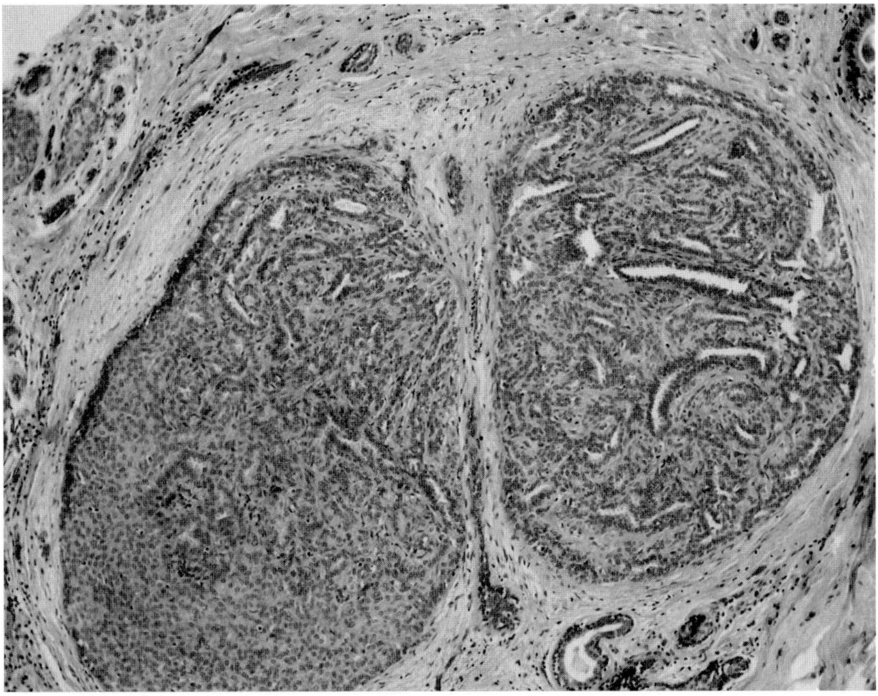

FIG. 4.35. Ductal hyperplasia/papillomatosis. A biphasic population is present. The slit-like extracellular lumens are lined by columnar cells, but the bulk of the lesion is made up of cuboidal myoepithelial cells that extend from the basement membrane to the columnar area.

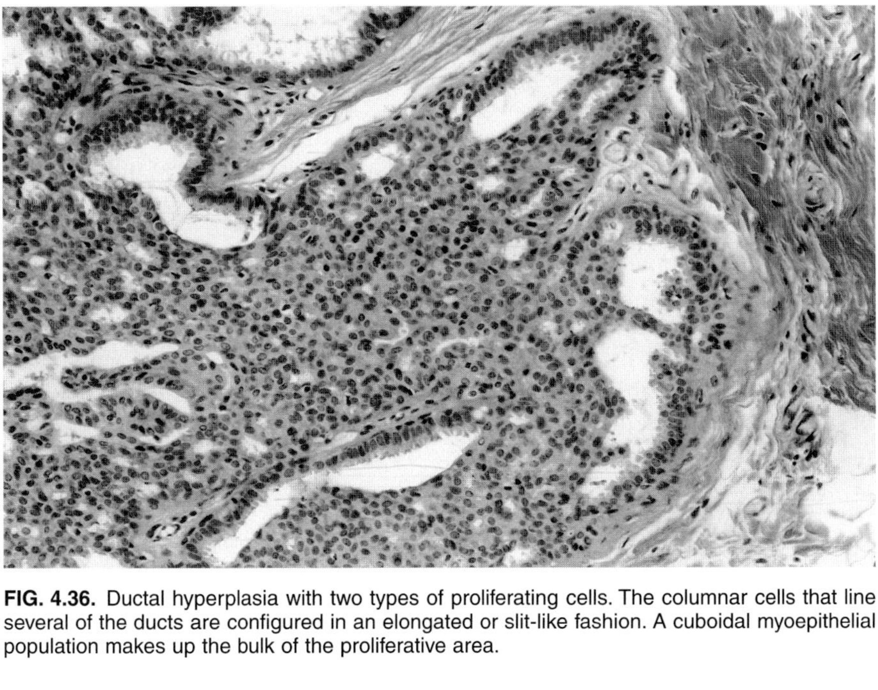

FIG. 4.36. Ductal hyperplasia with two types of proliferating cells. The columnar cells that line several of the ducts are configured in an elongated or slit-like fashion. A cuboidal myoepithelial population makes up the bulk of the proliferative area.

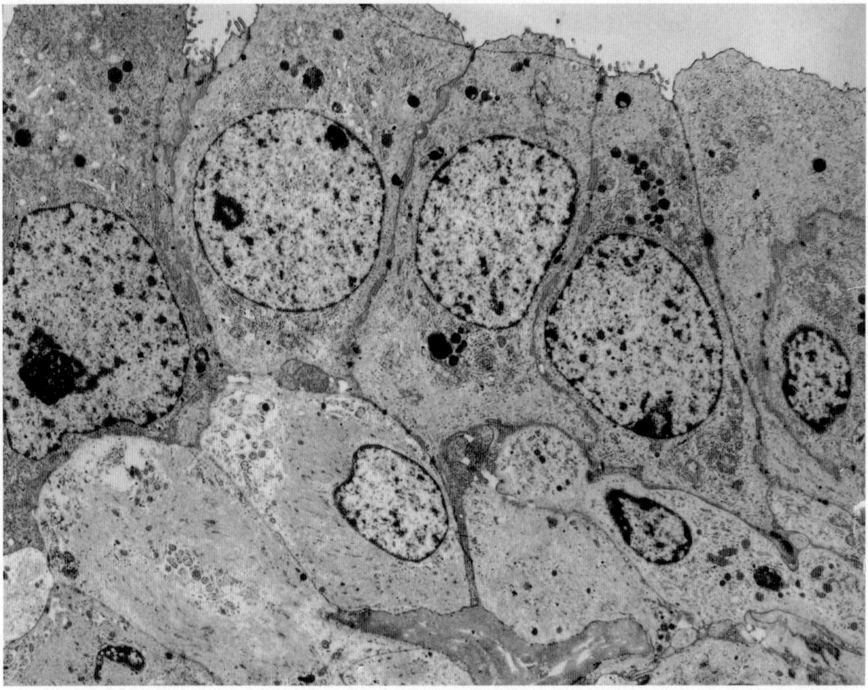

FIG. 4.37. Ductal hyperplasia. By electron microscopy, this proliferative duct has prominent columnar cells with secretory granules and microvilli that extend into the extracellular lumen. There is also a population of large active clear cells with intermediate filaments close to the basement membrane, indicative of their myoepithelial differentiation.

lobular carcinoma *in situ*/lobular neoplasia or ADH. Black et al. (56) described a grading system for ductal atypia and found a fivefold increase in the risk of cancer in patients with high-grade atypia, compared with patients who had changes characterized as normal or hyperplastic.

There have been several studies of the precancerous significance of the various benign epithelial proliferations of the breast that are associated with fibrocystic disease. Foote and Stewart (57) started this discussion in a comparison of proliferations in breasts that contained cancers with those that did not contain cancer. Black et al. (56), Jensen et al. (60), and Wellings et al. (63) suggested that atypical epithelial proliferative lesions were associated with an increased risk of breast cancer. Monson et al. (62) showed an increased risk of 1.7 to 5 times that of the population at large for proliferative breast disease. This is consistent with the findings of most of the other authors, although Devitt (64) found no increased risk.

Page et al. (65) reviewed the histology of benign breast biopsy specimens from 1,058 women and correlated each feature with the appearance of carcinoma during the follow-up period. The authors found no significant increase

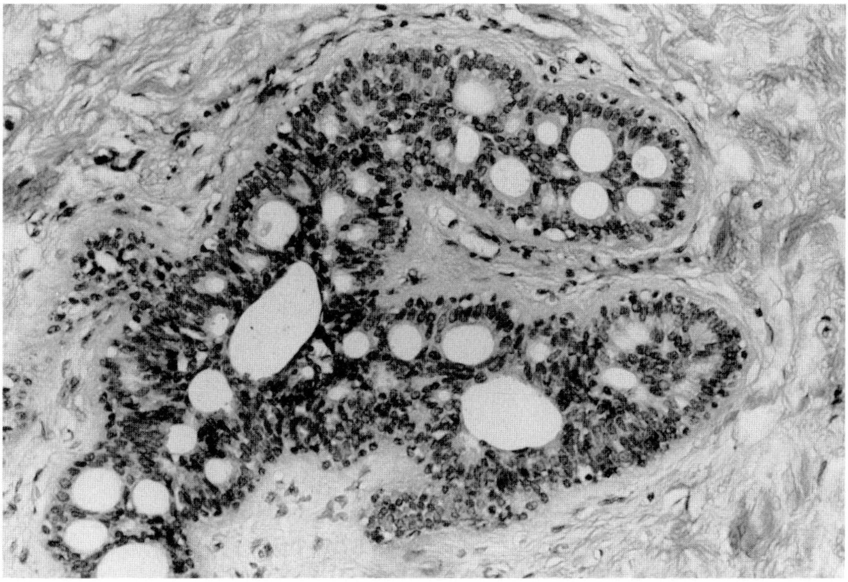

FIG. 4.38. Regular ductal hyperplasia in a small duct. Nuclei are small, touching, and without pattern, although there is a regularity to the extracellular lumens.

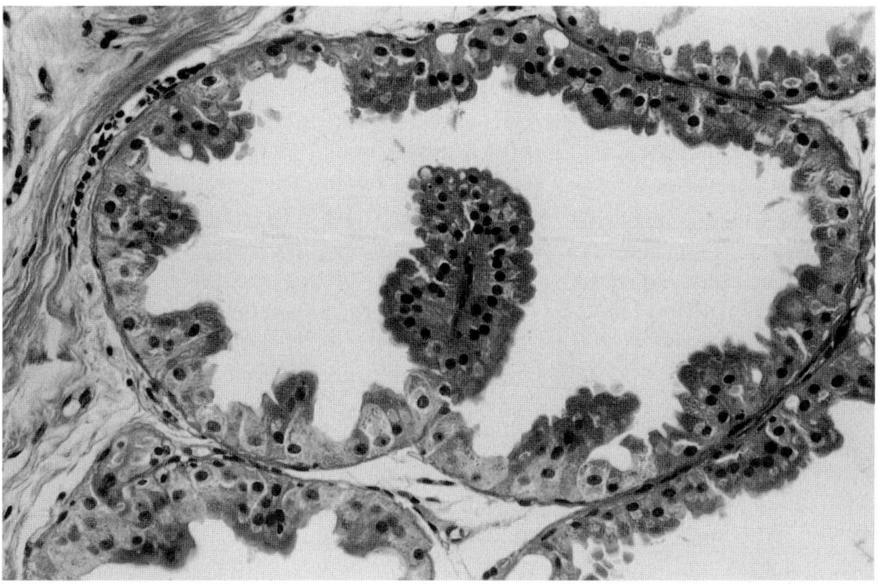

FIG. 4.39. Ductal hyperplasia with a simple micropapillary pattern that is composed of cells with apocrine metaplasia.

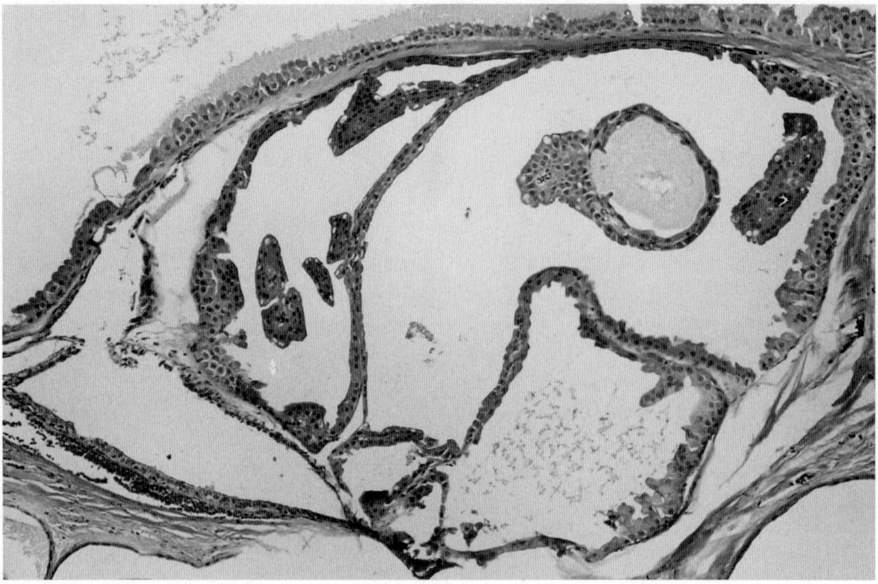

FIG. 4.40. Ductal hyperplasia in a large duct with irregular proliferation of a population that is rich in apocrine cells.

over the expected incidence of cancer in women with cystic disease, ductal ectasia, cysts, sclerosing adenosis, or fibroadenoma. Patients with DH or papillary apocrine hyperplasia in biopsy specimens that were taken before the age of 45 years had no increased risk, but the same lesions observed in women who were older than 45 years were associated with a twofold increase in the number of observed cancers. In this earlier and smaller study, ADH was not different from DH without atypia. Atypical lobular hyperplasia was associated with a sixfold increase in observed cancers when found in biopsy specimens from women under age 45 years, but only a threefold increase when seen in an older age group.

In 1993, Dupont et al. (66) reported on the Breast Cancer Detection Demonstration Project cases and confirmed the increased risk of breast cancer in the presence of proliferative disease and proliferative disease with atypia. Using as a reference population a group of patients who underwent breast biopsy and were found not to have proliferative disease, the study found a relative risk of 1.3 for carcinoma of the breast for proliferative disease without atypia and a relative risk of 4.3 for proliferative disease with atypical hyperplasia. Other studies have shown a range of relative risk of 1.3 to 1.9 for proliferative disease without atypia and of 3.7 to 13 for atypical hyperplasia. The study by Palli et al. (67) showed the highest risk for atypical hyperplasia at 13-fold. The study by London et al. (68) presented a relative risk of 1.6 and 3.7 for typical and atypical hyper-

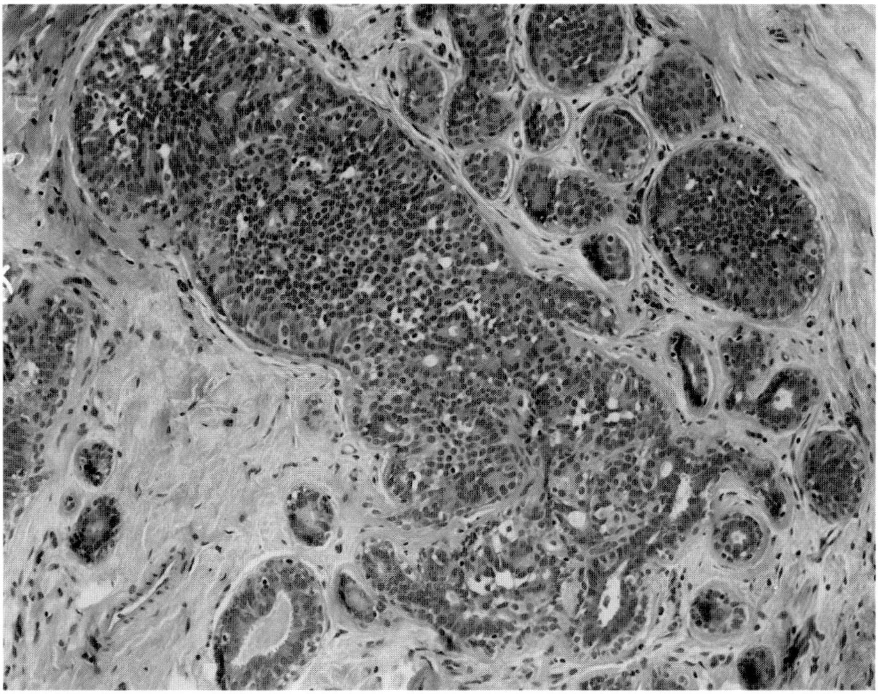

FIG. 4.41. Ductal hyperplasia. The large duct has irregular placement of nuclei and extracellular lumens with no consistent pattern. The smaller duct at the 2 o'clock position has atypical ducal hyperplasia.

plasia, respectively, and the previous study of Page et al. (65) reported 1.9 and 5.3 for relative risk of typical and atypical hyperplasia, respectively. Atypical hyperplasia, combined with a family history of breast cancer, had a relative risk of 22 for subsequent development of cancer of the breast, whereas atypical hyperplasia, without a family history, still had a relative risk of 4.2. A family history with no proliferative disease had a relative risk of 3.6. The presence of cysts in the breast had a relative risk of 1.9, whereas the presence of cysts with a family history of breast cancer had a relative risk of 4.2. These data indicate the importance of both atypical hyperplasia and family history in the prediction of the likelihood of development of cancer of the breast. Crissman et al. (69) studied the DNA content of 25 atypical hyperplasias and 35 intraductal carcinomas of the breast. The authors found DNA aneuploidy in 71% of the cases of DCIS and in 36% of the cases of ADH. The aneuploidy in DCIS correlated with a high nuclear grade and poor architectural differentiation. Aneuploidy was found in 63% of the nuclear grade 2 cases of DCIS and in 93% of the nuclear grade 3 cases. Thirty-eight percent of the cases of cribriform DCIS were aneuploid, whereas 82% of the solid variants of DCIS had an abnormal DNA histogram.

Summary

DH is much more common and has far more histologic variation than DCIS. In hyperplasia, both myoepithelial and epithelial cells proliferate and the latter often undergo focal apocrine metaplasia. The pattern of cells and their nuclei are irregular and unpredictable and small nuclei touch, overlap, and swirl. Extracellular lumina are slit-like, and the proliferating cells are spaced in an irregular way with overlapping nuclei (Table 4.1). ADH has a more regular pattern in part of the duct and generally lacks a prominent myoepithelial layer, but it lacks a consistent pattern and clearly malignant nuclei.

In DCIS, one cell type dominates, nuclei are regularly spaced, and the extracellular lumina may be rounded and tend to be more similar in size and more regular in distribution; however, regularity or mosaicism in the placement of nuclei is greater than the regularity of the low-power appearance of the proliferative pattern. A prominent fibrovascular papillary stalk is more often seen in DH (papillomatosis). The nuclei may be cytologically malignant in DCIS, but cytology is not the only guide to the diagnosis.

LOCALIZED INTRADUCTAL LESIONS

Localized intraductal lesions present as grossly evident tumorous masses and include IPC, solitary papillomas, multiple papillomas, and juvenile papillomatosis.

Papillary Carcinomas

Four categories of papillary carcinoma of the breast have been distinguished: (a) the previously described variants of DCIS, a noninvasive carcinoma extending into the medium and smaller ducts throughout the breast tissue, which is not evident grossly as a single tumor and may be papillary or micropapillary; (b) IPC, a large (greater than 3 mm in diameter) grossly evident tumor that is confined to a cystically dilated duct; (c) invasive papillary carcinoma, a rare form of invasive carcinoma characterized by a papillary structure and frequently associated with one of the noninvasive forms. Two or all three of these forms may coexist; and (d) a fourth type of papillary carcinoma is the micropapillary form of invasive carcinoma, often with angiolymphatic invasion (Chapter 8).

Papillary carcinomas of the breast are rare lesions that are classified in a variety of ways by different authors. Stewart (70) used the term noninfiltrating papillary carcinoma to refer to a lesion "limited to the mammary duct system and affecting the large, medium, or small radicals" and separately described intracystic carcinoma. McDivitt et al. (71) used the term noninfiltrating papillary carcinoma synonymously with intraductal carcinoma, *in situ* ductal carcinoma, and intraductal papillary carcinoma; however, the authors also described intracystic carcinoma separately. A number of authors have distinguished diffuse intraductal carcinoma or DCIS from the localized, so-called IPCs. Most authors distinguish between noninvasive and invasive papillary carcinomas, and Fisher et al. (72) reported a series of invasive papillary carcinomas. An invasive micropapillary carcinoma has also been described (73).

Intracystic Papillary Carcinoma

IPCs are rare, accounting for 0.5% to 1% of breast cancers. They are usually found in older women, may be bulky lesions, and are usually located away from the nipple. Grossly, they are circumscribed, cystic, and often necrotic (Fig. 4.42 and efigs. 4.113 and 4.114). Microscopically, they have a papillary configuration with fibrovascular cores that are covered by a single or multiple layer of cells; however, other patterns may also be present (Figs. 4.43 to 4.54 and efigs. 4.115 to 4.129). The older literature on this topic is confusing. Gatchell et al. (74) reported 48 such cases, but included 15 tumors in which invasive cancer was present in the breast, its veins, and/or its lymphatics. Sixteen percent of these patients were dead within 5 years, but it is not clear from the discussion whether they were the patients with invasive carcinomas. Czernobilsky (75) described 14 patients with intracystic carcinoma, but, in 5 patients, there was invasion outside of the cyst wall and, in 12 patients, the cyst wall was invaded. Two of these patients had axillary lymph node metastases and two other patients died of disease 9 and 10 years after simple mastectomy. McKittrick et al. (76) described 16 cases of IPC. How-

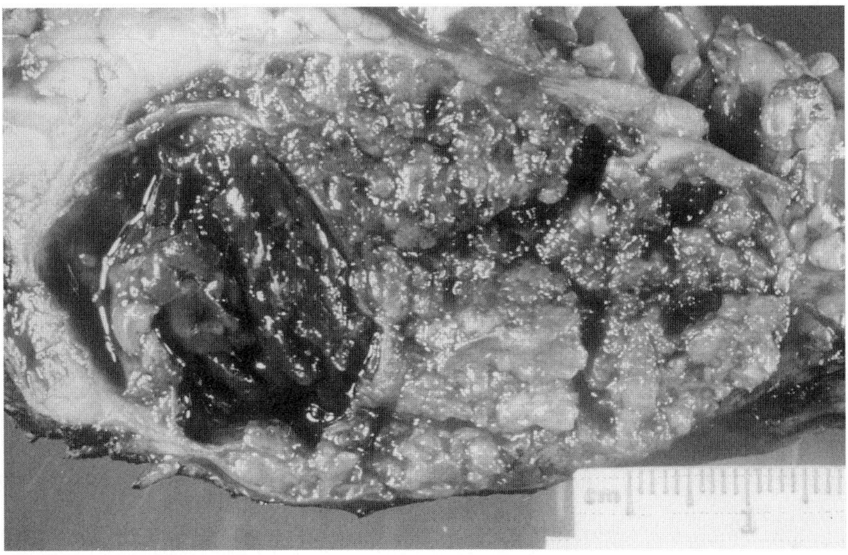

FIG. 4.42. Intracystic papillary carcinoma. This gross photograph illustrates a 6-cm intracystic mass that is markedly hemorrhagic and necrotic. Although there is no size that is diagnostic of malignancy in papillary neoplasms, the larger tumors are more likely to be malignant.

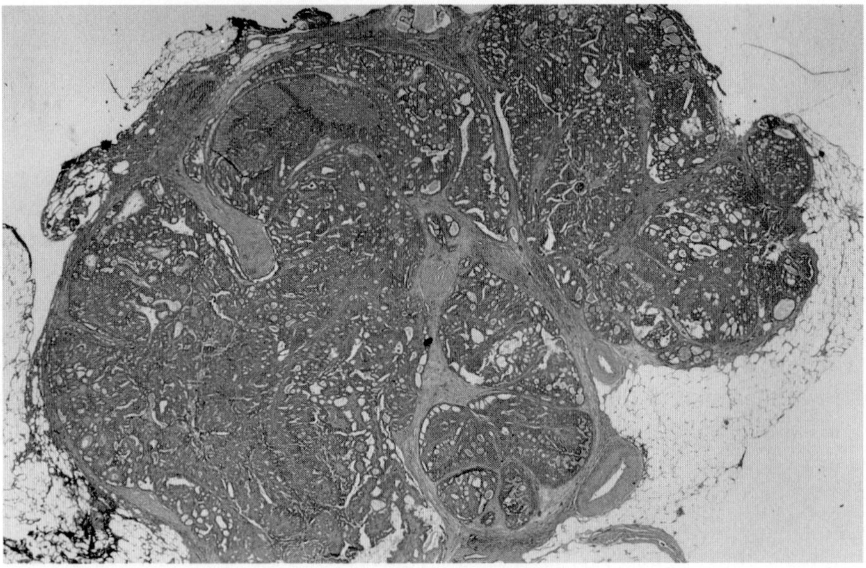

FIG. 4.43. Intracystic papillary carcinoma. This intracystic papillary lesion is markedly hypercellular at low magnification. It appears to be semisolid in some areas, but comprised of regular proliferations in others. It does not extend beyond the duct.

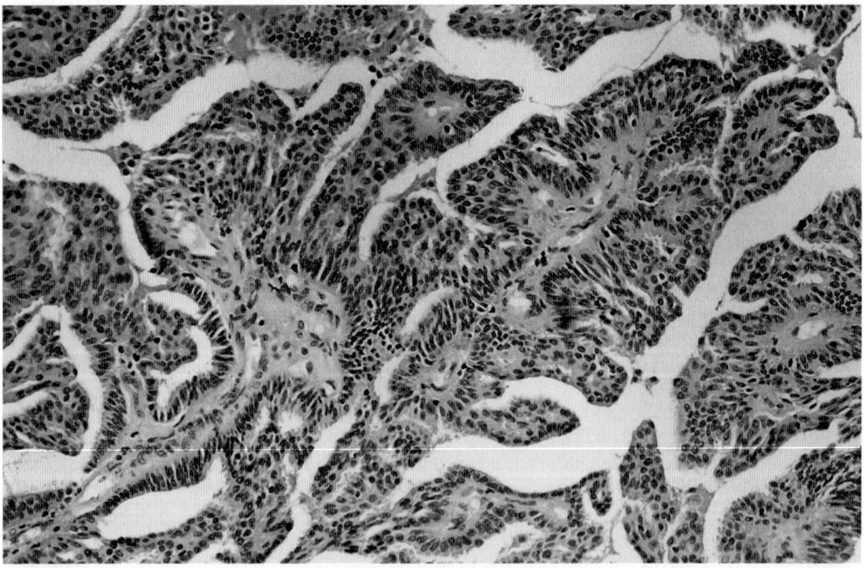

FIG. 4.44. Intracystic papillary carcinoma. A dense fibrovascular core is suggestive of a benign proliferation, but closer inspection shows that a single columnar cell population is proliferating perpendicular to the capillaries.

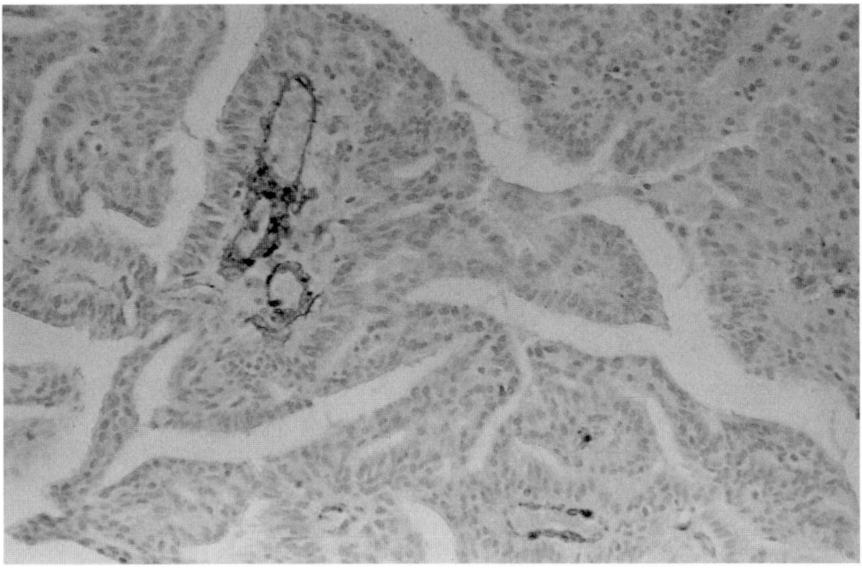

FIG. 4.45. Intracystic papillary carcinoma (IPC). The IPC shown in the preceding photomicrograph has been immunostained for smooth muscle actin. The smooth muscle associated with the blood vessels in the central cores is clearly decorated, but no myoepithelial layer is present on these fibrovascular cores. This is characteristic of carcinoma.

ever, in five of the cases, the entire breast was involved, suggesting that these were massive lesions in which invasion was probably present. Four of the 11 patients who had axillary lymph node dissections were found to have metastatic disease. Hunter and Sawyers (77) reported seven cases of IPC. One of them metastasized to axillary lymph nodes, bone, and viscera, but the definition of IPC they used is not clear. Squires and Betsill (78) described the cytology of IPC.

Most of the patients with IPC are of advanced age and have a prolonged duration of symptoms prior to surgery. Kraus and Neubecker (79) carefully described 21 patients with papillary carcinoma, using classic criteria (Table 4.5, see page 144). However, 2 of the 8 criteria used by the authors for the recognition of papillary carcinoma are epithelial invasion of stroma and intraductal carcinoma in adjacent ducts. Multiple separate foci were present in 2 of the 7 cases that were studied for this feature, and 47% of the carcinomas showed a cribriform pattern of DCIS in ducts adjacent to the grossly evident tumor. The overall prognosis in that group was not good, and radical mastectomy was recommended for those patients. Four of 6 patients treated with local

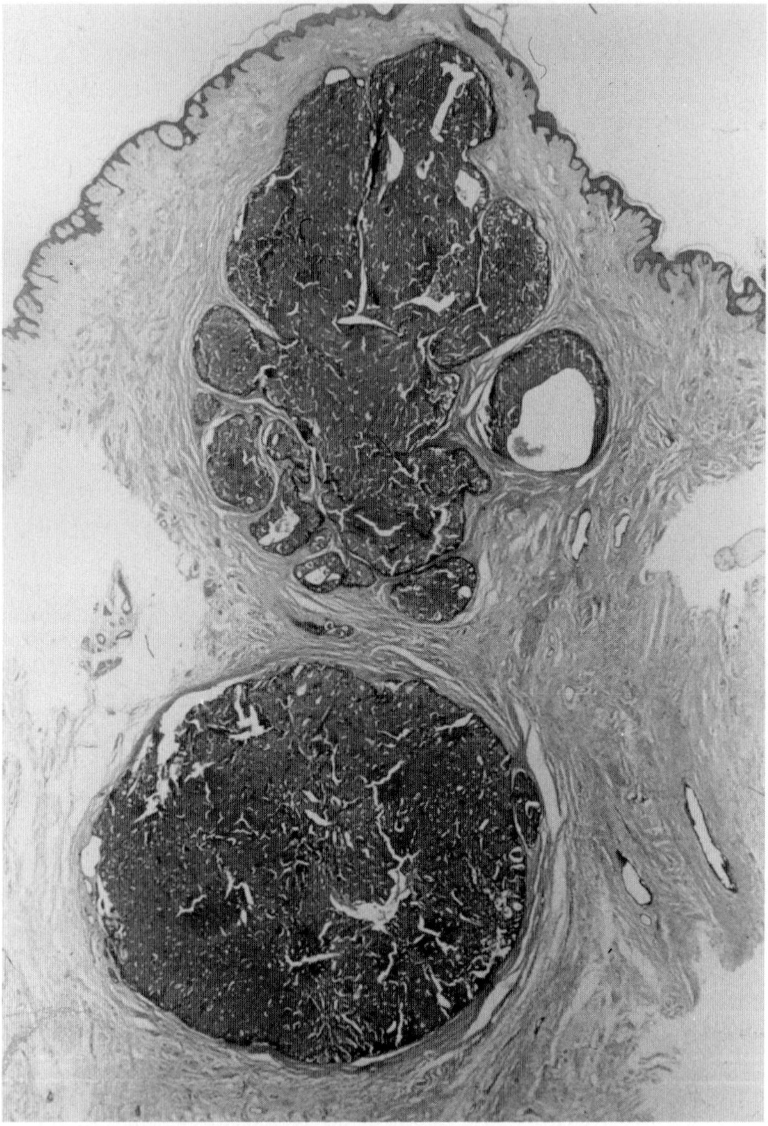

FIG. 4.46. Intracystic papillary carcinoma alone. Unusual in its location within the nipple, this lesion presents as a large intracystic papillary mass confined to the lactiferous ducts. The branching segmental collecting ducts are not involved.

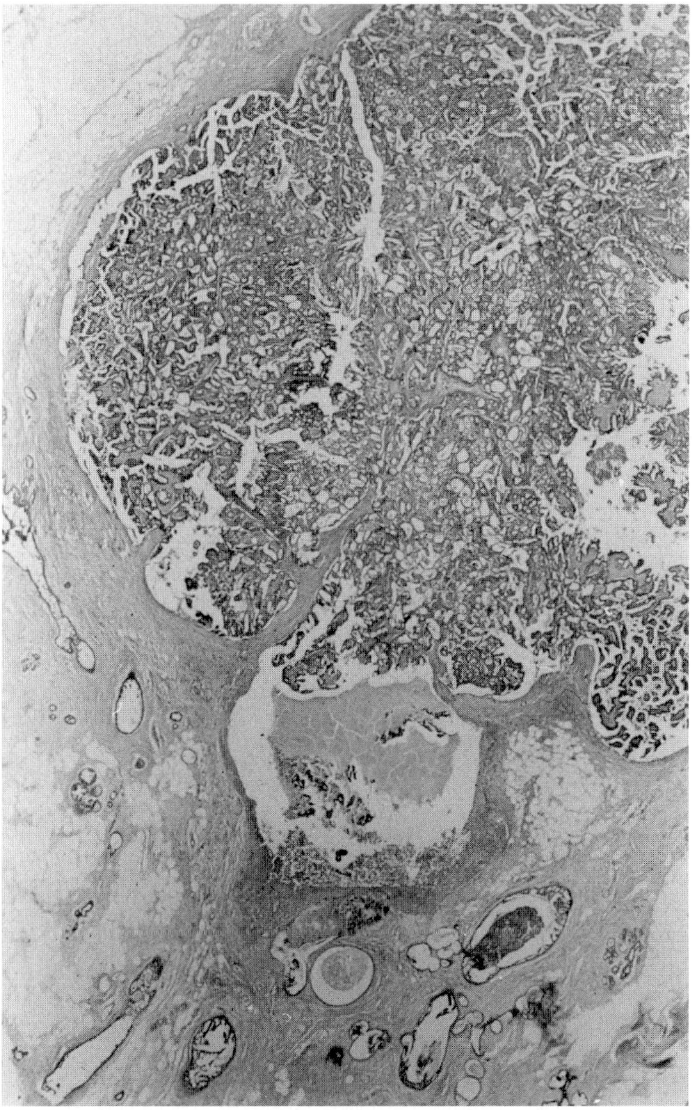

FIG. 4.47. Intracystic papillary carcinoma (IPC) with ductal carcinoma *in situ*. In this intracystic and intraductal lesion, one can see extensive micropapillary intraductal carcinoma in the medium-sized ducts (**lower half**) around the IPC.

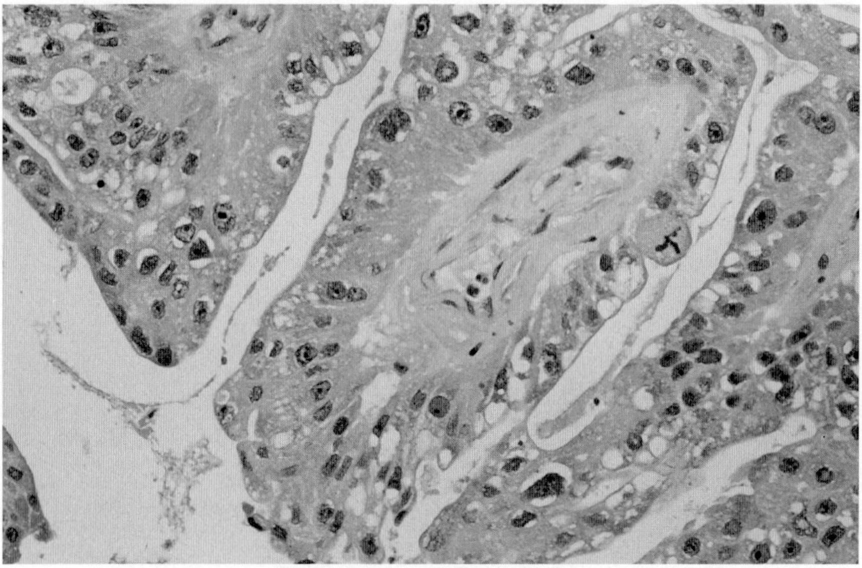

FIG. 4.48. Intracystic papillary carcinoma. The predominant pattern is papillary. Note the tripolar mitotic figure.

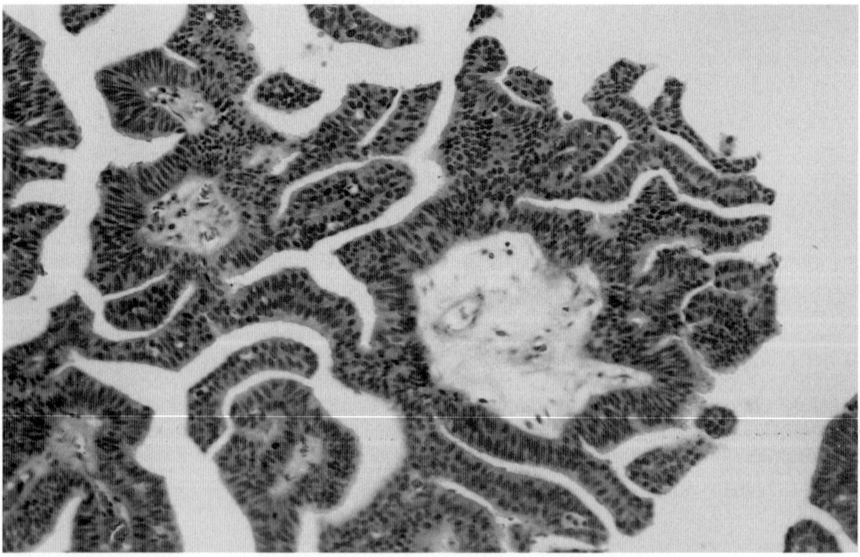

FIG. 4.49. Intracystic papillary carcinoma. Micropapillary pattern with minimal fibrovascular core. Note the proliferation of a single columnar cell type on either side of the central core. This picket fence configuration is characteristic of a malignant lesion. The cytologic features of the cells are of nuclear grade 1.

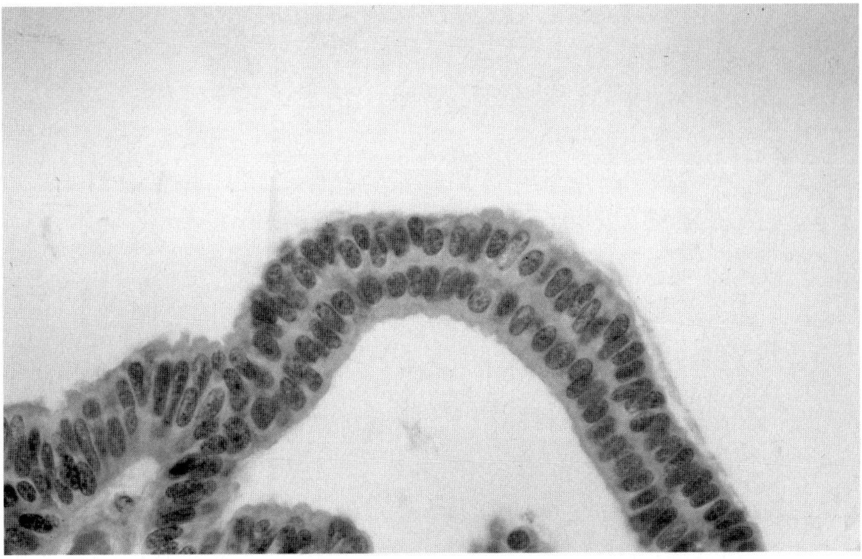

FIG. 4.50. Intracystic papillary carcinoma. At higher magnification, picket fence orientation of the columnar cells without a myoepithelium is evident.

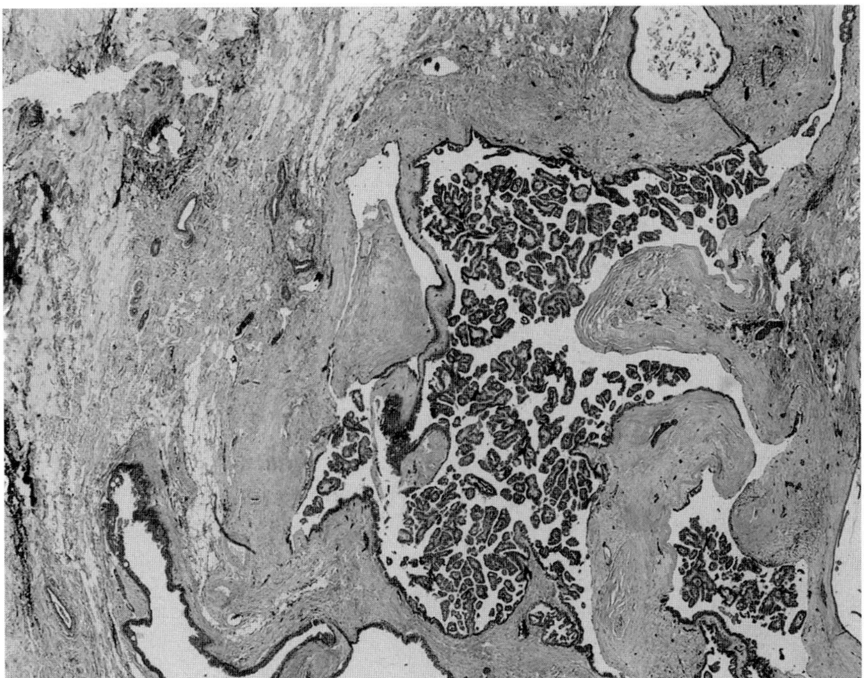

FIG. 4.51. Intracystic papillary carcinoma (IPC). The predominant feature is the scar that extends around and into the duct. Entrapment of papillary areas in the central portion of this IPC does not indicate aggressive behavior, but infiltration at the periphery of the cyst must be viewed with considerable concern.

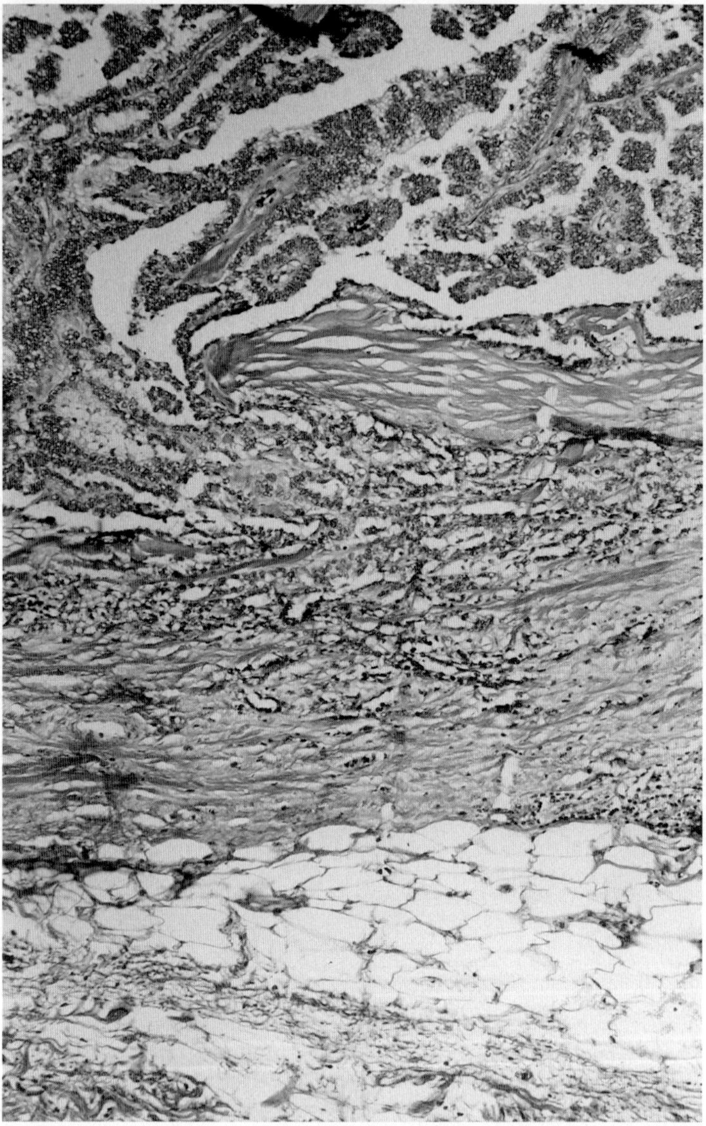

FIG. 4.52. Intracystic papillary carcinoma (IPC) with invasion. The IPC has a dense fibrous wall infiltrated by the carcinoma, which extends approximately two-thirds through its wall (**upper part**). The presence of areas such as this should be a source of concern and indicates invasion.

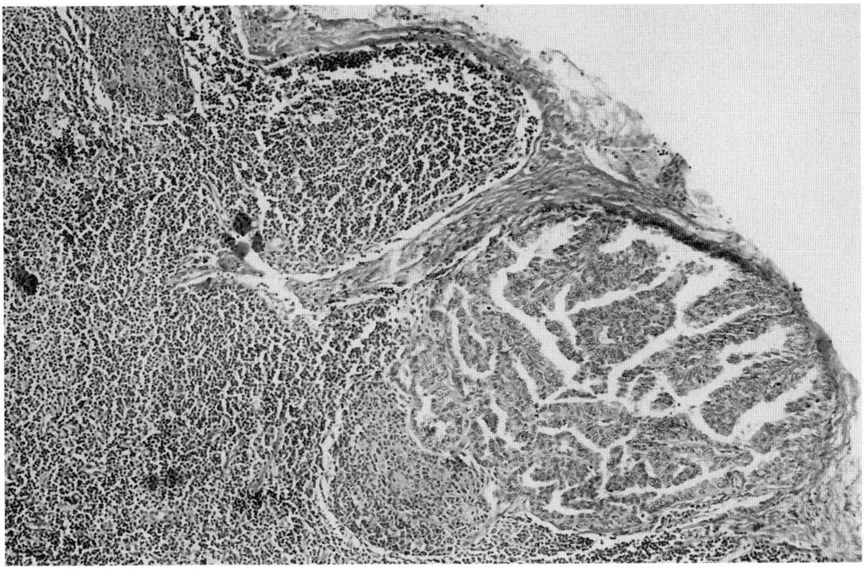

FIG. 4.53. Metastatic papillary carcinoma in an axillary lymph node. In the case shown in Fig. 4.52, a low axillary lymph node dissection was carried out and this subcapsular deposit of papillary carcinoma was present in one of the nodes.

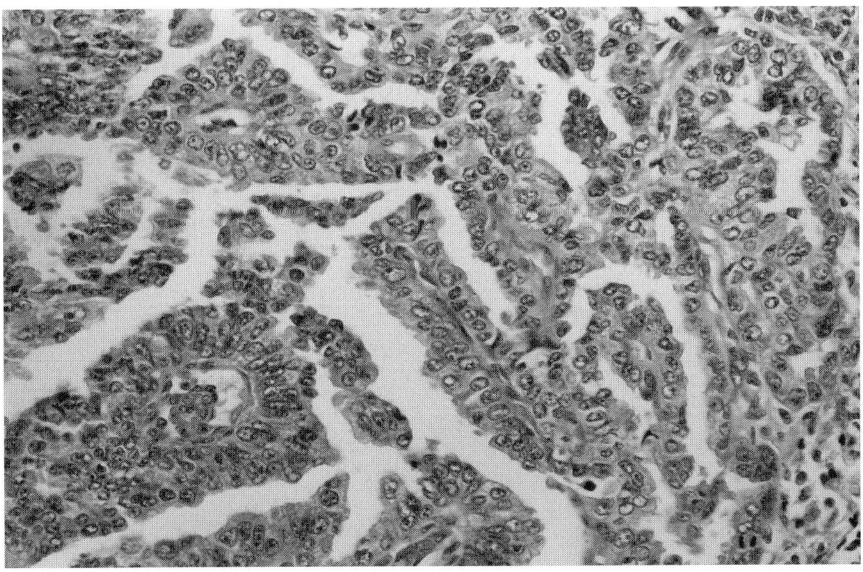

FIG. 4.54. Metastatic papillary carcinoma. At higher magnification, the papillary nature of the carcinoma, with its thin fibrovascular cores covered by single or multiple layers of a monomorphous proliferation of malignant cells with nuclear grade 2, is evident. This patient had no evidence of spread beyond the axillary lymph nodes.

TABLE 4.5. *Criteria for the diagnosis of papillary breast tumors*

Papilloma	Papillary carcinoma
Two cell types	One
Nuclei normal	Abnormal
Apocrine metaplasia	None
Complex pattern	Papillary or cribriform
Fibrovascular core	Less prominent
Entrapment in cyst	Invasion of cyst
Ductal hyperplasia	Ductal carcinoma *in situ*

From Kraus FT, Neubecker RD. The differential diagnosis of papillary tumors of the breast. *Cancer* 1962;15:444–455, with permission.

excision, 2 of 5 patients treated by simple mastectomy, and 3 of 10 patients treated by radical mastectomy had recurrences or metastases.

Carter et al. (80) reported a group of 41 cases of IPCs that were categorized as IPC alone, IPC with DCIS, and IPC with invasive carcinoma and distinguished from the DCIS and/or invasive carcinoma that often accompanies them. Among 15 patients treated by mastectomy for IPC associated with invasive ductal carcinoma, lymph node metastases were found in one-third of the cases in which lymphadenectomy was performed, and two of those patients died of breast cancer at 60 to 84 months. Eleven of these 15 patients had IPC, DCIS, and invasive ductal carcinoma. Twenty-nine patients with IPC without invasive cancer were treated by mastectomy and/or radiotherapy, and none of them died of disease. In 11 patients with lymph node dissections, there was no lymph node metastasis. IPC was separated into IPC alone (Fig. 4.46 and efig. 4.123), IPC with DCIS (Figs. 4.47 and efig. 4.124), and IPC with invasive cancer (Fig. 4.52 and efigs. 4.125 and 4.126).

In 11 cases of IPC, no mastectomy or radiotherapy was carried out after the biopsy was performed. Four patients with IPC, combined with DCIS, subsequently developed ipsilateral invasive carcinoma, but none of the seven patients with IPC without associated DCIS developed invasive carcinoma. Conversely, all of the patients who subsequently developed recurrence or invasive breast cancer had DCIS in association with the IPC. Seven patients with IPC, in the absence of DCIS, were treated by local excision and had no recurrence of disease after follow-up of 7 to 14 years. This study documents the association of IPC with DCIS and invasive carcinoma. It also reinforces the notion that intraductal carcinoma is a significant preinvasive lesion, but distinguishes the rare completely IPCs that may be an indolent tumor, in much the same way as papillary carcinoma of the bladder. The pathologist can therefore interpret completely intracystic papillary tumors as carcinoma with caution, as they are not terribly aggressive lesions. Conversely, the significance of the DCIS lesion is not to be underestimated.

Lefkowitz et al. (81) described 77 cases of IPC of the breast and also distinguished the cases into three categories: IPC alone, IPC associated with DCIS, and IPC associated with invasive carcinoma. Among the 35 cases of IPC alone and the 22 cases of IPC with DCIS, there were no recurrences and none of the patients developed distant metastases. Among the 20 patients with IPC and invasive carcinoma, 6 patients developed chest-wall recurrence and 3 developed distant metastases. The authors reported an age range of 34 to 92 years, with a mean age of 67 years. Only 9 of the 77 patients were 50 years of age or younger. Only 24 of the 77 patients had subareolar or central tumors. The tumor sizes ranged from 4 mm to 7.5 cm.

Leal et al. (82) reported on 29 additional cases of IPC divided as IPC alone, IPC with DCIS, and IPC with invasive carcinoma. The median age of the patients was 75 years, and most of their IPCs had low or intermediate nuclear grade, strongly expressed ER, and were negative for c-erbB-2. Lymph node metastasis was found in only one case and that patient had associated invasive carcinoma. The authors concluded that IPC is a low-grade carcinoma with overall good prognosis, but with a high frequency of associated DCIS or invasive carcinoma and that the associated carcinomas of higher grade determine the prognosis (Table 4.6).

Does IPC invade and metastasize? Yes, but rarely. Figures 4.53 and 4.54 and efig. 4.127 show a case with invasion of the cyst wall by IPC with axillary lymph node metastasis. It appears that the area where there is concern about true invasion is the capsule and not the central stalk, in which ducts are entrapped by the fibrovascular stroma.

There has been discussion in the literature about whether IPC arises in preexisting benign papillomas, and it is unlikely that this question can be definitively answered. Diagnosis of a benign papilloma requires examination of the entire lesion and therefore precludes follow-up. There is no good evidence to suggest that this transformation occurs often. McDivitt et al. (83) found no excisions of papillomas before the appearance of papillary carcinoma, and Carter (84) found no papillary carcinoma during the follow-up of benign papillomas. Some (about 20%) IPCs have areas with the features of a benign papilloma, which makes interpretation of the lesion difficult and also raises the pos-

TABLE 4.6. *Intracystic papillary carcinoma in three series categorized by associated lesions*

	Alone	With ductal carcinoma *in situ*	With invasion
Carter (80)	21 (0)	19 (0)	15 (2)
Lefkowitz (81)	35 (0)	22 (0)	20 (9)
Leal (82)	>9 (0)	>9 (0)	>11 (1)
	>65 (0)	>50 (0)	>46 (12)

Numbers in parentheses (column 1) indicate reference; numbers in columns 2–4 indicate number of cases; numbers in parentheses indicate recurrence or lymph node metastasis.

sibility that a morphologically benign papillary tumor preceded the appearance of the malignant one.

Intraductal Papillomas

IPs are 6 times as common as IPCs and 10 times as common as IPCs that are not associated with DCIS. The differential diagnosis of papillomas from IPCs is compounded by the relative rarity and the relatively benign clinical course of the IPC. Papillomas occur in all age groups, in all areas of the breast, and present as lumps, bloody nipple discharge, or both. They can best be found by dissection of the ductal system from which blood is expressed, if no mass is present. Grossly, they may be associated with large- or medium-sized ducts to which they are confined (Fig. 4.55 and efig. 4.130). Microscopically, they usually have prominent fibrovascular cores, but they may be quite cellular and irregular (Fig. 4.56, 4.57, and efigs. 4.130 to 4.146), and they may have all the patterns shown as DH. Papilloma may be associated with radial scar (Fig. 4.58) (Chapter 6) and may contain atypical hyperplasia.

In addition to the difficulties and controversy over the diagnosis of IP and, perhaps, in part because of these difficulties, controversy persists over the significance of IPs as precancerous lesions. Most authors believe that IPs of the breast are rarely associated with invasive carcinoma during the follow-up period. Kraus and Neubecker (79), Hendrick (85), Haagensen et al. (86), Hart (87), and

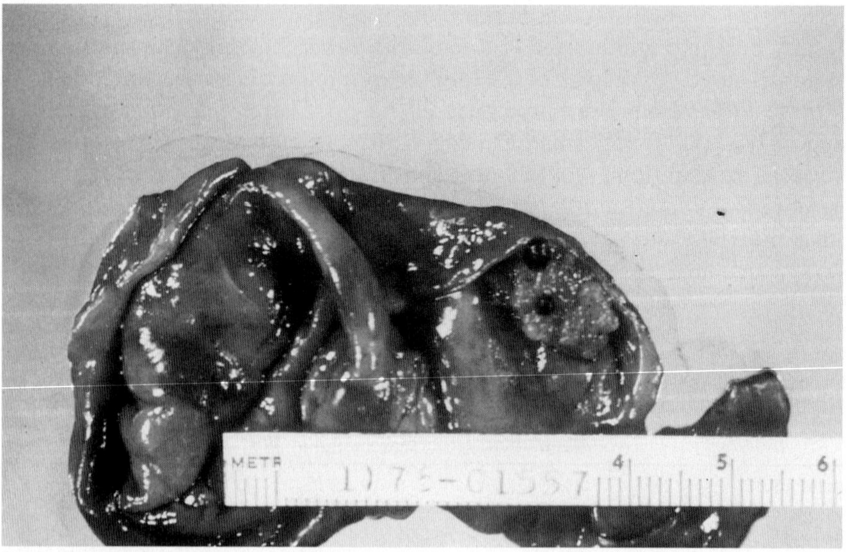

FIG. 4.55. Intracystic papilloma. This distended duct filled with blood contains a 7-mm nodule attached to its inner surface.

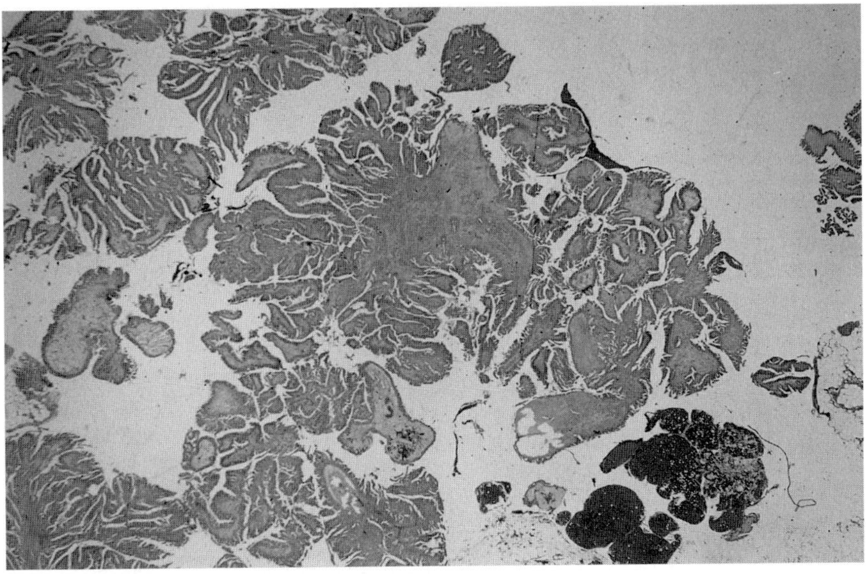

FIG. 4.56. Papilloma. The intracystic papillary proliferation is characterized by a dense fibrovascular core on which there is a modest proliferation.

Lewison and Lyons (88) reported a total of 427 cases of IPs of the breast in which carcinoma developed during the follow-up period in only two patients (0.4%), during a follow-up that, in most studies, ranged from 5 to 22 years. This is much less than the incidence of breast cancer in the general population and therefore raises some questions. Three other series of papillomas—those by Buhl-Jorgensen et al. (89), Moore et al. (90), and Kilgore et al. (91)—showed the development of cancer in 19 of 235 cases during a follow-up period of 4 months to 16 years. This is an incidence of 8%, which is closer to what might be anticipated. Such a large discrepancy suggests that some other factors are operative. Immediately, one might question if different diagnostic criteria had been used. Moore et al. (90) invited three expert pathologists to review seven papillary lesions (of 125) that were followed by invasive cancer. Three of the lesions were judged to have been papillary carcinomas from the beginning, but four lesions were not. Carter (84) reported on 64 cases of IPs of the breast, followed for a period of 5 to 17 years. Six lesions recurred as papillomas, and six patients went on to develop breast cancer. Two of the patients who developed carcinoma of the breast were among six patients with multiple papillomas, a lesion that Haagensen et al. (86) regarded as a precancerous condition. In 14 patients, there was distinct hyperplasia or papillomatosis of the associated ducts. Two of these patients developed breast cancer. Among 44 patients in whom there were only nonproliferative cystic changes or fibroadenomas, only 5% developed carci-

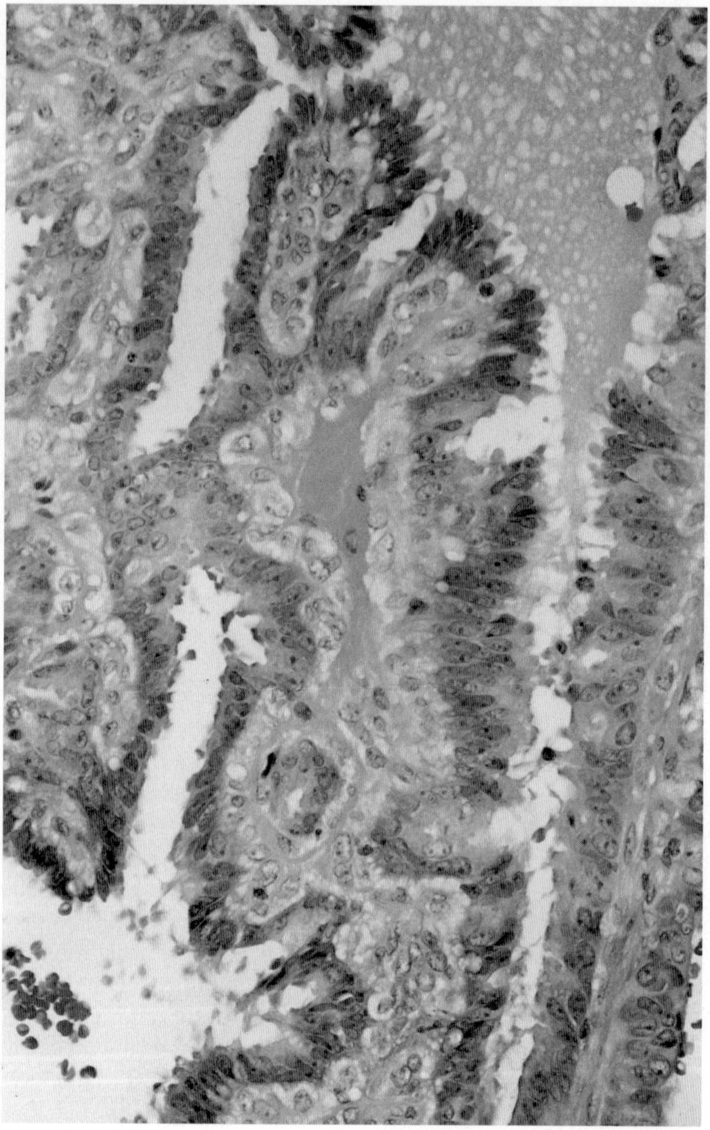

FIG. 4.57. Papilloma. At higher magnification, the papillary epithelial prominence is the result of proliferation of both myoepithelial and epithelial layers. The hyperplasia of the myoepithelial layer is striking in this area and is a strong indication that the lesion is benign.

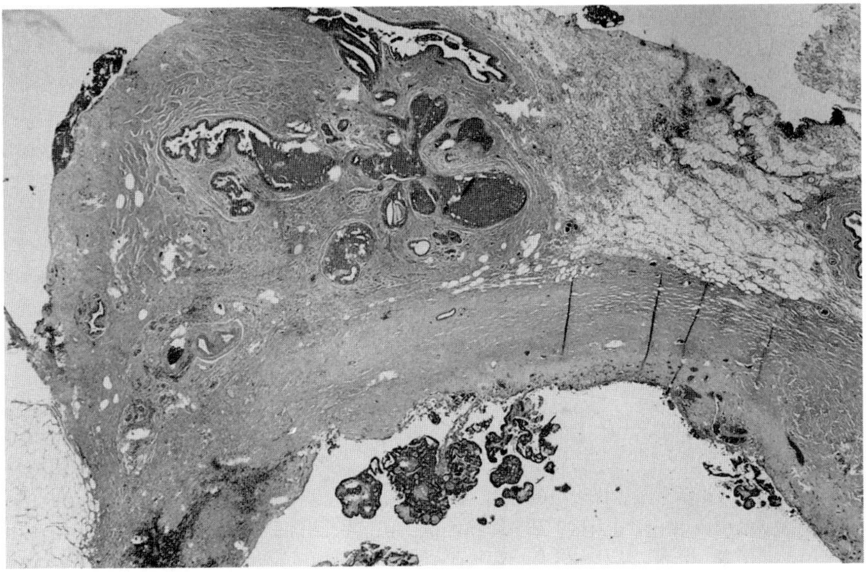

FIG. 4.58. Intracystic papilloma with associated radial scar. There is a dense scar in the wall of a dilated duct, from which a papilloma is proliferating (**lower half**). Immediately adjacent to the cyst wall, there is a radial scar (Chapter 6). The association of radial scar with papilloma occurs more often than by chance and suggests that some radial scars arise from papillomas. It also demonstrates that pseudoinfiltrative lesions may be part of the cyst wall and must be analyzed independently of the intracystic papillary tumor.

noma. The incidence of carcinoma in that series, although small, is different from that reported from one institution (Johns Hopkins) by Hart (87) and Lewison and Lyons (88), covering a period from 1895 to 1941. Among that group of 127 cases, 82 were treated by simple or radical mastectomy for the papillary tumors, which were histologically diagnosed as benign. Mastectomy obviously precludes ipsilateral breast cancer recurrence. A similar finding was evident in the series reported by Haagensen et al. (86), in which 32 of 108 patients with IP underwent mastectomy for the lesion. Papillomas must be distinguished from IPC, but one can be conservative with this diagnosis and in the treatment of IPC when it is found in the absence of DCIS.

Ciatto et al. (92) described 339 cases of benign IP that were followed for an average of 6.6 years. Ten breast cancers developed during this follow-up period, which was 10 times the expected number and was calculated to present a relative risk of 3.33 for the presence of IP. All of the breast cancers observed occurred in the same breast as the papilloma. No difference in relative risk was observed between single and multiple papillomas.

Rosen (93) reviewed the literature of 612 solitary papillomas that were treated by excision and found 11 ipsilateral carcinomas (2%), 10 contralateral carcinomas (2%), and 3 bilateral carcinomas (0.3%) in follow-up. The author concluded that solitary papillomas were not precancerous. Page et al. (94) conducted a case control study of women with papillomas that contained areas of atypical hyperplasia and found them to have a fourfold increased risk of cancer, compared to women with excision of papillomas that lacked atypia. Raju et al. (95) compared 20 women with papillomas that contained areas of DCIS (evident by lack of a myoepithelial component) with 60 women with histologically benign papillomas. In the group with focal DCIS, two women developed DCIS in the same breast and two women developed invasive carcinoma in the contralateral breast. Among the patients with histologically benign papillomas, there was one ipsilateral and two contralateral carcinomas observed in follow-up.

Azzopardi and Salm (96) described a sclerotic papilloma of large ducts, in which there was marked scarring with distortion of entrapped ducts that simulated invasive ductal carcinoma. Positive stains for myoepithelial cells were useful in identifying their benign nature. The authors used the term "ductal adenoma." Lammie and Millis (97) reported on 15 cases of ductal adenomas and concluded that they evolved by sclerosis of benign IPs. Ductal adenomas are much more difficult to correctly identify on core needle biopsies where they simulate invasive carcinoma to a marked degree (efigs. 4.141 to 4.146).

MULTIPLE PAPILLOMAS

Although only a few cases of multiple papillomas have been reported, there is a strong suggestion from this limited literature that they are significantly precancerous lesions. Haagensen (86) considered multiple IPs to be precancerous. Murad et al. (98) reported a high rate of recurrence and malignant transformation in women with multiple papillomas, compared to no cancer and only one recurrence among 73 women with solitary papilloma. Ohuchi et al. (99) described 3-dimensional serial reconstructions of breasts with papillomas in which solitary papillomas were found that originated in large ducts, whereas multiple papillomas arose in association with terminal duct/lobular units. Six of 16 (37.5%) of the peripheral or multiple papilloma cases were associated with carcinomas, but none of the 9 solitary papillomas that originated centrally was associated with carcinoma. Papotti et al. (100) reported finding carcinoembryonic antigen (CEA) immunopositivity in both multiple papillomas and in DCIS, but not in solitary papillomas.

Multiple papilloma cases are rare, but deserve special attention and further study. To distinguish them from microscopic papillomatosis, a size cutoff is necessary. I have defined papilloma as a grossly evident lesion that is usually at least 3 mm in diameter (Figs. 4.59 and 4.60 and efigs. 4.147 and 4.148). Recurrence of papillomas, even when they are histologically benign, should raise a suspicion for heightened risk of nonpapillary invasive carcinoma.

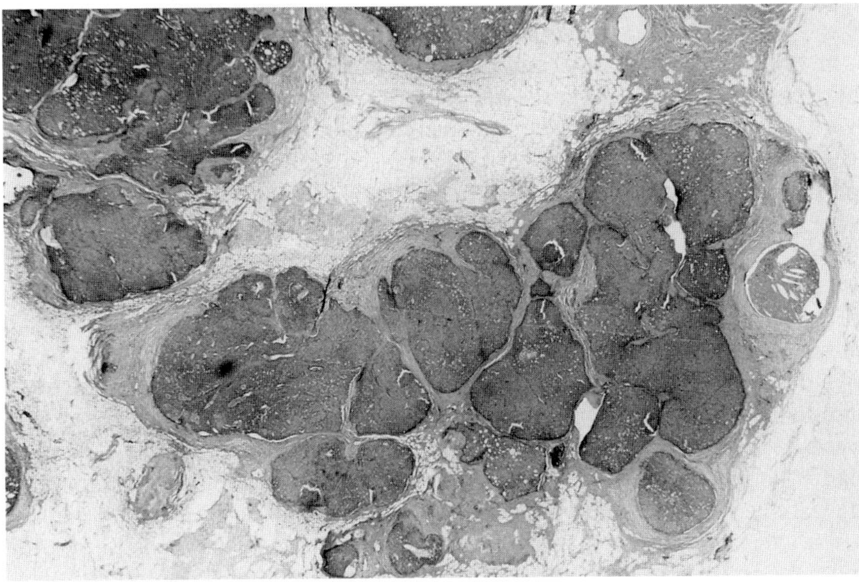

FIG. 4.59. Multiple papillomas. This low magnification photomicrograph shows multiple large ducts filled with papillary and solid growths.

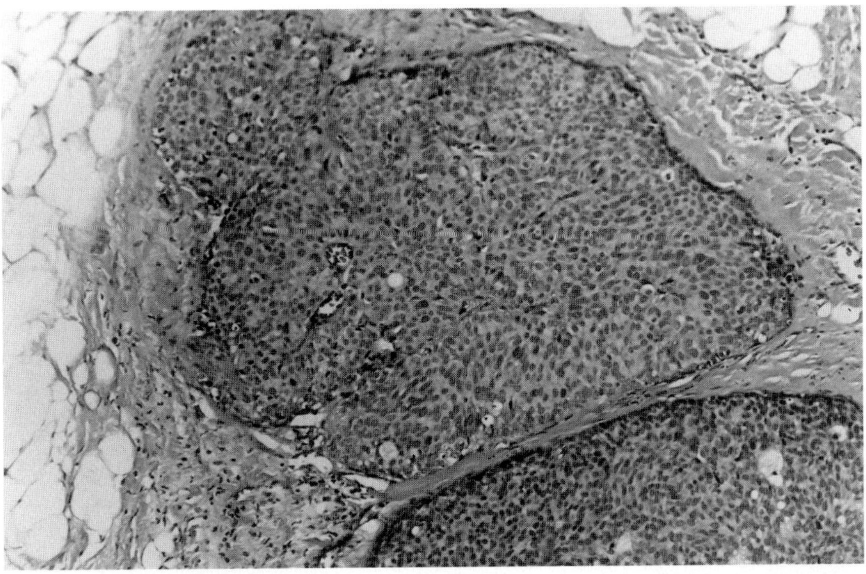

FIG. 4.60. Multiple papillomas. One of the intracystic tumors with a solid, but histologically benign appearance.

Juvenile Papillomatosis

In 1980, Rosen et al. (101) described 37 cases of juvenile papillomatosis of the breast in which the average age was 19 years, with a range from 10 to 44 years. The patients presented with localized multinodular masses that microscopically were characterized by the presence of numerous papillomas, somewhat severe cytologic atypia, and the presence of numerous dilated cysts that were so impressive that the lesion was referred to as Swiss cheese disease of the breast. Sclerosing adenosis often accompanied the papillomas. In 1982, Rosen et al. (102) described 41 patients with juvenile papillomatosis, followed for a median of 14 years. Age of diagnosis ranged from between 15 and 35 years, with a median of 19 years. Fifty-eight percent of the patients had a positive family history for breast carcinoma and six patients had bilateral juvenile papillomatosis. Of the four patients who subsequently developed breast cancer, all had bilateral disease originally, a recurrence of the juvenile papillomatosis after primary excision, and a family history of breast cancer. None of the patients with nonrecurrent unilateral unicentric juvenile papillomatosis was found to have subsequently developed carcinoma of the breast (Figs. 4.61 and 4.62 and efigs. 4.149 to 4.153). Bazzocchi et al. (103) reported on 13 cases of juvenile papillomatosis, with an average age of 25 years. A family history of breast cancer was reported in 33% of the cases. Coexistent carcinoma was found in 15% of the cases. Nonomura et al. (104) reported on a case

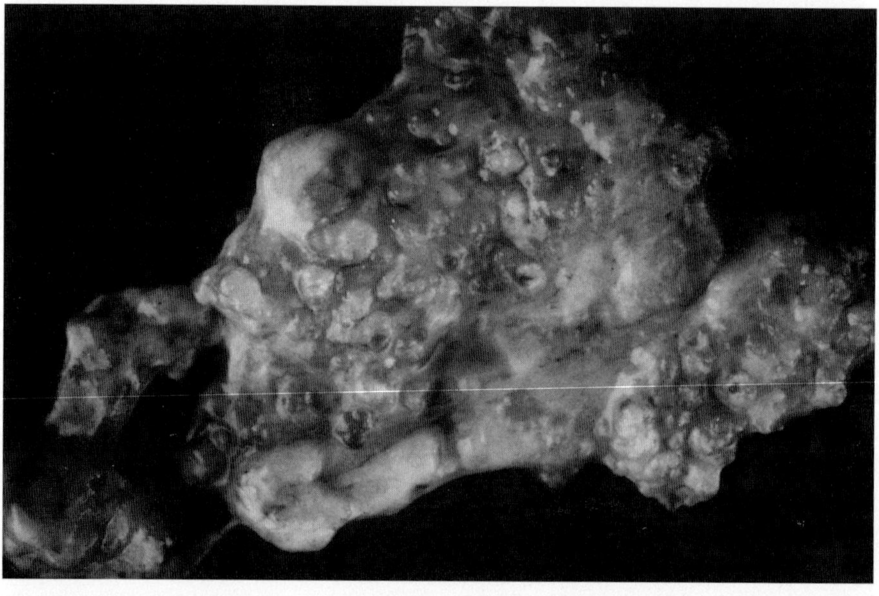

FIG. 4.61. Juvenile papillomatosis. This gross photograph shows a localized lesion in which the ducts are distended and filled with proliferating tissue.

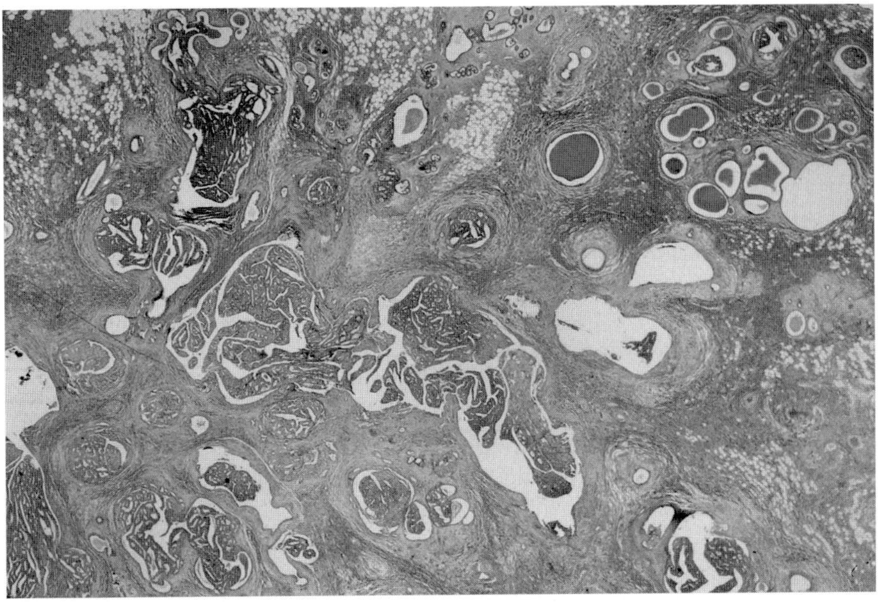

FIG. 4.62. Juvenile papillomatosis. In this low power photomicrograph, one can see two types of distended ducts, papillary proliferation and cystic ducts surrounded by dense scars, some of which are filled with secretory material. The empty ducts have been the source of the name Swiss cheese disease for juvenile papillomatosis. The papillary areas resemble a papilloma and the open ducts resemble fibrocystic changes with duct ectasia.

of secretory carcinoma in association with juvenile papillomatosis in a 12-year-old girl.

Summary: Papillary Tumors

IPC, without DCIS or invasion, is an unusual and low-grade carcinoma. Distinction from papilloma is based on the principles useful in distinguishing papillomatosis from DCIS and relies heavily on the demonstration of a pervasive myoepithelial layer in papillomas. IPCs are associated with DCIS in one-third of cases, indicating that they are malignant tumors. DCIS and invasive carcinoma that are associated with IPC take priority over the IPC diagnosis in determining outcome. IPC may show foci of papilloma (or papillomas may show foci of DCIS) that is indicative of transformation of benign papillomas, but this is probably a rare event. IPC that invades the cyst (ductal) wall may be associated with lymph node metastasis. Pseudoinfiltration of either the stalk or the cyst wall by papilloma may be a difficult problem in differential diagnosis, but it is not of clinical consequence. Ductal adenoma may mimic invasive carcinoma, especially on core needle biopsy. Multiple papillomas arise in association with the terminal duct/lobular unit and are precancerous. Juvenile papillomatosis has a high association with familial breast cancer and is associated with carcinoma.

NIPPLE LESIONS

Paget's Disease

Paget's disease of the nipple presents clinically as a persistent eczematous pruritic lesion of the nipple and surrounding areola (105). Histologically, it is characterized by the presence of large clear cells that occur individually or in small groups that are spread throughout the layers of the epidermis of the nipple (Figs. 4.63, 4.64, and 4.66 and efigs. 4.156, 4.157, and 4.160). These cells usually express HER2/neu (Fig. 4.68 and efig. 4.154) and often also stain for mucus, CEA, and epithelial membrane antigen (EMA) (Fig. 4.67 and 4.161). They are variably positive for keratin, although they are somewhat less intensely stained than the surrounding keratinocytes. S-100 protein is usually negative and HMB-45 is negative, which helps to distinguish Paget's disease from melanoma, a morphologically similar lesion that rarely, if ever, occurs in the nipple. The most reliable guide to diagnosis is the presence of scattered large cells with abundant

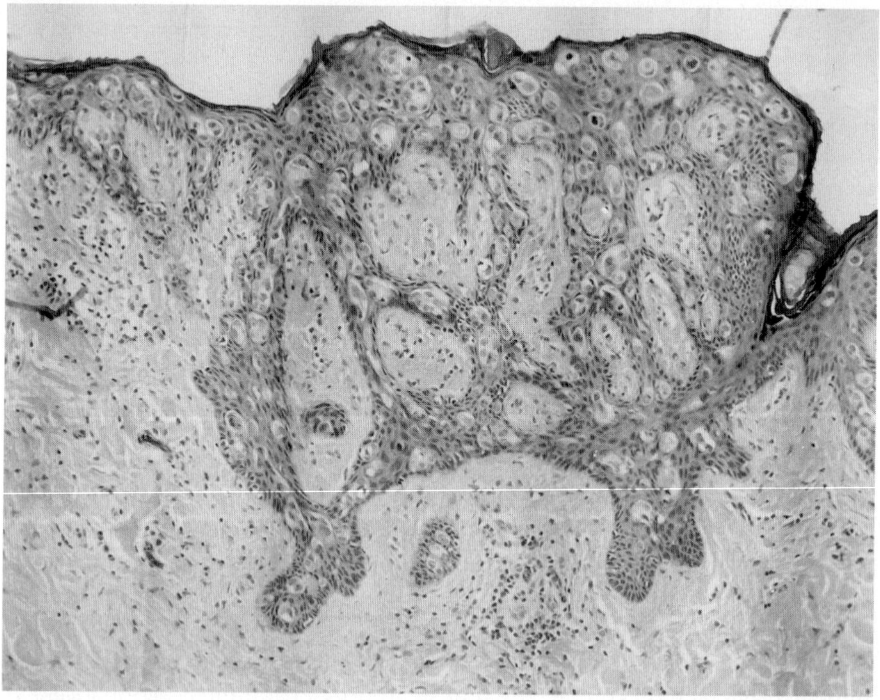

FIG. 4.63. Paget's disease. The Paget's cells are evident as individual large clear cells.

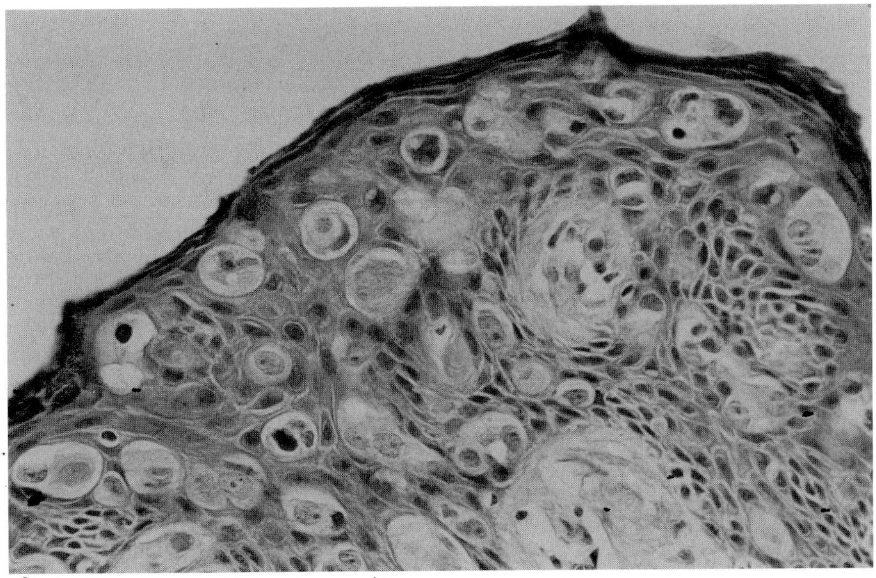

FIG. 4.64. Paget's disease. At higher magnification, the malignant nature of the cells becomes evident. A mitotic figure is present. The basal and keratinized layers are intact.

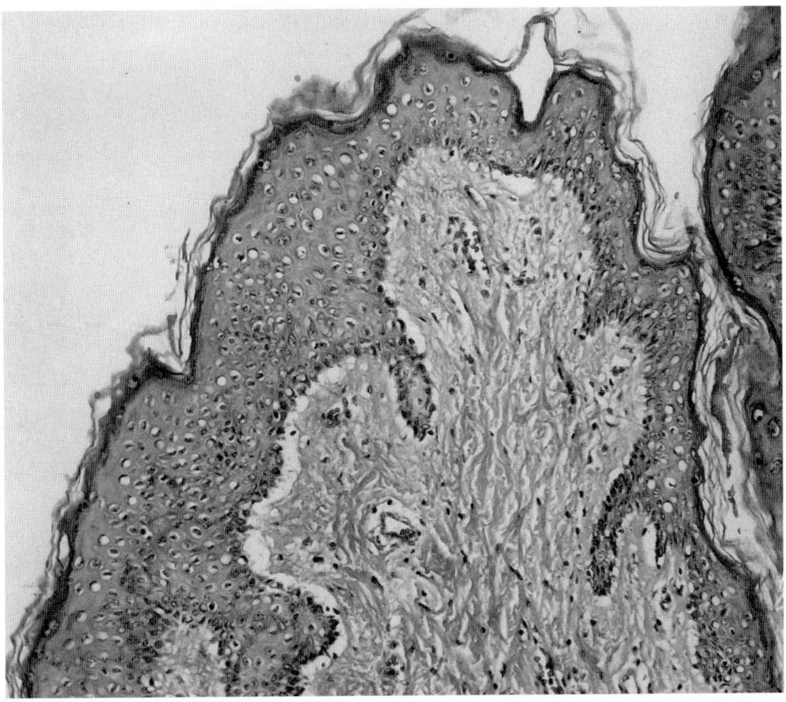

FIG. 4.65. Clear "Toker" cells of the epidermis of the nipple. These clear cells of the nipple epidermis are commonly seen and they are identified from their benign appearing nuclei.

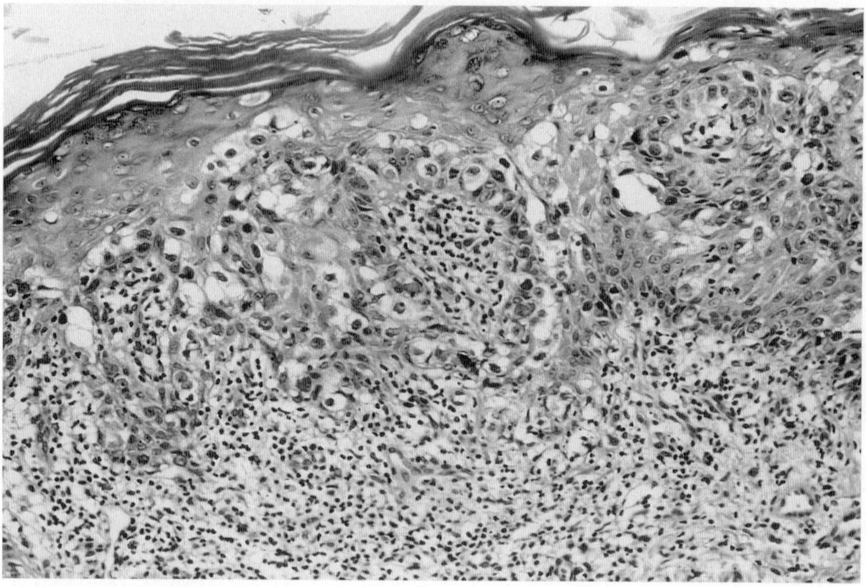

FIG. 4.66. Paget's disease. The Paget's cells are present from the basal layer to the midzone of the epidermis. The differential diagnosis includes Paget's disease, melanoma, and Bowen's disease.

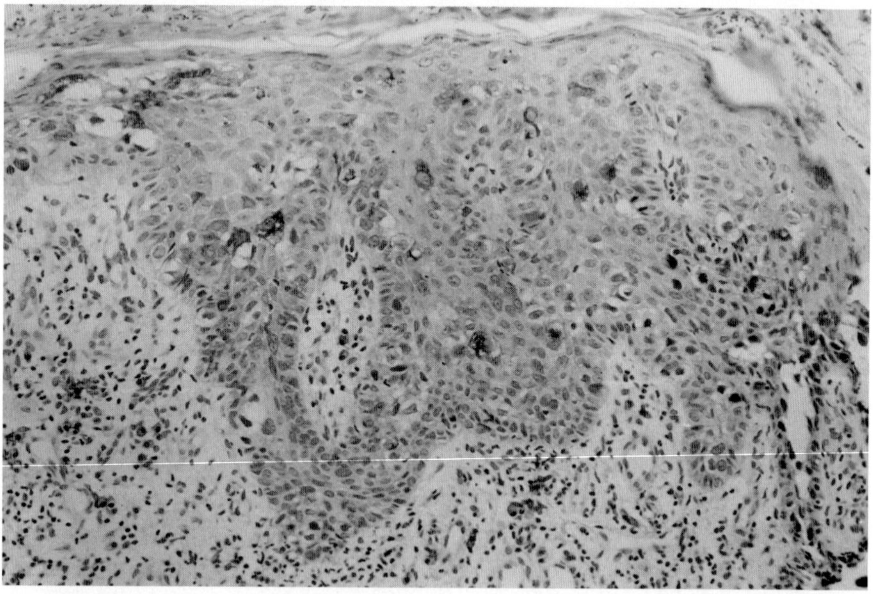

FIG. 4.67. Paget's disease. An immunostain for epithelial membrane antigen decorates the individual abnormal cells, indicative of Paget's disease and against a diagnosis of melanoma or Bowen's disease.

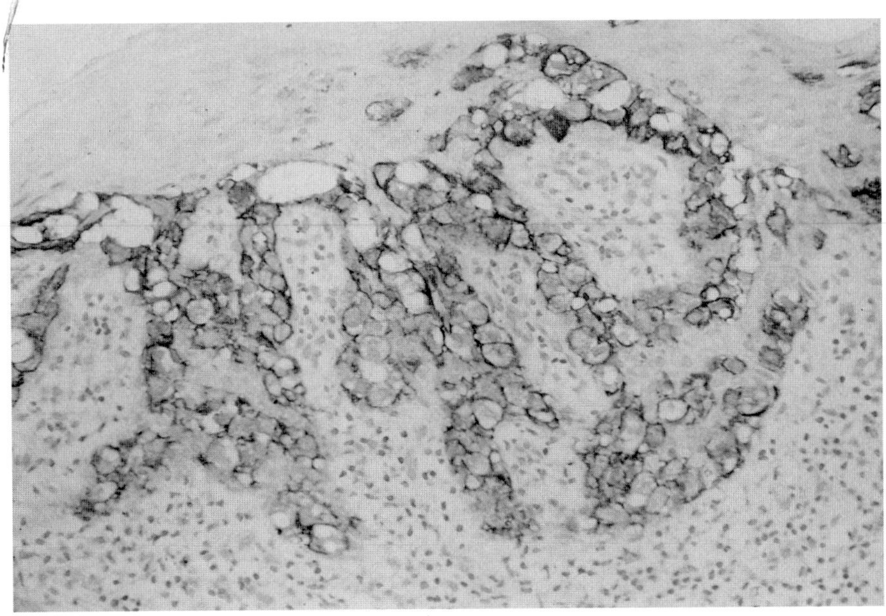

FIG. 4.68. Paget's disease. An immunostain for HER2/neu with its membrane staining pattern is diagnostic of mammary Paget's disease.

clear cytoplasm and malignant nuclei in the epidermis of the nipple. The diagnosis is confirmed by HER2/neu staining.

Smaller benign clear "Toker" cells are often present in the epidermis of the nipple (Fig. 4.65 and efig. 4.154); however, they have no known clinical significance. Yao et al. (106) reported immunohistochemical staining of the Toker cells in cases of histologically normal nipple epidermis and of nipples with Paget's disease. CK7 positive cells were found in 44% of the normal nipples and in 95% of nipples with Paget's disease. CAM5.2 stained epidermal cells in 42% of the normal nipples and in 94% of those with Paget's disease. HER2/neu labeled 68% of the Paget's disease cases and none of the normal nipple cases. The authors interpreted these changes as indicative of spread of normal lactiferous duct cells into the nipple epidermis.

Controversy over the origin of Paget's cells persists. It has been suggested that the cells represent an extension onto the epidermal surface by the intraductal component of the tumor, as is occasionally seen in the Pagetoid spread along the ducts of carcinoma cells in DCIS or LCIS. Vielh et al. (107) studied 44 cases of Paget's disease of the nipple and found Paget's cells to be PAS positive and diastase resistant in 32% and alcian blue positive at pH 2.5 in 18% of cases. In all cases, the Paget's cells were positive for EMA, and 84% were positive when stained for c-erbB-2. The authors suggested that these two histochemical and two immunohistochemical stains may be useful in distinguishing Paget's disease from Bowen's disease and eczema, which stain with none of these, and from nipple adenoma, which exhibits strong staining for EMA, but no staining for c-erbB-2. Keatings et al. (108) found staining for c-erbB-2 in all 12 cases of mammary Paget's disease and in all 9 cases of the underlying intraductal carcinoma in which this was studied. In 8 of the 9 cases, the *in situ* component was comedocarcinoma or a solid type. Extramammary Paget's disease stained positively for c-erbB-2 in only 4 of 10 cases, and the staining was less intense in these 4 cases than it was in the mammary Paget's disease. Wolber et al. (109) found positive membrane staining for c-erbB-2 in 15 of 19 cases of mammary Paget's disease, but in only 30% of vulvar Paget's disease and in none of 8 cases of scrotal Paget's disease or 5 cases of perianal Paget's disease. An underlying intraductal carcinoma was available for study in 14 of the 19 patients with mammary Paget's disease; 12 of those 14 intraductal carcinomas were positive for c-erbB-2. Ordonez et al. (110) also described differences between mammary and extramammary Paget's disease cells. Evidence that Paget's cells are connected to the surrounding keratinocytes by desmosomes, as demonstrated by Sagabiel (111) and Sagami (112), provides an opposing view. Others have suggested that they are derived from either melanocytes or keratinocytes and that they undergo differentiation toward glandular cells. Although the origin of the cells has yet to be resolved, it seems that Paget's disease arises in the nipple, in association with, but sometimes anatomically separately from, intraductal carcinoma in the underlying ducts of the breast. The evidence for this is the occasional absence of an underlying carcinoma, the more frequent anatomic separation of DCIS from Paget's disease, and finally the linkage of the Paget's cells to the surrounding keratinocytes. While controversy about the nature of Paget's cells may continue, there is a consensus that their presence constitutes an indication for additional diagnosis and treatment of the breast for carcinoma.

Paget's disease is almost invariably associated with underlying carcinoma of the breast, either *in situ* or invasive. In the large series of 214 histologically proven cases of Paget's disease reported by Ashikari et al. (113), 96 patients presented with the epidermal lesion that was not associated with a mass in the breast. Sixty-three of those patients had intraductal carcinoma, and the other 33 patients had infiltrating ductal carcinoma. The 5-year survival rate of patients with Paget's disease, with no palpable mass and negative axillary lymph nodes, was 97%, and the 10-year survival rate was 95%. Overall survival of patients with Paget's disease, with no palpable mass, was 92% at 5 years and 87% at 10 years. Survival was diminished significantly in patients with positive axillary lymph nodes, particularly in those with axillary lymph node metastases in the mid axilla and apex. Among 113 patients with palpable breast masses associated with Paget's disease, 20 patients had no clinical evidence of Paget's disease, but the diagnosis was retrospectively made after microscopic examination of the mastectomy specimen. The overall 5-year survival rate was 41%, and the 10-year survival rate was 38% for patients with palpable masses that were associated with Paget's disease. The 5-year survival rate for patients with Paget's disease that was associated with a palpable mass and negative axillary lymph nodes was 73%. For patients with lymph node metastases in the middle and upper levels of the axilla that was associated with a palpable mass, 5-year survival was only 20%. In six cases (3%) of histologically verified Paget's disease, no carcinoma was found in the mastectomy specimen. Although most of the carcinomas associated with Paget's disease were ductal cancers, either intraductal or infiltrating, there were six cases of lobular carcinoma. Two cases were infiltrating lobular carcinoma and four cases were lobular carcinoma *in situ*.

Paone and Baker (114) described 50 cases of Paget's disease of the nipple that were treated surgically, with underlying cancer present in all 50 cases. Among 19 patients with Paget's disease that was confined to the nipple and with no palpable breast mass, there were no axillary lymph node metastases and no deaths. Among the 31 patients with a palpable breast mass that was associated with Paget's disease, 19 patients died of metastatic disease, for a cumulative 10-year survival rate of 33%. Invasive carcinoma with negative lymph nodes was associated with a 10-year survival rate of 44%, whereas invasive carcinoma that was associated with positive axillary lymph nodes was associated with only a 10-year survival rate of 10%.

Bijker et al. (115) reported on 61 patients with Paget's disease of the nipple who were treated by complete excision of the nipple–areolar complex, including the underlying breast tissue, with free tumor margins followed by external irradiation. Ninety-seven percent of the patients presented with Paget's disease without an associated palpable mass; 93% of those patients had underlying DCIS in the underlying tissues, but, in 7% of patients, there was no underlying DCIS found. At a median follow-up of 6.4 years, 4 of the 61 patients developed recurrence in the treated breast (1 patient with DCIS and 3 patients with invasive carcinoma). The 5-year local recurrence rate was 5.2%. One of the patients who developed an invasive local recurrence died of disseminated breast cancer. Fu et al. (116) studied 14 cases of Paget's disease and found c-erb-2 staining in 93%, cyclin-D-1 in 100%, Ki-67 in 86%, bcl-2 in 14%, p53 overexpression in 43%, and 29% were positive for ER and progesterone receptor (PR). The rate of expression of these markers was similar in Paget's cells and in the underlying intraductal carcinoma.

Dixon et al. (117) reported on 48 patients with Paget's disease of the nipple in whom DCIS was found in 45 operative patients. The DCIS was predominantly solid or comedocarcinoma in type. Eight of the patients had associated invasive carcinoma. Thirty-seven of the patients underwent mastectomy, and only two patients developed local regional recurrences. Both of these patients had invasive foci in a mastectomy specimen and both remained disease-free at 8 years postoperatively. Ten patients had a cone excision of the nipple–areola complex; 4 of these 10 patients developed a local recurrence and 2 patients developed systemic metastases. The authors suggested that cone excision is not appropriate treatment for Paget's disease.

It is clear that Paget's disease is an important early warning of the very high likelihood of intraductal or invasive cancer in the underlying breast and it is therefore a strong indication for additional diagnostic studies and treatment. When Paget's disease is the sole indication for surgery, the likelihood of a cure is great. If a palpable mass in the breast and enlarged axillary lymph nodes are present, the likelihood of a cure decreases according to stage (118–123).

Papillary Adenoma of the Nipple (Erosive Adenomatosis)

Jones (124) described "florid papillomatosis of the nipple ducts" in 1955, and Shapiro and Karpas (125) described the lesion in 1965. Other names for this lesion include papillary adenoma of the nipple, erosive adenomatosis of the nipple, and subareolar papillomatosis. This lesion or group of lesions may mimic Paget's disease clinically, primarily because of its mass effect and the ulceration that may occur, as the name erosive adenomatosis used by Smith (126) and Smith and Jones (127) suggests. It is a lesion that microscopically has been diagnosed as invasive carcinoma of the breast.

The age range of patients with this lesion varies from 9 to 75 years, with most patients in their 40s, when breast cancer is an important consideration. Microscopically, the lesion is circumscribed, but it may grow directly onto the epidermal surface. It is composed of papillary fronds and ducts, which proliferate in a way that is similar to that seen in sclerosing adenosis deeper in the breast. The surface and some of the glandular spaces may be lined by squamous epithelium, and there may be an inflammatory component present (Figs. 4.69 to 4.75 and efigs. 4.162 to 4.170). Mitoses may be frequent, but do not, by themselves, indicate malignancy.

There are two keys for the recognition of nipple adenoma. First, the lesion is always in the nipple and does not involve the deeper mammary parenchyma. True carcinoma rarely involves the nipple without involving the breast, unless it is a recurrence. The previous diagnosis of carcinoma should then be known. In large adenomas, the distinction between nipple and breast involvement may be less evident. Second, the myoepithelial layer is prominent, although this may not be apparent on frozen section. If there is a question of adenoma (or papilloma), deferral of the frozen section of a nipple lesion may be the most prudent course. The clear, or myoepithelial, layer is usually apparent on paraffin sections and may be verified with an immunohistochemical stain with antibodies to smooth muscle actin. Bilateral adenomas of the nipple have been reported. Rosen and Caicco (128) reported cancer in the follow-up period of 9 of 51 cases of nipple adenoma. In two of the cases, carcinoma seemed to arise from the adenoma. This must be a rare occurrence, but the author also observed the apparent transition (Figs. 4.74 and 4.75 and efigs. 4.169 and 4.170). For this reason and to prevent recurrence, nipple adenomas should be completely excised, and it may be difficult to preserve the nipple in accomplishing an adequate excision.

The largest group of adenomas of the nipple was reported by Perzin and Lattes (129), who discussed the features of 65 cases. The authors stressed its pseudoinfiltrative nature and the proliferation of medium and small ducts, as is seen in

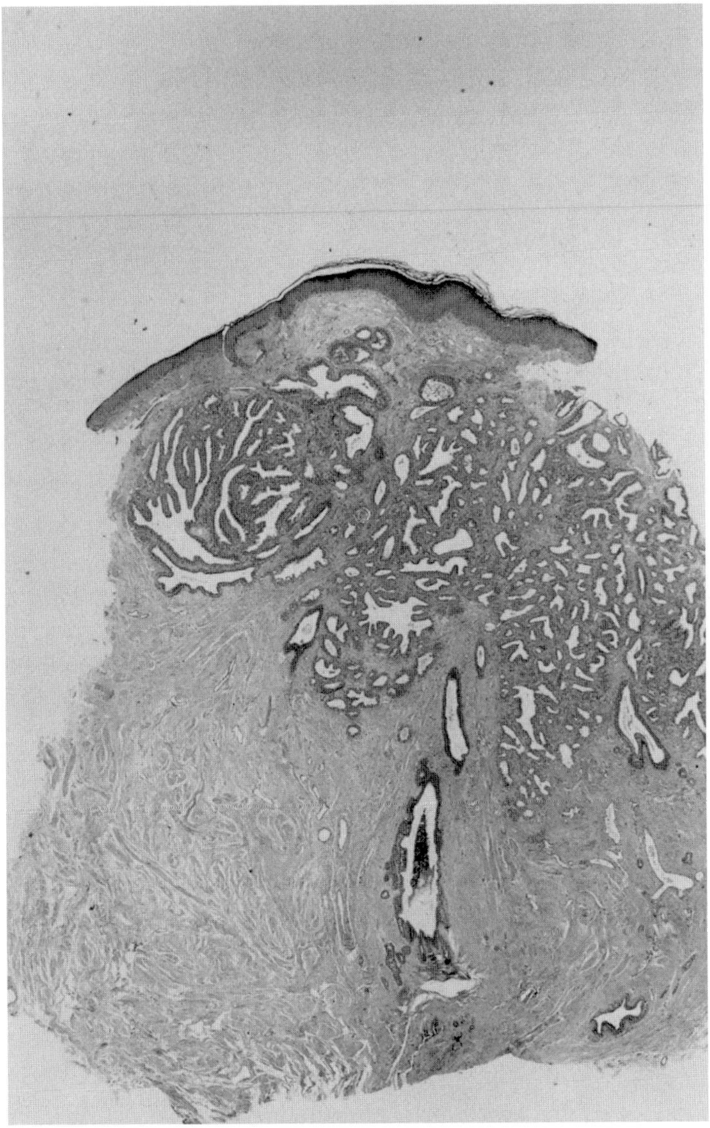

FIG. 4.69. Nipple adenoma. The location of the lesion in the nipple is a strong indication for considering a diagnosis of nipple adenoma (erosive adenomatosis).

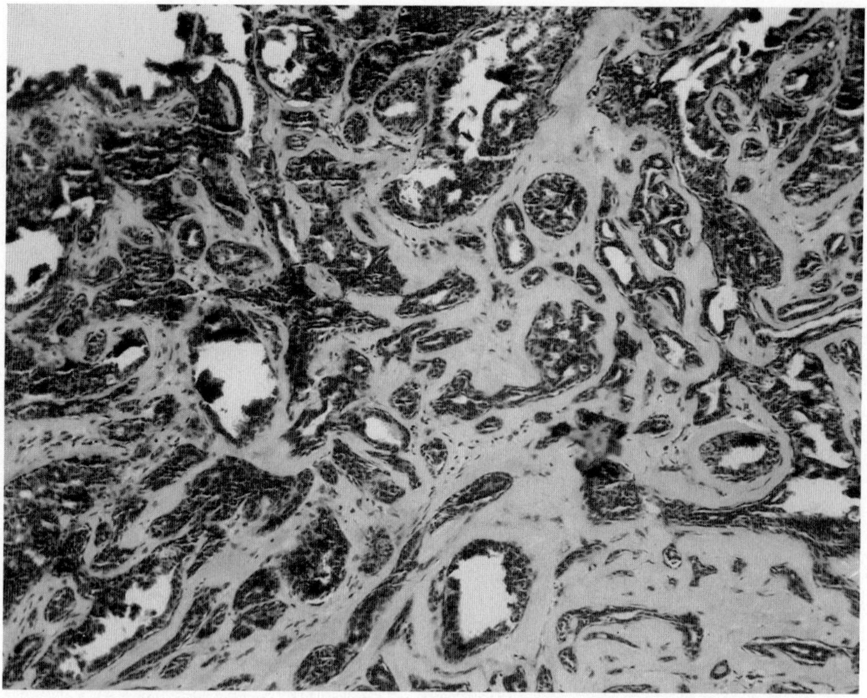

FIG. 4.70. Nipple adenoma, sclerotic type. At about the 11 o'clock position (**upper part**), there is a duct opening onto the nipple surface. The sclerotic tumor has areas suggestive of syringomatous differentiation (**lower part**).

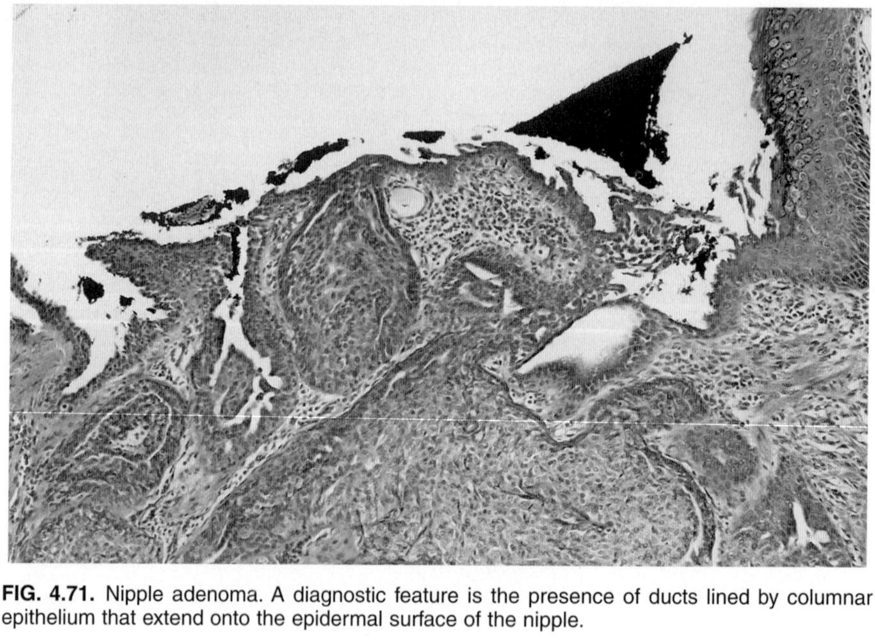

FIG. 4.71. Nipple adenoma. A diagnostic feature is the presence of ducts lined by columnar epithelium that extend onto the epidermal surface of the nipple.

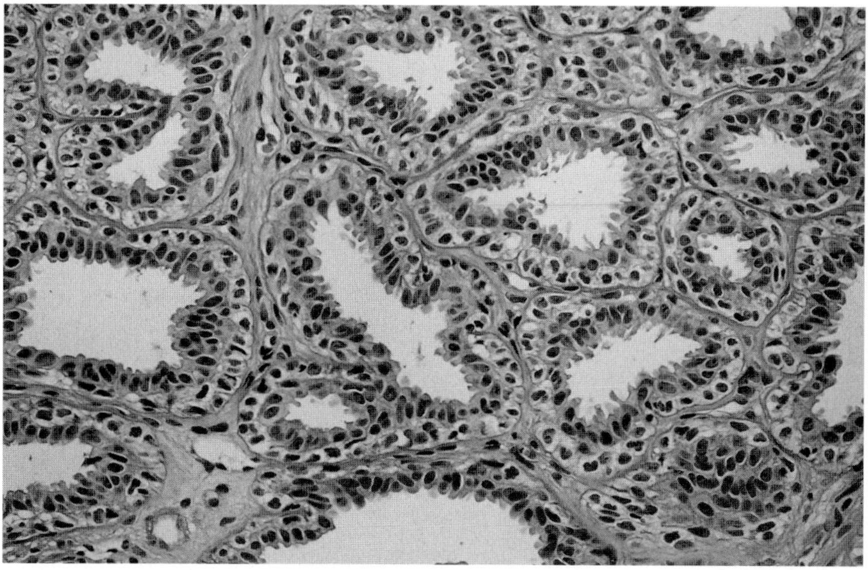

FIG. 4.72. Nipple adenoma. The proliferating ducts have a biphasic appearance with prominence of myoepithelial and columnar layers.

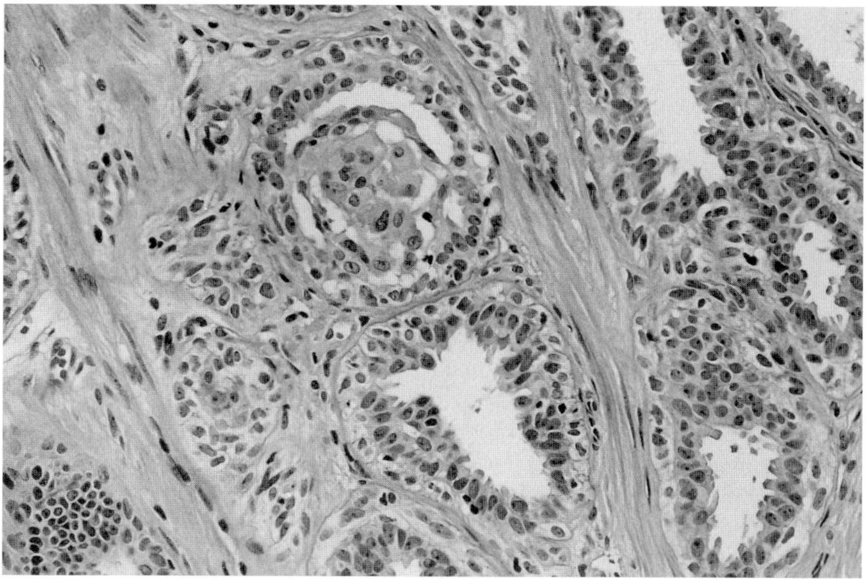

FIG. 4.73. Nipple adenoma. Nodules of squamous epithelium may form in a morule-like pattern within the proliferating ductal structures deep in the nipple.

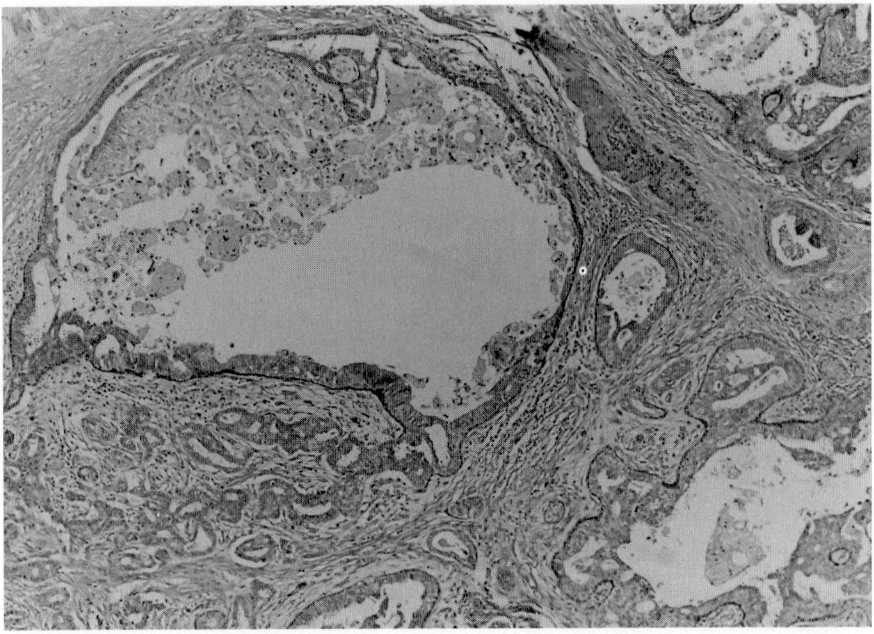

FIG. 4.74. Carcinoma arising in a nipple adenoma. Distended ducts that are characterized by a proliferation of epithelial cells with a clearly evident, if not proliferative, layer of myoepithelium present (upper part of photomicrograph). There is an infiltration of ducts into the stroma (**lower left corner**).

adenosis and sclerosing adenosis. A papillary proliferation also may be present. As noted above, mitoses may be frequent, but necrosis is rarely seen. In the 12 cases that were serially sectioned, a typical IP was found in one of the major nipple ducts deep to the adenoma, and the authors suggested that this may be part of the genesis of the lesion. Other authors (30,125,130,131) suggested that the tumor resembles syringocystadenoma papilliferum. All authors reporting on this tumor have noted the presence of the double cell layer with both myoepithelial and epithelial cells proliferating. This, in addition to the presence of the lesion directly in the nipple, is the most useful clue in distinguishing papillary adenoma of the nipple from invasive carcinoma. Among 29 patients who were treated by local excision, partial resection of the nipple, or total resection of the nipple, only one patient with a local excision (regarded as incomplete) had local recurrence during an average follow-up of 5.9 years.

Jones and Tavassoli (132) reported on five patients who had both nipple duct adenoma and carcinoma in the same breast. Two of the four invasive carcinomas were adjacent to the adenoma and immediately beneath the surface epithelium of the nipple. ADH was present in one of the two nipple duct adenomas. The other three patients, two with invasive carcinoma and one with intraductal carcinoma, had noncontiguous adenoma and carcinoma. Diaz et al. (133) evaluated

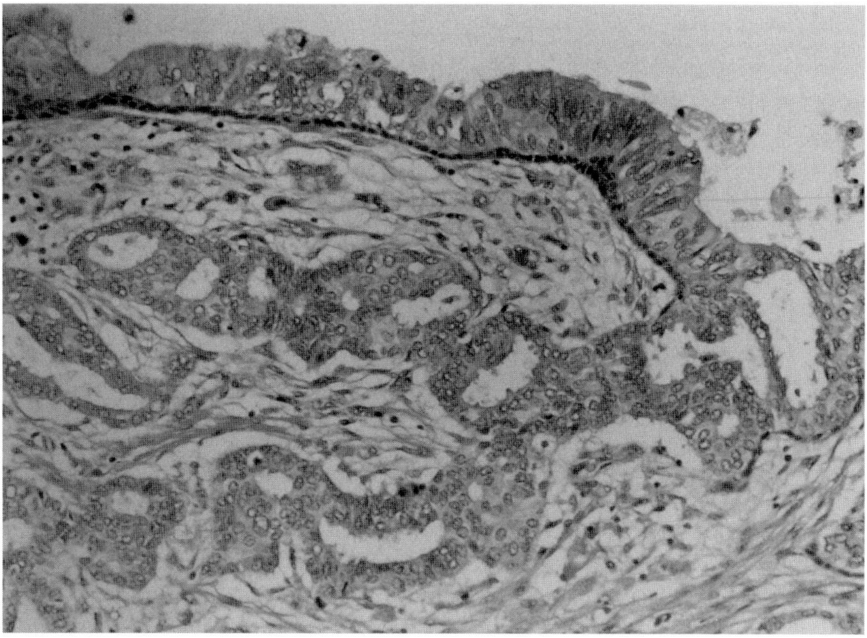

FIG. 4.75. Carcinoma arising in nipple adenoma. At higher magnification, the invasive ductal carcinoma is shown. The distinction between ducts lined by a myoepithelium and ducts invading the stroma is evident.

ten cases of nipple adenoma (erosive adenomatosis of the nipple) and demonstrated staining for cytokeratin, muscle-specific actin, vimentin, and glial fibrillary acidic protein in the myoepithelial layer and staining for CK uniformly and CEA focally in the epithelial layer.

Myers et al. (134) described the immunohistochemical and flow cytometric analysis of two cases of florid papillomatosis of the nipple (adenoma of the nipple). In both cases, the lesions were diploid, but had high S-phase fractions of 10.9% and 34.4%, respectively, consistent with the observed high mitotic rate. One was focally positive for gross cystic disease fluid protein 15 (GCDFP-15), but the other was not. In both instances, there was a continuous myoepithelial layer between the epithelium and the basement membrane and, in one case, this was confirmed by staining for muscle-specific actin with electron microscopic confirmation.

SYRINGOMA

Syringomatous adenoma of the nipple is similar to syringoma, which is seen elsewhere in the skin adnexa. Microscopically, it is composed of tubular, duct-like structures with an attenuated myoepithelial component. Some of the epithe-

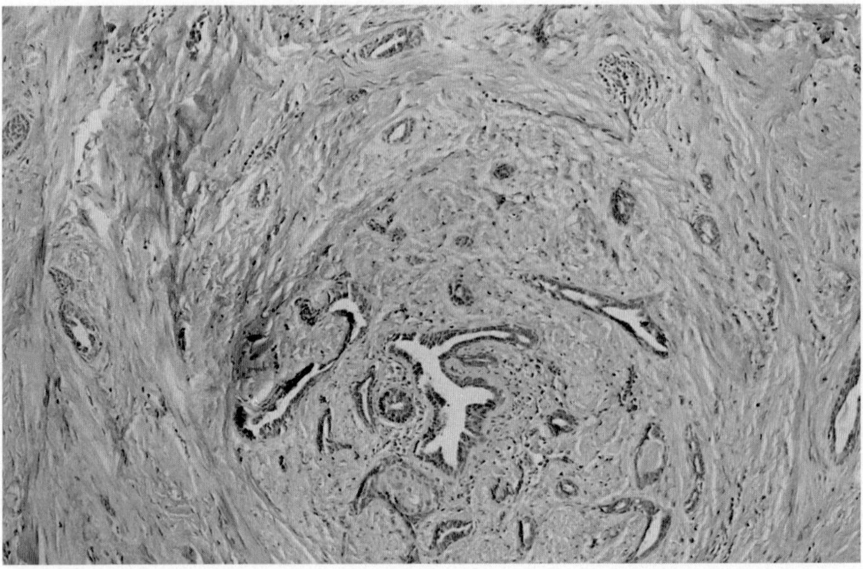

FIG. 4.76. Syringoma of the nipple. The normal central lactiferous collecting ducts of the nipple are normal, but are surrounded by small elongated comma-shaped ductal structures that suggests an infiltrative tumor.

lial cells may keratinize, (Figs. 4.76 to 4.78 and efigs. 4.171 to 4.174). Some of the comma-shaped structures appear to invade the erector smooth muscle bundles of the nipple (efigs. 4.175 and 4.176) and, less commonly, adjacent breast parenchyma.

Rosen (135) described five cases of syringoma of skin adnexal origin in the nipple, four cases of which were seen in women between the ages of 28 and 41 years. The lesion was solitary and unilateral in all cases. Two of the lesions were widely excised and the patients were free of recurrence at 2 and 2.5 years after nipple resection. A third patient was treated by mastectomy and was disease-free at 3 years. A fourth patient with incomplete excision had persistence and slow enlargement of the syringoma over the course of 22 years. Eventual partial mastectomy was required. No metastases were found. Suster et al. (136) described four cases of syringomatous squamous tumors in women aged 37 to 70 years. In one case, the lesion was found in the vicinity of a large cyst. All four patients were treated by local excision, with no evidence of recurrence over a follow-up period of 1 to 6 years.

Jones et al. (137) reported on 11 cases of infiltrating syringomatous adenoma of the nipple. The authors stressed the lack of ulceration, but the invasion of dermis, smooth muscle, underlying mammary parenchyma, and, rarely, the perineural space. The small ducts or strands of epithelium invaded irregularly into a cellular, edematous, and collagenized stroma. The ducts were often teardrop- or comma-shaped and varied from tubular to squamous, with either type predomi-

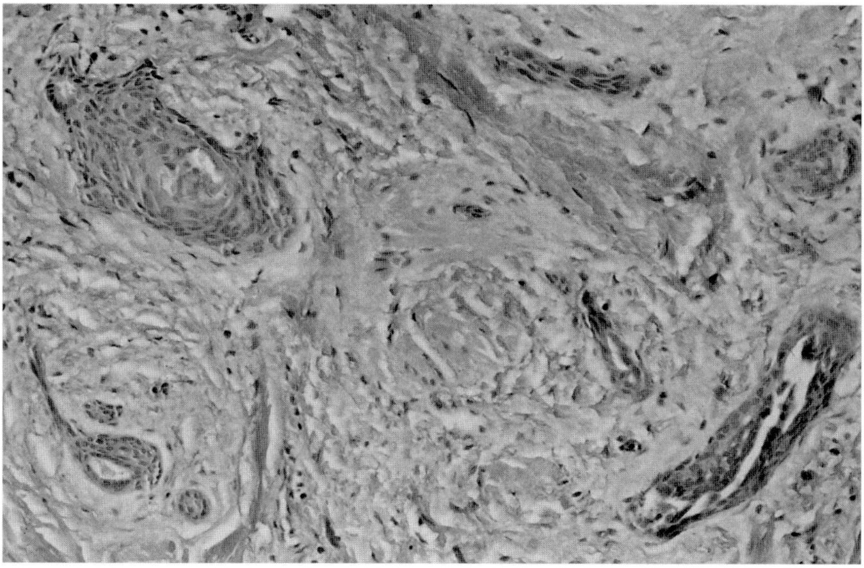

FIG. 4.77. Syringoma of the nipple. At higher magnification, some of the ductal structures are focally differentiated as squamous epithelium and other ducts have the epithelial-myoepithelial differentiation characteristic of benign lesions of the breast.

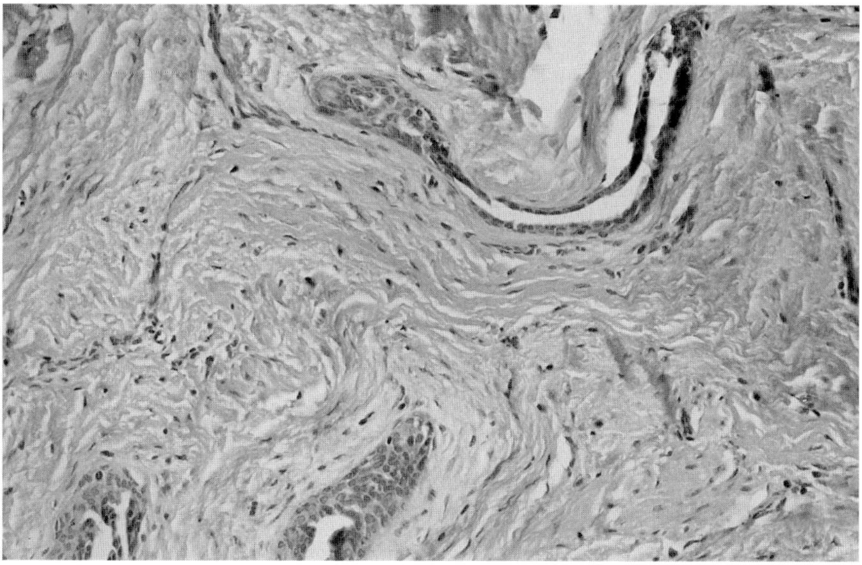

FIG. 4.78. Syringoma of the nipple. The elongated comma shape of the duct is characteristic and unlike structures formed by ductal carcinoma.

nating. A myoepithelial layer was prominent and it was highlighted immunohistochemically with antibodies to actin. Ten patients were treated by local excision and four of them had recurrence, with one patient requiring three reexcisions. One patient had a subcutaneous mastectomy, but had recurrence in the nipple. Follow-up of 3 months to 10 years (average of 3.3 years) was available in nine patients. All patients were well and none had developed metastases.

INVASIVE BREAST CANCER INVOLVING THE NIPPLE

Invasive ductal carcinoma of the breast may also invade the nipple. Lambert et al. (138) reported on 54 nipple positive carcinomas among 803 breast cancer patients. Tumor stage, size, lymph node status, histologic grade, and location were all significant predictors of nipple involvement. Luttges et al. (139) reported finding nipple involvement in 38% of 166 patients who underwent mastectomy, investigated by giant sections of the breast and small sections from the nipple. Multifocal carcinoma was present in 76 of the 166 patients and multicentric carcinomatous foci were found in 36 patients with affected nipples. The authors concluded that multicentricity and multifocality of breast cancer, in addition to advanced tumor stage and subareolar location of the carcinoma, correlated with nipple involvement.

REFERENCES

1. Fisher ER, Costantino J, Fisher B, et al. Pathologic findings from the National Surgical Adjuvant Breast Project (NSABP) Protocol B-17: intraductal carcinoma (ductal carcinoma *in situ*). *Cancer* 1995;75:1310–1319.
2. Tavassoli FA, Norris HJ. Intraductal apocrine carcinoma: a clinicopathologic study of 37 cases. *Mod Pathol* 1994;7:813–818.
3. Leal C, Henrique P, Lopes C, et al. Apocrine ductal carcinoma-*in-situ* of the breast: histologic classification and expression of biologic markers. *Hum Pathol* 2001:487–493.
4. Azzopardi J. Problems in breast pathology. Major problems in pathology. Philadelphia: WB Saunders, 1979:II.
5. Guerry P, Erlandson RA, Rosen PP. Cystic hypersecretory hyperplasia and cystic hypersecretory duct carcinoma of the breast: pathology, therapy, and follow-up of 39 patients. *Cancer* 1988;61:1611–1620.
6. Tsang WYW, Chan JKC. Endocrine ductal carcinoma *in situ* (E-DCIS) of the breast: a form of low-grade DCIS with distinctive clinicopathologic and biologic characteristics. *Am J Surg Pathol* 1996;20:921–943.
7. Betsill WL, Rosen PP, Lieberman P, et al. Intraductal carcinoma: long term follow-up after treatment by biopsy alone. *JAMA* 1978;239:1863–1867.
8. Carter D, Smith RR. Carcinoma *in situ* of the breast. *Cancer* 1977;40:1189–1193.
9. Shah JP, Rosen PP, Robbins GF. Pitfalls of local excision in the treatment of carcinoma of the breast. *Surg Gynecol Obstet* 1973;136:721–725.
10. Ashikari R, Hajdu SI, Robins GF. Intraductal carcinoma of the breast. *Cancer* 1971;28:1182–1187.
11. Ozello L, Sanpitak P. Epithelial–stromal junction of intraductal carcinoma of the breast. *Cancer* 1970;26:1186–1198.
12. Barsky SH, Siegal GP, Jannotta F, et al. Loss of basement membrane components by invasive tumors but not by their benign counterparts. *Lab Invest* 1983;49:140–147.
13. Patchefsky AS, Schwartz GF, Finklestein SD. Heterogeneity of intraductal carcinoma of the breast. *Cancer* 1989;63:731–741.
14. Lagios MD, Margolin FR, Westdahl PR, et al. Mammographically detected duct carcinoma *in situ*:

frequency of local recurrence following tylectomy and prognostic effect of nuclear grade on local recurrence. *Cancer* 1989;63:618–624.
15. Bellamy COC, McDonald C, Salter DM, et al. Noninvasive ductal carcinoma of the breast: the relevance of histologic categorization. *Hum Pathol* 1993;24:16–23.
16. Poller D, Silverstein M, Galea M, et al. Ductal carcinoma *in-situ* of the breast: a proposal for a new simplified histological classification association between cellular proliferation and C-erb B2 protein expression. *Mod Pathol* 1994;7:257–262.
17. Holland R, Peterse JL, Millis RR, et al. Ductal carcinoma *in situ*: a proposal for a new classification. *Semin Diagn Pathol* 1994;11:167–180.
18. Bobrow LGH, Gregory WM, Springall RD, et al. The classification of ductal carcinoma *in situ* and its association with biological markers. *Semin Diagn Pathol* 1994;11:199–207.
19. Lennington WJJ, Dalton LW, Page DL. Ductal carcinoma *in situ* of the breast: heterogeneity of individual lesions. *Cancer* 1994;73:118–124.
20. Eusebi V, Foschini MP, Cook MG, et al. Long term follow-up of *in situ* carcinoma of the breast with special reference to clinging carcinoma. *Semin Diagn Pathol* 1989;6:165–173.
21. Cataliotti L, Distante V, Ciatto S, et al. Intraductal breast cancer: review of 183 consecutive cases. *Eur J Cancer* 1992:28A:917–920.
22. Baird RM, Worth A, Hislop G. Recurrence after lumpectomy for comedo-type intraductal carcinoma of the breast. *Am J Surg* 1990;159:479–481.
23. O'Malley FP, Page DL, Nelson EH, et al. Ductal carcinoma *in situ* of the breast with apocrine cytology: definition of a borderline category. *Hum Pathol* 1994;25:164–168.
24. Abati AD, Kimmel M, Rosen PP. Apocrine mammary carcinoma: a clinicopathologic study of 72 cases. *Am J Clin Pathol* 1990;94:371–377.
25. Van de Vijver MJP, Mooi WJ, Wisman P, et al. Neu-protein overexpression in breast cancer. Association with comedo-type ductal carcinoma *in situ* and limited prognostic value in stage II breast cancer. *N Engl J Med* 1988;319:1239–1245.
26. Varley JM, Swallow JE, Brammar WJ, et al. Alterations to either c-erbB-2 (neu) or c-myc proto-oncogenes in breast carcinomas correlate with poor short-term prognosis. *Oncogene* 1987;1: 423–430.
27. Liu ET, Thor A, Barcos M, et al. The HER2 (c-erB-2) oncogene is frequently amplified *in situ* carcinomas of the breast. *Oncogene* 1992;7:1027–1032.
28. Lodato RF, Maguire HCJ, Greene MI, et al. Immunohistochemical evaluation of c-erbB-2 oncogene expression in ductal carcinoma *in situ* and atypical ductal hyperplasia of the breast. *Mod Pathol* 1990;3:449–454.
29. Somerville JEC, et al. c-erbB-2 overexpression and histological type of *in situ* and invasive breast carcinoma. *J Clin Pathol* 1992;45:16–20.
30. Aasmundstad T, Haugen O. DNA ploidy in intraductal breast carcinomas. *Eur J Cancer* 1990;26: 956–959.
31. Ohuchi N, Furuta A, Mori S. Management of ductal carcinoma *in situ* with nipple discharge: intraductal spreading of carcinoma is an unfavorable pathologic factor for breast-conserving surgery. *Cancer* 1994;74:1294–1302.
32. Guidi AJ, Fischer L, Harris JR, et al. Microvessel density and distribution of ductal carcinoma *in situ* of the breast. *J Natl Cancer Inst* 1994;86:614–619.
33. Tsang WYC, Chan JKC. Neural invasion in intraductal carcinoma of the breast. *Hum Pathol* 1992;23:202–204.
34. Schwartz GF, Patchefsky AS, Finklestein SD, et al. Nonpalpable *in situ* ductal carcinoma of the breast. Predictors of multicentricity and microinvasion and implications for treatment. *Arch Surg* 1989;124:29–32.
35. Schwartz GF, Finkel GC, Garcia JC, et al. Subclinical ductal carcinoma *in situ* of the breast: treatment by local excision and surveillance alone. *Cancer* 1992;70:2468–2474.
36. Badve S, A'Hern RP, Ward AM, et al. Prediction of local recurrence of ductal carcinoma *in situ* of the breast using five histological classifications: a comparative study with long follow-up. *Hum Pathol* 1998;29:915–923.
37. Consensus conference on the classification of ductal carcinoma *in situ* (Editorial). *Hum Pathol* 1997;28:1221–1225.
38. AJCC Cancer Staging Manual, 5th Edition, Raven, Philadelphia, 1997.
39. Rosner D, Lane WW, Penetrante R. Ductal carcinoma *in situ* with microinvasion: a curable entity using surgery alone without need for adjuvant therapy. *Cancer* 1991;67:1498–1503.

40. Prasad ML, Osborne MP, Hoda SA. Observations on the histopathologic diagnosis of microinvasive carcinoma of the breast. *Anat Pathol* 1998;3:209–232.
41. Zavotsky J, Hansen N, Brennan MB, et al. Lymph node metastasis from ductal carcinoma *in situ* with microinvasion. *Cancer* 1999;85:2439–2443.
42. Wong JH, Kopald KH, Morton DL. The impact of microinvasion on axillary node metastases and survival in patients with intraductal breast cancer. *Arch Surg* 1990;125:1298–1301; discussion 1301–1302.
43. Silver SA, Tavassoli FA. Mammary ductal carcinoma *in situ* with microinvasion. *Cancer* 1998; 82:2382–2390.
44. Kinne DW, Petrek JA, Osborne MP, et al. Breast carcinoma *in situ*. *Arch Surg* 1989;124:33–36.
45. Hardman PD, Worth A, Lee U, et al. The risk of occult invasive breast cancer after excisional biopsy showing *in situ* ductal carcinoma of comedo pattern. *Can J Surg* 1989;32:56–60.
46. Lagios MD, Westdahl PR, Margolin FR, et al. Duct carcinoma *in situ*. Relationship of extent of noninvasive disease to the frequency of occult invasion, multicentricity, lymph node metastases, and short-term treatment failures. *Cancer* 1982;50:1309–1314.
47. Schnitt S. Microinvasive carcinoma of the breast: a diagnosis in search of a diagnosis. *Adv Anat Pathol* 1998;5:367–372.
48. Page D, Dupont WD, Rogers LW, et al. Atypical hyperplastic lesions of the female breast: a long term follow-up study. *Cancer* 1985;55:2698–2708.
49. Tavassoli FA, Norris HJ. A comparison of the results of long-term follow-up for atypical intraductal hyperplasia and intraductal hyperplasia of the breast. *Cancer* 1990;65:518–529.
50. O'Connell P, Pekkel V, Fuqua SA, et al. Analysis of loss of heterozygosity in 399 premalignant breast lesions at 15 genetic loci. *J Natl Cancer Inst* 1998;90:697–703.
51. Rosai J. Borderline epithelial lesions of the breast. *Amer J Surg Pathol* 1991;15:209–221.
52. Schnitt SJ, Connolly JL, Tavassoli FA, et al. Interobserver reproducibility in the diagnosis of ductal proliferative breast lesions using standardized criteria. *Am J Surg Pathol* 1992;16:1133–1143.
53. Bodian CA, Perzin KH, Lattes R, et al. Reproducibility and validity of pathologic classifications of benign breast disease and implications for clinical applications. *Cancer* 1993;71:3908–3913.
54. Eliasen C, Optiz LM, Vamvakas EC, et al. Flow cytometric analysis of DNA ploidy and S-phase fraction in breast cancer using cells obtained by *ex vivo* fine-needle aspiration: an optimal method for sample collection. *Mod Pathol* 1991;4:196–200.
55. Rosen PP. Proliferative breast "disease": an unresolved diagnostic dilemma. *Cancer* 1993;71: 3798–3807.
56. Black MM, Barclay THC, Cutler SJ, et al. Association of atypical characteristics of benign breast lesions with subsequent risk of cancer. *Cancer* 1972;29:338–343.
57. Foote FW, Stewart FW. Comparative studies of cancerous versus noncancerous breasts. *Ann Surg* 1945;121:197–222.
58. Gallagher HS, Martin JE. Early phases in the development of breast cancer. *Cancer* 1969;24: 1170–1178.
59. Hutchinson WB, Thomas DB, Hamlin WB, et al. Risk of breast cancer in women with benign breast disease. *J Natl Cancer Inst* 1980;65:13–20.
60. Jensen JM, Rice JR, and Wellings SR. Preneoplastic lesions in the human breast. *Science* 1976;191: 295–297.
61. Kern WH, Brooks RN, Atypical epithelial hyperplasia associated with breast cancer and fibrocystic disease. *Cancer* 1969;24:668–675.
62. Monson RR, Yen S, MacMahon B. Chronic mastitis and carcinoma of the breast. *Lancet* 1976;2: 224–226.
63. Wellings SR, Jensen HM, Marcum RG. An atlas of subgross pathology of the human breast with special reference to possible precancerous lesions. *J Natl Cancer Inst* 1971;55:231–273.
64. Devitt JE. Fibrocystic disease of the breast is not premalignant. *Surg Gynecol Obstet* 1972;134:803.
65. Page DL, Zwaag RV, Rogers L, et al. Relation between component parts of fibrocystic disease complex and breast cancer. *J Natl Cancer Inst* 1978;61:1055–1063.
66. Dupont WD, Parl FF, Hartmann WH, et al. Breast cancer risk associated with proliferative breast disease and atypical hyperplasia. *Cancer* 1993;71:1258–1265.
67. Palli D, Roselli del Turco M, Simoncini R, et al. Benign breast disease and breast cancer: a case control study in a cohort in Italy. *Int J Cancer* 1991;47:703–706.
68. London SJ, Connolly JL, Schnitt SJ, et al. A prospective study of benign breast disease and breast cancer. *JAMA* 1992;267:941–944.

69. Crissman JD, Visscher DW, Kubus J. Image cytophotometric DNA analysis of atypical hyperplasias and intraductal carcinomas of the breast. *Arch Pathol Lab Med* 1990;114:1249–1253.
70. Stewart FW. *Atlas of tumor pathology*, fasc. 34. Washington: Armed Forces Institute of Pathology, 1950:18 and 53.
71. McDivitt RW, Stewart FW, Berg JW. *Atlas of tumor pathology*, fasc. 2, 2nd series. Washington: Armed Forces Institute of Pathology, 1967.
72. Fisher ER, Palekar AS, Redmond C, et al. Pathologic findings from the National Surgical Adjuvant Breast Project (Protocol No. 4). VI. Invasive papillary cancer. *Am J Clin Pathol* 1980;73:313–322.
73. Siriaunkgul S, Tavassoli F. Invasive micropapillary carcinoma of the breast. *Mod Pathol* 1993;6:660–662.
74. Gatchell FG, Dockerty MB, Claggett OT. Intracystic carcinoma of the breast. *Surg Gynecol Obstet* 1958;106:347–352.
75. Czernobilsky B. Intracystic carcinoma of the female breast. *Surg Gynecol Obstet* 1967;124:93–98.
76. McKittrick JE, Doane WA, Failing RM. Intracystic papillary carcinoma of the breast. *Am Surg* 1969; 35:195–202.
77. Hunter CE Jr, Sawyers JL. Intracystic papillary carcinoma of the breast. *South Med J* 1980;73: 1484–1486.
78. Squires JE, Betsill WLJ. Intracystic carcinoma of the breast: a correlation of cytomorphology, gross pathology, microscopic pathology and clinical data. *Acta Cytol* 1981;25:267–271.
79. Kraus FT, Neubecker RD. The differential diagnosis of papillary tumors of the breast. *Cancer* 1962;15:444–455.
80. Carter D, Orr SL, Merino MJ. Intracystic papillary carcinoma of the breast. After mastectomy, radiotherapy or excisional biopsy alone. *Cancer* 1983;52:14–19.
81. Lefkowitz M, Lefkowitz W, Wargotz ES. Intraductal (intracystic) papillary carcinoma of the breast and its variants: a clinicopathologic study of 77 cases. *Hum Pathol* 1994;25:802–809.
82. Leal C, Costa I, Fonseca D, et al. Intracystic (encysted) papillary carcinoma of the breast: a clinical, pathological, and immunohistochemical study. *Hum Pathol* 1998;29:1097–104.
83. McDivitt RW, Steward FW, Berg JW. *Atlas of tumor pathology*, fasc. 2, 2nd series. Washington: Armed Forces Institute of Pathology, 1968:22–48.
84. Carter D. Intraductal papillary tumors of the breast: a study of 78 cases. *Cancer* 1977;39:1689–1692.
85. Hendrick JW. Intraductal papilloma of the breast. *Surg Gynecol Obstet* 1957;105:215–223.
86. Haagensen CC, Stout AP, Phillips JS. The papillary neoplasms of the breast. I. Benign intraductal papilloma. *Ann Surg* 1951;133:18–36.
87. Hart D. Intracystic papillomatous tumours of the breast. *Arch Surg* 1927;14:793–835.
88. Lewison EF, Lyons JG Jr. Relationship between benign breast disease and cancer. *Arch Surg* 1953; 66:94–114.
89. Buhl-Jorgensen SE, Fischermann K, Johansen H, et al. Cancer risk in intraductal papilloma and papillomatosis. *Surg Gynecol Obstet* 1968;127:1307.
90. Moore SW, Pearce J, Ring F. Intraductal papilloma of breast. *Surg Gynecol Obstet* 1961;112:153–158.
91. Kilgore AR, Fleming R, Ramos N. The incidence of cancer with nipple discharge and the risk of cancer in the presence of papillary disease of the breast. *Surg Gynecol Obstet* 1953;96:649–660.
92. Ciatto S, Cirillo A, Bonarki R, et al. The risk of breast cancer subsequent to histologic diagnosis of benign intraductal papilloma follow-up study of 339 cases. *Tumori* 1991;77:41–43.
93. Rosen PP. Arthur Purdy Stout and papilloma of the breast. Comments on the occasion of his 100th birthday. *Am J Surg Pathol* 1986;10:100–107.
94. Page DL, Salhany KE, Jensen RA, et al. Subsequent breast carcinoma risk after biopsy with atypia in a breast papilloma. *Cancer* 1996;78:258–266.
95. Raju UB, Lee MW, Zarbo RJ, et al. Papillary neoplasia of the breast: immunohistochemically defined myoepithelial cells in the diagnosis of benign and malignant papillary breast neoplasms. *Mod Pathol* 1989;2:569–576.
96. Azzopardi JG, Salm R. Ductal adenoma of the breast: a lesion which can mimic carcinoma. *J Pathol* 1984;144:15–23.
97. Lammie GA, Millis RR. Ductal adenoma of the breast—a review of fifteen cases. *Hum Pathol* 1989; 20:903–908.
98. Murad TM, Contesso G, Mouriesse H. Papillary tumors of large lactiferous ducts. *Cancer* 1981;48:122–133.
99. Ohuchi N, Abe R, Kasai M. Possible cancerous change of intraductal papillomas of the breast. A 3-D reconstruction study of 25 cases. *Cancer* 1984;54:605–611.

100. Papotti M, Eusebi V, Bussolati G. Immunohistochemical analysis of benign and malignant papillary lesions of the breast. *Am J Surg Pathol* 1983;7:451–461.
101. Rosen PP, Cantrell B, Mullen DL, et al. Juvenile papillomatosis (Swiss cheese disease) of the breast. *Am J Surg Pathol* 1980;4:3–12.
102. Rosen PP, Lyngholm B, Kinne DW, et al. Juvenile papillomatosis of the breast and family history of breast carcinoma. *Cancer* 1982;49:2591–2595.
103. Bazzocchi F, Santini D, Martinelli G, et al. Juvenile papillomatosis (epitheliosis) of the breast. A clinical and pathologic study of 13 cases. *Am J Clin Pathol* 1986;86:745–748.
104. Nonomura A, Kimura A, Mizukami Y, et al. Secretory carcinoma of the breast associated with juvenile papillomatosis in a 12-year-old girl. A case report. *Acta Cytol* 1995;39:569–576.
105. Paget J. On disease of the mammary areola preceding cancer of the mammary gland. St. Bartholomew Hospital Report, 1874;10:87–89.
106. Yao D, Hoda S, Ying L, et al. Intraepidermal cytokeratin 7 reactive cells in non-neoplastic nipple represent interepithelial extension of lactiferous duct cells. *Mod Pathol* 2001;14:42A.
107. Vielh P, Validire P, Kheirallah S, et al. Paget's disease of the nipple without clinically and radiographically detectable breast tumor. Histochemical and immunohistochemical study of 44 cases. *Pathol Res Pract* 1993;189:150–155.
108. Keatings L, Wright C, Corbett IP, et al. c-erB-2 oncoprotein expression in mammary and extramammary Paget's disease: an immunohistochemical study. *Histopathology* 1990;17:243–247.
109. Wolber RAD, Wick MR. Expression of c-erB-2 oncoprotein in mammary and extramammary Paget's disease. *Am J Clin Pathol* 1991;96:243–247.
110. Ordonez NG, Awalt H, Mackay B. Mammary and extramammary Paget's disease: an immunocytochemical and ultrastructural study. *Cancer* 1987;59:1173–1183.
111. Sagabiel RW. Ultrastructural observations on epidermal cells in Paget's disease of the breast. *Am J Pathol* 1969;57:49–64.
112. Sagami S. Electron microscopic studies in Paget's disease. *Med J Osaka Univ* 1963;14:173–188.
113. Ashikari R, Park K, Huvos AG, et al. Paget's disease of the breast. *Cancer* 1970;26:680–685.
114. Paone JF, Baker RR. Pathogenesis and treatment of Paget's disease of the breast. *Cancer* 1981;48: 825–829.
115. Bijker N, Rutgers EJ, Duchateau L, et al. Breast-conserving therapy for Paget disease of the nipple: a prospective European Organization for Research and Treatment of Cancer study of 61 patients. *Cancer* 2001;91:472–477.
116. Fu W, Lobocki CA, Silberberg BK, et al. Molecular markers in Paget disease of the breast. *J Surg Oncol* 2001;77:171–178.
117. Dixon ARG, Ellis IO, Elston CW, et al. Paget's disease of the nipple. *Br J Surg* 1991;78:722–723.
118. Freund H, Maydovnik M, Laufer N, et al. Paget's disease of the breast. *J Surg Oncol* 1977;9:93–98.
119. Kister SJ, Haagensen CD. Paget's disease of the breast. *Am J Surg* 1970;119:606–609.
120. Maier WP, Rosemond GPH, Al-Saleem TI, et al. Paget's disease of the female breast. *Surg Gynecol Obstet* 1969;128:1253–1263.
121. Nance FC, Deloach DH, Welsh RA, et al. Paget's disease of the breast. *Am Surg* 1970;171:864.
122. Ridenhour CE, Perez-Mesa C, Hori JM. Paget's disease of the nipple. *Cancer Bull* 1969;21:15–16.
123. Rissanen PM, Holsti P. Paget's disease of the breast. *Oncology* 1969;23:209–216.
124. Jones DB. Florid papillomatosis of the nipple ducts. *Cancer* 1955;8:315–319.
125. Shapiro L, Karpas CM. Florid papillomatosis of the nipple. *Am J Clin Pathol* 1965;44:155–159.
126. Smith EJ, Kron SD, Gross PR. Erosive adenomatosis of the nipple. *Arch Dermatol* 1970;102:330–332.
127. Smith NP, Jones EW. Erosive adenomatosis of the nipple. *Clin Exp Dermatol* 1977;2:79–84.
128. Rosen PP, Caicco JA. Florid papillomatosis of the nipple. A study of 51 patients, including nine with mammary carcinoma. *Am J Surg Pathol* 1986;10:87–101.
129. Perzin KH, Lattes R. Papillary adenoma of the nipple (florid papillomatosis, adenoma, adenomatosis). A clinicopathologic study. *Cancer* 1972;29:996–1009.
130. Handly RW, Thackery AC. Adenoma of the nipple. *Br J Cancer* 1962;16:187.
131. Nichols FC, Dockerty MB, Judd JE. Florid papillomatosis of the nipple. *Surg Gynecol Obstet* 1958; 107:471.
132. Jones MW, Tavassoli FA. Coexistence of nipple duct adenoma and breast carcinoma: a clinicopathologic study of five cases and review of the literature. *Mod Pathol* 1995;8:633–636.
133. Diaz NM, Palmer JO, Wick MR. Erosive adenomatosis of the nipple: histology, immunohistology, and differential diagnosis. *Mod Pathol* 1992;5:179–184.

134. Myers JL, Mazur MT, Urist MM, et al. Florid papillomatosis of the nipple: immunohistochemical and flow cytometric analysis of two cases. *Mod Pathol* 1990;3:288–293.
135. Rosen PP. Syringomatous adenoma of the nipple. *Am J Surg Pathol* 1983;7:739–745.
136. Suster S, Moran CA, Hurt MA. Syringomatous squamous tumors of the breast. *Cancer* 1991;67: 2350–2355.
137. Jones MW, Norris HJ, Snyder RC. Infiltrating syringomatous adenoma of the nipple: a clinical and pathologic study of 11 cases. *Am J Surg Pathol* 1989;13:197–201.
138. Lambert PA, Kolm P, Perry RR. Parameters that predict nipple involvement in breast cancer. *J Am Coll Surg* 2000;191:354–359.
139. Luttges J, Kalbfleisch H, Prinz P. Nipple involvement and multicentricity in breast cancer. A study on whole organ sections. *J Cancer Res Clin Oncol* 1987;113:481-487.

5

Lobular Lesions

The terminal duct lobular unit (TDLU) is the physiologically active tissue in the breast. This unit has the most active cell turnover rate and is the site of origin of most of epithelial neoplasms of the breast (Fig. 5.1). Epithelial proliferation is maximal in the late luteal phase and becomes markedly enhanced if pregnancy ensues; however, it is followed by apoptosis 3 days after mitosis, if the breast returns to the resting state (1). Changes in the TDLU stroma and epithelium during the menstrual cycle and with aging are described in Chap-

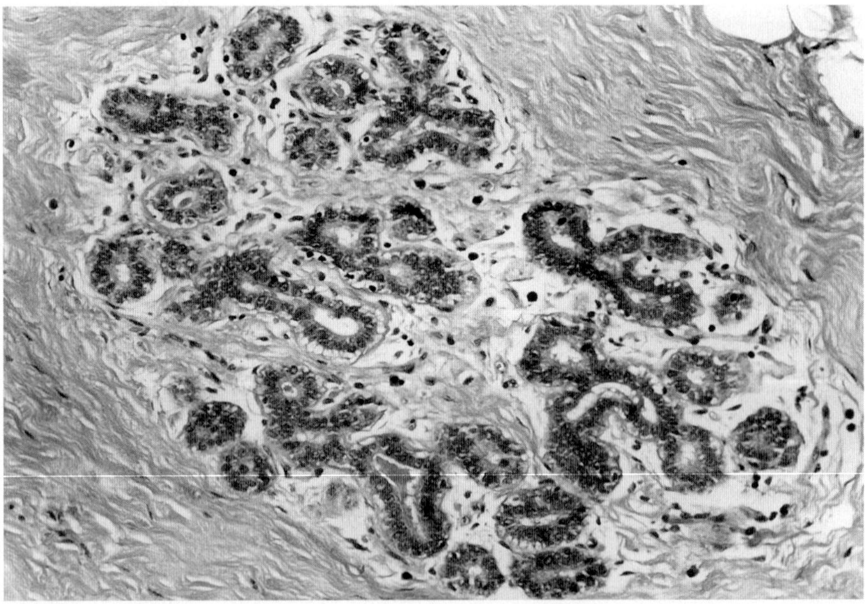

FIG. 5.1. Lobular unit. Terminal ducts are distributed through the loose stroma of the lobule and are characterized by two cell layers: a centrally placed epithelial layer around a patent lumen and a peripheral clear myoepithelial layer.

ter 1. During pregnancy, the epithelial cells proliferate, enlarge, and differentiate to lactational forms; the myoepithelial layer becomes markedly attenuated; and the stroma becomes inapparent by light microscopy. The responses among the lobules may vary, and an occasional lactating lobule may be found in biopsies that are taken in various phases of the menstrual cycle. This may reflect the clonal status of lobules. Segmental and collecting ducts are morphologically unchanged during lactation.

Physiologic changes may be significant and there are also abnormal changes in the structure of the lobule that are commonly observed in association with fibrocystic changes in the larger ducts. Allred et al (2) have described the changes as an unfolding of the lobular units with associated early genetic changes of neoplastic transformation, without morphologic abnormality. As noted in Chapter 1, clonality has been shown by Humara and loss of heterozygosity studies in microdissected normal lobules, which suggests that the cells of a lobule develop from a single progenitor, which makes molecular recognition of the earliest neoplastic changes difficult. Atrophy with myoid metaplasia of the myoepithelial cells may occur (Fig. 5.2 and efig. 5.1). Clear cell change of no known clinical significance also may be seen (efigs. 5.2 and 5.3).

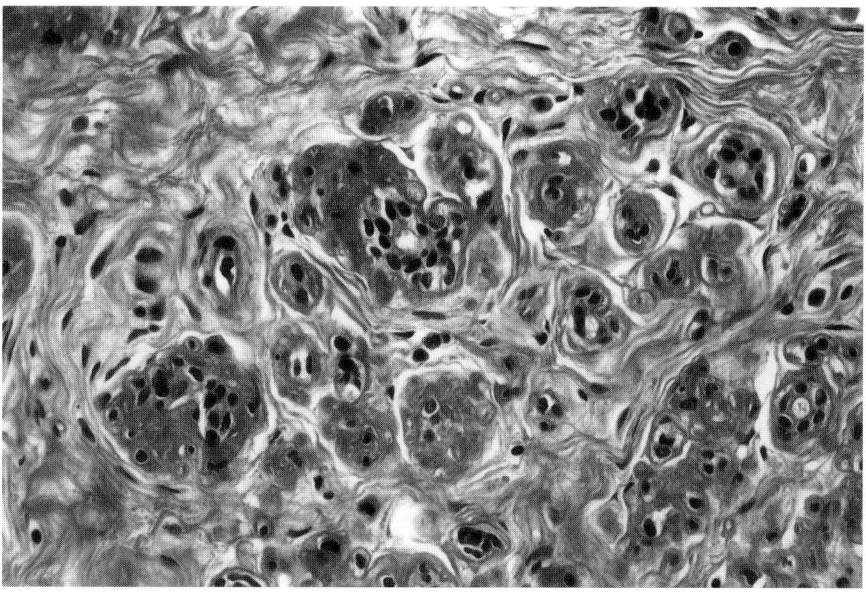

FIG. 5.2. Sclerotic lobule. Epithelial elements are atrophic and the myoepithelial layer has undergone myoid hyperplasia that resembles smooth muscle bundles.

BLUNT DUCT ADENOSIS

Blunt duct adenosis (BDA) is a term used to denote a lobular configuration of distended terminal ducts that have a columnar epithelium lining the central extracellular lumen and a normal lining of myoepithelial cells adjacent to the basement membrane area. The lobular stroma may be normal or fibrosed and basement membranes may be thickened (Figs. 5.2 and 5.3 and efigs. 5.6 and 5.7). Calcium phosphate microcalcifications are often found clustered in these distended ducts. Foote and Stewart (3) and Rosen and Oberman (4) used this term. Occasionally, the distended terminal ducts may simulate a tubular carcinoma, and are to be distinguished from microglandular adenosis in which the lobular pattern is not present and myoepithelial cells are inapparent. BDA is not grossly evident and is observed as part of a biopsy that is done for another lesion, unless the biopsy is done for clustered calcifications, in which case BDA may be the site of the calcification.

Columnar Alteration with Apocrine Snouts and Secretins (CAPSS)

Fraser et al. (5) reviewed 100 consecutive breast biopsies that were performed for microcalcifications and found 42 cases in which the terminal ducts of the lobule had undergone columnar alteration, with the appearance of prominent

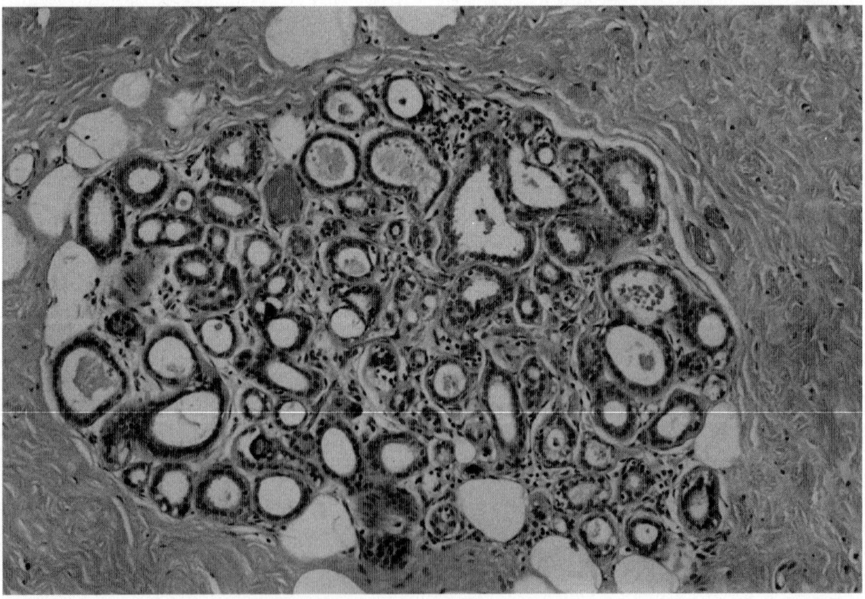

FIG. 5.3. Blunt duct adenosis. This lobule is characterized by dilated ducts, lined by a columnar epithelium. Lobular stroma is sclerotic.

apical snouts extending into the luminal border and with secretions in the extracellular lumen (Figs. 5.4 and 5.5 and efigs. 5.8 to 5.13). Calcifications were found in 74% of the cases of CAPSS. These calcifications were round, frequently psammomatous, and appeared dense and rounded on mammography. Within the 42 cases was a spectrum of change that ranged from the lesion described as CAPSS to one with atypia, to columnar epithelial tufting with bridges and micropapillations, and finally to atypical ductal hyperplasia, borderline for ductal carcinoma *in situ* (DCIS). Although the CAPSS lesion was found with similar frequency in biopsies with and without DCIS, the CAPSS associated with DCIS were more often of the histologically low grade and micropapillary, or cribriform, pattern than in cases without associated CAPSS. Anatomically, CAPSS and DCIS were frequently found close together in the same or adjacent TDLUs. Goldstein and O'Malley (6) described a similar lesion in 17 of 293 cases, of which 80 were fibrocystic change, 32 were tubular carcinomas, 41 were invasive grade I ductal carcinomas with DCIS, 40 were invasive grade I ductal carcinomas without DCIS, 40 were grade III invasive ductal carcinomas, 40 were invasive lobular carcinomas, and 20 were well differentiated DCIS without invasive cancer. Fourteen of the 17 cases of atypical ductal cells with apocrine snouts were found in association with tubular carcinomas and 3 cases were found with invasive grade I ductal carcinomas.

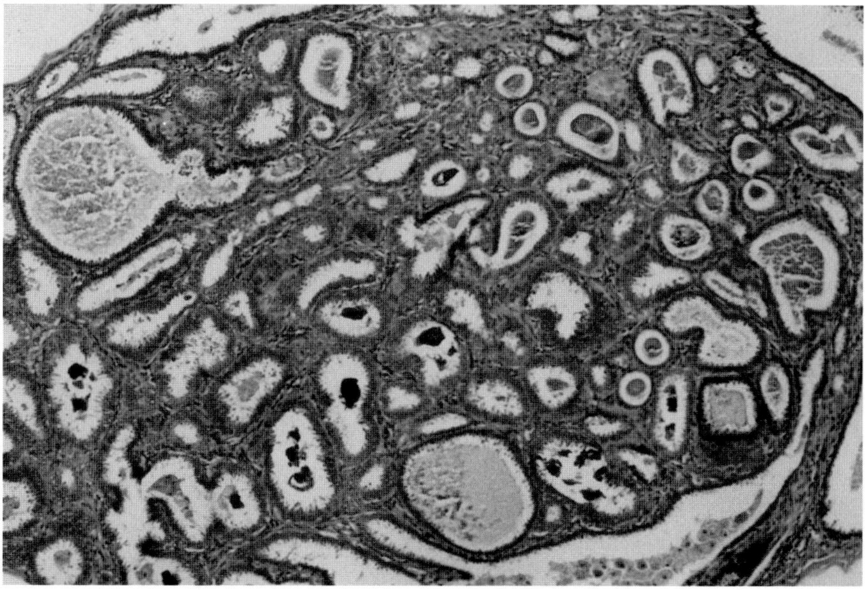

FIG. 5.4. Columnar alteration with apocrine snouts and secretions. The ducts in this lobule are dilated and lined by a columnar epithelium with what appears to be a micropapillary pattern. Secretions and calcifications are in the lumens and the lobular stroma is sclerotic.

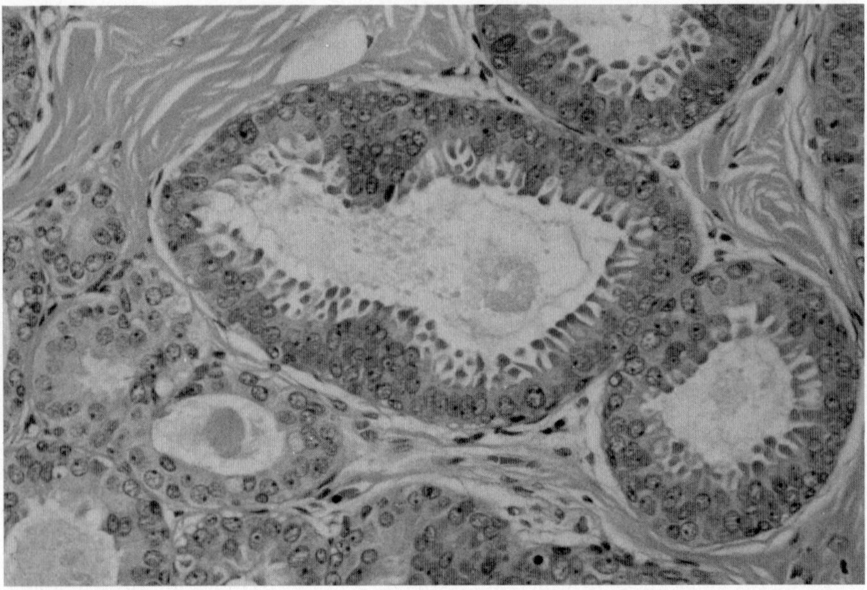

FIG. 5.5. Columnar alteration with apocrine snouts and secretions. These dilated ducts are lined by cells with elongated apocrine snouts that mimic a micropapillary proliferation.

Pregnancy-like Hyperplasia

Shin and Rosen (7) described a pregnancy-like or pseudolactational hyperplasia of the breast as an incidental finding. Calcifications were present in 10 of the 12 cases studied. Cystic hypersecretory hyperplasia also was present in five of the cases and merged with the pseudolactational hyperplasia. Atypia was associated with the change in 4 of the 12 specimens. Differential diagnosis from cystic hypersecretory hyperplasia, cystic hypersecretory carcinoma *in situ*, and secretory carcinoma was based primarily on lack of atypia in the cells of pseudolactational hyperplasia (efigs. 5.4 and 5.5).

NEOPLASTIC LOBULAR CELLS

A spectrum of change can be observed from the normal resting lobular architecture through lobular hyperplasia (LH) (Figs. 5.6 to 5.8 and efigs. 5.16 to 5.18) to atypical lobular hyperplasia (ALH) (Figs. 5.9 to 5.11 and efigs. 5.19 to 5.21) to lobular neoplasia/lobular carcinoma *in situ* (LCIS) (Figs. 5.12 to 5.16 and efigs. 5.22 to 5.25, 5.28, and 5.30). Dividing lines among these diagnoses are not sharp. The differences are more quantitative in character

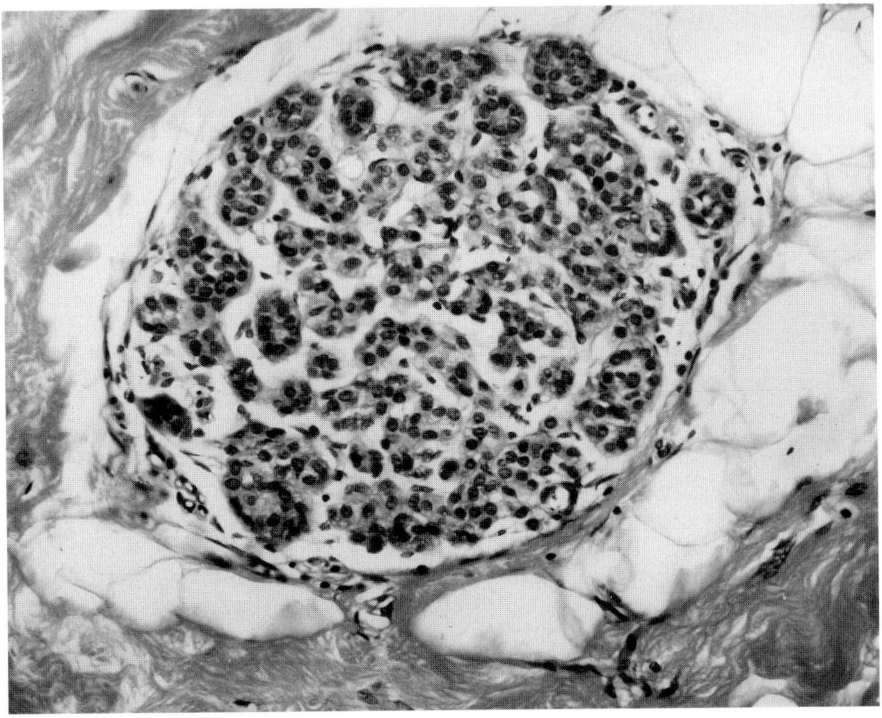

FIG. 5.6. Lobular hyperplasia. There is a proliferation of cells in the terminal ducts of this lobule and the central lumen is correspondingly diminished. Some profiles are oval.

than in the spectrum of proliferative lesions that occur in larger ducts, in which the changes are more qualitative and pattern oriented. The neoplastic lobular cells are seen as monomorphous, bland, and frequently detached cuboidal cells under the epithelial layer. The "lobular" cells have abundant cytoplasm, a polygonal shape, and fit together in a regular pattern. Many of the cells contain clear intracytoplasmic spaces, similar to vacuoles in their light microscopic appearance, which distort the bland, round, hyperchromatic, centrally placed, and usually amitotic nuclei. In both ALH and LCIS, these cells may proliferate out of the lobule into larger ducts, where they distend the zone between the epithelial cells and the basement membrane in a Pagetoid fashion, sometimes leaving the epithelium that lines the extracellular lumen intact.

Electron microscopy of neoplastic lobular cells (8) shows them to be similar in size and polygonal in shape. The clear spaces within the cytoplasm, which appear to be vacuoles by light microscopy and frequently stain for

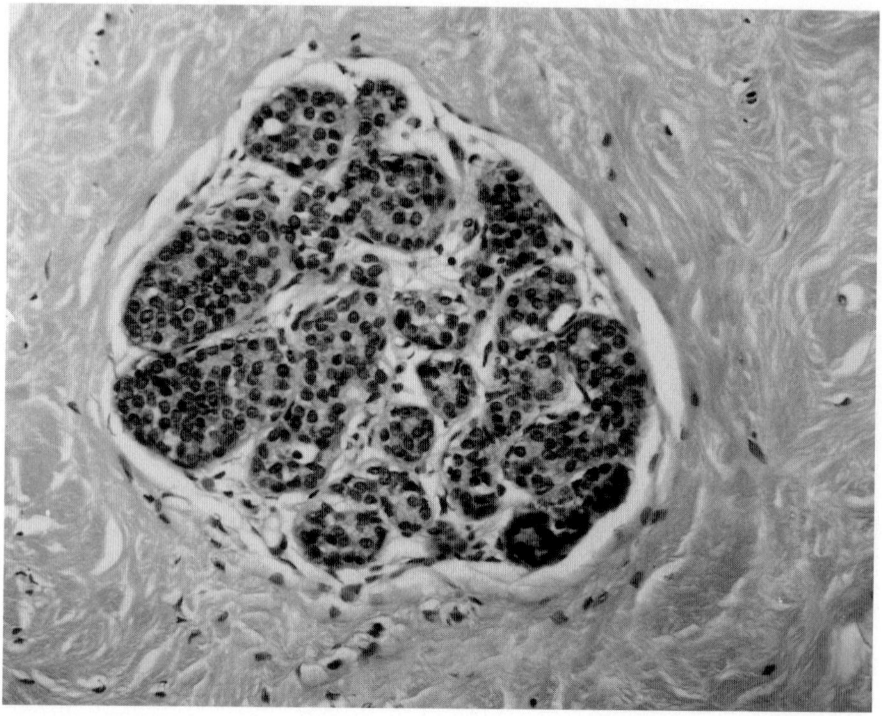

FIG. 5.7. Lobular hyperplasia. There is more proliferation of the cells and less distinction between the epithelial and myoepithelial layers in this lobule. Most profiles are round and those **(on the left)** are distended, but the cells are irregularly spaced. The nuclei are larger, but round and hyperchromatic. Lumina are present, but it is difficult to be certain they are extracellular.

mucus, are actually intracytoplasmic lumina. Secretory material usually is not evident in these intracytoplasmic lumina, which have not been shown to communicate with the extracellular space (Figs. 5.17 to 5.19 and efigs. 5.26 and 5.27). The cytoplasm of many of the lobular cells is filled with intermediate filaments, which have been considered to be myofilaments, keratin, or both. They may stain immunohistochemically with antibodies to low- or high-molecular weight keratin, smooth muscle actin, or all of these. Some cells have both intracytoplasmic lumina and intermediate filaments, and cells attached to the basement membrane by hemidesmosomes may contain intracytoplasmic lumina (Fig. 5.18). Normal epithelial and myoid cells are much less evident.

In their original description of LCIS, Foote and Stewart (9) argued that the cells of LCIS were myoepithelial, because the "lobular" cells resembled the

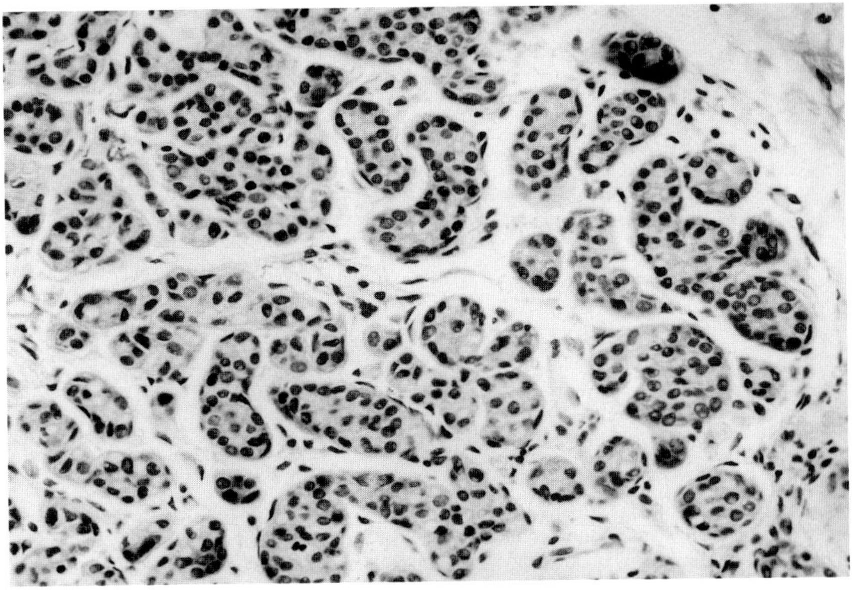

FIG. 5.8. Lobular hyperplasia. Extracellular lumens are not evident in any of these terminal ducts, but nearly all of the profiles are elongated, indicating lack of distention (hence limited proliferation). The cells seem to be all of one type, but most seem to have nuclei polarized to an antiluminal location.

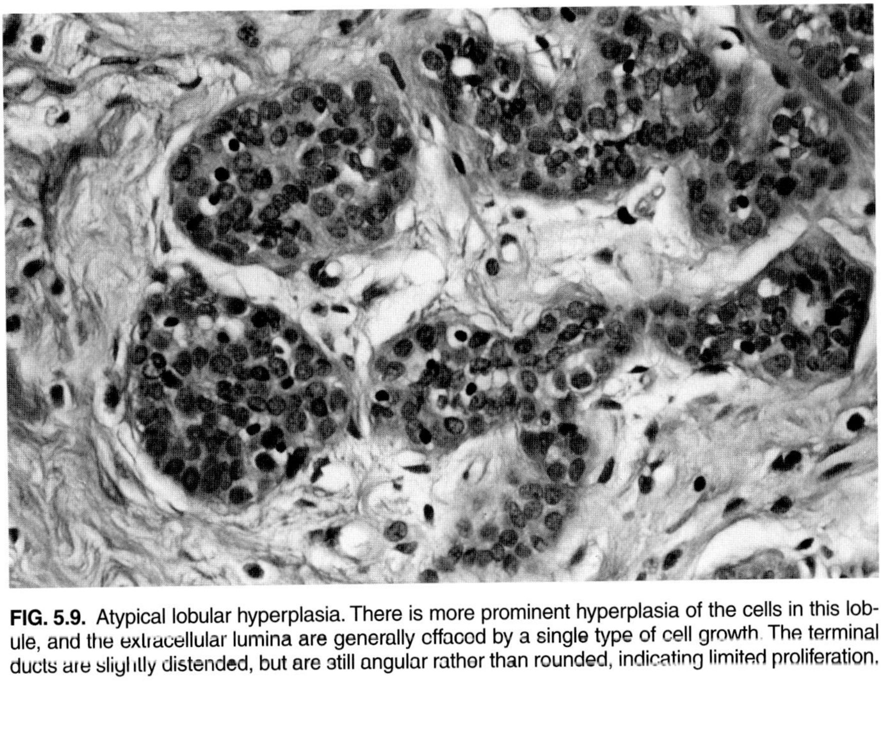

FIG. 5.9. Atypical lobular hyperplasia. There is more prominent hyperplasia of the cells in this lobule, and the extracellular lumina are generally effaced by a single type of cell growth. The terminal ducts are slightly distended, but are still angular rather than rounded, indicating limited proliferation.

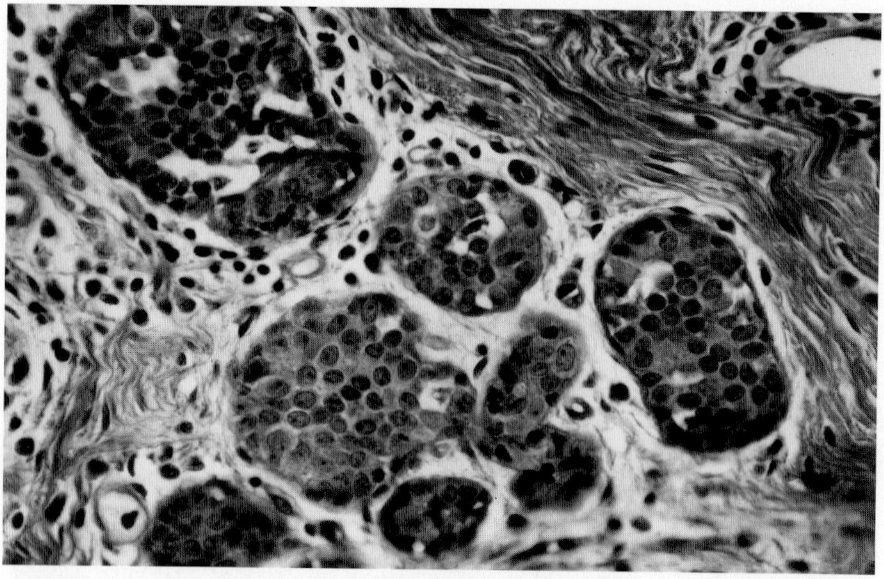

FIG. 5.10. Atypical lobular hyperplasia. The terminal ducts of this lobule are distended by abnormal cells of a single type and the central lumens have been effaced, but most profiles retain an angular configuration. This is borderline atypical lobular hyperplasia/lobular carcinoma *in situ*.

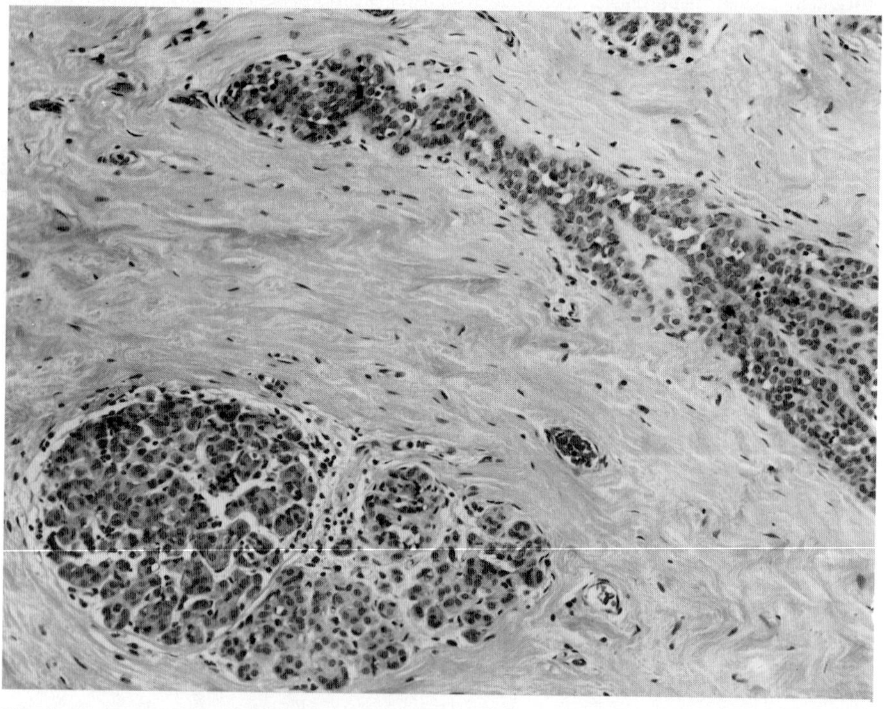

FIG. 5.11. Atypical lobular hyperplasia. The proliferating cells involve the lobule, the terminal ducts, and the larger duct (**upper half**). An extracellular lumen is present throughout much of this large duct.

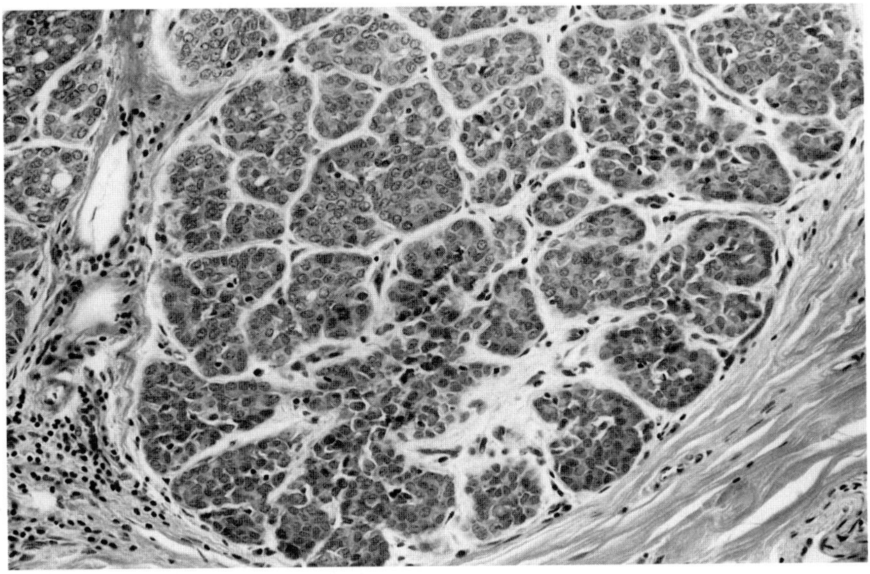

FIG. 5.12. Borderline lobular carcinoma *in situ.* The terminal ducts in this lobule are filled by a single type of cell that is proliferating and that distends the terminal ducts with five or six cells across to form rounded profiles. Extracellular lumens are effaced.

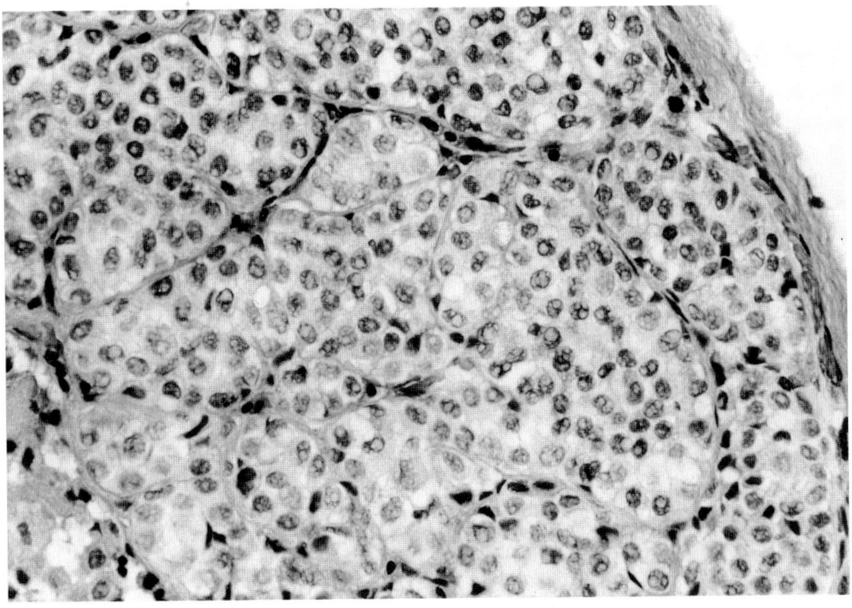

FIG. 5.13. Lobular carcinoma *in situ.* The terminal ducts are markedly distended by a proliferation of monomorphous cells that have effaced the lumen. The nuclei are round, regular, and evenly spaced. Intracellular lumens are present. The stroma is thinned.

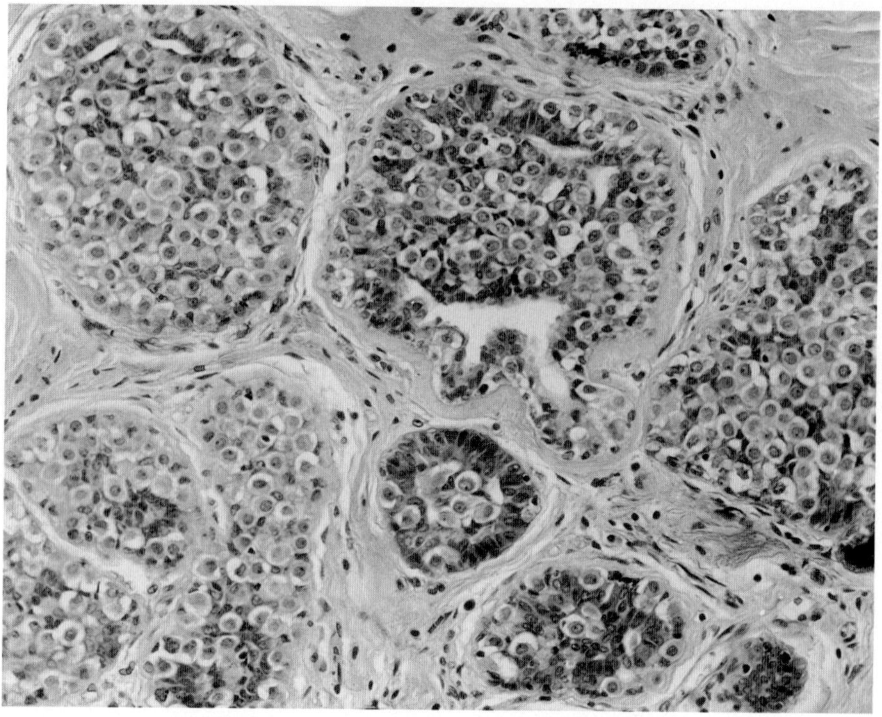

FIG. 5.14. Lobular carcinoma *in situ.* The terminal ducts are distended by cells that have a distinctly Pagetoid appearance. They form a mosaic pattern as they proliferate within the round, markedly distended, terminal ducts. The central lumens are effaced in most.

clear or basket cells and were seen near the basement membrane by light microscopy. Others have argued that the cells are epithelial in nature. Regardless of their origin, the cells are abnormal, seem to have some characteristics of both types of cells found in the resting terminal duct, and are distinctive by light and electron microscopy.

A proliferation of lobular cells in the zone closest to the basement membrane, normally occupied by myoepithelial cells, characterizes LH. A progressive filling of the duct by the same cells, with eventual effacement of the extracellular lumen, characterizes ALH. The terminal ducts are distended by this proliferation of abnormal cells, and the shape of the terminal ducts changes from oval to round in LCIS.

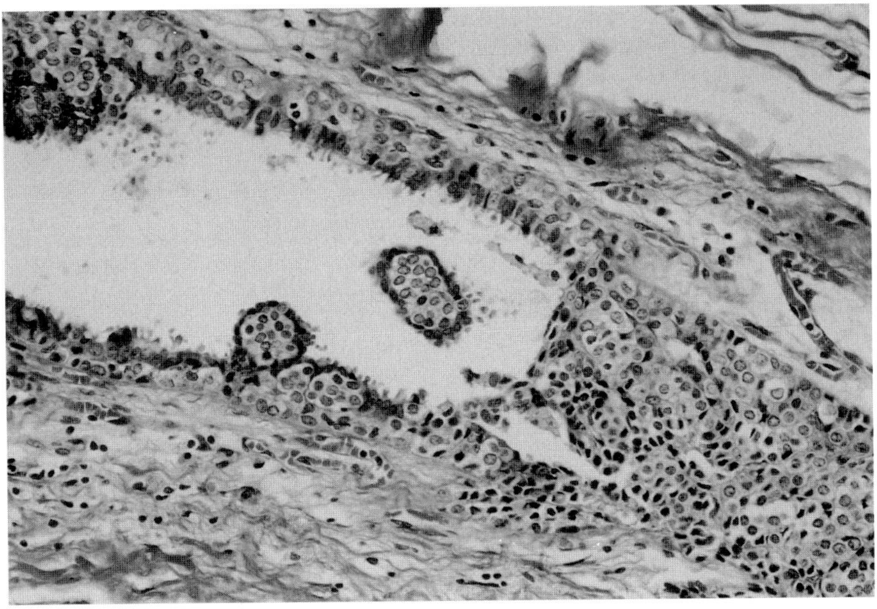

FIG. 5.15. Lobular carcinoma *in situ* (LCIS) in an extralobular duct. Just as ductal carcinoma *in situ* may involve lobules, LCIS may extend into the larger duct and fill the lumen (**right**). LCIS is found in the area between the basement membrane and the columnar cells that line the lumen, which is usually occupied by myoepithelial cells (**left**). LCIS in larger ducts can be recognized from the cellular appearance.

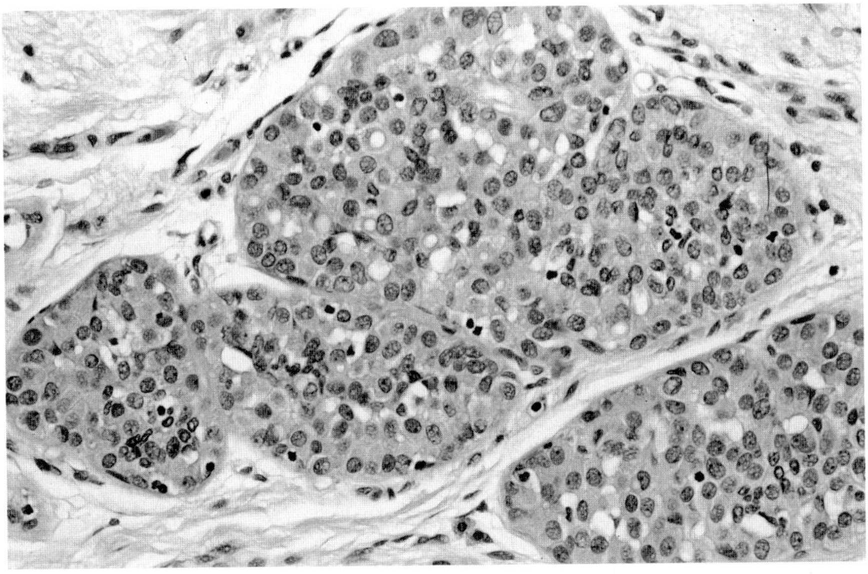

FIG. 5.16. Lobular carcinoma *in situ* (LCIS) with prominent intracellular lumina. In this full-blown case of LCIS, there are spaces within the cytoplasm of many of the cells producing a signet ring pattern in some of them. These spaces are intracellular lumens, not mucinous or secretory vacuoles.

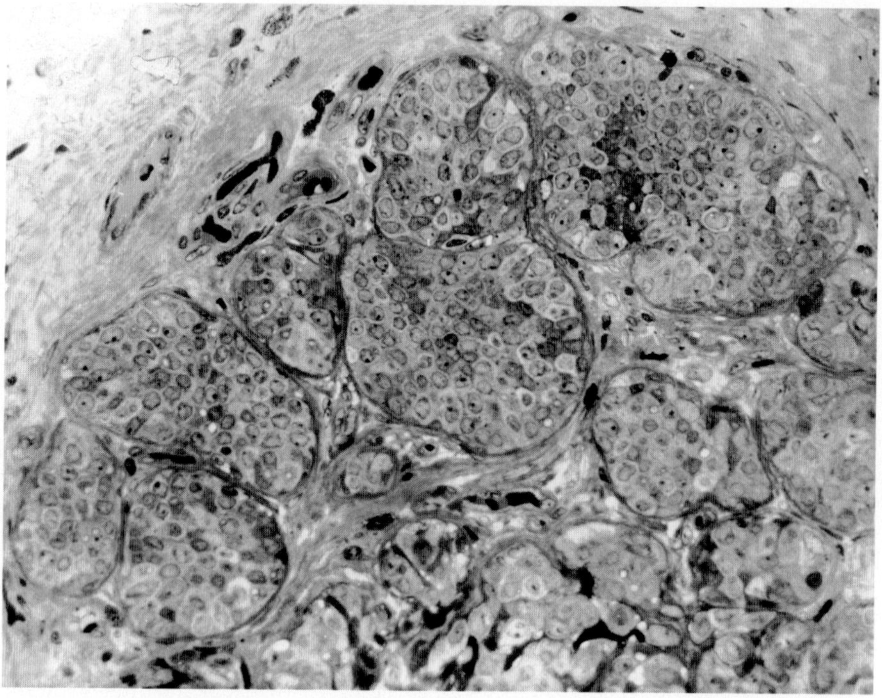

FIG. 5.17. Lobular carcinoma *in situ*. A thin section displays the distention of the terminal ducts by the abnormal cells. Intracellular lumens are present in both central and peripheral cells.

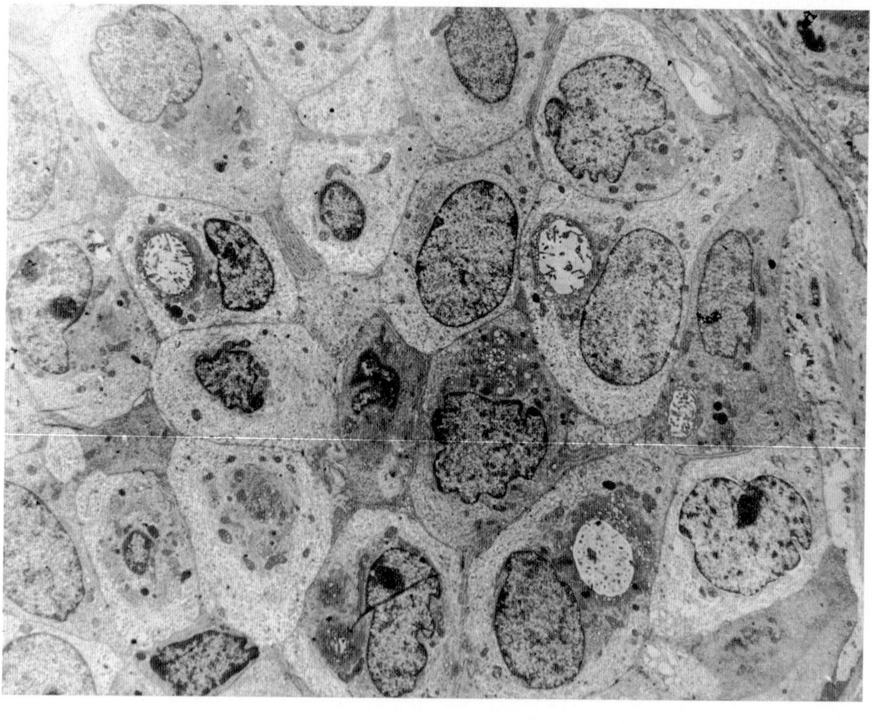

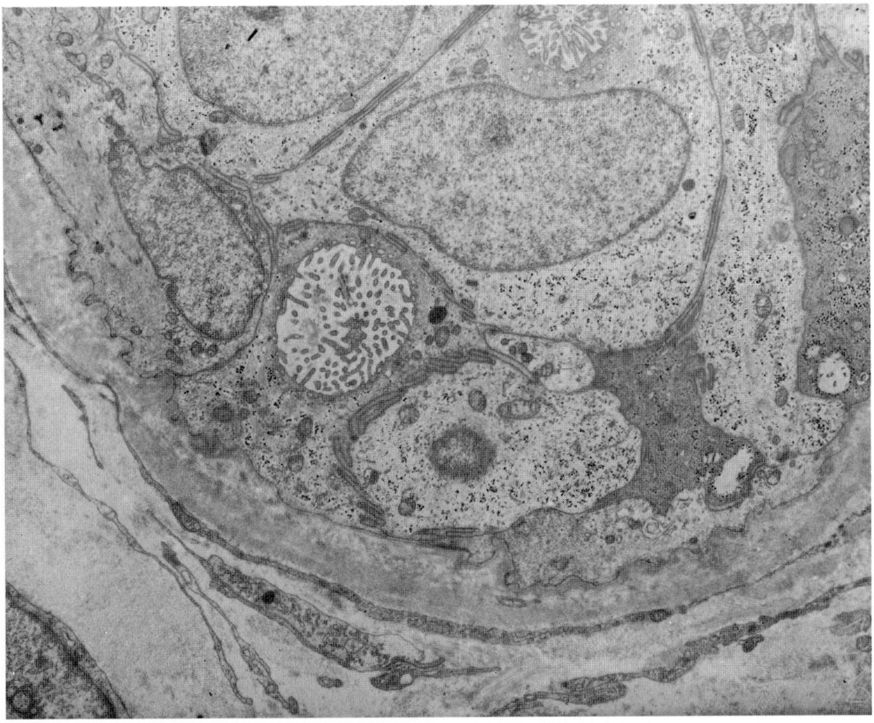

FIG. 5.19. Lobular carcinoma *in situ* with intracellular lumen. In this electron micrograph, a prominent intracellular lumen is evident in a cell attached to the basement membrane. Prominent microvilli characterize the intracellular lumen and distinguish it from a secretory or mucinous vacuole.

ATYPICAL LOBULAR HYPERPLASIA

Page et al. (10–12) and Dupont and Page (13) defined LCIS as the complete filling, distortion, and distention of at least half of the terminal ducts in one or more lobular units by evenly spaced cells with round monotonous hyperchromatic nuclei and cuboidal or polygonal cytoplasm. ALH "will fail to meet at least one of the preceding criteria." The criterion most often missing is distension of the terminal ducts, but the lumens may not be effaced and only a few of the terminal ducts may be affected. This description was confirmed in 1990 (12). Using this definition, the authors found 126 cases of ALH among 10,542 benign breast biopsy specimens (1.2%). Sixteen (13%) of these 126 patients developed invasive carcinoma during a follow-up period that averaged 12 years and ranged from 4.6 to 21.9 years. Eleven

←

FIG. 5.18. Lobular carcinoma *in situ* (LCIS). In this electron micrograph of LCIS, the cells proliferate and fill a terminal duct. Three of the cells have prominent intracellular lumens into which microvilli project, and two other cells appear to show portions of an intracellular lumen. Some of the cells also display prominent intermediate filaments.

of the 16 carcinomas were ipsilateral and 1 carcinoma was bilateral. The histology of the carcinomas was varied, with two invasive lobular carcinomas, one atypical medullary carcinoma; the remainder of the carcinomas was of the ductal type. The relative risk of developing invasive carcinoma in either breast after the diagnosis of ALH was 4.2 times the risk in a control group. In women with both ALH and a family history of breast cancer in a mother, sister, or daughter, the relative risk was 8.4 times that of the control group. All of the patients who subsequently developed carcinoma were younger than 55 years at the time of their biopsies, which were shown to contain ALH. Dupont and Page (13) reported that the incidence of invasive cancer after the diagnosis of atypical hyperplasia was constant from year to year. Since the risk of breast cancer increases with age for the entire population, the relative risk drops with time from diagnosis.

Unfortunately, the dividing lines between the histology of LH, ALH, lobular neoplasia, and LCIS are not clearly drawn, although the consensus seems to be as stated and illustrated. Rosai (14) and Schnitt et al. (15) have demonstrated how difficult the borderline cases may be.

In distinguishing typical LH from ALH, the pathologist should bear in mind that only 1.2% of over 10,000 benign breast biopsy specimens were considered ALH by Page and Dupont (12). The reader is referred to that report for its illustrations. ALH is an unusual lesion with significant implications. The term lobular neoplasia was intended to be synonymous with LCIS; however, it has been used by some to be more or less the same as ALH or to indicate the whole spectrum from ALH to LCIS.

The significance of the quantitative aspects of LCIS is not clear. LCIS was described by Foote and Stewart (9) as multifocal and often bilateral, and that is how some authors regard it. Hutter and Foote (16) insisted on this finding, whereas others, notably Wheeler et al. (17), however, argued that the morphologic diagnosis of cancer is not made on quantitative grounds in other organs and that a single focus was diagnostic of LCIS. There are serious students of this lesion, however, who reject the term LCIS and use the term neoplasia instead. Carter and Smith (18) suggested that increasing amounts of LCIS, especially when found bilaterally, correlates with increasing risk of invasive cancer, and Page et al. (19) came to a similar conclusion; however, the careful studies of larger groups of cases, with longer follow-ups, by Rosen et al. (20) and Haagensen et al. (21) did not support this view.

LOBULAR CARCINOMA *IN SITU*/LOBULAR NEOPLASIA

LCIS and ALH are not grossly evident lesions and they are detected incidentally in biopsies done for another lesion. It is unusual for them to be the site of calcification in a needle localization that is done for clustered calcifications. The histologic appearance has been defined above. Much of the significance of the histologic findings in the debate between the group of pathologists and surgeons who supported the concepts of Foote and Stewart (9) in viewing lobular lesions as carcinoma *in situ* and the group that supported the views of Haagensen et al. (22), who considered the lesion lobular neoplasia, apparently ended in 1978 when the two groups published major works with similar results and conclusions.

Rosen et al. (20) reported on the long-term follow-up of 99 patients with LCIS. The overall frequency of LCIS in biopsy specimens from patients without concurrent invasive carcinoma was 1.3%. The average length of follow-up, including patients who died before maximal potential follow-up (25 to 35 years), was 24 years. LCIS was divided equally between the two breasts, but simultaneous bilateral LCIS was not found. It was found most commonly in the upper outer quadrant, as had been shown previously by Lambird and Shelley (23). The average age at diagnosis was 45 years, with a range from 28 to 78 years. Only five of the patients were considered postmenopausal. A variety of other proliferative changes were found in many of the biopsy specimens with LCIS. Thirty-eight patients had papillomatosis, 30 had atypical LH, 23 had sclerosing adenosis, 15 had LH, 16 had fibroadenomas, and 11 had atypical papillomatosis. In 39 patients, the lobules with LCIS were approximately normal in size, whereas in the other 60 patients, the lobules were distended to twice the normal size or larger. Extralobular terminal ducts were involved in 64 cases. In approximately one-half of the cases, the cells were of small size; in the other half of cases, the cells were larger or they were a combination of small and large cells. None of these factors correlated with subsequent development of invasive cancer.

Thirty-two percent of the patients were subsequently treated for 36 breast carcinomas. Twenty patients had infiltrating ductal carcinoma and 13 patients had infiltrating lobular carcinoma. One patient had colloid carcinoma and one patient had tubular carcinoma. Five patients were found to have intraductal carcinoma and 10 patients were subsequently found to have LCIS. The difference in the risk of developing ipsilateral and contralateral carcinoma was quite small. Twelve patients had ipsilateral carcinoma, 9 had contralateral carcinoma, and 7 had bilateral carcinoma. The interval between the original diagnoses of LCIS was 2 to 31 years in those patients who developed ipsilateral breast cancer and 3 to 30 years in those with contralateral breast cancer. Approximately 38% of the patients who subsequently developed carcinoma did not have evidence of the disease until at least 20 years after LCIS was found. Thirteen patients had ipsilateral mastectomy and lymphadenectomy; 54% of these patients had axillary lymph node metastases and 47% had lymph node metastases from contralateral carcinomas. Sixteen of the 32 patients with breast carcinoma died of the disease. The risk of developing cancer in the breast was 9 times normal and the risk of death, as a result of breast cancer, was 10 times normal in this group of patients. The authors reviewed the family history of breast cancer, history of pregnancy, biopsy size, presence of associated cysts, number of lobules involved, lymphocytic reaction, degree of lobular distention, terminal duct involvement, and cell type involved, but they found no predictive value among any of these variables. Nine patients were treated immediately with ipsilateral mastectomy. None of these patients subsequently developed cancer in the contralateral breast. Thirteen patients were considered to have not LCIS, but atypical LH. Follow-up information was available for only seven of these patients. One of those seven patients developed invasive carcinoma in the ipsilateral breast.

Haagensen et al. (21) reported on 211 patients with lobular lesions; these were defined and illustrated the same as LCIS, but they were termed lobular neoplasia by the authors. The length of follow-up varied from 1 to 42 years, with a mean of 14 years. A total of 9.8% of patients developed carcinoma in the ipsilateral breast and 9.8% developed carcinoma in the contralateral breast, for a total of 17.1% patients developing breast carcinoma. (Some patients developed carcinoma in both breasts.) Six patients died of breast cancer. In all six of these patients, the original lobular lesion had not been recognized and the patients were not followed systematically at 4-month intervals. The age distribution of this series was similar to that of the series of Rosen et al. (20). Both groups of authors commented that the incidence of lobular lesions is considerably diminished after menopause and they consider this to suggest regression. Data collected in this series suggest that the disease was restricted to the terminal ducts of the lobules in premenopausal women much more frequently than in postmenopausal women, in whom both terminal and larger ducts were more often involved. The interval between the diagnosis of lobular neoplasia and the development of subsequent carcinoma was a long one, in this series as well; 14 of the 38 carcinomas observed developed after a 10-year interval.

The authors of both these series have extensively cited the pertinent literature (17,24–33) and they present their views of the significance of this lesion, but its fundamental nature still remains to be decided. It seems from these two studies that it is not productive to think of the lobular lesions as cancer cells that attempt to break through the basement membrane to invade the stroma. Microinvasion is rarely, if ever, observed in association with LCIS, whereas with DCIS, the problem of microinvasion is often presented. The variety of invasive carcinomas with which LCIS is associated, and the fact that both breasts are at approximately equal risk of developing invasive cancer, further substantiates the view that LCIS indicates that some of the conditions required for the development of invasive carcinoma are present.

If these are not cancer cells attempting to break through the basement membrane, what are they? My own view is that they indicate an underlying change in the mammary tissue that enhances the likelihood that a malignant transformation within an epithelial cell of the breast will go on to form an invasive cancer. The perimenopausal age distribution of the majority of cases suggests that hormonal influences are important in its causation. Mouse mammary tumors require a susceptible strain, a virus, and an appropriate hormonal environment. Without all three factors, tumors do not develop. Although this analysis is certainly too simplistic for human carcinomas, it does lend itself to the suggestion that the recognition of LCIS/lobular neoplasia (and ALH) is a warning that all of the mammary tissue is at risk. How this occurs remains to be determined. The decreased incidence in postmenopausal women indicates spontaneous regression. Are patients with regressed LCIS at higher risk? In this regard, it is interesting to note from the series by Rosen et al. (20) that only 17 of the 32 patients who subsequently developed invasive carcinoma still had associated residual LCIS.

In 1993, Ottesan et al. (34) reported a series from Denmark of 69 cases of LCIS that were followed for an average of 5 years. Eight patients developed invasive carcinoma, four patients developed DCIS and LCIS, one patient was found to have DCIS, and eight patients were shown to have residual LCIS in the ipsilateral breast.

Higher nuclear size and number of involved lobules correlated with higher risk of invasive cancer, which was overall 11 times that of the reference population.

Page et al. (19) reported 39 cases of florid LCIS, followed for 19 years, that was shown to have a relative risk of 8 for developing invasive carcinoma (17% absolute risk at 15 years), compared to a fourfold to fivefold risk for ALH. In this series, level of risk was not affected by either family history or post-menopausal estrogen replacement. Five of the 10 recurrences were ipsilateral, three recurrences were contralateral, and one recurrence was bilateral.

Beute et al. (35) and Sonnenfeld et al. (36) described the mammographic association of LCIS with microcalcifications, although the calcifications may not be in the lobules involved. LCIS is regarded as an incidental finding for mammographically detected lesions. Oberman and Markey (37) reported eight cases of LCIS that involved sclerosing adenosis—a combination that is easily mistaken for invasive carcinoma, especially on core needle biopsy (Figs. 5.20 to 5.22).

LCIS/lobular neoplasia is:

1. Usually found during the perimenopausal period.
2. Inapparent clinically and found incidentally in biopsies that were done because of other lesions.
3. Associated with an increase in the risk of developing invasive breast cancer of any type, in either breast and usually many years later.

The treatment or follow-up of this lesion should take all of these factors into consideration. Careful follow-up is an absolute minimum, however, since Carter

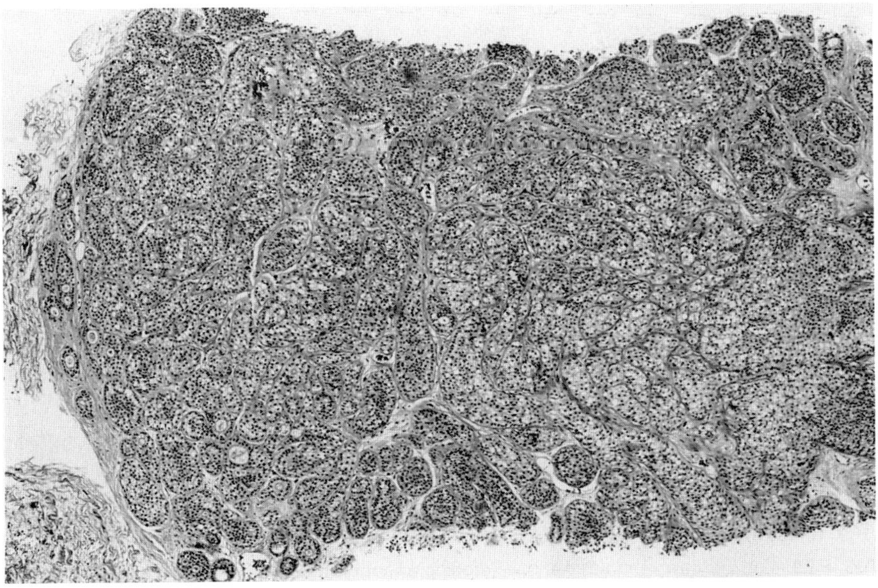

FIG. 5.20. Lobular carcinoma *in situ* in sclerosing adenosis. In this core needle biopsy specimen, there is a large volume of epithelium that, at first glance, appears to represent invasive carcinoma

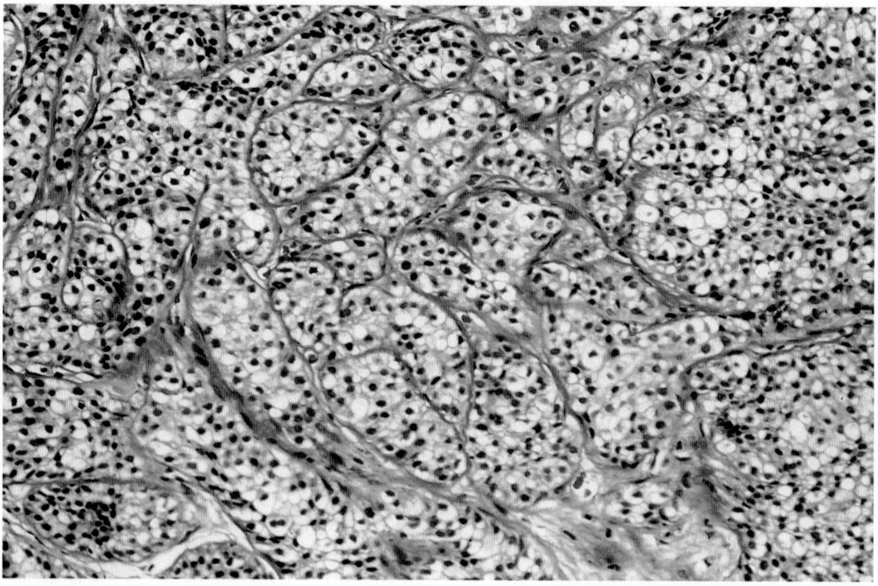

FIG. 5.21. Lobular carcinoma *in situ* in sclerosing adenosis. At higher magnification, it is evident that the epithelial structures are filled and distended by a monomorphous proliferation of cells, some of which have intracellular spaces, but many of which have a clear cytoplasm. The resemblance to invasive carcinoma is striking.

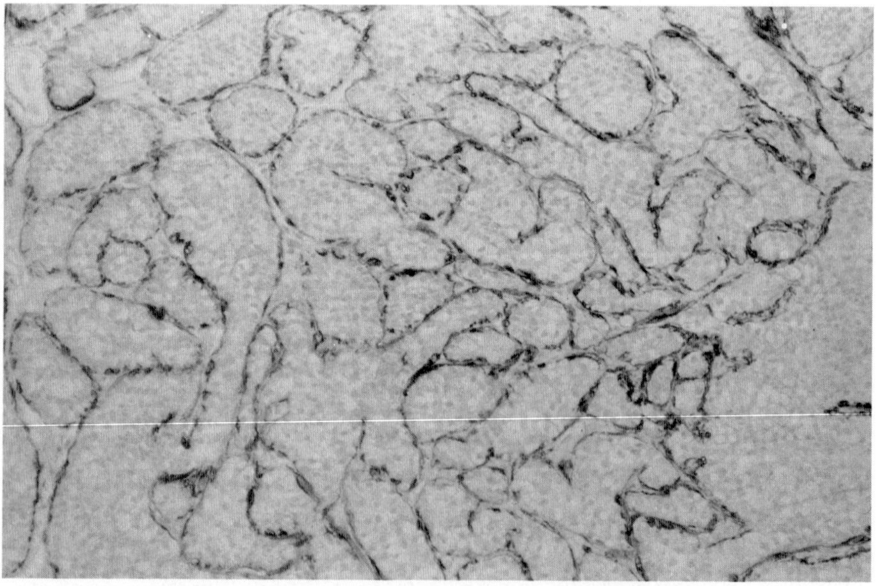

FIG. 5.22. Lobular carcinoma *in situ* in sclerosing adenosis immunostained for type IV collagen demonstrates that all of the structures are bounded by basement membrane, indicating that this is not invasive carcinoma, but a proliferation within ducts.

TABLE 5.1. *Comparison of atypical lobular hyperplasia, lobular carcinoma in situ, and lobular neoplasia*

	Atypical lobular hyperplasia[a]	Lobular carcinoma *in situ*[b]	Lobular neoplasia[c]
Patients (no.)	126	99	211
Invasive cancer (no./%)	16 (13%)	32 (32%)	36 (17%)
Interval (yr;mean)	4.6–21.9 (12)	2–31 (24)	1–42 (14)
Ipsilateral	69%	37%	50%
Relative risk	4.2–8.4	9	—
Risk	Yes	No	No family history

[a]From Page, et al. Atypical hyperplastic lesions of the female breast: a long-term follow-up study. *Cancer* 1985;55:2698–2708, with permission.

[b]From Rosen PP, Lieberman PH, Brown DW Jr, et al. Lobular carcinoma *in situ* of the breast: detailed analysis of 99 patients with average follow-up of 24 years. *Am J Surg Pathol* 1978;2: 225–235, with permission.

[c]From Haagensen CC, Lane N, Lattes R, et al. Lobular neoplasia (so-called lobular carcinoma *in situ*) of the breast. *Cancer* 1978;42:737–769, with permission.

and Smith (18) found invasive carcinoma "incidentally" in 3 of 49 mastectomies that were done for LCIS.

Table 5.1 summarizes the data for the studies on ALH, LCIS, and lobular neoplasia. Note that relative risk was not calculated in the same way by Page et al. (10) and Rosen et al. (20).

Lobular Carcinoma *In Situ* Versus Ductal Carcinoma *In Situ*

LCIS must be distinguished from DCIS involving the lobules by so-called "retrograde cancerization" because of the difference in clinical management. LCIS is followed, whereas DCIS is usually treated with additional surgery and/or radiation. Cytologically, DCIS usually has more anaplastic, irregular, and mitotically active nuclei and variation in the cytoplasm, which generally lacks the intracytoplasmic lumina described above (Fig. 5.23 and efigs. 5.31 to 5.36). Lobules in which retrograde cancerization has occurred are usually surrounded by a dense infiltrate of chronic inflammatory cells with distorting fibrosis, and there is often a question of microinvasion by the DCIS (Chapter 4). Neither is true for LCIS.

However, lesions in which the TDLU is filled with bland low-grade cells, without a pattern, present a problem in differential diagnosis (Fig. 5.24 and efig. 5.37). Immunohistochemistry may offer help in this differential diagnosis. LCIS is almost invariably estrogen receptor (ER) and progesterone receptor (PR) positive and rarely, if ever, positive for HER2/neu. DCIS, may, however, be ER and PR positive and HER2/neu may be negative, especially in cases of solid low nuclear grade DCIS, which is the problem in differential diagnosis with LCIS. Acs et al. (38) studied 198 cases of CIS with staining for E-cadherin and reported staining of all cases of DCIS, but staining of only 3 of 53 cases of LCIS. Cases with mixed LCIS/DCIS features did not stain for E-cadherin. Goldstein et

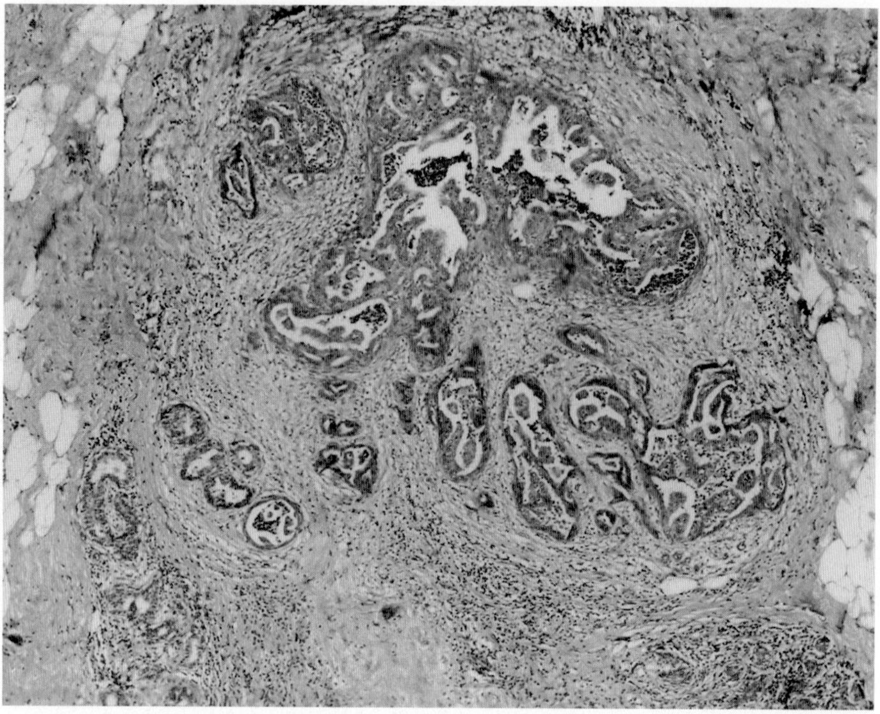

FIG. 5.23. Ductal carcinoma *in situ* in a lobule. The micropapillary pattern and marked fibrosis of the lobular stroma differ from lobular carcinoma *in situ.*

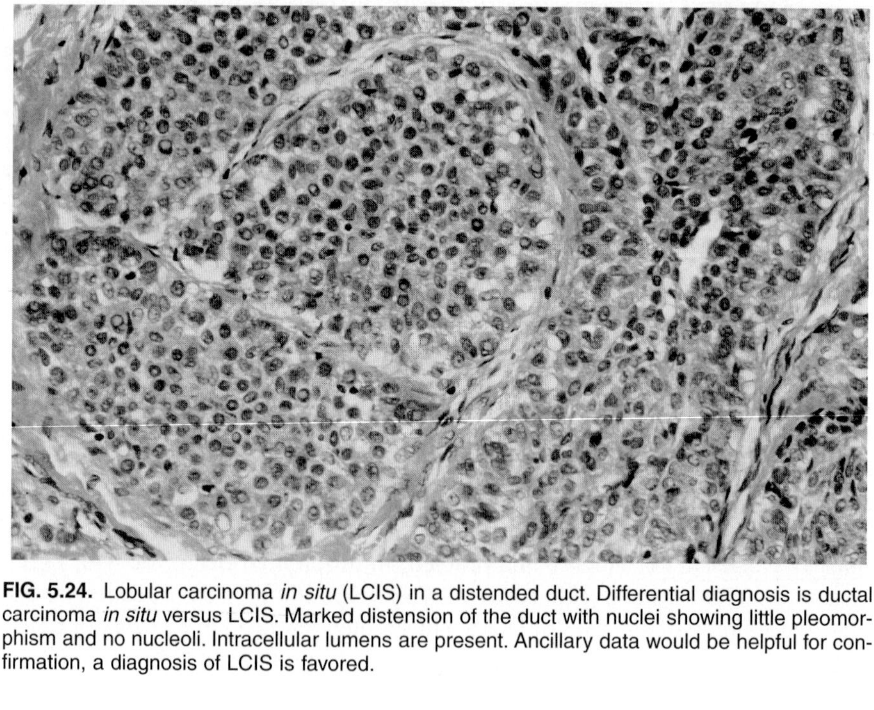

FIG. 5.24. Lobular carcinoma *in situ* (LCIS) in a distended duct. Differential diagnosis is ductal carcinoma *in situ* versus LCIS. Marked distension of the duct with nuclei showing little pleomorphism and no nucleoli. Intracellular lumens are present. Ancillary data would be helpful for confirmation, a diagnosis of LCIS is favored.

al. (39) reported 82 cases of LCIS with no other malignancy and long-term follow-up. Sixteen patients developed 21 cancers (9 ipsilateral, 2 contralateral, and 5 bilateral) in the 21.6-year mean follow-up period. Nine of the 82 cases of LCIS had focal E-cadherin immunostaining and these patients developed ipsilateral invasive carcinoma in higher frequency and in a shorter interval than the patients with E-cadherin negative LCIS. Jacobs et al. (40) studied 28 cases of LCIS and 33 cases of DCIS with antibodies to E-cadherin and reported negativity in all cases of LCIS and positivity in all cases of DCIS. Maluf et al. (41) studied 12 cases of *in situ* carcinoma with ductal and lobular features, with antibodies to E-cadherin. The authors reported that all E-cadherin positive *in situ* lesions were associated with invasive carcinomas, with ductal features, and that 5 of 6 E-cadherin negative CIS lesions were associated with invasive lobular carcinomas. The use of some (or a combination) of these antibodies may be a useful adjuvant in the differential diagnosis of LCIS from DCIS.

A pleomorphic variant of invasive lobular carcinoma has been described (Chapter 8). A pleomorphic variant of LCIS (PLCIS) has also been recognized, primarily in association with its invasive counterpart. PLCIS is difficult to distinguish from DCIS, if it occurs in the absence of invasive carcinoma, as has been suggested; however, fortunately, this is a rare occurrence and its clinical significance has not been established. Middleton et al. (42) described 38 cases of invasive pleomorphic lobular carcinoma, in which 8 patients had classic LCIS and 17 had PLCIS with non-cohesive large pleomorphic cells with abundant eosinophilic cytoplasm filling and distending terminal ducts. Immunohistochemical analysis of the cases revealed ER positivity in 81% of cases, PR positivity in 67%, and HER2/neu positivity in 81%. Consistent with the notion that invasive PLCIS has apocrine features, 71% of the PLCIS stained with GCDFP-15. Thus, PLCIS has a much higher incidence of HER2/neu staining and a lower incidence of ER and PR positivity than classic LCIS.

SUMMARY

The terminal ducts may display a spectrum of changes from LH to ALH to lobular neoplasia/LCIS. With the exception of LH, these changes are unusual. Criteria for distinguishing these diagnoses and the significance of doing so are somewhat problematic, but the clinical management of the diagnosis of either ALH or LCIS is the careful follow-up of both breasts and not additional surgery, which should allow further studies to clarify this issue. Tamoxifen has been suggested for use in patients who have increased risk of breast cancer. Those with either ALH or LCIS are considered in the group with increased risk and are therefore eligible for treatment (43). In 2001, Fisher et al. (44) reported the results from the National Surgical Adjuvant Breast and Bowel (NSABP) phase 1 trial that showed a 50% reduction in invasive carcinoma in women with ADH and LCIS, as well as a reduction in the incidence of ADH and LCIS in women who had not been diagnosed with those lesions after the administration of tamoxifen.

REFERENCES

1. Anderson TJ. Normal breast: myths, realities, and prospects. *Mod Pathol* 1998;11:115–119.
2. Allred DC, Mohsin SK, Fuqua SA. Histological and biological evolution of human premalignant breast disease. *Endocr Relat Cancer* 2001;8:47–61.
3. Foote FW, Stewart FW. Comparative studies of cancerous versus noncancerous breasts. *Ann Surg* 1945;121:197–222.
4. Rosen PP, Oberman HA. *Atlas of tumor pathology*, 3rd series. Washington: Armed Forces Institute of Pathology, 1993.
5. Fraser JL, Raza S, Chorny K, et al. Columnar alteration with prominent apical snouts and secretions: a spectrum of changes frequently present in breast biopsies performed for microcalcifications. *Am J Surg Pathol* 1998;22:1521–1527.
6. Goldstein N, O'Malley B. Cancerization of small ectatic ducts of the breast by ductal carcinoma *in situ* cells with apocrine snouts. *Am J Clin Pathol* 1997;107:561–566.
7. Shin SJ, Rosen PP. Pregnancy-like (pseudolactational) hyperplasia: a primary diagnosis in mammographically detected lesions of the breast and its relationship to cystic hypersecretory hyperplasia. *Am J Surg Pathol* 2000;24:1670–1674.
8. Carter D, Yardley JH, Shelley WM. Lobular carcinoma of the breast: an ultrastructural comparison with certain duct carcinomas and benign lesions. *Johns Hopkins Med J* 1969;125:25–43.
9. Foote FW Jr, Stewart FW. Lobular carcinoma *in situ*: a rare form of mammary cancer. *Am J Pathol* 1941;17:491–496.
10. Page D, Dupont WD, Rogers LW. Atypical hyperplastic lesions of the female breast: a long term follow-up study. *Cancer* 1985;55:2698–2708.
11. Page DL. Cancer risk assessment in benign breast biopsies. *Hum Pathol* 1986;17:871–874.
12. Page DL, Dupont WD. Anatomic markers of human premalignancy and risk of breast cancer. *Cancer* 1990;66:1326–1335.
13. Dupont WD, Page DL. Relative risk of breast cancer varies with time since diagnosis of atypical hyperplasia. *Hum Pathol* 1989;20:723–725.
14. Rosai J. Borderline epithelial lesions of the breast. *Am J Surg Pathol* 1991;15:209–221.
15. Schnitt SJ, Connolly JL, Tavassoli FA, et al. Interobserver reproducibility in the diagnosis of ductal proliferative breast lesions using standardized criteria. *Am J Surg Pathol* 1992;16:1133–1143.
16. Hutter RVP, Foote FW Jr. Lobular carcinoma *in situ*: long term follow-up. *Cancer* 1969;24: 1081–1085.
17. Wheeler JE, Enderline HT, Roseman JM, et al. Carcinoma *in situ* of the breast: long term follow-up. *Cancer* 1974;34:554–563.
18. Carter D, Smith RR. Carcinoma *in situ* of the breast. *Cancer* 1977;40:1189–1193.
19. Page DL, Kidd JE, Dupont WD. Lobular neoplasia of the breast: higher risk for subsequent invasive cancer predicted by more extensive disease. *Hum Pathol* 1991;22:1232.
20. Rosen PP, Lieberman PH, Brown DW Jr, et al. Lobular carcinoma *in situ* of the breast: detailed analysis of 99 patients with average follow-up of 24 years. *Am J Surg Pathol* 1978;2:225–235.
21. Haagensen CC, Lane N, Lattes R, et al. Lobular neoplasia (so-called lobular carcinoma *in situ*) of the breast. *Cancer* 1978;42:737–769.
22. Haagensen CD, Lane N, Bodian C. Coexisting lobular neoplasia and carcinoma of the breast. *Cancer* 1983;51:1468.
23. Lambird PA, Shelley WM. The spatial distribution of lobular *in situ* mammary carcinoma. *JAMA* 1969;210:689–693.
24. Andersen JA. The basement membrane and lobular carcinoma *in situ* of the breast: a light microscopical study. *Acta Pathol Microbiol Scand* 1975;83:245–250.
25. Andersen JA. Lobular carcinoma *in situ* of the breast. *Cancer* 1977;39:2597–2602.
26. Anderson JA. Lobular carcinoma *in situ* of the breast with ductal involvement: frequency and possible influence on prognosis. *Acta Pathol Microbiol Scand* 1974;82:655–662.
27. Anderson JA. Lobular carcinoma *in situ*: a long term follow-up in 52 cases. *Acta Pathol Microbiol Scand* 1974;82:519–533.
28. Benfield JR, Jacobson M, Warner NW. *In situ* lobular carcinoma of the breast. *Arch Surg* 1965;91:130–135.
29. Fechner RE Lobular carcinoma *in situ*: a rare form of mammary cancer. *Am J Pathol* 1971;17: 491–496.
30. Giordano JM, Klopp CT. Lobular carcinoma *in situ*: incidence and treatment. *Cancer* 1973;31:105–109.

31. Godwin JT. Chronology of lobular carcinoma in the breast: report of a case. *Cancer* 1952;5:259–266.
32. Lewison EF, Finney GG Jr. Lobular carcinoma *in situ* of the breast. *Surg Gynecol Obstet* 1968;126: 1280–1286.
33. McDivitt RW, Hutter RVP, Foote FW Jr, et al. *In situ* lobular carcinoma: a prospective follow-up study indicating cumulative patient risks. *JAMA* 1967;201:8–86.
34. Ottesan GL, Graverson HP, Blichert-Toft M, et al. Lobular carcinoma *in situ* of the female breast. Short-term results of a prospective nationwide study. *Am J Surg Pathol* 1993;17:14–21.
35. Beute BJ, Kalisher L, Hutter RVP. Lobular carcinoma *in situ* of the breast: clinical, pathologic and mammographic features. *Am J Roentgenol* 1991;157:257.
36. Sonnenfeld MR, Frenna TH, Weidner N, et al. Lobular carcinoma *in situ*: mammographic-pathologic correlation of results of needle-directed biopsy. *Radiology* 1991;181:363–367.
37. Oberman HA, Markey BA. Noninvasive carcinoma of the breast presenting in adenosis. *Mod Pathol* 1991;4:31–35.
38. Acs G, Lawton TJ, Rebbeck TR, et al. Differential expression of E-cadherin in lobular and ductal neoplasms of the breast and its biologic and diagnostic implications. *Am J Clin Pathol* 2001;115:85–98.
39. Goldstein NS, Bassi D, Watts JC, et al. E-cadherin reactivity of 95 noninvasive ductal and lobular lesions of the breast. Implications for the interpretation of problematic lesions. *Am J Clin Pathol* 2001;115:534–542.
40. Jacobs TW, Pliss N, Kouria G, et al. Carcinomas *in situ* of the breast with indeterminate features: role of E-cadherin staining in categorization. *Am J Surg Pathol* 2001;25:229–236.
41. Maluf HM, Swanson PE, Koerner FC. Solid low-grade *in situ* carcinoma of the breast: role of associated lesions and E-cadherin in differential diagnosis. *Am J Surg Pathol* 2001;25:237–244.
42. Middleton LP, Palacios DM, Bryant BR, et al. Pleomorphic lobular carcinoma: morphology, immunohistochemistry, and molecular analysis. *Am J Surg Pathol* 2000;24:1650–1656.
43. Vogel VG. Reducing the risk of breast cancer with tamoxifen in women at increased risk. *J Clin Oncol* 2001;19:87S–92S.
44. Fisher B, Land S, Mamounas E, et al. Prevention of invasive breast cancer in women with ductal carcinoma *in situ*: an update of the national surgical adjuvant breast and bowel project experience. *Semin Oncol* 2001;28:400–418.

6

Pseudoinfiltrative Lesions

A wide variety of pseudoinfiltrative lesions, which may be difficult to distinguish from invasive, low grade, or tubular carcinoma, are found in association with cystic changes in the breast. Some of these have been described and named, but others have yet to be clearly defined. The lesions share three characteristics: distortion of normal architecture, stromal change, and proliferation of epithelial elements. Recognition of the overall pattern is often a helpful feature in the interpretation of the epithelial elements, and recognition of the benign nature of the epithelium is usually the conclusive observation. Immunohistochemistry, with application of antibodies to basement membrane and the myoepithelium, are useful in the identification of normal acinar structures that have dual layers lying within basement membranes, which are often thickened. Examination "off Köhler" illumination may also outline basement membranes. The described lesions include sclerosing adenosis, atypical apocrine sclerosing lesion (AASL), blunt duct adenosis (BDA), microglandular adenosis (MGA), and radial scar (RS). Sclerosing adenosis, AASL, and BDA are recognized from their lobular configuration. MGA is a nonlobular lesion and RS is an interlobular lesion with lobules apparently drawn into it. Some of their features are compared to those of tubular carcinoma in Table 6.1.

TABLE 6.1. *A comparison of sclerosing adenosis, atypical apocrine sclerosing lesion, microglandular adenosis, radial scar, and tubular carcinoma*

	Epithelium	Myoepithelium	Basement membrane
SA	Varied	Prominent	Thick
AASL	Apocrine	Present	Thick
MGA	Clear, S-100+	?Absent	Present
RS	Open ducts	Present	Present
TC	Open ducts	Absent	Absent

SA, sclerosing adenosis; AASL, atypical apocrine sclerosing lesion; MGA, microglandular adenosis; RS, radial scar; TC, tubular carcinoma.

SCLEROSING ADENOSIS

Sclerosing adenosis is the largest and least well-defined group of pseudoinfiltrative lesions, with several patterns and a range of sizes. It is usually multiple and may coexist with RSs. Clusters of fine microcalcification often point out these lesions mammographically. In general, the lesions are smaller than 5 mm, and most are microscopic. The border is more rounded than in RSs, and the overall configuration is that of an expanded distorted lobule with extensive fibrosis, usually without evident fibroblastic proliferation, which markedly distorts internal lobular architecture. The small ducts are more numerous and denser (adenosis) than expected in a lobule. Basement membranes may be so markedly thickened that they merge with the fibrosis and become inapparent, although careful examination of the lesion, aided by immunohistochemical staining for type IV collagen and electron microscopy (1), has demonstrated that the basement membranes are increased in thickness (Figs. 6.1 to 6.7 and efigs. 6.1 to 6.6). This may be especially helpful in a core needle biopsy of sclerosing adenosis (Fig. 6.8). The ducts vary in appearance from compressed atrophic-appearing structures to markedly proliferative distended examples of ductal or lobular hyperplasia. A myoepithelial layer may be relatively inapparent on H&E, but it is shown to be a prominent or even predominant feature when antibodies to smooth muscle actin or calponin are employed. Lee et al. (2) described a variant of sclerosing adenosis, which they termed tubular

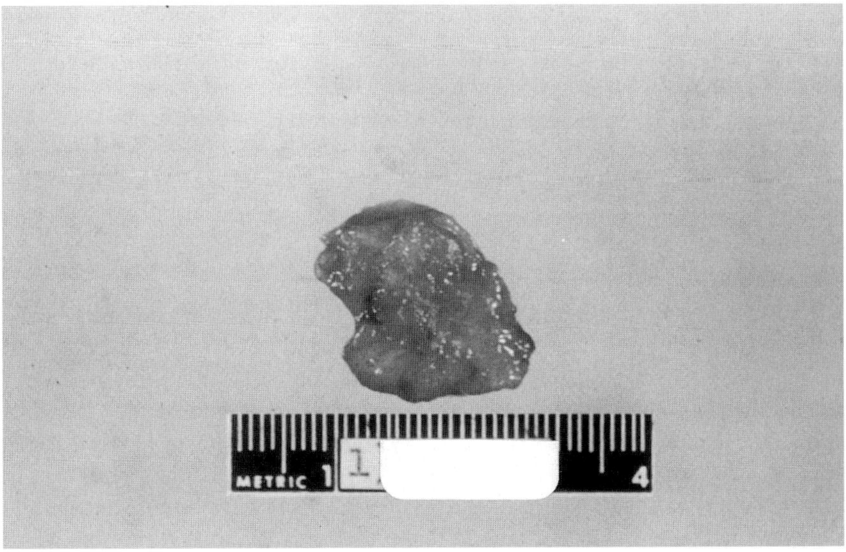

FIG. 6.1. Sclerosing adenosis. The gross appearance of sclerosing adenosis is a firm white rounded lesion that blends with the stroma at its margin.

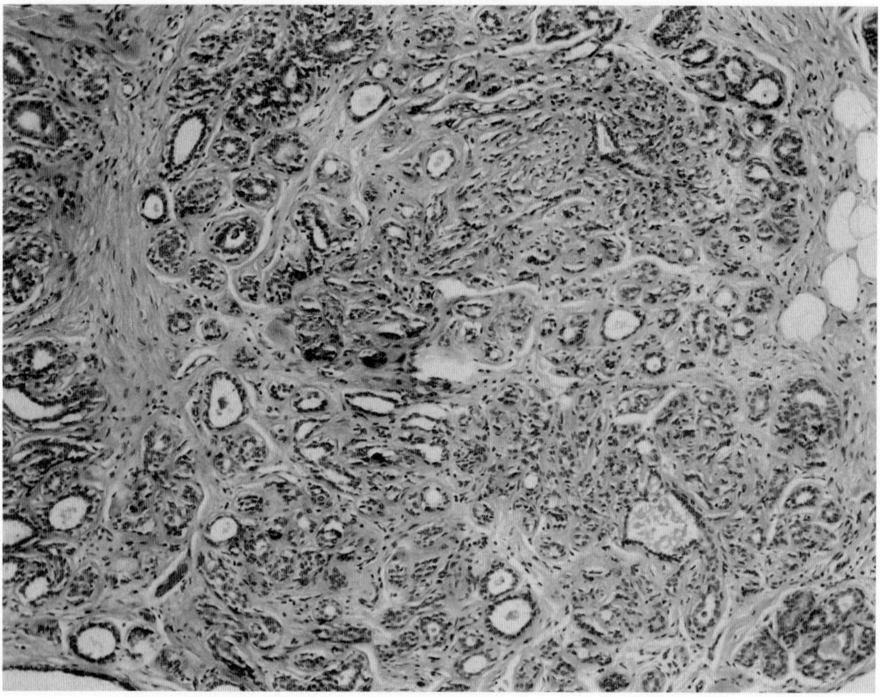

FIG. 6.2. Sclerosing adenosis. The expanded lobular architecture has been distorted by a fibrosing process that has entrapped the terminal ducts, which are more numerous than in normal lobules. This suggests that a proliferative process (adenosis) has occurred. The low power view shows the usual size of this lesion, which is approximately two to three times that of a normal lobule. Ducts within this process show various shapes. Most are so compressed that they have no evident lumen, but some are open and distended.

adenosis, due to the elongation of the terminal ducts. (Fig. 6.9 and efigs. 6.7 and 6.8).

Small ducts of sclerosing adenosis, which have been shown to be benign by both morphology and clinical follow-up, have been found in perineural spaces (Fig. 6.10 and efig. 6.13) (3). Compare Fig. 6.10 and efig. 6.13 with the carcinoma in the perineural space in Fig. 6.11 and efig. 6.12. Rarely, lobular units have been seen under the peripheral sinus of an axillary lymph node (4) in association with sclerosing adenosis. Atypical lobular hyperplasia (ALH), lobular carcinoma *in situ* (LCIS) (Fig. 6.12 and efigs. 6.9 and 6.10) (5), and, less frequently, ductal carcinoma *in situ* (DCIS) (efig. 6.11) may be present within a sclerosing adenosis lesion and may mimic invasive carcinoma. Although the proliferation has features of cancer, basement membranes remain intact or thickened. Eusebi et al. (6) reported on five cases of LCIS and two cases of DCIS in

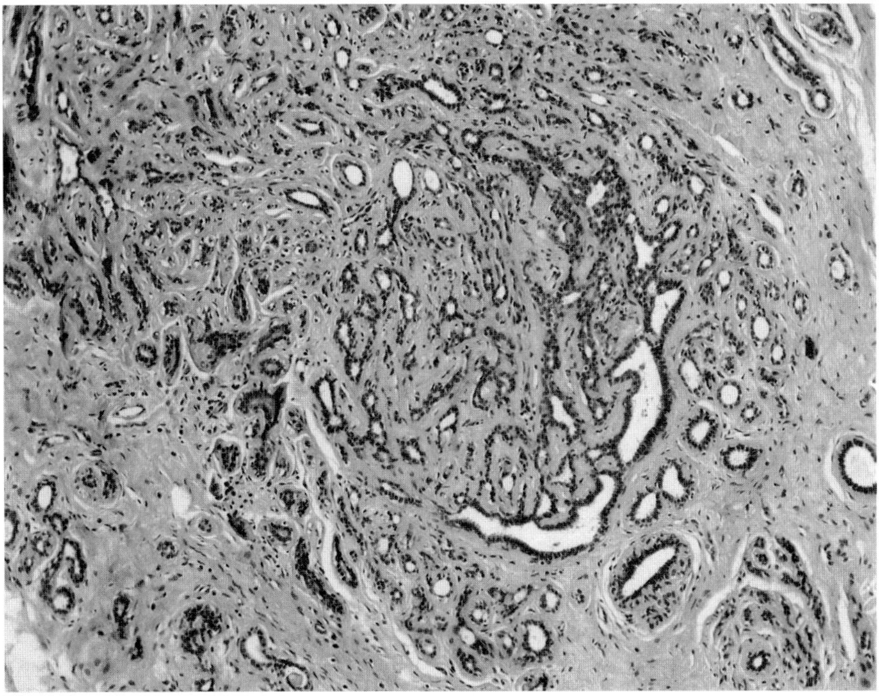

FIG. 6.3. Sclerosing adenosis. This circumscribed lesion is two to three times normal lobular size. There is marked distortion of all the terminal ducts in this lobule, most of which are slit-like in configuration, but several are open and rounded.

sclerosing adenosis in which frozen section diagnosis of invasive cancer was given in two cases. Invasive carcinoma also may involve lobules with sclerosing adenosis (Figs. 6.13 and 6.14). Jensen et al. (7) reported a twofold risk of invasive carcinoma in patients with sclerosing adenosis, primarily because of its frequent association with ALH (but not with atypical ductal hyperplasia). Sclerosing adenosis also correlated with perimenopausal age, microcalcifications, and a family history of breast cancer. Sclerosing adenosis, without atypical hyperplasia, was found to have a relative risk of 1.7 for the development of invasive breast cancer.

ADENOSIS TUMOR

Nielsen (8) described 27 cases of adenosis tumor that were similar to sclerosing adenosis microscopically; however, they were large enough to present grossly as a tumor mass, measuring 6 to 23 mm in diameter, with a mean diam-

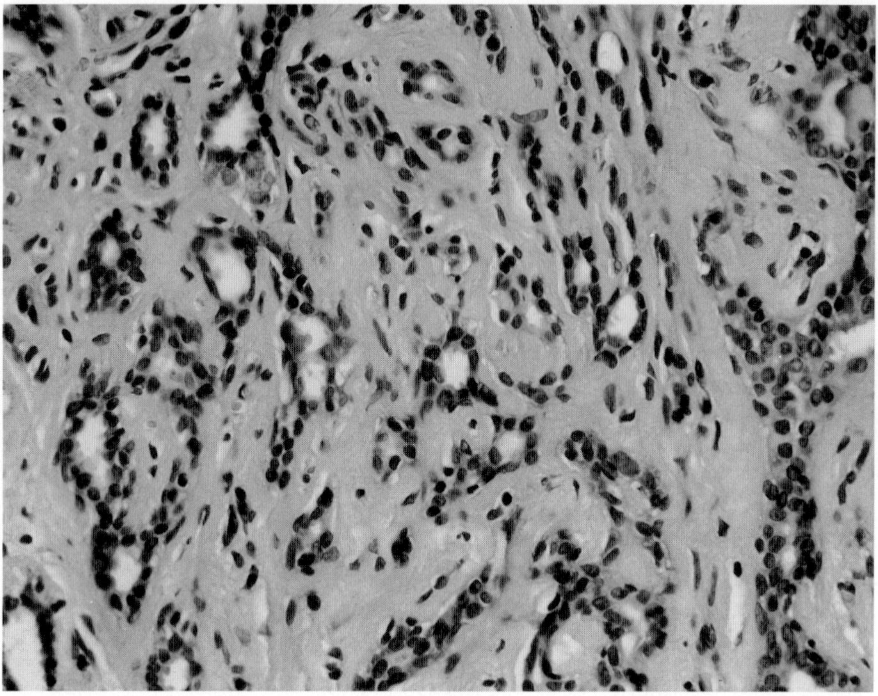

FIG. 6.4. Sclerosing adenosis. At higher magnification, the central area of sclerosing adenosis shows the entrapped distorted terminal ducts, some of which show both epithelial and myoepithelial cells, but others present a pseudoinfiltrative pattern within the lobular stroma. The dense eosinophilic sclerotic material between the terminal ducts can be shown to contain markedly thickened basement membrane material and stains positively for type IV collagen.

eter of 13 mm. Twenty of the 27 cases were poorly circumscribed. A mixture of histologic patterns was present, with classic sclerosing adenosis, microcysts, apocrine metaplasia, and luminal histiocytes commonly seen. Epithelial atypia was found in 26% of the cases and fat or nerve infiltration was seen in 30% of cases. None of the 18 pure adenosis tumors had recurred. Fat invasion is a poor criterion for carcinoma because the fibrous stroma of a normal lobule may be replaced with fat, especially with aging. Often, the fat is invading the area around the epithelium. Absence of a desmoplastic reaction is a strong indication of a benign pseudoinfiltrative process.

ATYPICAL APOCRINE METAPLASIA IN SCLEROSING LESIONS

Apocrine metaplasia may occur in sclerosing adenosis, as it does in numerous other benign lesions of the breast epithelium (Fig. 6.15 and efig. 6.14). The appearance of apocrine cells may add a feature that is even more worrisome than

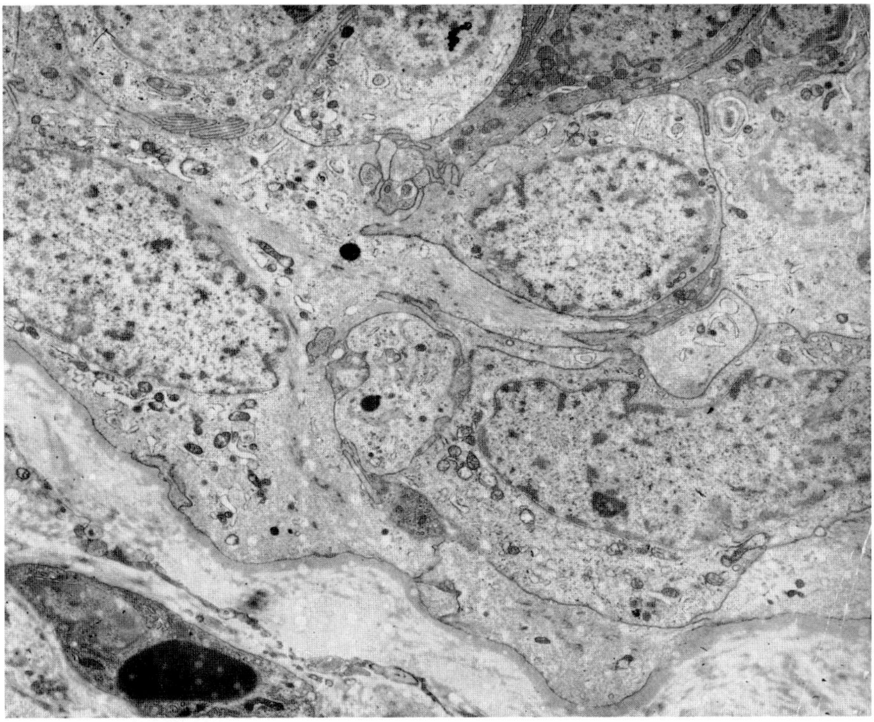

FIG. 6.5. Sclerosing adenosis. Electron micrograph of a distorted duct, taken from an area such as that shown in Fig. 6.4. The thickened basement membrane remains intact around this distorted duct, and the myoepithelial nature of most cells is evident.

the appearance of sclerosing adenosis (Fig. 6.16 and efig. 6.15). When the appearance of the nuclei becomes markedly atypical, this lesion may closely simulate and easily be mistaken for an invasive carcinoma (Figs. 6.17 and 6.18 and efigs. 6.15 to 6.20). Carter and Rosen (9) described 51 patients with this combination of features. The lesions were incidentally found during biopsies that were done for other palpable or mammographically evident abnormalities. The average age at diagnosis was 58 years. The AASLs were usually less than 1 cm in diameter, but, in one-third of the cases, they were between 1 and 2 cm in greatest dimension. Microscopically, they were characterized by a sclerosing adenosis pattern in which the proliferating cells had the eosinophilic granules of apocrine metaplasia; however, large nuclei with very prominent nucleoli, lent a degree of atypia to the microscopic appearance of the lesion. Basement membranes and myoepithelial cells were present. Follow-up of the patients, however, failed to reveal that this atypia had any precancerous implication, as it does in the other lesions that were designated atypical. Seidman et al. (10) reported an

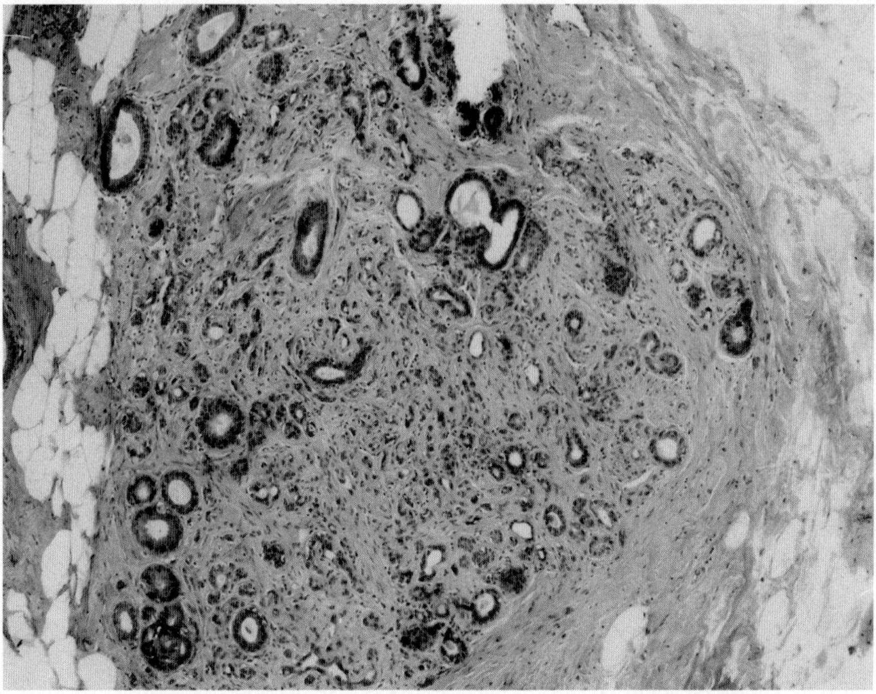

FIG. 6.6. Sclerosing adenosis. There is marked variation among the ducts present in the proliferating fibrous stroma. Many ducts are open and have the residual architecture of normal resting terminal ducts, but others are markedly compressed and mimic invasive cancer.

extremely high association between AASL and carcinoma, but this observation has not been confirmed and is not a generalized experience.

DCIS of an apocrine type may be found in AASL and, of course, has the significance of DCIS (efigs. 6.21 to 6.22).

BLUNT DUCT ADENOSIS

BDA is a term used to indicate dilatation of terminal ducts in a lobule where the epithelium of columnar and myoepithelium is intact. It is a common site for clustered fine calcifications that are detected mammographically (Chapter 5). Rarely, BDA may simulate a tubular carcinoma (Figs. 6.19 and 6.20 and efigs. 6.23 to 6.26).

FIG. 6.8. Sclerosing adenosis. A stereotactically directed needle biopsy has obtained a core of sclerosing adenosis. Careful attention to the outline and configuration of ducts and the judicious use of immunohistochemical stains for basement membrane and myoepithelium will help avoid misinterpretation as carcinoma.

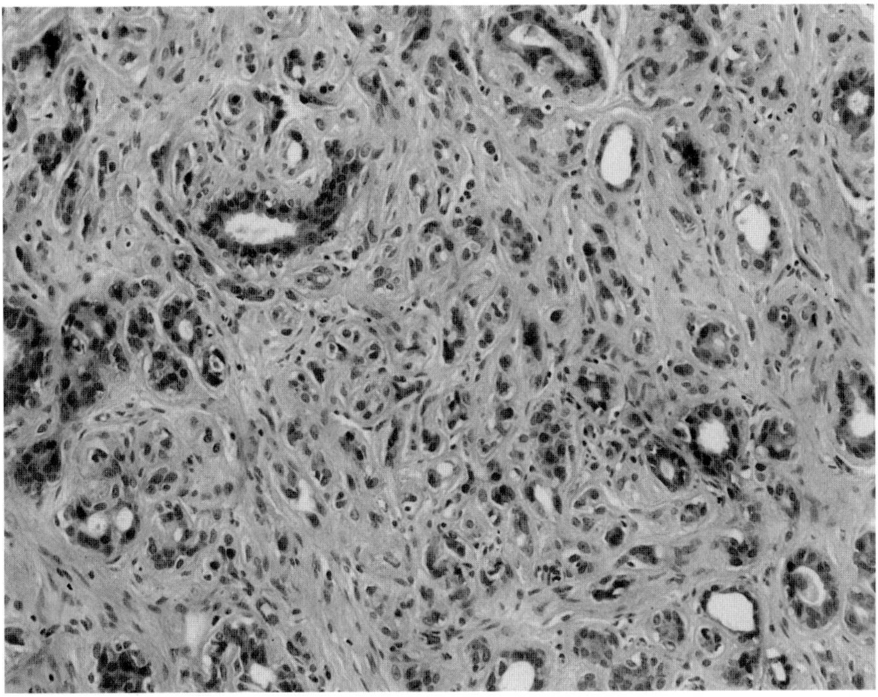

FIG. 6.7. Sclerosing adenosis. In this higher power photomicrograph, the entrapped ducts mimic invasive carcinoma. The small groups of cells are highly compressed terminal ducts with prominent basement membranes, but they might be mistaken for small islands of invasive carcinoma.

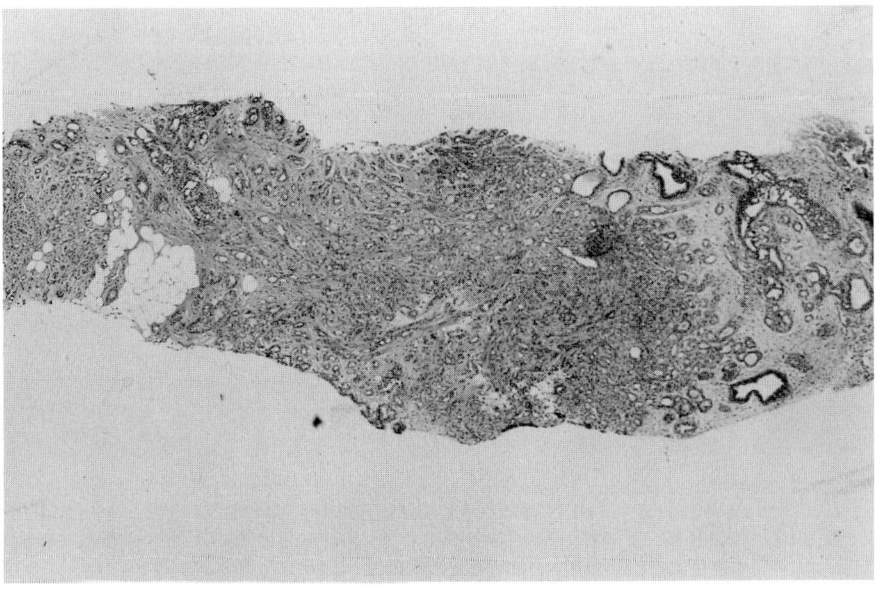

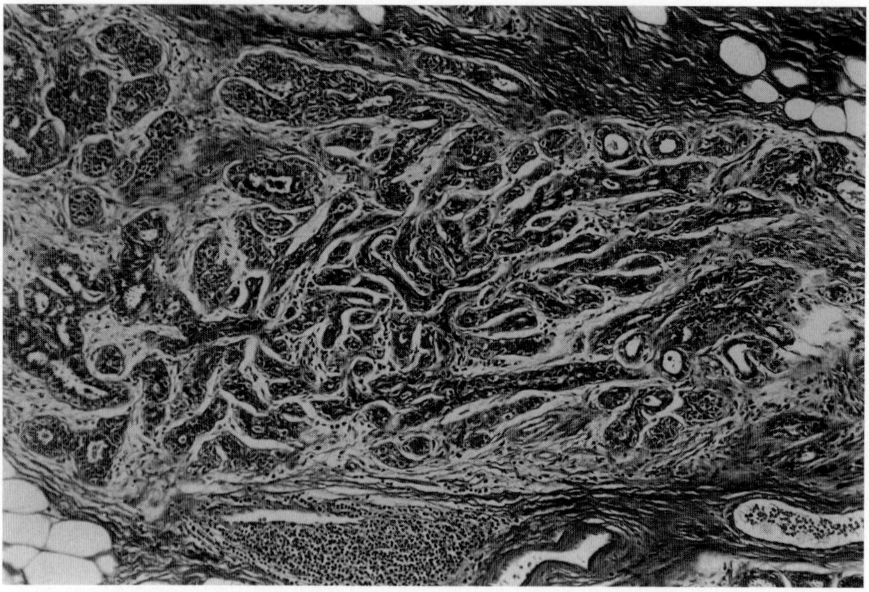

FIG. 6.9. Tubular adenosis. This lobular lesion has elongated ducts in a setting of sclerosing adenosis.

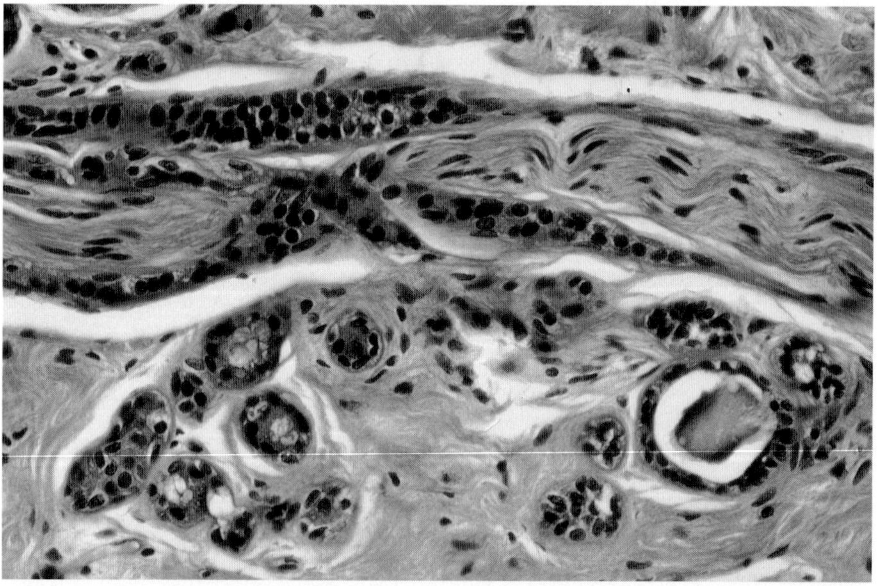

FIG. 6.10. Sclerosing adenosis. Proliferating ducts of sclerosing adenosis may infiltrate into the perineural space, in the absence of carcinoma and in patients with the benign course characteristic of sclerosing adenosis. Ductal epithelium also has been rarely found in the peripheral sinuses of axillary lymph nodes in association with sclerosing adenosis (Chapter 9).

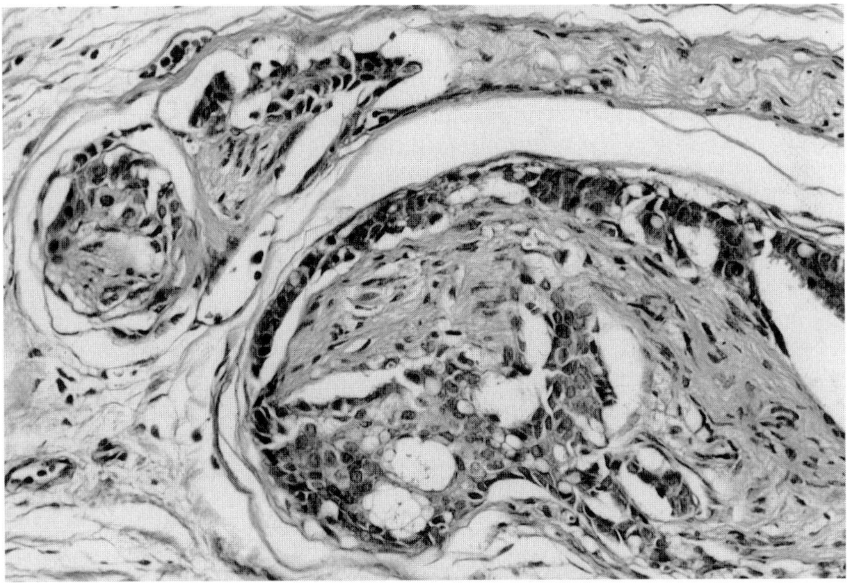

FIG. 6.11. Carcinoma with perineural invasion. Carcinoma is the lesion usually found in perineural spaces. The cells are clearly malignant, compared to the cells seen in Fig. 6.10.

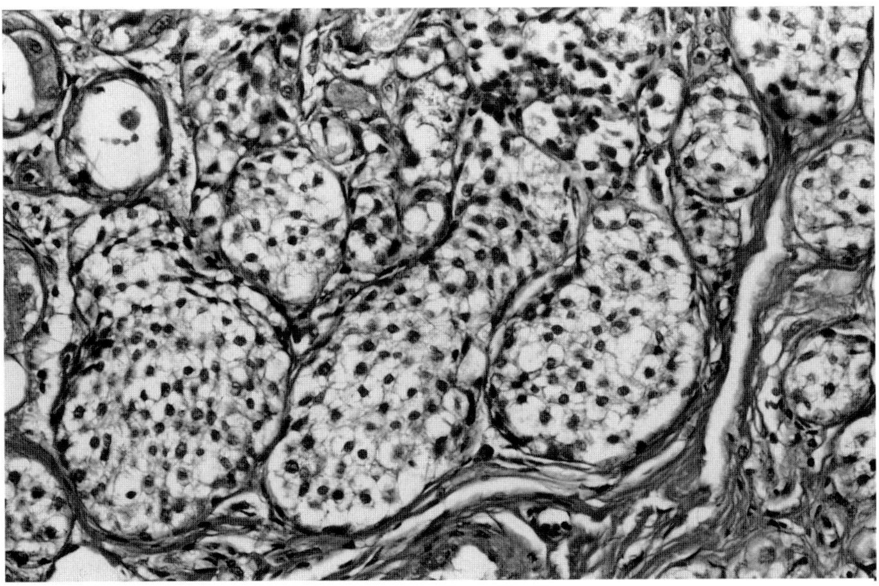

FIG. 6.12. Lobular carcinoma *in situ* in sclerosing adenosis. When distorted by sclerosing adenosis, this proliferative lesion may mimic invasive carcinoma.

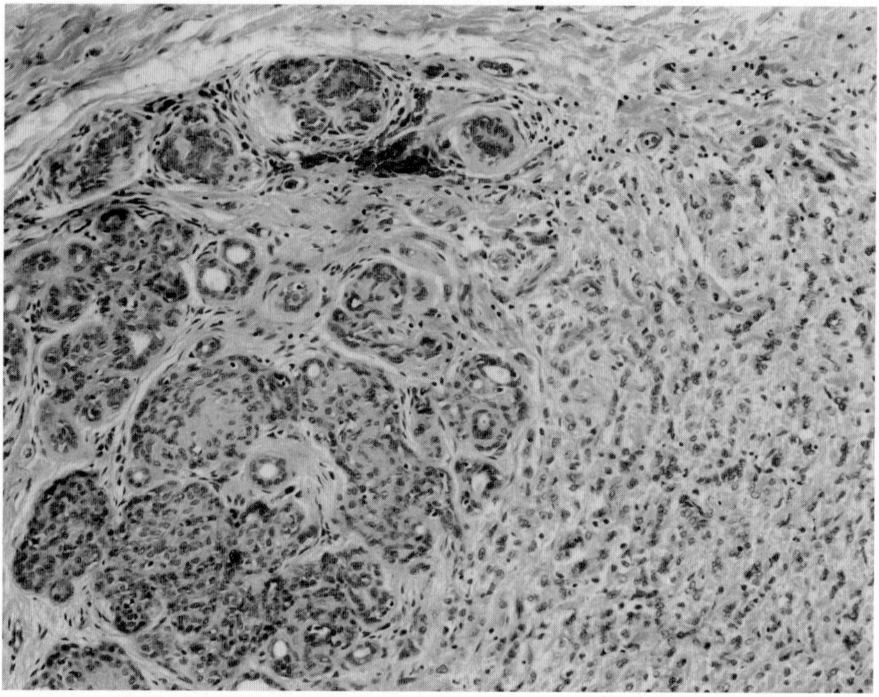

FIG. 6.13. Invasive lobular carcinoma in sclerotic lobule. The **left half** of the photomicrograph is a lobule that is distorted by sclerosing adenosis with prominent basement membranes around many of the terminal ducts. Single files of cells that are characteristic of infiltrating lobular carcinoma are shown (**right**).

MICROGLANDULAR ADENOSIS

Rosen (11) described 13 cases of MGA as a proliferation of terminal ducts that seem to be separated from any lobular organization, spreading through the stroma in seemingly random fashion. The poorly circumscribed areas vary in overall dimensions from 1 to 5 cm. The low-power appearance is of numerous closely packed ducts, usually small and relatively uniform in size, which seem to wander randomly through a stroma that is less sclerotic than in either sclerosing adenosis or RS. Characteristically, there is a single layer of large clear cells in the ducts, but a double layer of normal-appearing cells or a range of ductular or lobular hyperplasias may be present (Figs. 6.21 to 6.26 and efigs. 6.27 to 6.33). In the 13 cases described by Rosen (11), LCIS was present in 2 cases, and DCIS was present in another 2 cases. Two other patients developed invasive carcinoma at 6- and 18-year intervals, respectively. Clement and Azzopardi (12) described 6 similar cases.

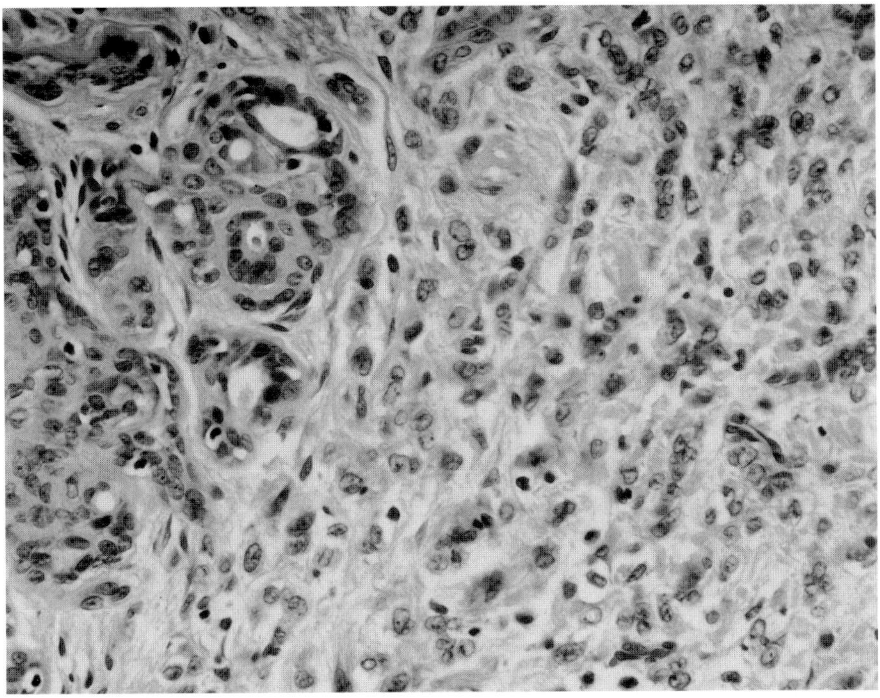

FIG. 6.14. Invasive lobular carcinoma in sclerotic lobule. At higher magnification, the single cells and single files of cells with nuclear molding distinguish this infiltrating lobular carcinoma from the entrapped terminal ducts shown in Fig. 6.7.

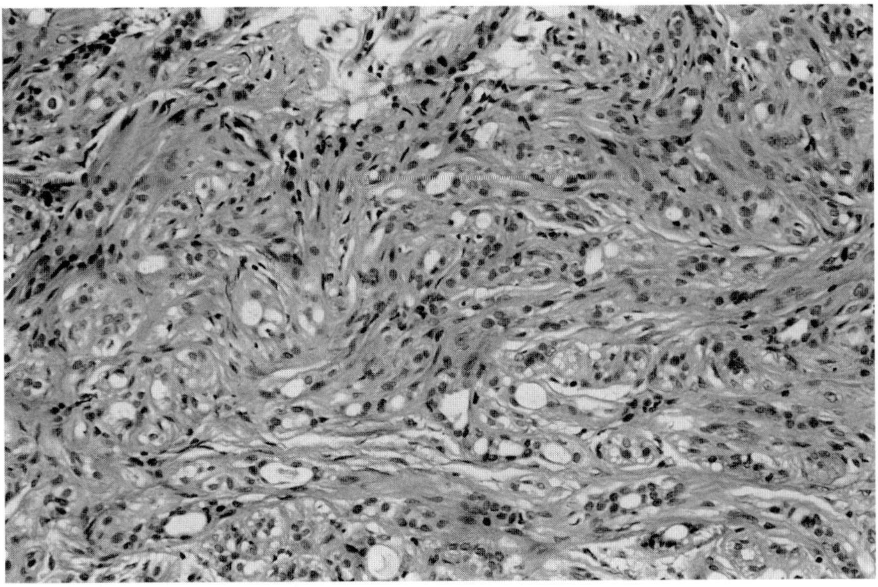

FIG. 6.15. Sclerosing adenosis. In this photomicrograph, the sclerotic process entraps terminal ducts with normal nonsecretory cytoplasm.

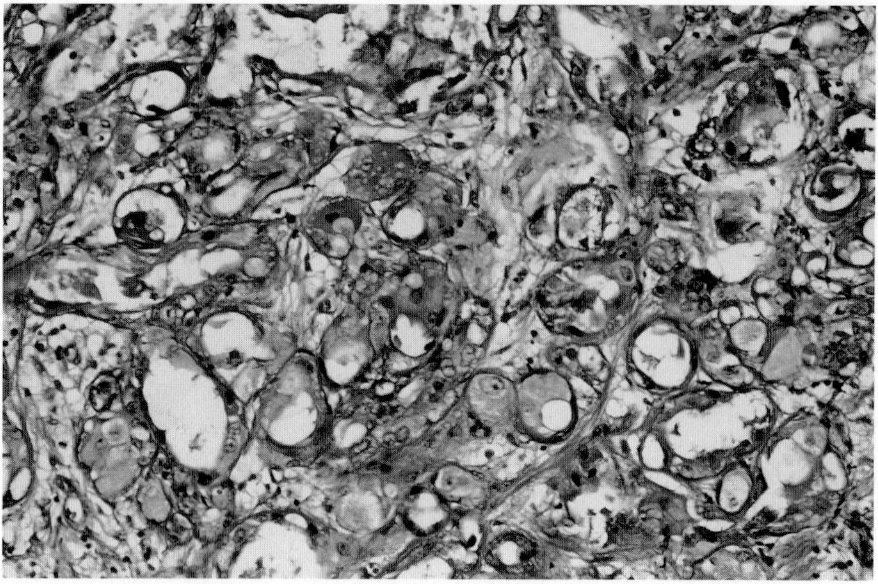

FIG. 6.16. Atypical apocrine sclerosing lesion. The ducts in this area of sclerosing adenosis exhibit cytoplasm with apocrine change and large nuclei with prominent nucleoli.

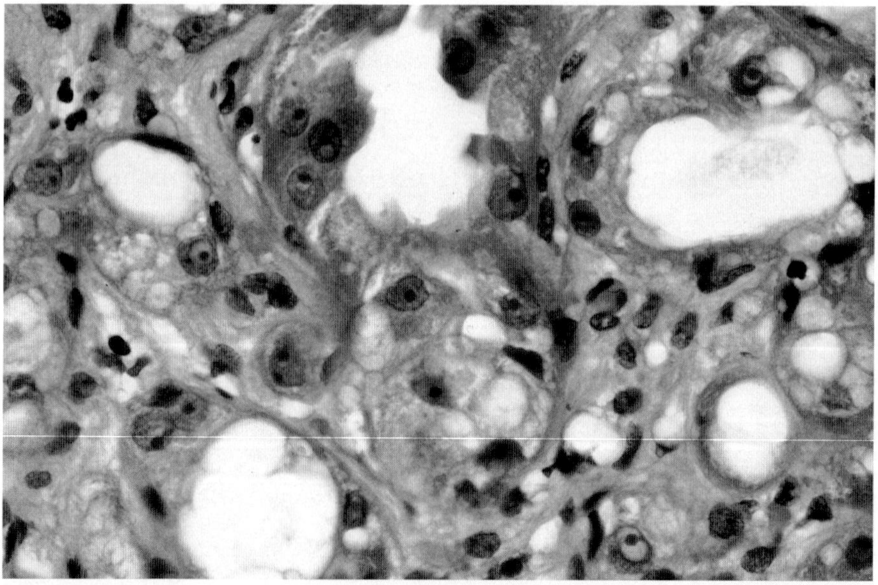

FIG. 6.17. Atypical apocrine sclerosing lesion. At higher magnification, the ducts show the features of apocrine metaplasia with granular eosinophilic cytoplasm and large nuclei with prominent nucleoli.

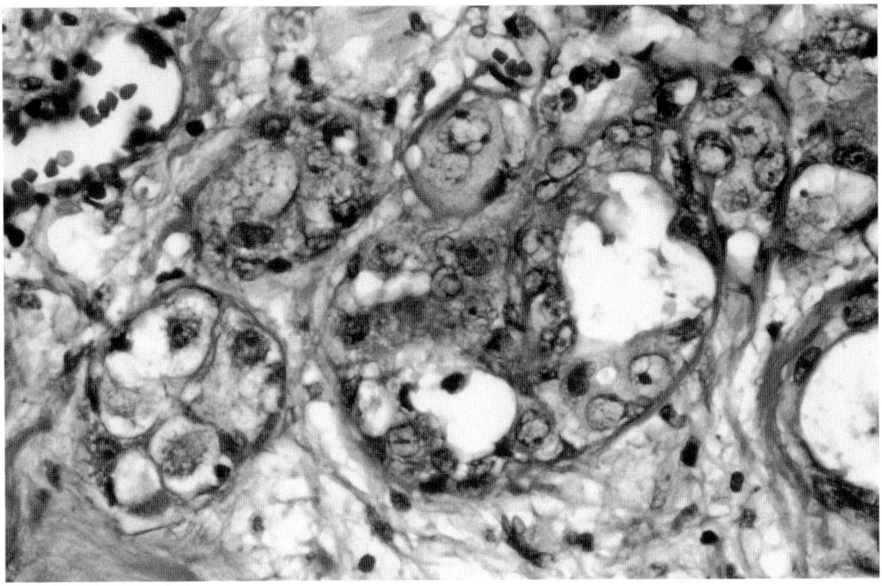

FIG. 6.18. Atypical apocrine sclerosing lesion. These epithelial cells display apocrine metaplasia with large nuclei with unusually large and prominent nucleoli. Although probably a degenerative change, the appearance may mimic that of invasive carcinoma.

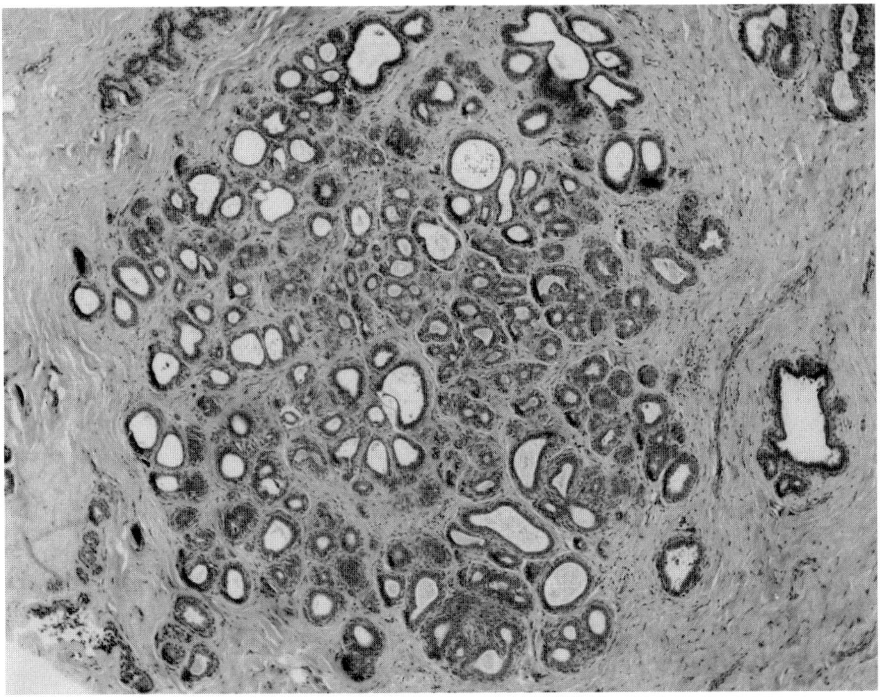

FIG. 6.19. Blunt duct adenosis. This circumscribed lobule has undergone some sclerotic distortion, but the noticeable feature is the roundness of its terminal ducts, which produces a superficial resemblance to tubular carcinoma.

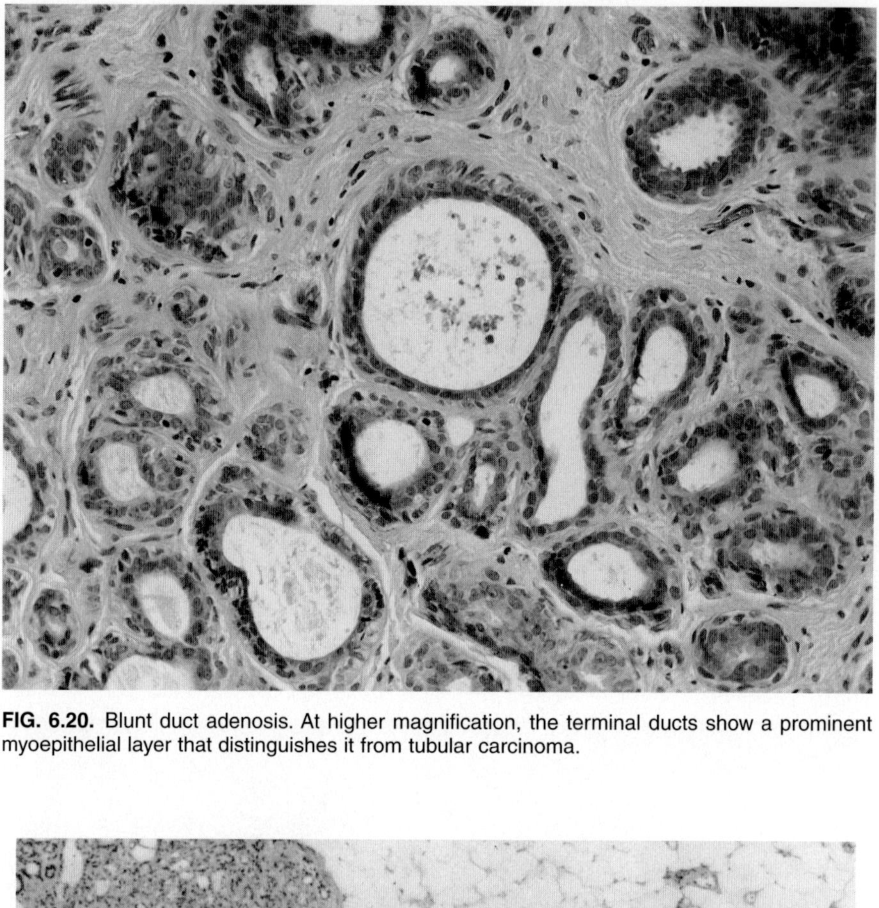

FIG. 6.20. Blunt duct adenosis. At higher magnification, the terminal ducts show a prominent myoepithelial layer that distinguishes it from tubular carcinoma.

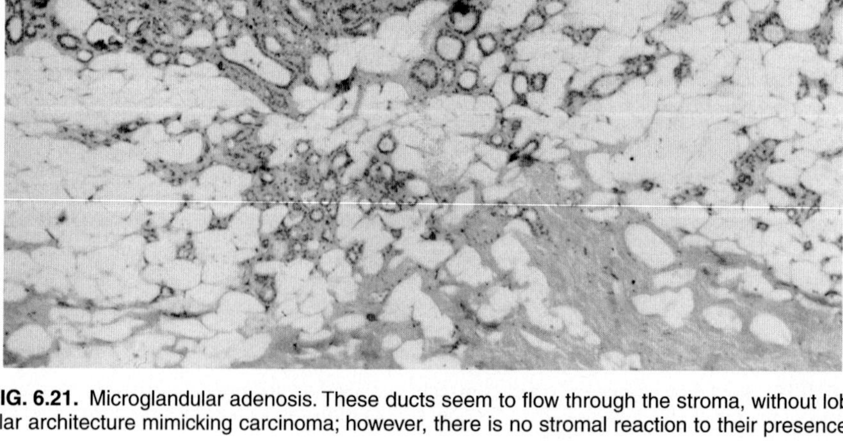

FIG. 6.21. Microglandular adenosis. These ducts seem to flow through the stroma, without lobular architecture mimicking carcinoma; however, there is no stromal reaction to their presence.

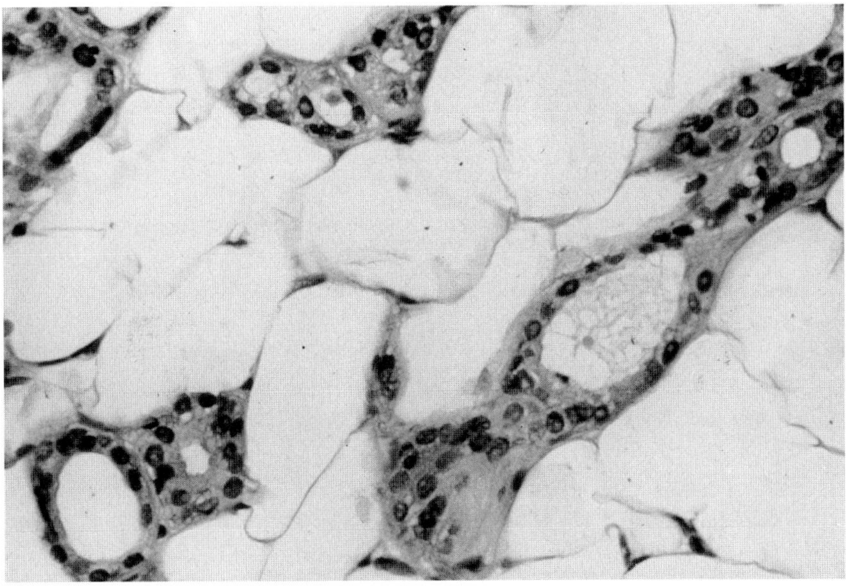

FIG. 6.22. Microglandular adenosis. At higher magnification, the ducts are surrounded by a nonreactive fatty stroma. The cells of these ducts have a clear-to-granular cytoplasm and are a monolayer.

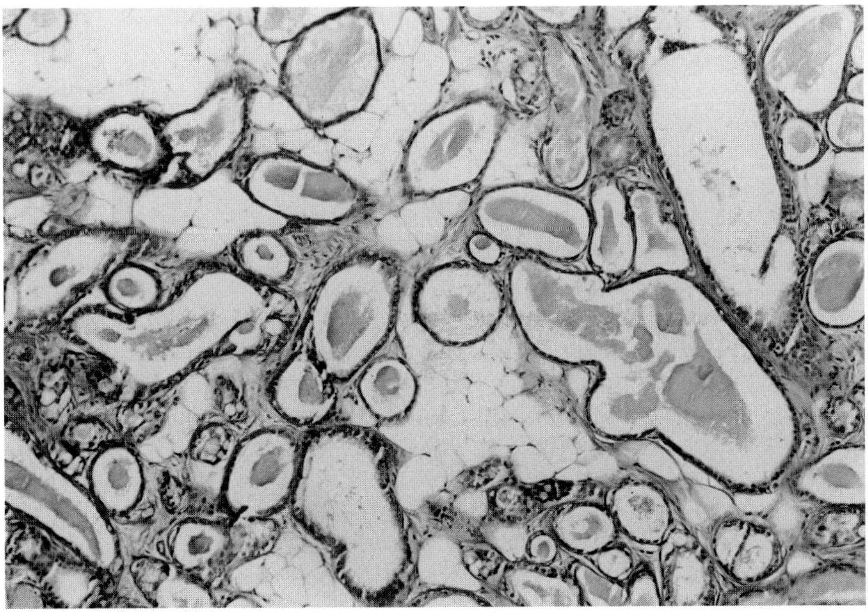

FIG. 6.23. Microglandular adenosis. Dilated ducts lined by a monolayer of cells and filled with secretory material spread through the nonreactive fatty stroma. The ducts lack a lobular configuration or any other organization.

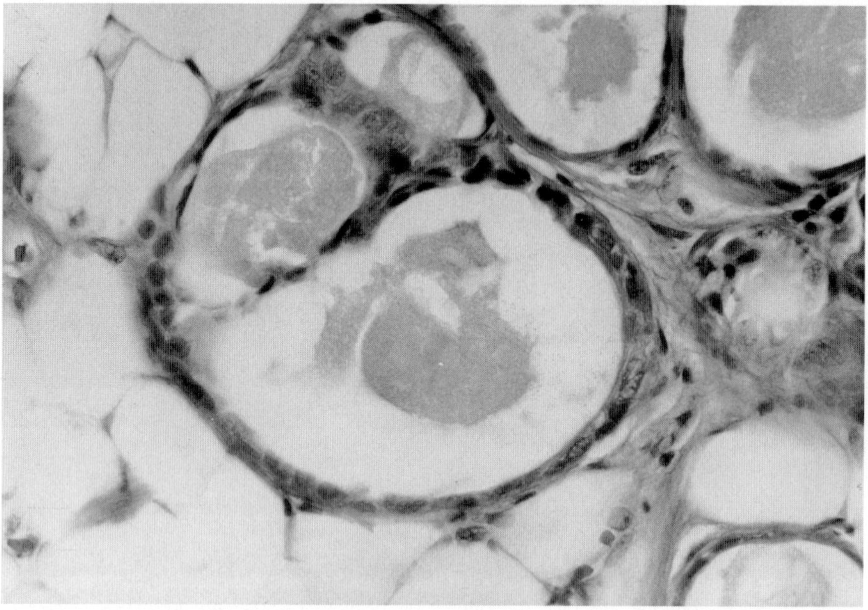

FIG. 6.24. Microglandular adenosis. At higher magnification, the ducts contain secretory material and are lined by a single layer of atrophic epithelial cells.

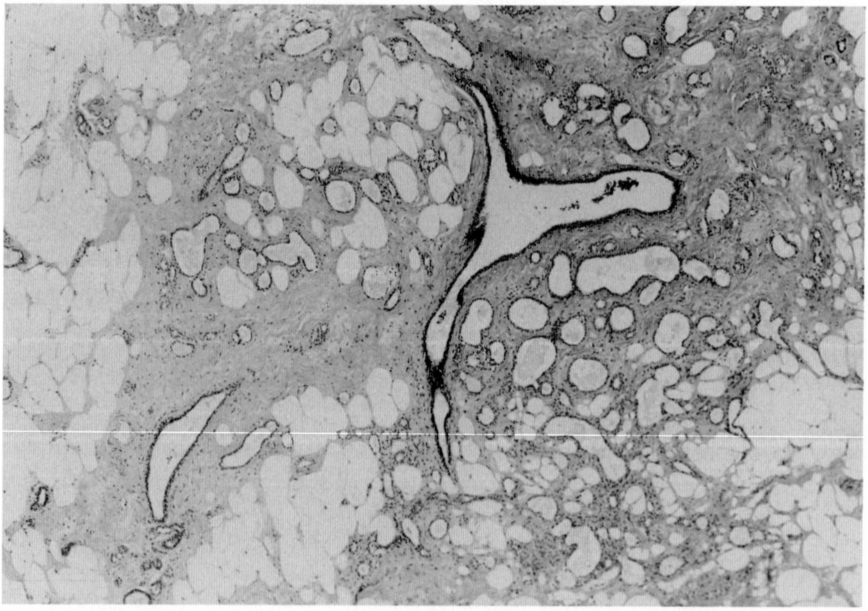

FIG. 6.25. Microglandular adenosis. This proliferation of ducts seems to arise in a lobule and flows through interlobular stroma without causing a reaction.

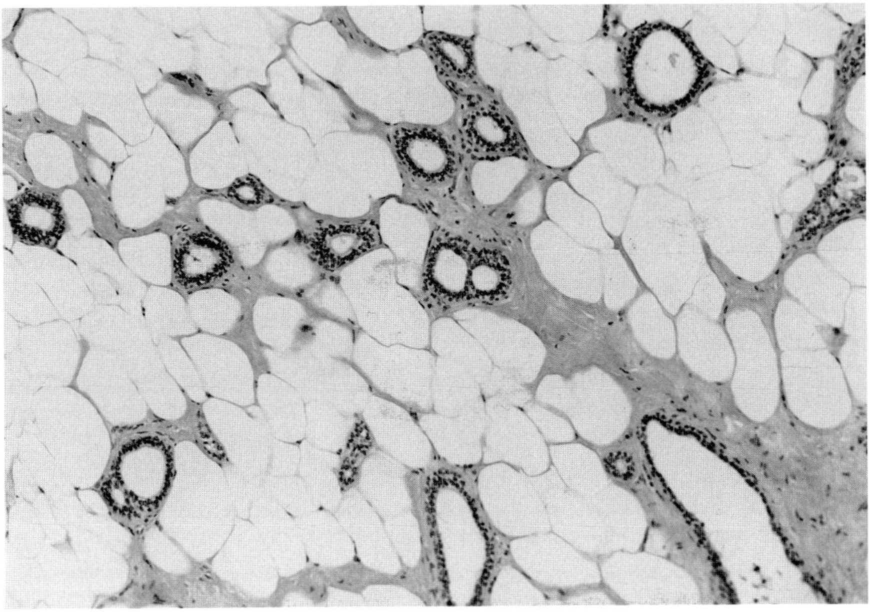

FIG. 6.26. Microglandular/adenomyoepithelial adenosis. Ducts appear to wander through the fatty stroma without apparent relationship to a duct or lobular system and without a stromal reaction.

Kay (13) studied the ultrastructure of MGA from a 75-year-old woman and reported a remarkable degree of villous interdigitation between epithelial cells, as well as an abundance of apical lysosomal granules. A thick basement membrane surrounded the gland in this case. Tavassoli and Norris (14) recorded the ultrastructure of 11 cases of MGA. The authors reported that a prominent epithelial layer was present; however, there was no myoepithelial layer. A thick basement membrane was present around the ductal structures. In contrast, tubular carcinoma had neither myoepithelial cells nor a basement membrane, whereas sclerosing adenosis had both a myoepithelial layer and a dense basement membrane. Subsequently, Tavassoli and Bratthauer (15) reported on the immunohistochemical evaluation of 12 cases of MGA and confirmed the absence of a myoepithelial layer, the presence of a dense basement membrane, and a strikingly positive staining of the epithelial cells for S-100 protein. All 12 cases studied also were found to be negative for progesterone receptors. Eusebi et al. (16) reported that MGA lacked a myoepithelial layer, but Diaz et al. (17) found a myoepithelial layer in 9 of 10 cases of MGA, but no myoepithelium in 10 cases of tubular carcinoma. Immunostaining for S-100 protein, carcinoembryonic antigen, estrogen receptors, and gross cystic disease fluid protein 15 were positive in both MGA and tubular carcinoma. Basement membranes invested MGA, but not tubular carcinoma. Kiaer et al.

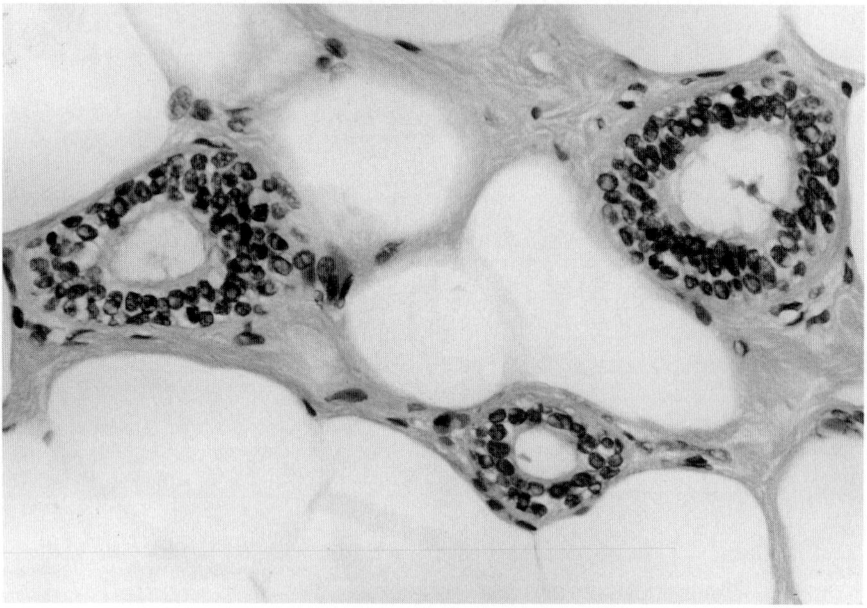

FIG. 6.27. Adenomyoepithelial adenosis. Unlike microglandular adenosis, these ducts have two cell layers, with an outer layer of clear myoepithelial cells.

(18) and Lee et al. (2) used the term "adenomyoepithelial adenosis" to describe a lesion that had the random pseudoinfiltrative features of MGA, but ducts that contained both epithelial and myoepithelial components (Fig. 6.27 and efigs. 6.34 to 6.37).

Rosenblum et al. (19) described seven cases of carcinoma that arose in association with MGA. The authors traced a morphologic spectrum of atypia to carcinoma from the adenosis into the carcinoma. However, these authors recommend only a careful follow-up for MGA and MGA with atypia. James et al. (20) described a similar series. Koenig et al. (21) described 20 cases of MGA with atypia, with progression of 7 cases to intraductal carcinoma, 5 cases to *in situ* and invasive carcinoma, and 7 cases to invasive carcinoma without an *in situ* component. The carcinoma tended to be solid with nuclear grade 2 to 3. CK7 was positive and CK 903 was negative in all cases. Most of the cases were also immunostained for α-1-antitrypsin, α-1-antichymotrypsin, and antichymotrypsin, but this is not unique among breast or other carcinomas. Some lesions combine features of MGA, sclerosing adenosis, and BDA (Fig. 6.28).

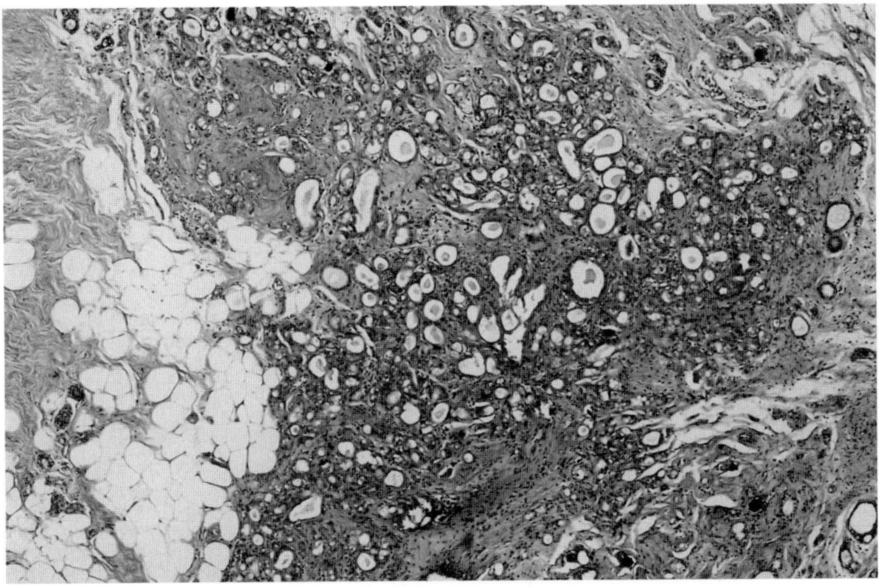

FIG. 6.28. Pseudoinfiltrative lesion. This benign lesion combines features of sclerosing adenosis with focal apocrine metaplasia, blunt duct adenosis, and microglandular adenosis. Analysis of the individual components prevents overinterpretation as carcinoma.

RADIAL SCAR (PAPILLARY SCLEROSING LESION)

Radial scars (RS) have a daisy shape with a densely fibrotic and elastotic core that contains entrapped terminal ducts and a stellate periphery of ducts and lobules in which proliferation may range from hyperplasia to carcinoma *in situ*. They are usually 2 to 15 mm in diameter. The relatively small core may appear or disappear on levels or cutdowns of the lesion. Grossly and mammographically, RS resembles a small stellate carcinoma. Orel et al. (22) found them to contain clustered microcalcifications. Microscopically, the center of the RS may resemble tubular carcinoma (Figs. 6.29 to 6.34 and efigs. 6.38 to 6.47).

Fenoglio and Lattes (23) described sclerosing papillary proliferations, most of which have the configuration of RS. One of their cases was a papilloma that had undergone sclerosis, as described and illustrated in Chapter 4. The authors likened the sclerotic papilloma to the other sclerosing papillary proliferations (RS) in their report (efigs. 6.48 to 6.53). In 1975, Hamperl (24) described a sclerosing lesion and referred to it as RS (*strahlige narben*). The microscopic description was essentially identical to that of Fenoglio and Lattes (23). In 1979, Fisher et al. (25) described a similar lesion, using the term "nonencapsulated sclerosing lesion." Azzopardi (26) described the lesion as infiltrating epitheliosis. In 1980, Eusebi (27) described the same lesion and used the term of Fisher, et al. (25), "nonencapsulated sclerosing lesion." In 1980, Linell et al. (28)

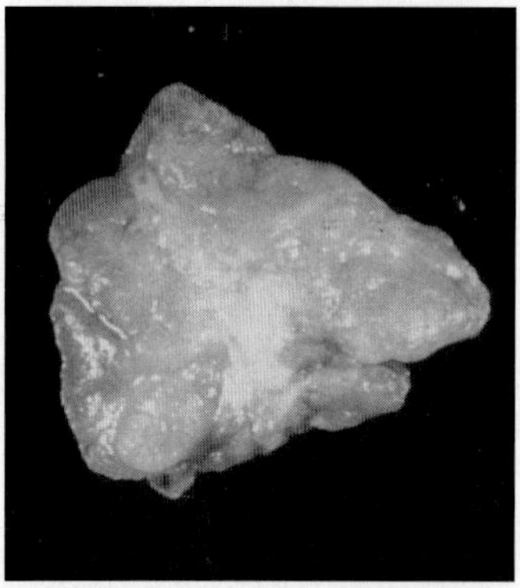

FIG. 6.29. Radial scar. This gross photograph shows a small radial scar that has the stellate appearance of a small invasive carcinoma.

described a series of RSs and, solely from morphologic observation without follow-up information, suggested that the RS core contained the earliest phases of invasive ductal carcinoma and that many breast cancers had their origins in similar circumstances. Some authors have repeated his conclusion without critical review of the paper and have perpetuated the notion, erroneously I believe, that RSs contain small carcinomas. In 1981, Rickert et al. (29) described a similar lesion and used the term "indurative mastopathy." Rosen (30) used the term

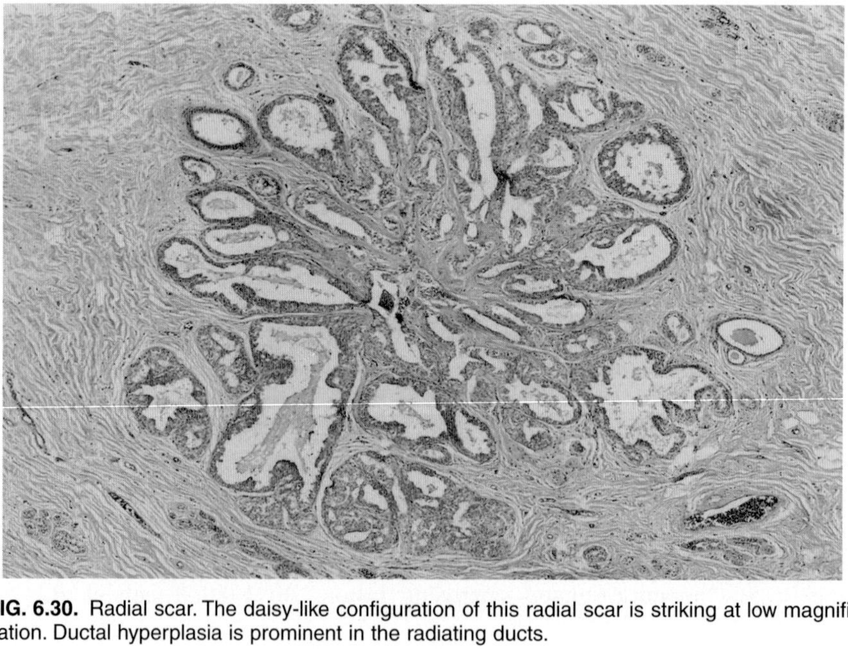

FIG. 6.30. Radial scar. The daisy-like configuration of this radial scar is striking at low magnification. Ductal hyperplasia is prominent in the radiating ducts.

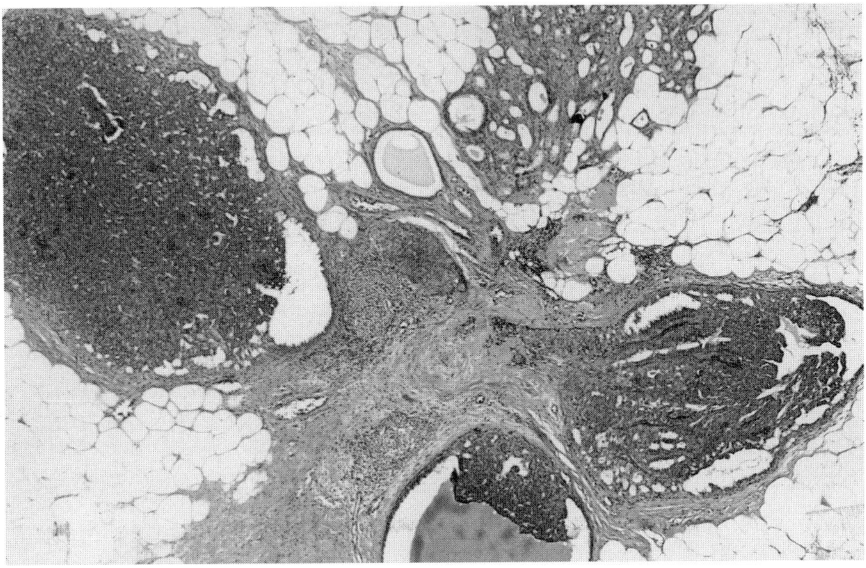

FIG. 6.31. Radial scar. The stellate configuration of this lesion is enhanced by ductal hyperplasia in the large ducts that make up the peripheral component, which seems to focus attention on the elastotic core.

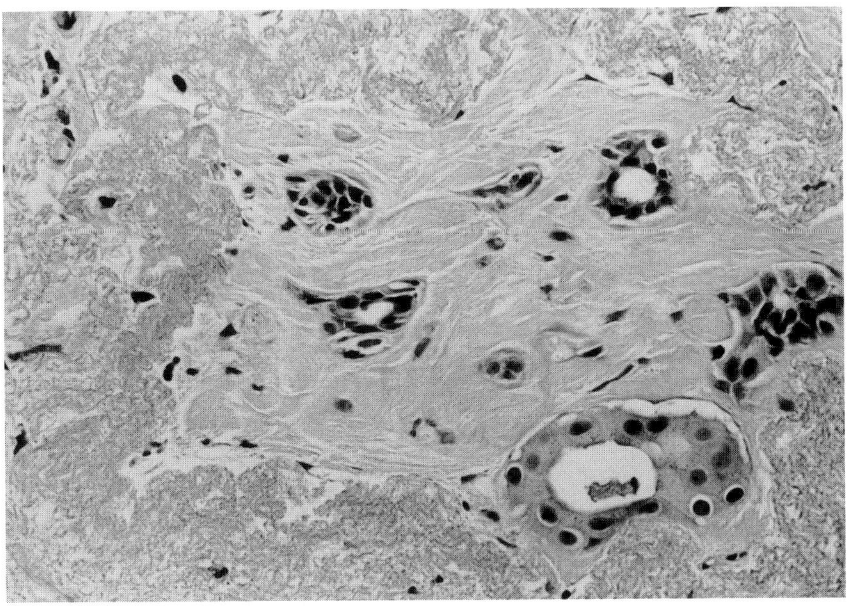

FIG. 6.32. Radial scar. The central elastotic core of the radial scar contains a few small ducts that appear to be compressed by the stroma. Three ducts have a two-cell population and one duct shows apocrine metaplasia.

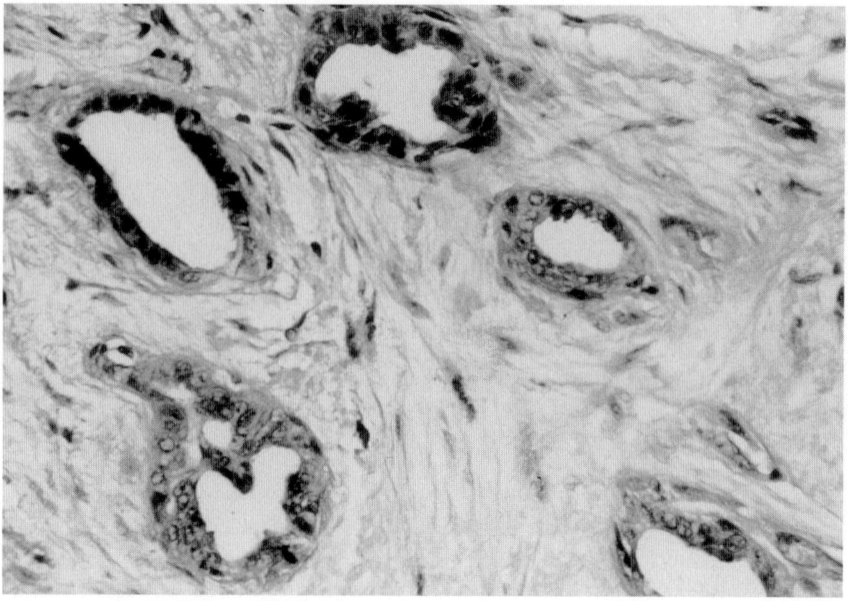

FIG. 6.33. Radial scar. These ducts in the elastotic core of a radial scar appear more ominous. Two ducts show a double cell population, but the other ducts do not. Some of these individual ducts are histologically indistinguishable from those seen in a tubular carcinoma.

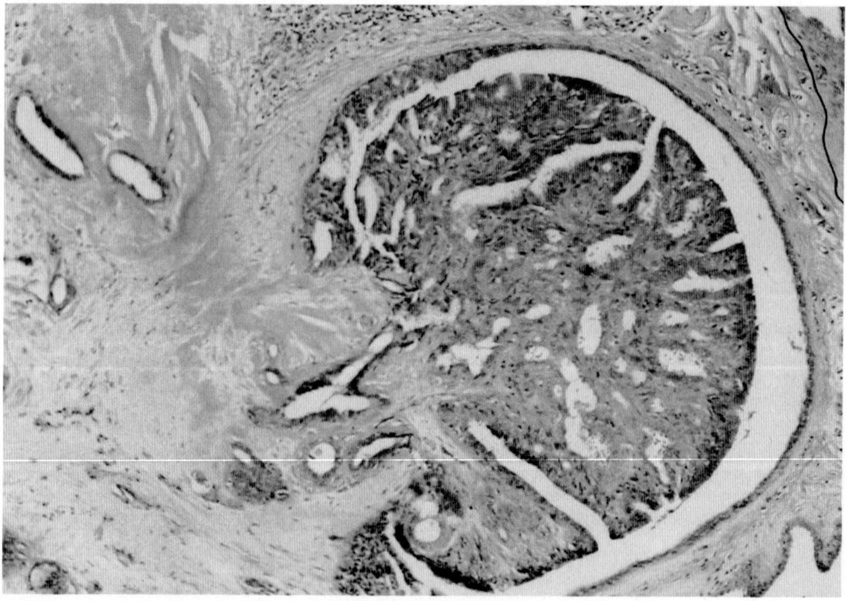

FIG. 6.34. Radial scar. A central elastotic core containing small ducts similar to those seen in Fig. 6.33 is shown here **(left)** and a sclerotic papilloma is depicted **(right)**. The association of radial scars with papillomas such as this suggests a possible histogenetic relationship.

"subareolar sclerosing duct hyperplasia" to describe 12 cases of RS-like lesions in the subareolar area. Despite the variety of names, all of these authors have essentially described the same lesion. RS is the shortest and perhaps most descriptive of the terms.

Battersby and Anderson (31) noted the contribution of myofibroblasts to the proliferation within the central portion of the RS in early, but not late, phases. In 1993, de la Torre et al. (32) described the presence of hyaluronic acid in both RSs and invasive tubular carcinomas.

RSs are seen fairly frequently and are often multiple. Linell et al. (28) found from 1 to 25 RSs in 16% of the mastectomies that were done for carcinoma of the breast. Wellings and Alpers (33) found from 1 to 13 RSs in 14% of benign breast biopsies and from 1 to 31 RSs in 26% of mastectomies that were done for invasive carcinoma of the breast. Nielsen et al. (34) found RSs in the contralateral breast of 35 of 84 autopsy specimens from patients with invasive breast cancer; however, the authors found no excess of RSs among cases with carcinoma, compared to controls, and concluded that RSs were not premalignant. Anderson and Battersby (35) came to the same conclusion from studying 68 autopsy specimens.

Both LCIS and DCIS may be found in association with RSs and presumably they have the significance of carcinoma *in situ* that is found elsewhere. Sloane and Mayers (36) studied 126 RSs that were removed from 91 women and reported the presence of carcinoma in radiographically detected RSs that were larger than 7 mm and found in women older than 50 years. Among 74 internal cases at Royal Marsden Hospital, the authors found 6 cases each of atypical ductal hyperplasia and DCIS and 2 cases each of ALH and LCIS. There was 1 case of invasive ductal carcinoma. Among 52 referred cases, the incidence of those lesions was more than doubled. No relationship was found between cancer in RSs and in the surrounding breast. The authors recommended excision of detected RS and considered RSs that were 7mm or larger to have a relationship to carcinoma; however, those RSs smaller than 7mm did not have a relationship to carcinoma. The relationship of size to carcinoma demonstrated a threshold at 7mm and not a curve. I report the size of the largest RS found in nonmalignant cases.

The pathogenesis of RS is not known. Linell et al. (28) suggested that RS is an important precursor of carcinoma, but follow-up studies by Andersen and Gram (35), Fisher et al. (25), and Fenoglio and Lattes (23) showed no increase in the incidence of invasive cancer following biopsies that contained RSs. Excision of the RS is required for diagnosis, which is simultaneously therapeutic. Reexcision for RS is not indicated. If carcinoma accompanies RS, then treatment for that type of carcinoma must be considered (37).

The primary interest usually is not in the proliferative changes in the corona of the RS, but rather it is in the small ducts that are found in its fibroelastic core. These ducts are identifiable as benign when they contain both epithelial and myoepithelial layers, but, occasionally, some of them may not show two layers of cells (Figs. 6.32 to 6.34 and efigs. 6.44 to 6.47). This appearance, plus the associated fibroelastic core, closely mimics the histology of tubular carcinoma (efigs. 6.54 to 6.55) and forms the basis for the suggestion that RSs contain early cancers. Willebrand et al. (38) reported an intact basement membrane around all epithelial structures in 16 RSs that were studied by immunohistochemistry for type IV collagen, but Battersby and Anderson (31) reported loss of basal lamina by electron microscopic study in early RSs. The clinical difference between RS and a less than 1-mm tubular carcinoma is not measurable because tubular carcinomas of that size are not expected to be associated with metastasis. Fisher et al. (25) found no treatment failures among their nonencapsulated sclerosing lesions (RS), which was not statistically different from the 1 treatment failure among 14 tubular carcinomas. Taylor and Norris (39) found only 1 fatal case among 81 tubular carcinomas. Scanning lens recognition of the RS, with its central fibroelastotic core and corona of ducts or lobules, is helpful in providing perspective for any tubular carcinoma-like structures in the core.

Jacobs et al. (40) performed a case control study of 1,396 women who had undergone breast biopsies and found a 1.8 relative risk of breast cancer among women with RS, compared to those without RS. The breast cancers were not found arising in RS, however. Denley et al. (41) reported five cases of low-grade adenosquamous carcinomas with glandular and squamous epithelial differentiation in a spindle cell background, coexisting with, but anatomically distinct from, RS, which they termed "complex sclerosing lesion." The size of the lesions varied from 7 to 24 mm, with a mean of 16mm, and the age range of the cases was 49 to 68 years, with a mean of 62 years, which is consistent with the features of size and age that were described by Sloane et al. (36).

REFERENCES

1. Jao W, Recant W, Swerdlow MA. Comparative ultrastructure of tubular carcinoma and sclerosing adenosis of the breast. *Cancer* 1976;38:180–186.
2. Lee K, Chan J, Gwi E. Tubular adenosis of the breast: a distinctive lesion mimicking invasive carcinoma. *Am J Surg Pathol* 1996;20:46–54.
3. Taylor HB, Norris HJ. Epithelial invasion of nerves in benign disease of the breast. *Cancer* 1967;20: 2245–2249.
4. Edlow D, Carter D. Heterotopic epithelium in axillary lymph nodes: report of a case and review of the literature. *Am J Clin Pathol* 1973;59:666–668.
5. Fechner RE. Lobular carcinoma *in situ* in sclerosing adenosis. A potential source of confusion with invasive carcinoma. *Am J Surg Pathol* 1981;5:233–239.
6. Eusebi V, Collina G, Bussolati G. Carcinoma *in situ* in sclerosing adenosis of the breast: an immunocytochemical study. *Semin Diagn Pathol* 1989;6:146–152.
7. Jensen RA, Page DL, Dupont WD, et al. Invasive breast cancer risk in women with sclerosing adenosis. *Cancer* 1989;64:1977–1983.
8. Nielsen BB. Adenosis tumour of the breast—a clinicopathological investigation of 27 cases. *Histopathology* 1987;11:1259–1275.
9. Carter DJ, Rosen PP. Atypical apocrine metaplasia in sclerosing lesions of the breast: a study of 51 patients. *Mod Pathol* 1991;4:1–5.
10. Seidman JD, Ashton M, Lefkowitz M. Atypical apocrine adenosis of the breast: a clinicopathologic study of 37 patients with 8.7 year follow-up. *Cancer* 1996;77:2529–2537.
11. Rosen PP. Microglandular adenosis. A benign lesion simulating invasive mammary carcinoma. *Am J Surg Pathol* 1983;7:137.
12. Clement PB, Azzopardi JG. Microglandular adenosis of the breast: a lesion simulating tubular carcinoma. *Histopathology* 1983;7:169.

13. Kay S. Microglandular adenosis of the female mammary gland: study of a case with ultrastructural observations. *Hum Pathol* 1985;16:637.
14. Tavassoli FA, Norris HJ. Microglandular adenosis of the breast. A clinicopathologic study of 11 cases with ultrastructural observations. *Am J Surg Pathol* 1983;7:731.
15. Tavassoli FA, Bratthauer GL. Immunohistochemical profile and differential diagnosis of microglandular adenosis. *Mod Pathol* 1993;6:318–322.
16. Eusebi V, Foschini MP, Betts CM, et al. Microglandular adenosis, apocrine adenosis, and tubular carcinoma of the breast. An immunohistochemical comparison. *Am J Surg Pathol* 1993;17:99–109.
17. Diaz NM, McDivitt RW, Wick MR. Microglandular adenosis of the breast: an immunohistochemical comparison with tubular carcinoma. *Arch Pathol Lab Med* 1991;115:578–582.
18. Kiaer H, Nielson B, Paulsen S, et al. Adenomyoepithelial adenosis and low grade adenomyoepithelioma of the breast. *Virchows Arch* 1984;405:55–67.
19. Rosenblum MK, Purrazzella R, Rosen PP. Is microglandular adenosis a precancerous disease? A study of carcinoma arising therein. *Am J Surg Pathol* 1986;10:237.
20. James BA, Cranor ML, Rosen PP. Carcinoma of the breast arising in microglandular adenosis. *Am J Clin Pathol* 1993;100:507–513.
21. Koenig C, Dadmanesh F, Bratthauer G, et al. Carcinoma arising in microglandular adenosis: an immunohistochemical analysis of 20 intraepithelial and invasive neoplasms. *Int J Surg Pathol* 2000;8:303–315.
22. Orel SG, Evers K, Yeh IT, et al. Radial scar with microcalcifications: radiologic-pathologic correlation. *Radiology* 1992;183:479–482.
23. Fenoglio C, Lattes R. Sclerosing papillary proliferations in the female breast. A benign lesion often mistaken for carcinoma. *Cancer* 1974;33:691–700.
24. Hamperl H. Strahlige narben und obliterierende mastopathy. *Virchows Arch* 1975;369:55–68.
25. Fisher ER, Palekar AS, Kotwal N, et al. A nonencapsulated sclerosing lesion of the breast. *Am J Clin Pathol* 1979;71:240–246.
26. Azzopardi J. Problems in breast pathology. Major problems in pathology. Philadelphia: WB Saunders, 1979, II.
27. Eusebi V. Nonencapsulated sclerosing lesion of the breast. *Am J Clin Pathol* 1980;73:456.
28. Linell F, Ljungberg O, Anderson I. Breast carcinoma: aspects of early stages, progression and related problems. *Acta Pathol Microbiol Scand* 1980;(A):[Suppl]272.
29. Rickert RR, Kalisher L, Hutter RVP. Indurative mastopathy: a benign sclerosing lesion of the breast with elastosis which may stimulate carcinoma. *Cancer* 1981;47:561–571.
30. Rosen PP. Subareolar sclerosing duct hyperplasia of the breast. *Cancer* 1987;59:1927–1930.
31. Battersby S, Anderson TJ. Myofibroblast activity of radial scars. *J Pathol* 1985;147:33–40.
32. de la Torre M, Wells AF, Bergh J, et al. Localization of hyaluronan in normal breast tissue, radial scar, and tubular breast carcinoma. *Hum Pathol* 1993;24:1294–1297.
33. Wellings SR, Alpers CE. Subgross pathologic features and incidence of radial scars in the breast. *Hum Pathol* 1984;15:475.
34. Nielsen M, Jensen J, Andersen JA. An autopsy study of radial scar in the female breast. *Histopathology* 1985;9:287.
35. Andersen JA, Gram JB. Radial scar in the female breast: a long term follow-up study of 32 cases. *Cancer* 1984;53:2557–2560.
36. Sloane JP, Mayers MM. Carcinoma and atypical hyperplasia in radial scars and complex sclerosing lesions: importance of lesion size and patient age. *Histopathology* 1993;23:225–231.
37. Andersen JA, Carter D, Linell F. A symposium on sclerosing lesions of the breast. *Pathol Ann* 1986; 21:145–179.
38. Willebrand D, Bosman FT, de Goeij AF. Patterns of basement membrane deposition in benign and malignant breast tumours. *Histopathology* 1986;10:1231–1241.
39. Taylor H, Norris HJ. Well differentiated carcinoma of the breast. *Cancer* 1970;25:687–692.
40. Jacobs TW, Byrne C, Colditz G, et al. Radial scars in benign breast biopsy-specimens and the risk of breast cancer. *N Engl J Med* 1999;340:430–436.
41. Denley H, Pinder S, Tan P, et al. Metaplastic carcinoma of the breast arising within complex sclerosing lesion: a report of five cases. *Histopathology* 2000;36:203–209.

7

Adnexal-type Tumors

The breast is an ectodermally derived exocrine secretory structure that has been described as a modified sweat gland, although in most respects the modifications are more significant than the similarities. Function, control, and proliferation in the breast are far more complex than in a sweat gland, but the breast shares basic structural similarities with skin adnexal and salivary glands (e.g., collecting ducts and draining lobules that are composed of acinar structures with an epithelial/myoepithelial configuration). Several neoplasms with features similar to those seen elsewhere in exocrine glands occur rarely in the breast. Histologic similarities between invasive ductal carcinoma and adnexal-type tumors bring them into differential diagnosis more often than their actual incidence. The adnexal prototype is adenomyoepithelioma (monomorphic adenoma), with pleomorphic adenoma (benign mixed tumor) occurring as the most frequent variant, and eccrine spiradenoma, syringocystadenoma, hidradenoma, and syringoma also rarely occurring in the breast. The most commonly seen member of the adnexal-type tumor group is adenoid cystic carcinoma, which must be distinguished from collagenous spherulosis (CS). Some other carcinomas have been reported to have a myoepithelial component, and there are rare examples of purely myoepithelial tumors of the breast.

ADENOMYOEPITHELIOMA (MONOMORPHIC ADENOMA)

Adenomyoepitheliomas are characterized by a biphasic proliferation of epithelial and myoepithelial cells. The myoepithelial element is usually the most prominent proliferating component (Figs. 7.1 to 7.6 and efigs. 7.1 to 7.9). Koyama et al. (1) measured the proliferative activity of two adenomyoepitheliomas by immunohistochemistry. The authors reported the MIB-1(Ki-67)/MSA positive cell index, which indicates the cycling rate of myoepithelium, as 19.2% and 17.7%, respectively, compared to the MIB-1/CAM5.2 index of epithelial cells as 10.2% and 9.5%, respectively. Rosen (2) described 18 adenomyoepitheliomas (0.8 to 2.5 cm in diameter) in women who ranged in age from 27 to 80 years (average age, 58 years). The tumors were firm and circumscribed with

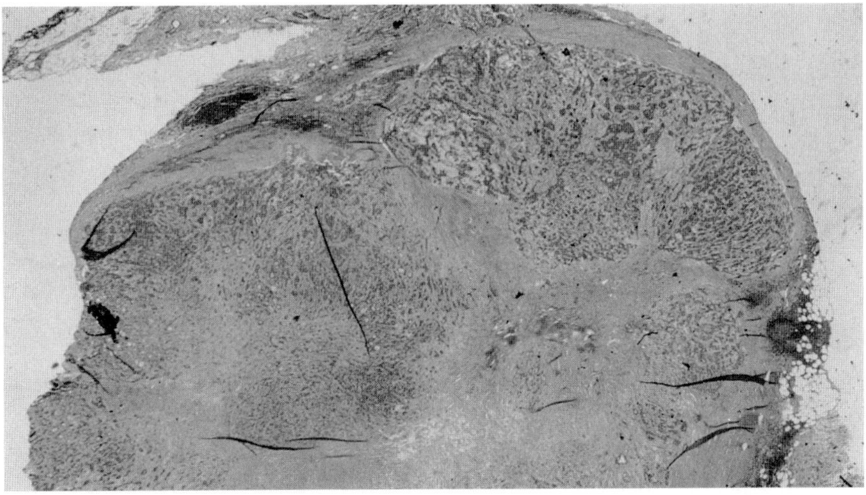

FIG. 7.1. Adenomyoepithelioma. The low power view of this lesion is of a cellular, but sharply circumscribed, tumor.

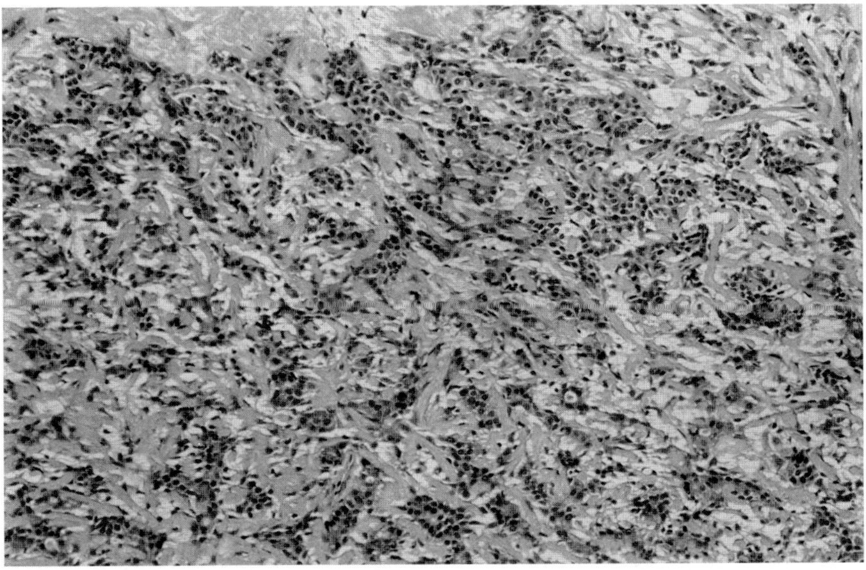

FIG. 7.2. Adenomyoepithelioma. Trabeculae of epithelial and myoepithelial structures infiltrate a fibrous stroma.

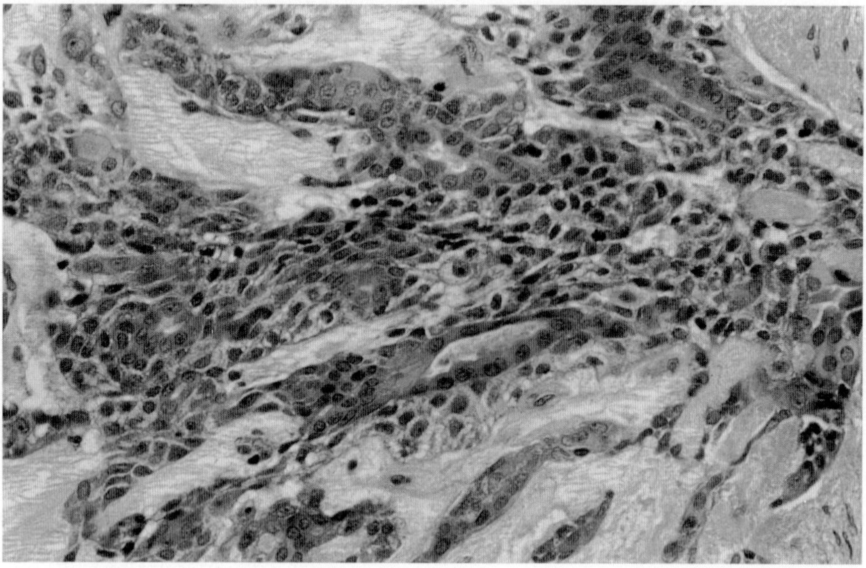

FIG. 7.3. Adenomyoepithelioma. Slit-like extracellular lumens of ducts are dominated by a proliferation of spindle and cuboidal myoepithelial cells.

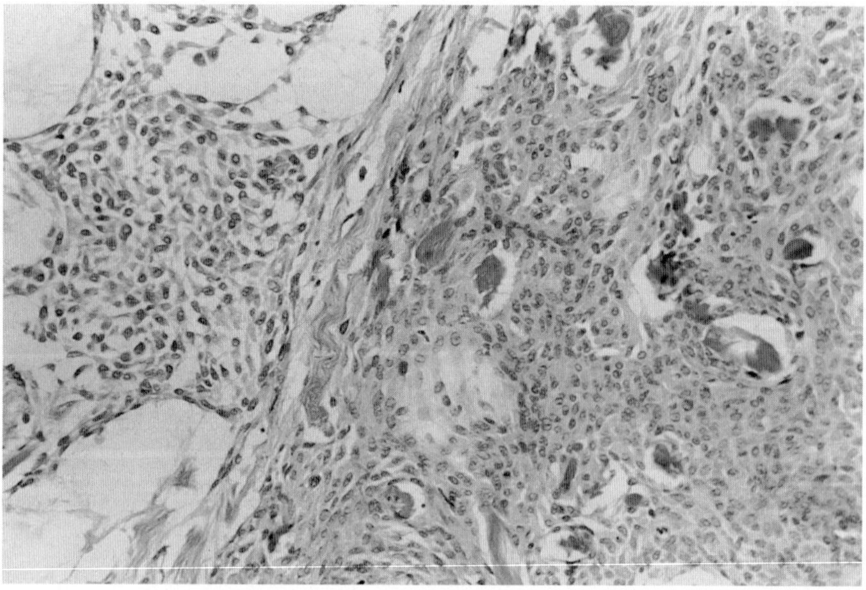

FIG. 7.4. Adenomyoepithelioma. Spindle and clear myoepithelial cells are the predominant features.

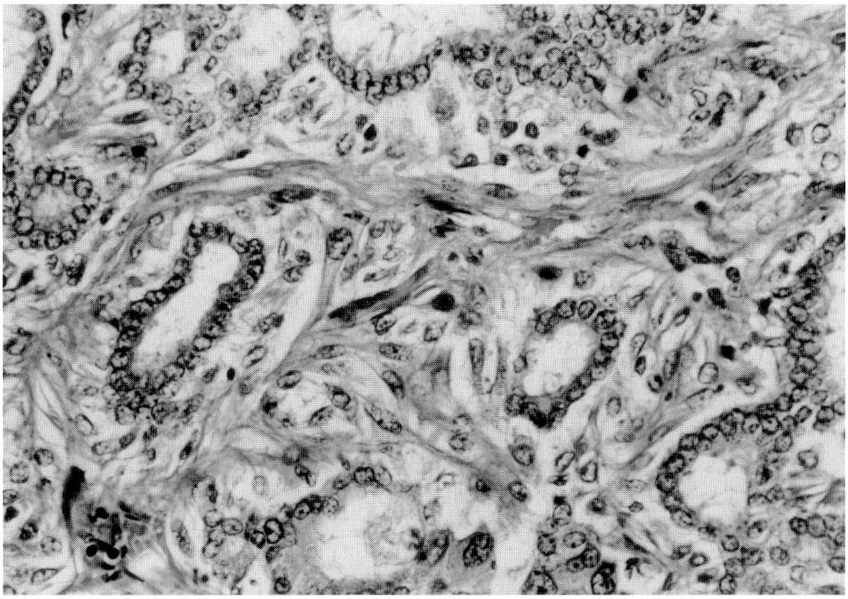

FIG. 7.5. Adenomyoepithelioma. Periluminal columnar cells are surrounded by unusually large and clear myoepithelial cells with small round regular nuclei.

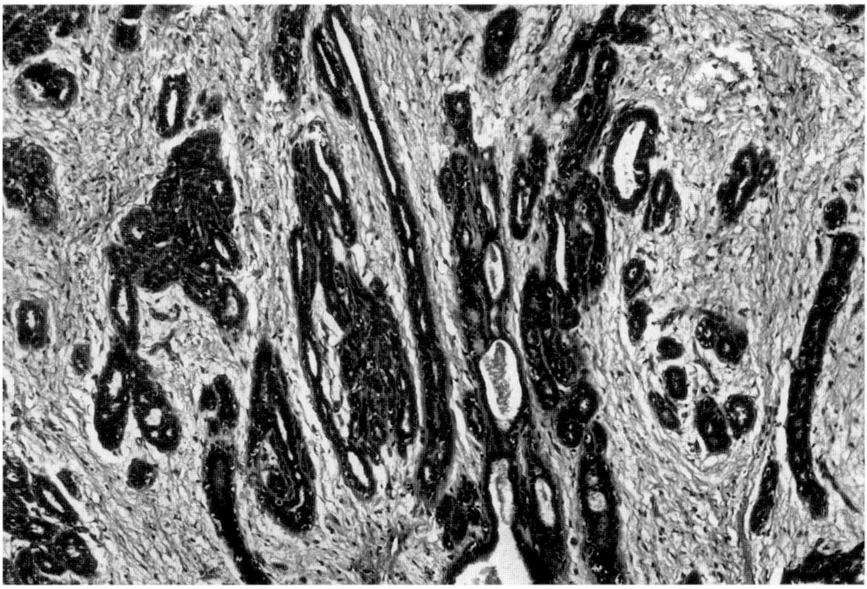

FIG. 7.6. Adenomyoepithelioma. Ductal structures with epithelial and myoepithelial components are surrounded by a proliferating fibrous stroma.

prominent myoepithelial and epithelial components. Clear and spindle myoepithelial cells were immunohistochemically marked for S-100 protein and muscle common antigen, but they were negative for epithelial membrane antigen (EMA), prekeratin, and carcinoembryonic antigen (CEA). The reverse was true for the epithelial cells, which were in varying states of proliferation, although some epithelial cells were stained for S-100 protein. Four of the six tumors that were studied expressed estrogen receptors. Intraductal papillary adenomyoepitheliomatous hyperplasia was present within the tumors and in surrounding ducts. Two patients who were treated by local resection suffered recurrence, but all patients were well at completion of follow-up. Jabi et al. (3) reported similar benign behavior.

Tavassoli (4) described three types of myoepithelial lesions of the breast: myoepitheliosis, adenomyoepithelioma, and myoepithelial carcinoma. All of these lesions were characterized by a prominence of myoepithelial cells that were located adjacent to the basement membrane, with clear cytoplasm and cytoplasmic smooth muscle that was evident on electron microscopy or by immunohistochemical stains. The author described 27 adenomyoepitheliomas that varied in size from 1 to 7 cm, with a median size of 2.5 cm. Most of them were sharply circumscribed. Histologically, the adenomyoepitheliomas were characterized by the presence of an extremely prominent myoepithelial layer and were stratified according to their histologic appearance into 7 predominantly spindle cell tumors, 8 tubular adenomyoepitheliomas, and 12 lobulated variants. The spindle cell type was composed of a predominantly spindled myoepithelial proliferation with admixed epithelium-lined spaces, some of which were cystic and many of which had apocrine metaplasia. The spindled cells were highly decorated when stained for S-100 protein, but there was little reaction for actin or cytokeratin. The tubular pattern was characterized by proliferation of rounded tubules that were surrounded by large numbers of myoepithelial cells. Lobulated adenomyoepitheliomas were composed of solid nests of clear eosinophilic myoepithelial cells that proliferated around compressed epithelial-lined spaces. One patient with a tubular-type adenomyoepithelioma, and another patient with a lobulated-type adenomyoepithelioma, developed a recurrence. The other patients remained well after surgical excision, which ranged from local to wide.

Young and Clement (5) described three cases of adenomyoepithelioma, one of which recurred, despite a bland cytologic and histologic appearance. The authors recommended wide local excision as primary treatment.

Weidner and Levine (6) reported on two patients with adenomyoepitheliomas. In both patients, a prominent spindled myoid component was immunoreactive for vimentin, but not for desmin. Ultrastructural examination showed the features of prominent myoepithelial cells, with intermediate filaments and dense bodies present throughout. Neither of the patients had recurrence or metastasis of the lesion. Zarbo and Oberman (7) reported a case of an extremely cellular adenomyoepithelioma that had a benign follow-up. Eusebi et al. (8) described adenomyoepitheliomas that had a predominance of solid clear cell myoepithelial proliferation in which the glandular luminal cells had extensive apocrine metaplasia. Both of the cases described were found in association with atypical apocrine sclerosing lesions (Chapter 6). Short-term follow up revealed no recurrence. Tamura et al. (9) described an adenomyoepithelioma in a 47-year-old man.

MALIGNANT ADENOMYOEPITHELIOMA

Although adenomyoepitheliomas are usually histologically benign and do not recur when locally excised, some have the histology of a malignant tumor (efigs.7.10 and 7.11) and some of these metastasize.

Loose et al. (10) described six cases of adenomyoepithelioma, of which two were malignant. Two of the four histologically benign adenomyoepitheliomas recurred after local resection at 48 and 60 months. In a fifth patient, an adenomyoepithelioma with an extremely high mitotic rate and nuclear atypicality of the myoepithelial component was treated by a mastectomy. There were no lymph node metastases, and the patient was well 18 months postoperatively. A sixth patient with an adenomyoepithelioma that showed markedly atypical and mitotically active myoepithelial cells had six local recurrences over a period of 52 months. The patient was treated by reexcisions and finally by mastectomy, but pulmonary metastases occurred at 54 months, brain metastases were found at 60 months, and she died 64 months after the appearance of the first lesion. In malignant adenomyoepitheliomas, extremely high mitotic rates, ranging from 11 to 14 per 10 high-power fields of myoepithelium, were observed. An infiltrative growth pattern was associated with local recurrence. Mitotic activity and nuclear atypia were quite limited in the myoepithelial cells in the four other tumors, but two of these recurred locally. The pulmonary metastasis showed both epithelial and myoepithelial cells by electron microscopy, although the predominant malignant component was myoepithelial in nature.

Trojani et al. (11) reviewed the literature on adenomyoepitheliomas and found that, in general, they behave in a benign fashion. Seven of the 60 previously reported cases had recurred, but only one of those cases had been reported to show involvement of an axillary lymph node. The authors reported a case of adenomyoepithelioma with lung metastasis that presented the same biphasic pattern as the primary tumor. The tumor presented as a mass in the upper outer quadrant of the breast of a 51-year-old woman. Initial excision revealed a cystic lesion with a thick wall and an intracystic vegetation with adenomyoepithelial features. The myoepithelial cells stained for α-smooth muscle actin and S-100 protein, but not for estrogen or progesterone receptors. The tumor recurred 1 year after surgery, with six 1-cm or smaller nodules in the original site. The patient was then treated with radiation and chemotherapy, but, 2 years after the first excision, three pulmonary nodules developed; these nodes were removed and shown to be histologically identical to the lesions removed from the breast. The predominant cell type in the metastasis was the myoepithelial cell. Michal et al. (12) described a 77-year old woman who had an adenomyoepithelioma of the breast that measured 10 × 8 × 8 cm. The adenomyoepithelioma had three distinctive components: tubular adenomyoepithelioma, a solid area in which there were features of both epithelial and myoepithelial cells and an anaplastic undifferentiated spindle cell carcinoma. The myoepithelial cells in the adenomyoepithelial component reacted strongly to muscle actin and were negative for cytokeratin. The solid cell component reacted negatively with all the antibodies. The undifferentiated carcinoma was also negative for cytokeratin and S-100 protein. Follow-up was not given on this case.

Rasbridge and Millis (13) reported on seven cases of adenomyoepithelioma with histologic features that were suggestive of malignancy with local recurrences. In two cases, the histology suggested ordinary infiltrating ductal carcinoma. Two histologic patterns were described: typical or benign adenomyoepithelioma, merging with areas of malignant cells, or architectural adenomyoepithelioma with cellular atypia and mitotic activity throughout. Both patterns were associated with a more aggressive course than the usual cytologically bland amitotic adenomyoepithelioma. Ahmad and Heller (14) reported on a case of adenomyoepithelioma with local invasion, severe cytologic atypia, and high mitotic count without metastasis. Simpson et al. (15) reported an adenomyoepithelioma that was associated with an osteosarcoma, which recurred twice, and disseminated with fatal outcome in 39 months. In the final recurrence, a separate small focus of invasive carcinoma was identified.

In summary, adenomyoepitheliomas with cellular atypia or a high mitotic rate are suspect for at least local recurrence and rarely metastasis. Recurrence may show carcinoma, sarcoma, malignant myoepithelioma, or biphasic malignancy with both carcinoma and myoepithelioma.

BENIGN MIXED TUMOR (PLEOMORPHIC ADENOMA)

Benign mixed tumor, with its varying proportions of proliferating duct-like structures, myoepithelial components, and cartilaginous stroma, is the most common canine mammary tumor (16), but pleomorphic adenomas are rare in women (17). These tumors have been mistaken for carcinoma, especially on frozen section, because of their cellularity, close association of epithelium with proliferating stromal elements, and the lack of recognition, by pathologists, of pleomorphic adenoma in the breast. As in most of the other benign lesions discussed previously, the keys to a correct diagnosis include familiarity with the entity, identification of a prominent myoepithelial component, and recognition of the variation of the ductal proliferation. Cartilaginous areas may be prominent and have been mistaken for mucoid carcinoma. Chondrocytes are present and are usually singly placed in lacunae (Figs. 7.7 to 7.12 and efigs. 7.12 to 7.21). The differential diagnosis includes invasive ductal, colloid, and metaplastic carcinoma, all of which lack a myoepithelial component and usually have more obviously malignant-appearing cells in larger groups. Metaplastic carcinomas have much more cellular and anaplastic cartilage, which may be associated with malignant osteoid.

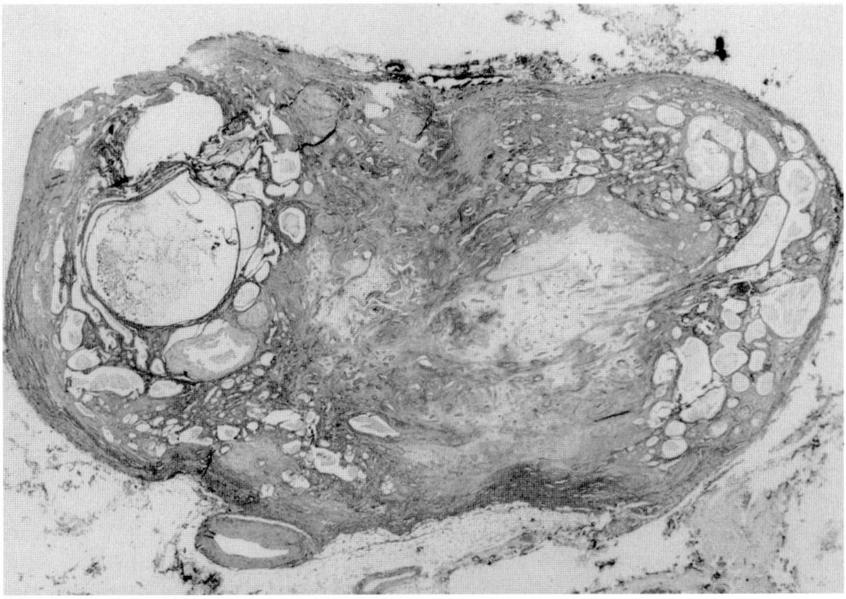

FIG. 7.7. Pleomorphic adenoma. This benign mixed tumor has rounded pushing contours. Areas are cystic and there is an island of cartilaginous differentiation at the 3 o'clock position.

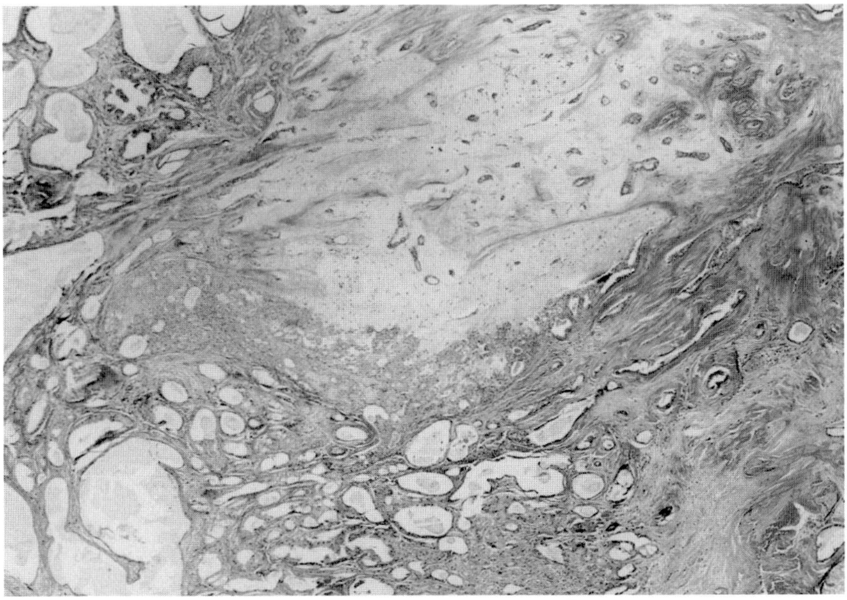

FIG. 7.8. Pleomorphic adenoma, benign mixed tumor. Epithelial elements are at the circumscribed periphery and chondroid stromal elements are in the center.

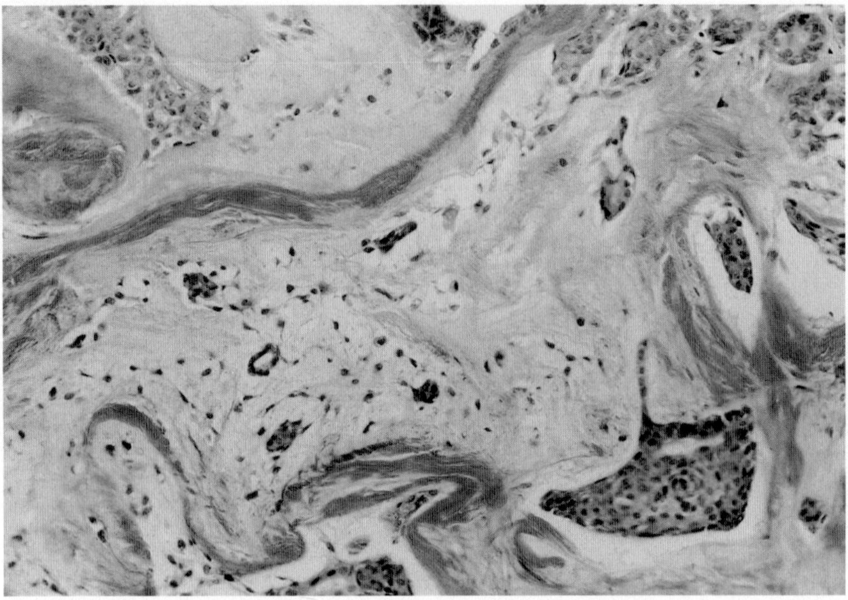

FIG. 7.9. Pleomorphic adenoma, benign mixed tumor. The cartilaginous matrix is characterized by chondrocytes in small lacunae in the cartilage, which distinguishes this lesion from the fibrous stroma of adenomyoepithelioma (Fig. 7.6).

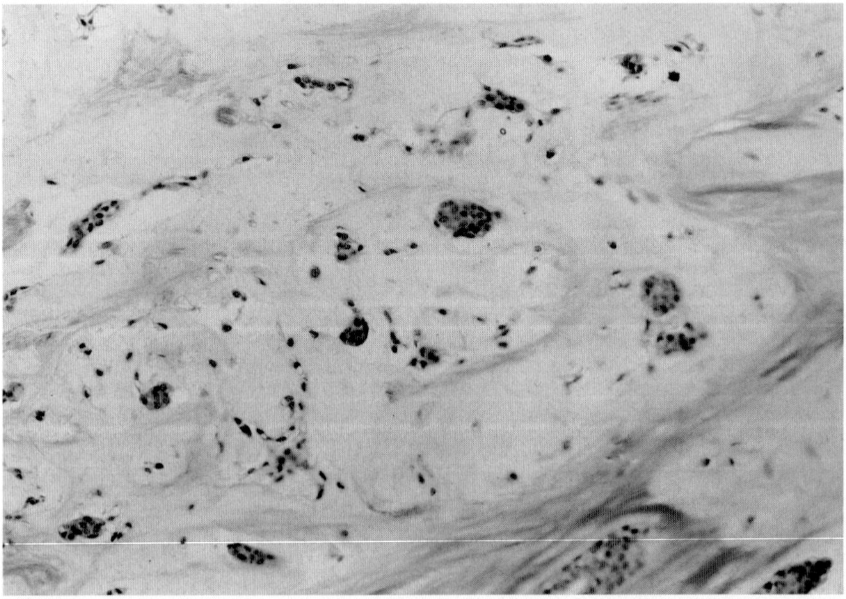

FIG. 7.10. Pleomorphic adenoma, benign mixed tumor. The cartilaginous matrix appears to arise directly from myoepithelium. The chondrocytes and the cartilage that they produce appear mature, distinct from the immature cartilage and malignant cells of metaplastic carcinoma (Chapter 8).

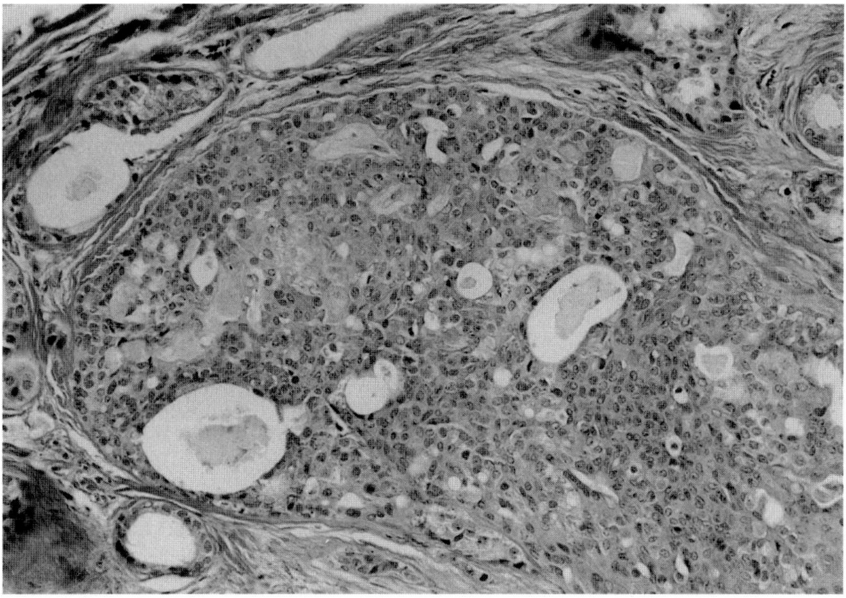

FIG. 7.11. Pleomorphic adenoma, benign mixed tumor. Ductal structures with prominent myoepithelium are the dominant features.

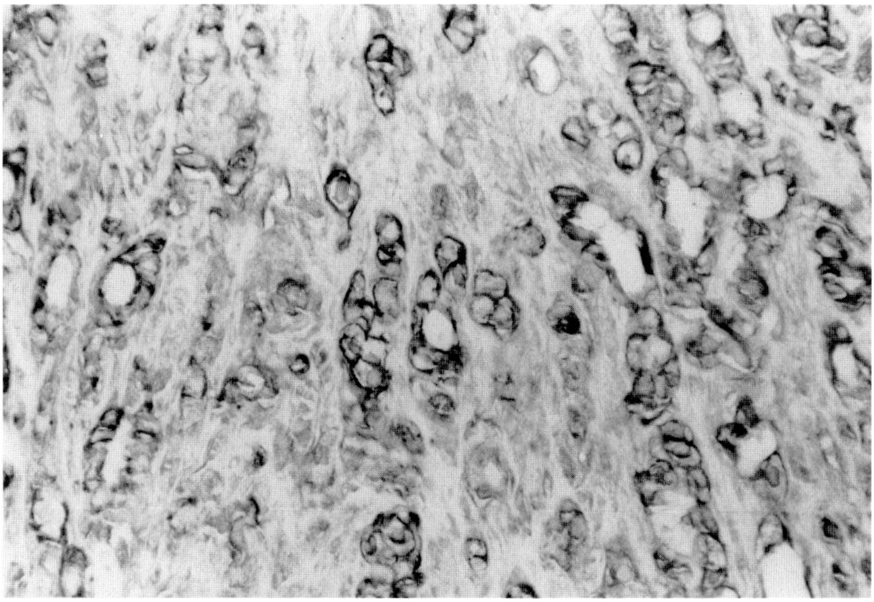

FIG. 7.12. Pleomorphic adenoma, benign mixed tumor. Epithelial elements immunostained for smooth muscle actin demonstrate the myoepithelial component.

First reported by Smith and Taylor (18), who considered them metaplastic papillomas, mixed tumors are rare, and follow-up has shown a uniformly good prognosis. Rarely, they are associated with intraductal papillomas (Fig. 7.13 and efigs. 7.22 to 7.27). Although the border is sharply circumscribed, it extends into the breast with knobby projections, as in the salivary gland mixed tumors. It is easy to visualize incomplete excision, but this apparently is unusual in the breast. Sheth et al. (19) reported a case and reviewed the literature. Size usually varies from 1 to 4 cm, although a 20-cm benign mixed tumor has been reported (18). Focal calcification of the chondroid matrix may be evident grossly and mammographically. The age range is from the third to eighth decades, with more patients in the older age range.

Moran et al. (20) reported six cases of mammary pleomorphic adenoma that ranged in size from 1 to 4 cm in diameter and were all histologically characterized by the admixture of benign glandular elements, myoepithelial elements, and cartilaginous or myxoid components. One of these tumors also contained abundant tyrosine-like crystals, which have been described in benign mixed tumors of the parotid gland. The tumors were grossly circumscribed, although microscopically they had pushing areas that extended into the parenchyma. Three of the lesions presented as palpable masses, two lesions were malignant-appearing masses on mammogram, and one lesion was incidental to the presence of an

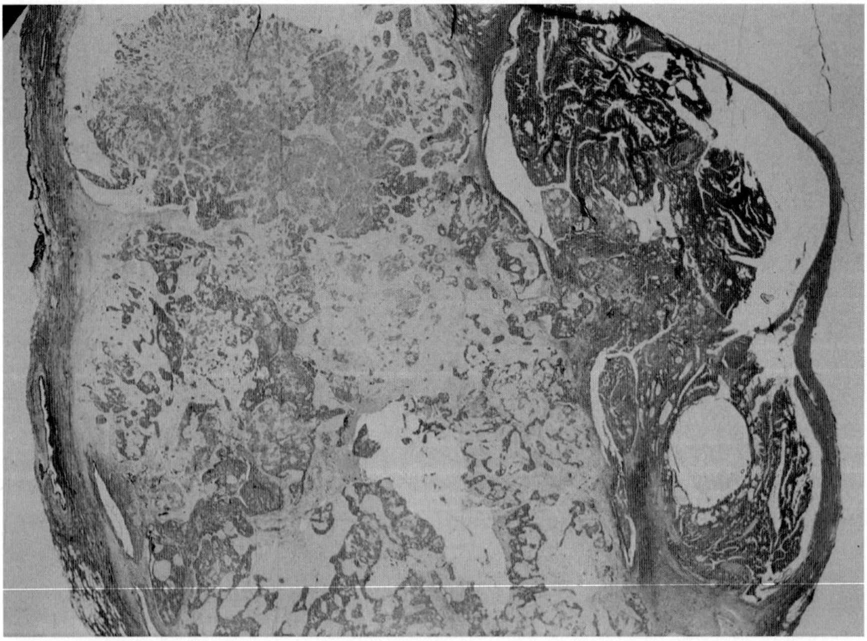

FIG. 7.13. Pleomorphic adenoma, benign mixed tumor. This benign mixed tumor (**left**) is adjacent to an intraductal papilloma (**right**).

infiltrating ductal carcinoma that was treated by mastectomy. Immunohistochemistry was performed for keratin, CEA, actin, GFAP, S-100 protein, and vimentin. CEA stained only the luminal contents of the ducts. The epithelium was stained for keratin and S-100 protein. The myoepithelial elements were stained for keratin, smooth muscle actin, S-100 protein, and vimentin. The spindle components displayed a staining pattern that was identical to that of the myoepithelial component, but also stained for GFAP. Cartilaginous areas stained in the same way as the spindle components. The five patients treated by excision alone did not suffer recurrence, during a follow-up period that varied from 1 to 7 years. The patient treated by mastectomy died of metastatic breast cancer, but had no evidence of recurrence of the pleomorphic adenoma.

Ballance et al. (21) described a 77-year-old woman with a 2-cm pleomorphic adenoma in the breast that showed the histologic appearance and the immunohistochemical profile of those described by Moran et al. (20). Electron microscopy revealed a predominance of cells that had intermediate filaments with dense bodies and intercellular junctions, which suggested the predominantly myoepithelial cell differentiation of the tumor. Flow cytometry demonstrated that the tumor was diploid. This patient was alive and well 14 months postoperatively. The authors reviewed 35 cases that were reported in the English literature and found that 31% of the cases had been treated by mastectomy, suggesting difficulty with the diagnosis, especially on frozen section. Three of the other cases had recurrence locally, but were adequately treated by reexcision or simple mastectomy, without subsequent reported recurrence.

Sugano et al. (22) reported on two cases of locally infiltrative adenomyoepithelioma with cartilagenous matrix that resembled pleomorphic adenoma. The adenomyoepitheliomas had a nontubular epithelial component and an associated comedocarcinoma. One tumor recurred locally at 6 months, but there was no evidence of metastasis in the short follow-up.

OTHER ADNEXAL TUMORS OF THE BREAST

SYRINGOMATOUS TUMORS

Suster et al. (23) described 4 cases of syringomatous squamous tumors in the parenchyma of the breast, which were not related to the overlying skin or nipple, in women whose ages ranged from 37 to 70 years. Three of the lesions presented on mammogram as stippled microcalcifications. All were 1.5 cm or less in diameter and were treated by local excision. Follow-up from 1 to 6 years showed no evidence of recurrence. Histologically, the tumors were relatively well circumscribed, but they were predominantly fibrous and composed of small nests of squamous cells that contained large cyst-like islands similar to those seen in syringomas in other parts of the skin.

Nipple syringomas are described and illustrated in Chapter 4. Rosen (24) described four cases of syringomatous adenoma of the nipple, which presented with firm nodules in the nipple that represented highly infiltrative tumors with epithelial and myoepithelial cells. Nests and cords of cytologically uniform squamous cells, which resembled those of the sweat gland duct, infiltrated the dermis, underlying breast tissue, and especially the smooth muscle bundles in the nipple. Follow-up of those patients revealed that they had been cured by local excision of the nipple and surrounding tissues. Ward et al. (25) described two additional cases, one of which measured 3.5 cm in greatest dimension. One was treated by simple mastectomy, following local excision, and no residual tumor was found in the mastectomy specimen. The other was treated by wide local excision, and both were free of disease at 12 and 9 months. In one case, there appeared to be connections between the neoplastic epithelium and the epidermis. A myxoid background and a prominent sclerotic collagenous stroma, invasion of perineural spaces, and the adventitia, but not the lumina of blood vessels, were seen in both cases. Staining for S-100 protein was seen in the tumor and in Langerhans cells. Jones et al. (26) described 11 syringomas of the nipple. Ten syringomas were treated by local excision and recurred; however, they were successfully managed by reexcision, and none metastasized. Syringoma closely simulates invasive carcinoma and should be considered in the differential diagnosis of that entity.

Other benign adnexal-like tumors have been described in the breast. Draheim et al. (27) described an eccrine spiradenoma similar to the basaloid adnexal tumor that is characterized by lobulation and a clear two-cell (epithelial and myoepithelial) population (Figs. 7.14 and 7.15 and efigs. 7.28 to 7.31). Panico et al. (28) reported on an eccrine spiradenoma that recurred 3 times following local excision. Estrogen and progesterone receptors were diffusely stained in the tumor. Saboo-

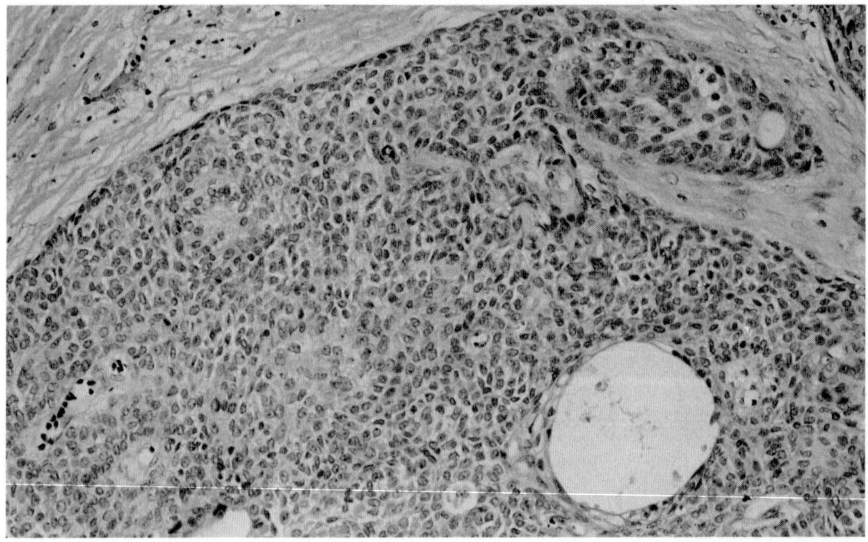

FIG. 7.14. Eccrine spiradenoma. This basaloid tumor in the breast has the lobulation and cystic dilatation of ducts of an eccrine spiradenoma.

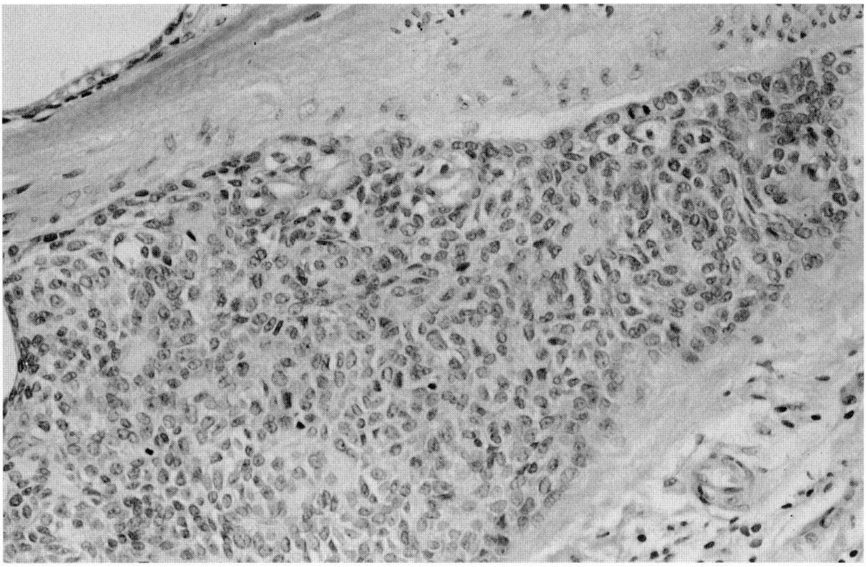

FIG. 7.15. Eccrine spiradenoma. At higher magnification, the spindling myoepithelial cells are evident, as is the basaloid orientation of cells adjacent to the stroma. Note the mitotic figure in the basal row of cells (**upper right**). This tumor was recurrent.

rian et al. (29) published a case of a 68-year-old woman who reported a 50-year history of a breast mass that suddenly grew, involved the skin, and was associated with nipple discharge. The eccrine spiradenoma pattern was associated with adenosquamous carcinoma, rhabdomyosarcoma, and osteosarcoma.

Finck et al. (30) described a clear cell hidradenoma in the breast similar to the adnexal lesion of that description. All of the cells of the clear cell hidradenoma were epithelial in character (efigs. 7.32 to 7.35). Subramony (31) described bilateral syringocystadenoma papilliferum of the nipple. This lesion is similar in many ways to the adenoma of the nipple (Chapter 4). Nowak et al. (32) reported on a 2-cm syringocystadenoma papilliferum in a 39-year-old man. Gokaslan et al. (33) reported on a solitary cylindroma that was incidentally found in an excision for invasive lobular carcinoma in the breast of a 61-year-old woman.

With the exception of hidradenoma, the key to the recognition of these adnexal tumors is identification of a prominent myoepithelial component, as part of a pattern seen more often in another exocrine gland. Adnexal tumors tend to be less aggressive than the carcinomas they mimic.

ADENOID CYSTIC CARCINOMA

Adenoid cystic carcinoma (ACC), which constitutes fewer than 1% of invasive cancers of the breast, is histologically similar to those seen in the skin adnexa and salivary glands; however, almost all authors have agreed that the prognosis of ACC of the breast is much better than that of ACC in the salivary glands (34–46). Although any metastasis from ACC of the breast is rare, bloodborne metastases to the lung (47) and other organs (48) have been described.

ACCs are usually small, but they have been reported as large as 8 cm in diameter. They are found predominantly in the mammary parenchyma, but may invade the skin, as does ductal carcinoma of the breast. Grossly, they are firm and well demarcated, but they may be locally invasive. Microscopically, they have the classic adenoid cystic appearance, with a "cylindroma" component in which hyalinized cores or cylinders of mucoid PAS-positive material are found within, and lining, the lumina in a characteristic cribriform pattern (Fig. 7.16 and efig. 7.36), at least focally. The small cells are uniform in size and have hyperchromatic nuclei (Fig. 7.17 and efig. 7.37). Perineural invasion may be seen (efig. 7.38). A trabecular or solid pattern may be found in association with the characteristic cylindromatous pattern. Perzin et al. (49) and Spiro et al. (50) showed that ACCs of the salivary glands have a more aggressive course when the trabecular or solid pattern dominates. The cylindromatous pattern is considered the best differentiated and therefore the most benign of the ACC group, certainly

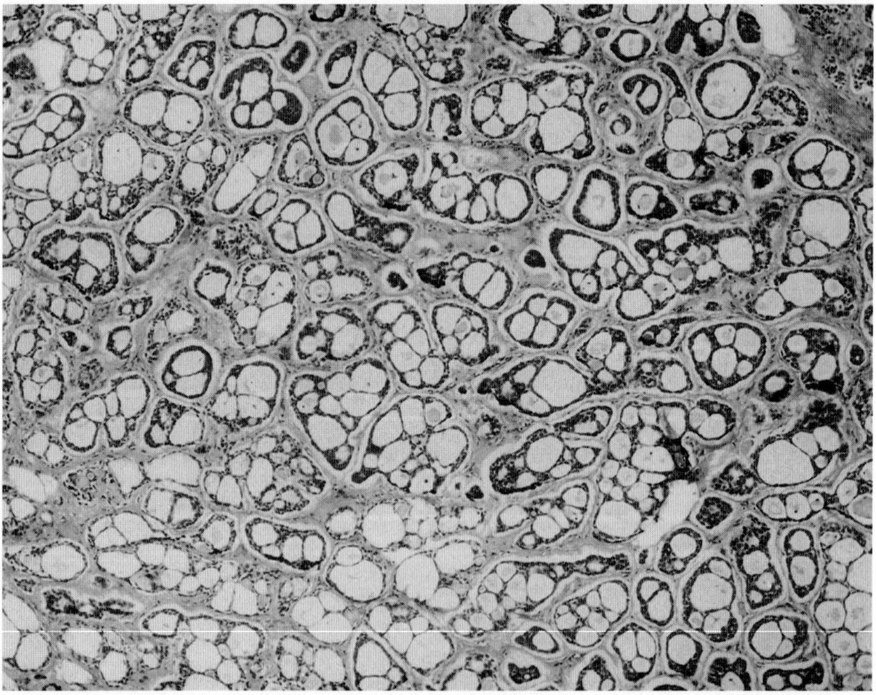

FIG. 7.16. Adenoid cystic carcinoma. Infiltrating adenoid cystic carcinoma with compound or cribriform glands that contain dense eosinophilic material in the extracellular lumina.

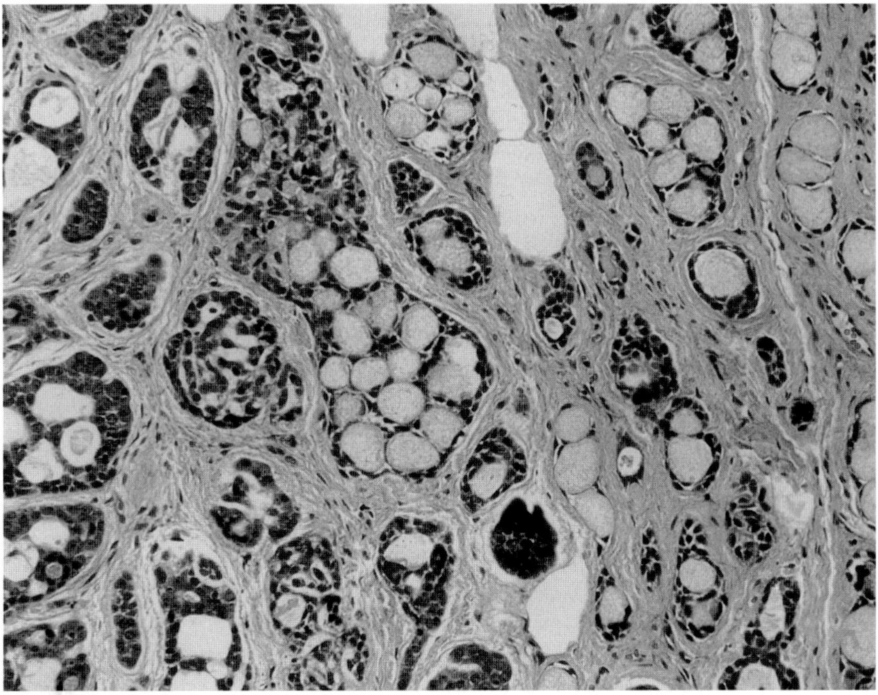

FIG. 7.17. Adenoid cystic carcinoma of the breast. At higher magnification, the regularity of the lumens of the invasive ducts of this carcinoma is apparent. The cells proliferate in a thin, usually single, layer around the lumens, which are distended with dense eosinophilic material that is responsible for the term cylindroma. The extracellular material stains positively with PAS and also stains for type IV collagen. The malignant cells may show features of myoepithelium and stain for smooth muscle actin.

within the breast. Kleer and Oberman (51) studied 31 cases of ACC of the breast, stratified according to histology. The patients reported on all patients who were alive, with no evidence of disease, after a median follow-up of 7 years. With universal survival, histology was not a prognostic indicator. Ten of 20 were subareolar, all were grossly circumscribed, but 12 of 20 also had focal infiltration. Five of the 19 cases studied expressed estrogen receptor protein.

Ro et al. (52) reported 12 cases of pure ACC of the breast and stratified them according to grades I, II, and III, as described for salivary gland ACC by Perzin et al. (49) and Spiro et al. (50). All 5 patients with grade I (cylindromatous) ACC were alive and free of disease, but 1 of the 6 patients with a grade II (cylindromatous and cribriform) ACC developed local recurrence 5 years after diagnosis. That patient subsequently developed pulmonary metastases and died of metastatic ACC 13 years after diagnosis. The patient with the grade III (predominantly solid) ACC had metastatic disease in the axillary lymph nodes at the time of mastectomy and died 2 years later.

Differential diagnosis is from the cribriform variant of intraductal and invasive ductal carcinoma (described in Chapters 4 and 8, respectively) and from CS, which is described below. Adenoid cystic differentiation may be seen in conjunction with other types of carcinoma of the breast, especially ductal carcinoma of the breast (53). When ductal carcinoma is present in association with ACC, the ductal component determines the behavior and it is generally worse than that of the ACC.

Due et al. (54) immunostained an ACC from the breast of a 78-year-old woman and found that the pseudocysts in the cylindromatous pattern were lined and filled by type IV collagen. The epithelium stained positively for EMA, whereas the proliferating myoepithelial component stained positively for vimentin. Stains for estrogen and progesterone receptors were negative. Trojani et al. (44) reported on five cases of ACC of the breast that were identified by the presence of myoepithelial cells stained for α-smooth muscle actin. In this series of cases, the size ranged from 1.2 to 2.5 cm and the margins were predominantly infiltrating. Three of the ACCs were tubular and cribriform and two of the ACCs were solid grade III lesions. Estrogen and progesterone receptors were negative in all four of the cases tested. Four of the patients were initially treated by tumorectomy. One patient had recurrence at 8 years after surgery, but was well 3 years later.

COLLAGENOUS SPHERULOSIS

Clement et al. (55) described 15 cases of CS that they found in the breasts of women aged 39 to 55 years. CS is an intraductal proliferation in which there were intraluminal clusters of eosinophilic spherules that measured from 20 to 100 μm in diameter (Fig. 7.18 and efigs. 7.39 to 7.41). The spherules are rich in collagen and contain PAS-positive and type IV collagen-positive basement membrane-like material, as is seen in ACC. The cells immediately surrounding the spherules stain positively for actin, which is indicative of myoepithelial differentiation. By follow-up, CS was benign. CS can be confused easily with ACC of the breast or with intraductal carcinoma of a cribriform type, but it is usually localized to one or a very few ducts and has the diagnostic features described above. Divaris et al. (56) described a unique case in which CS involved multiple lobules bound together by a proliferative fibrous stroma to form a palpable mass; however, the lesion remained noninvasive.

In summary, ACC should be distinguished from CS and intraductal and invasive cribriform carcinomas. The ACC has, at least focally, a cylindromatous pattern with central cores of dense eosinophilic material that is PAS-positive, stains for type IV collagen, and is lamina densa by electron microscopy. The cells that surround (and presumably elaborate) the basement membrane material have myoepithelial features by immunohistochemistry with staining for vimentin, smooth muscle actin, and keratin type 14. ACC is an invasive carcinoma. CS is almost always a small and incidental finding of cylindromatous changes that are limited to a duct and it is always noninvasive. Cribriform carcinomas have the

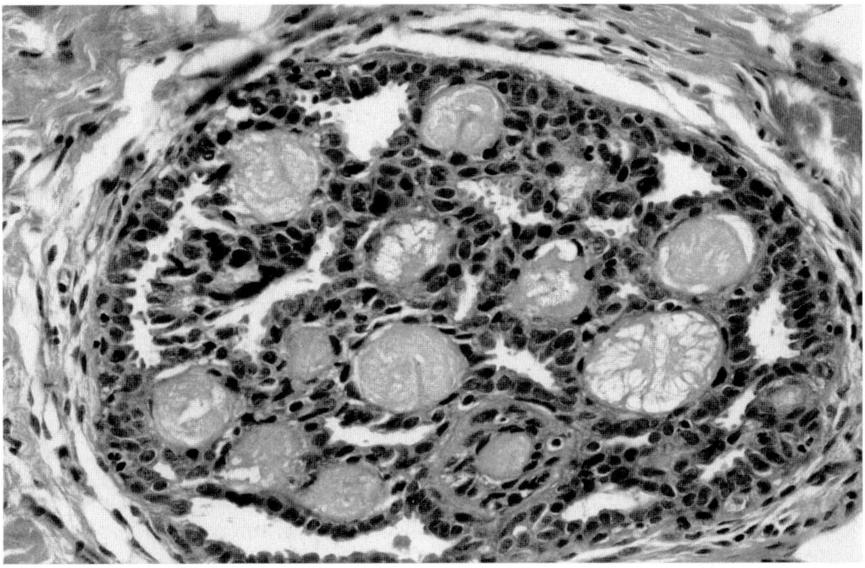

FIG. 7.18. Collagenous spherulosis. This small duct has a regular proliferation of small cells around the perfectly circular, dense extracellular material, which can be shown to contain type IV collagen. Only three ducts in a large biopsy specimen displayed this change.

regular shape of ACC and CS, but they lack the basement membrane-like material that is seen in those two lesions.

OTHER CARCINOMAS WITH A MYOEPITHELIAL COMPONENT

Foschini and Eusebi (57) listed low-grade adenosquamous (syringomatous) carcinoma and poorly differentiated myoepithelial-rich carcinomas as other malignancies of the breast with myoepithelial differentiation. Van Hoeven et al. (58) reported on 32 cases of low-grade adenosquamous carcinoma of the breast that displayed glandular and squamous differentiation that was ultrastructurally analogous to the acrosyringium of the eccrine sweat gland. The carcinomas ranged from 0.6 to 8.0 cm in diameter. Only 2 of 15 tested cases expressed estrogen receptor. One of 12 patients with examined axillary lymph nodes had a node that was positive for metastatic carcinoma. Another patient had pulmonary metastasis. Twenty patients had no recurrence and five patients treated initially by local excision had recurrence. One of those cases was fatal.

Three cases of poorly differentiated myoepithelial-rich carcinomas with spindle shaped myoepithelial cells intermingled with the epithelial component were described by Damiani et al. (59). The authors noted central necrosis as a major feature of the tumors. Tsuda et al. (60) described invasive ductal carcinomas with large central acellular zones, in which 16 of 20 had spindle cells that immunostained for S-100 protein, α-smooth muscle actin, and keratin 14, which was indicative of myoepithelial differentiation. Among 40 invasive ductal carcinomas without central acellular zones, only 6 of 40 cases had cells that expressed the myoepithelial phenotype. The myoepithelial component was a marker for lung and brain metastasis.

PURELY MYOEPITHELIAL TUMORS

Tavassoli (4) described three cases of myoepitheliosis in which a biphasic pattern with a predominant myoepithelial component was present in a localized lesion. Spindle-to-cuboid myoepithelial cells sometimes extended as nodules into small ducts, in much the same way as is seen in cellular fibroadenomas; however, the proliferating cells stained for both actin and S-100 protein. Erlandson and Rosen (61) described a spindle cell myoepithelioma that arose in the breast of a 60-year-old woman. It measured 2.8 cm in diameter, was composed of interlacing bundles of spindle cells that were arranged in a storiform pattern, and did not exhibit infiltration of the surrounding tissues. Electron microscopy showed spindled cells joined by mature desmosomes, encompassed by basal lamina, with intermediate filaments containing fusiform densities. Pinocytotic vesicles marked the cell surface. In other areas, prekeratin filaments indicated squamous metaplasia within the cells. The differential diagnosis was between a tumor of myofibroblasts, smooth muscle cells, and myoepithelial cells; the ultrastructural features of this lesion were those of a myoepithelioma. On frozen section, the lesion was called a metaplastic carcinoma, and a mastectomy was performed with low axillary dissection. Postoperative follow-up of 3 months revealed no recurrence. Estrogen and progesterone receptors were absent from the cells.

Malignant Myoepithelioma

Tavassoli (4) described a malignant myoepithelioma that was composed of infiltrating plump atypical spindle cells that stained for smooth muscle actin and S-100 protein, with numerous mitotic figures. Electron microscopy revealed pinocytic vesicles, myofibrils with dense bodies, thick aggregates of intermediate filaments, and patchy basal lamina. Tight junctions also were observed. The patient had wide local excision and was well 19 months after surgery. Thorner et al. (62) reported a malignant myoepithelioma of the breast in an 81-year-old woman. This mass measured 21 × 10 × 5 cm and eroded the overlying skin. A single axillary lymph node metastasis was present. The tumor cells were a monomorphous population of spindle cells, arranged in interlacing bundles with numerous mitotic figures and areas of necrosis. Skin and skeletal muscle were both invaded. There was no apparent epithelial differentiation in the light microscopic study. By electron microscopy, the cells had pinocytotic vesicles and intermediate filaments, and some of these intermediate filaments stained for cytokeratin and actin. This patient died of other causes 2 months after surgery, without evidence of spread. Chen et al. (63) described a myoepithelial carcinoma in a 54-year-old woman. This tumor was also large, measuring 17 × 11 × 6 cm, with a central necrotic cavity, and the tumor infiltrated the border with satellite nodules. The tumor cells were spindled in shape and anaplastic, with numerous mitotic figures. The cells stained positively for cytokeratin, S-100 protein, GFAP, and muscle-specific actin. By electron microscopy the cells possessed pinocytotic vesicles, basal lamina, tonofilaments, desmosomes, and numerous intermediate filaments with dense bodies. No epithelial component was evident. A modified radical mastectomy was performed, but, 3 weeks later, the patient developed a pathologic fracture of her left hip and was found to have metastases in the femoral neck, as well as the radius. The patient died 6 months later of widespread metastatic disease. Tamai (64) described a malignant myoepithelioma growing as an intraductal tumor with a solid and comedocarcinoma appearance, with spindle cells staining for S-100 protein and α-smooth muscle actin. Lakhani et al. (65) described a malignant myoepithelioma of the breast that was immunostained for CAM5.2, actin, vimentin, and cytokeratin 14, but not for cytokeratins 18 and 19. Recently, Van Dorpe et al. (66) and Shiraishi et al. (67) described similar malignant myoepitheliomas of the breast.

In summary, nearly all of the lesions in the breast that contain a prominent myoepithelial component are benign and the presence of this prominent myoepithelial component is usually a strong indication of a lack of malignancy. However, there are exceptions to every rule, and there are rare malignant myoepithelial tumors. One should be wary of biphasic or spindle cell tumors that have mitotically active myoepithelial cells. In the majority of cases, myoepitheliosis, adenomyoepithelioma, and myoepithelioma have been only locally invasive, but some tumors, especially large ones, have displayed a high level of malignancy with the ability to metastasize to lymph nodes, lungs, bone, and elsewhere.

REFERENCES

1. Koyama M, Kurotaki H, Yagihashi N, et al. Immunohistochemical assessment of proliferative activity in mammary adenomyoepithelioma. *Histopathology* 1997;31:134–139.
2. Rosen PP. Adenomyoepithelioma of the breast. *Hum Pathol* 1987;18:1232–1237.
3. Jabi M, Dardick I, Cardigos N. Adenomyoepithelioma of the breast. *Arch Pathol Lab Med* 1988;112: 73–76.
4. Tavassoli FA. Myoepithelial lesions of the breast: myoepitheliosis, adenomyoepithelioma and myoepithelial carcinoma. *Am J Surg Pathol* 1991;15:554–568.
5. Young RH, Clement PB. Adenomyoepithelioma of the breast. A report of three cases and review of the literature. *Am J Clin Pathol* 1988;89:308–314.
6. Weidner N, Levine JD. Spindle-cell myoepithelioma of the breast: a microscopic, ultrastructural and immunocytochemical study. *Cancer* 1988;62:1561–1567.
7. Zarbo RJ, Oberman HA. Cellular adenomyoepithelioma of the breast. *Am J Surg Pathol* 1983;7: 863–870.
8. Eusebi V, Casadei GP, Bussolati G, et al. Adenomyoepithelioma of the breast with a distinctive type of apocrine adenosis. *Histopathology* 1987;11:305–315.
9. Tamura G, Monma N, Suzuki Y, et al. Adenomyoepithelioma (myoepithelioma) of the breast in a male. *Hum Pathol* 1993;24:678–681.
10. Loose JH, Patchefsky AS, Hollander IJ, et al. Adenomyoepithelioma of the breast. A spectrum of biologic behavior. *Am J Surg Pathol* 1992;16:868–876.

11. Trojani M, Guiu M, Trouette H, et al. Malignant adenomyoepithelioma of the breast. An immunohistochemical, cytophotometric, and ultrastructural study of a case with lung metastases. *Am J Clin Pathol* 1994;101:598–602.
12. Michal M, Baumruk, L, Burger J, et al. Adenomyoepithelioma of the breast with undifferentiated carcinoma component. *Histopathology* 1994;24:274–276.
13. Rasbridge S, Millis R. Adenomyoepithelioma of the breast with malignant features. *Virchows Arch* 1998;432:123–130.
14. Ahmed A, Heller D. Malignant adenomyoepithelioma of the breast with malignant proliferation of epithelial and myoepithelial elements: a case report and review of the literature. *Arch Pathol Lab Med* 2000;124:632–636.
15. Simpson R, Cope N, Skalova A, et al. Malignant adenomyoepithelioma of the breast with mixed osteogenic, spindle cell and carcinomatous differentiation. *Am J Surg Pathol* 1998;22:631–636.
16. Allen AC. So-called mixed tumors of the mammary gland of dog and man, with special reference to the general problem of bone and cartilage formation. *Arch Pathol* 1940;29:589–624.
17. Makek M, Von Hochstetter AR. Pleomorphic adenoma of the human breast. *J Surg Oncol* 1980;14: 281–286.
18. Smith BH, Taylor HB. The occurrence of bone and cartilage in mammary tumors. *Am J Clin Pathol* 1969;51:610–618.
19. Sheth MT, Hathaway D, Petrelli M. Pleomorphic adenoma ("mixed" tumor) of human female breast mimicking carcinoma clinico-radiologically. *Cancer* 1978;41:659–665.
20. Moran CA, Suster S, Carter D. Benign mixed tumors (pleomorphic adenomas) of the breast. *Am J Surg Pathol* 1990;14:913–921.
21. Ballance WA, Ro JY, el-Naggar AK, et al. Pleomorphic adenoma (benign mixed tumor) of the breast. An immunohistochemical, flow cytometric, and ultrastructural study and review of the literature. *Am J Clin Pathol* 1990;93:795–801.
22. Sugano I, Nagao T, Tajima Y, et al. Malignant adenomyoepithelioma of the breast: a non-tubular and matrix-producing variant. *Pathol Int* 2001;51:193–199.
23. Suster S, Moran CA, Hurt MA. Syringomatous squamous tumors of the breast. *Cancer* 1991;67: 2350–2355.
24. Rosen PP. Syringomatous adenoma of the nipple. *Am J Surg Pathol* 1983;7:739–745.
25. Ward BE, Cooper PH, Subramony C. Syringomatous tumor of the nipple. *Am J Clin Pathol* 1989;92: 692–696.
26. Jones MW, Norris HJ, Snyder RC. Infiltrating syringomatous adenoma of the nipple: a clinical and pathologic study of 11 cases. *Am J Surg Pathol* 1989;13:197–201.
27. Draheim J, Neubecker RD, Sprinz H. An unusual tumor of the breast resembling eccrine spiradenoma. *Am J Clin Pathol* 1959;31:511–516.
28. Panico L, D'Antonio A, Chiacchio R, et al. An unusual, recurring breast tumor with features of eccrine spiradenoma: a case report. *Am J Clin Pathol* 1996;106:665–669.
29. Saboorian MH, Kenny M, Ashfaq R, et al. Carcinosarcoma arising in eccrine spiradenoma of the breast. Report of a case and review of the literature. *Arch Pathol Lab Med* 1996;120:501–504.
30. Finck FM, Schwinn CP, Keasbey LE. Clear cell hidradenoma of the breast. *Cancer* 1968;22:125–135.
31. Subramony C. Bilateral breast tumors resembling syringocystadenoma papilliferum. *Am J Clin Pathol* 1987;87:656–659.
32. Nowak M, Pathan A, Fatteh S, et al. Syringocystadenoma papilliferum of the male breast. *Am J Dermatopathol* 1998;20:422–424.
33. Gokaslan ST, Carlile B, Dudak M, et al. Solitary cylindroma (dermal analog tumor) of the breast: a previously undescribed neoplasm at this site. *Am J Surg Pathol* 2001;25:823–826.
34. Anthony PP, James PD. Adenoid cystic carcinoma of the breast: prevalence, diagnostic criteria and histogenesis. *J Clin Pathol* 1975;28:647–655.
35. Cavano FJ, Taylor HB. Adenoid cystic carcinoma of the breast. *Cancer* 1969;24:740–745.
36. Galloway JR, Woolner LB, Clagett OT. Adenoid cystic carcinoma of the breast. *Surg Gynecol Obstet* 1966;122:1289–1294.
37. Greiner TC, Robinson RA, Maves MD. Adenoid cystic carcinoma: a clinicopathologic study with flow cytometric analysis. *Am J Clin Pathol* 1989;92:711–720.
38. Greshong LE. Adenoid cystic carcinoma of the breast. *Arch Surg* 1966;92:424–427.
39. Hjorth S, Magnusson PH, Blomquist P. Adenoid cystic carcinoma of the breast. *Acta Chir Scand* 1977;143:155–158.

40. Koss LG, Brannan CD, Ashikari R. Histologic and ultrastructural features of adenoid cystic carcinoma of the breast. *Cancer* 1970;26:1271–1279.
41. Lim SK, Kovi J, Warner OG. Adenoid cystic carcinoma of the breast with metastasis: a case report and review of the literature. *J Natl Med Assoc* 1979;71:329–330.
42. Peters GN, Wolff M. Adenoid cystic carcinoma of the breast: report of 11 new cases. Review of the literature and discussion of biological behavior. *Cancer* 1983;52:680–686.
43. Tavassoli FA, Norris HJ. Mammary adenoid cystic carcinoma with sebaceous differentiation: a morphologic study of the cell types. *Arch Pathol Lab Med* 1986;110:1045–1053.
44. Trojani M, de Mascarel I, Coindre JM. Adenoid cystic carcinoma of the breast. Value of immunohistochemical study in diagnosis. *Tumori* 1991;77:130–135.
45. Verani R, Bel-Kahn J. Mammary adenoid cystic carcinoma with unusual features. *Am J Clin Pathol* 1973;59:653–658.
46. Zaloudek C, Oertel YC, Orenstein JM. Adenoid cystic carcinoma of the breast. *Am J Clin Pathol* 1984;81:297–307.
47. Wilson WB, Spell JP. Adenoid cystic carcinoma of the breast: a case with recurrence and regional metastasis. *Ann Surg* 1967;166:861–864.
48. Herzberg AJ, Bossen EH, Walther PJ. Adenoid cystic carcinoma of the breast metastatic to the kidney: a clinically symptomatic lesion requiring surgical management. *Cancer* 1991;68:1015–1020.
49. Perzin KH, Gullane P, Clairmond AC. Adenoid cystic carcinoma arising in salivary glands. *Cancer* 1978;42:265–282.
50. Spiro RH, Huvos AG, Strong EW. Adenoid cystic carcinoma of salivary origin. *Am J Surg* 1974;128: 512–520.
51. Kleer CG, Oberman HA. Adenoid cystic carcinoma of the breast: value of histologic grading and proliferative activity. *Am J Surg Pathol* 1998;22:569–575.
52. Ro JY, Silva EG, Gallager HS. Adenoid cystic carcinoma of the breast. *Hum Pathol* 1987;18: 1276–1281.
53. Harris M. Pseudoadenoid cystic carcinoma of the breast. *Arch Pathol Lab Med* 1977;101:307–309.
54. Due W, Herbst WD, Loy V, et al. Characterisation of adenoid cystic carcinoma of the breast by immunohistology. *J Clin Path* 1989;42:470–476.
55. Clement PB, Young RH, Azzopardi JG. Collagenous spherulosis of the breast. *Am J Surg Pathol* 1987;11:411–417.
56. Divaris DX, Smith S, Leask D, et al. Complex collagenous spherulosis of the breast presenting as a palpable mass: a case report with immunohistochemical and ultrastructural studies. *Breast J* 2000;6: 199–203.
57. Foschini MP, Eusebi V. Carcinomas of the breast showing myoepithelial cell differentiation. A review of the literature. *Virchows Arch* 1998;432:303–310.
58. Van Hoeven KH, Drudis T, Cranor ML, et al. Low-grade adenosquamous carcinoma of the breast. A clinicopathologic study of 32 cases with ultrastructural analysis. *Am J Surg Pathol* 1993;17:248–258.
59. Damiani S, Riccioni L, Pasquinelli G, et al. Poorly differentiated myoepithelial cell rich carcinoma of the breast. *Histopathology* 1997;30:542–548.
60. Tsuda H, Takarabe T, Hasegawa T, et al. Myoepithelial differentiation in high-grade invasive ductal carcinomas with large central acellular zones. *Hum Pathol* 1999;30:1134–1139.
61. Erlandson RA, Rosen PP. Infiltrating myoepithelioma of the breast. *Am J Surg Pathol* 1982;6: 785–793.
62. Thorner PS, Kahn HJ, Baumal R, et al. Malignant myoepithelioma of the breast. An immunohistochemical study by light and electron microscopy. *Cancer* 1986;57:745–750.
63. Chen PC, Chen CK, Nicastri AD, et al. Myoepithelial carcinoma of the breast with distant metastasis and accompanied by adenomyoepitheliomas. *Histopathology* 1994;224:543–548.
64. Tamai M. Intraductal growth of malignant mammary myoepithelioma. *Am J Surg Pathol* 1992;16: 1116–1125.
65. Lakhani SR, O'Hare MJ, Monaghan P, et al. Malignant myoepithelioma (myoepithelial carcinoma) of the breast: a detailed cytokeratin study. *J Clin Pathol* 1995;48:164–167.
66. Van Dorpe J, De Weer F, Bekaert J, et al. Malignant myoepithelioma of the breast. Case report with immunohistochemical study. *Arch Anat Cytol Pathol* 1996;44:193–198.
67. Shiraishi T, Nakayama T, Fukutome K, et al. Malignant myoepithelioma of the breast metastasizing to the jaw. *Virchows Arch* 1999;435:520–523.

8

Invasive Carcinomas

Although invasive carcinoma of the breast is often considered a single entity and is separated according to probability of metastasis at time of discovery by the staging schemes, a century of study has yielded separation of the following distinctive histologic subtypes: tubular carcinoma, cribriform carcinoma, papillary carcinoma, micropapillary carcinoma, medullary carcinoma (MC), colloid carcinoma, ductal carcinoma, carcinoma of no other specification (NOS), lobular carcinoma, apocrine carcinoma, lipid-rich carcinoma, histiocytoid carcinoma, neuroendocrine carcinoma, metaplastic carcinoma of heterologous or homologous type, spindle cell carcinoma, squamous cell carcinoma, mucoepidermoid carcinoma, and adenosquamous carcinoma. Because of their distinctive histologic appearances, these entities are important to pathologists and many have unique clinical presentation and behavior as well.

Tubular, cribriform, papillary, medullary, and colloid carcinoma are considered favorable subtypes, but they account for fewer than 15% of breast cancers. Haffty et al. (1) reported on a series of 1,008 patients who were treated by conservative surgery, without axillary dissection, followed by radiation therapy at Yale-New Haven Hospital between 1970 and 1990. Twenty-one patients had tubular carcinoma, 17 had MC, and 16 had mucinous carcinoma. With a median follow-up of 10.5 years in these 54 patients, only two developed distant disease. One tubular carcinoma patient was thought to have metastasized from a nonbreast primary; however, the other patient did develop a metastasis from a colloid (mucinous) carcinoma. Five of 17 patients with MC suffered breast relapses, but none of the patients with tubular or mucinous carcinoma had local recurrence.

Other histologic types account for the great majority of cases and nearly all the deaths from breast cancer. Stalsberg and Thomas (2) reported that the age-specific incidence rates showed a marked shift toward mucinous, papillary, and signet ring cell carcinomas between the ages of 50 and 85 years, compared with the premenopausal period. Rosen et al. (3) reported that lobular carcinoma was most often associated with a family history of breast cancer, whereas MC was least often associated, with a sister of the patient having had carcinoma of the breast. Somerville et al. (4) reported that c-erbB-2 overexpression was found in 20% of invasive ductal carcinomas; however, it was found in only 1 of 24 infiltrating lobular carcinomas and in 1 of 7 MCs. These data suggest that histology does separate subtypes of invasive carcinoma that have biological and clinically relevant differences.

TUBULAR CARCINOMAS

Tubular carcinoma (TC) is unusual in the general population, but its incidence may rise to as high as 10% in mammographically detected carcinomas (5). TC presents serious problems in differential diagnosis from some benign pseudoinvasive lesions (Chapter 6) and can be histologically overestimated among invasive carcinomas. Although TC is a distinctive form in its pure state, a significant number are associated with infiltrating ductal carcinoma of a higher grade. In the mixed tubular/ductal carcinoma group, the infiltrating ductal carcinoma detracts from the prognosis. It is therefore important to strictly define TC.

McDivitt et al. (6) redefined and reemphasized the characteristics of TC. TCs have stellate or infiltrative borders, unlike the rounded borders of sclerosing adenosis. The infiltrating carcinoma is composed of small, oval, or round glands that are separated from one another by abundant stroma, which is reactive, frequently with production of elastin. The malignant glands branch or anastomose minimally and are open and distended, without compression, by the adjacent stroma or by proliferation of the epithelial cells into multiple layers. The cancer cells are arranged in a monolayer of cells with grade 1 nuclei around the open glandular lumina, with no myoepithelial layer or basement membrane (Figs. 8.1 to 8.4 and efigs. 8.1 to 8.4). The authors emphasized that at least 75% of the carcinoma's composition must be of the tubular type, in order for the carcinoma to have the good prognosis of TC. Oberman and Fidler (5) summarized the literature on TC in 1979 and found that only 1 of the 81 TC patients previously reported had died of carcinoma; that particular patient had bilateral TCs, as reported by Taylor and Norris (7).

Late local recurrence is a problem, however. In 1982, McDivitt et al. (6) reported on 135 cases of TC that varied in size from 0.2 to 2.5 cm, with a mean diameter of approximately 1 cm. This size is consistent with the variation reported in the literature. *In situ* carcinoma was often associated with TC and it was usually low nuclear grade micropapillary or cribriform in type. Other authors have noted the occasional association of lobular carcinoma *in situ* (LCIS) with TC. In the series by McDivitt et al. (6), 12 of 109 patients with axillary dissections were found to have lymph node metastases. Four percent of these patients developed recurrent or disseminated metastatic disease during a mean follow-up period of 7.2 years, and two of those patients died of breast cancer. In 9% of the cases, carcinoma occurred in the contralateral breast. Of 17 patients treated by less than mastectomy, only 1 patient had a recurrence, but among the 120 patients treated by mastectomy, 27.5% had residual carcinoma in

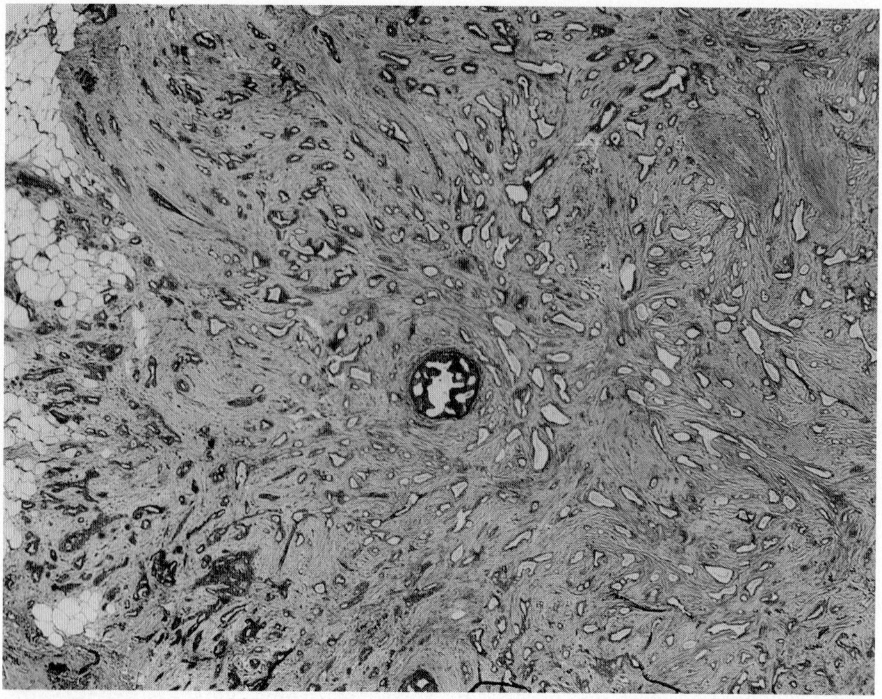

FIG. 8.1. Tubular carcinoma. The stroma is infiltrated by numerous open ductal structures that form a stellate nonlobular pattern.

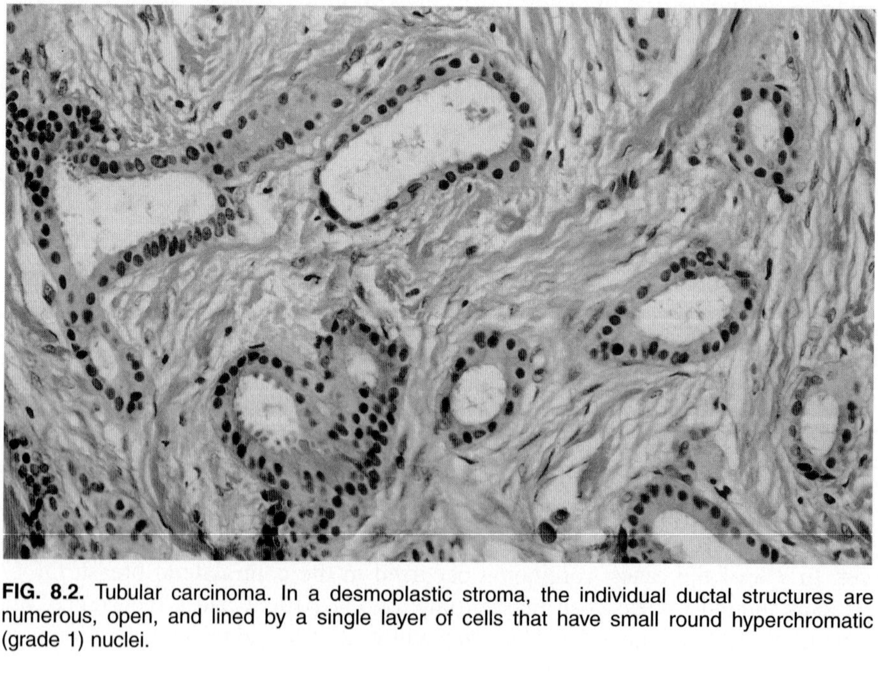

FIG. 8.2. Tubular carcinoma. In a desmoplastic stroma, the individual ductal structures are numerous, open, and lined by a single layer of cells that have small round hyperchromatic (grade 1) nuclei.

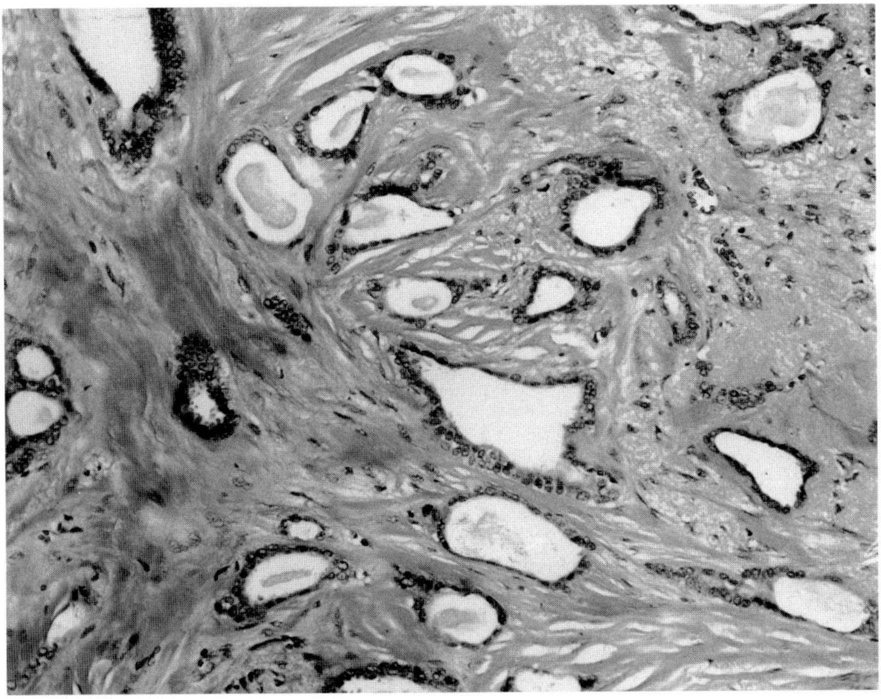

FIG. 8.3. Tubular carcinoma. Some of the distended ducts are angular, but they are lined by a monolayer of small cells with grade 1 nuclei.

the mastectomy specimen. Lagios et al. (8) also noted multicentricity. In 20 of 33 patients with residual carcinoma, there was residual TC at the biopsy site and, in 6 patients, there was invasive carcinoma remote from the biopsy site. Multicentric *in situ* carcinoma was present in 7 patients with intraductal in 4 and LCIS in 3 patients. Van Bogaert and Maldague (9) and Parl and Richardson (10) reported similar findings.

Deos and Norris (11), reporting on a large group of TC, emphasized the importance of dividing the pure TC from TC that were mixed with the ordinary infiltrating ductal carcinomas. Axillary lymph node metastases occurred in only 6% of the pure TC, but it occurred in 29% of the patients with the mixed carcinomas. The 5-year actuarial survival for the pure TC and mixed groups was 100% and 93%, respectively. Fifty percent of patients with pure TC who were treated by excisional biopsy alone recurred locally and 28% of mastectomy specimens in the pure TC group had residual carcinoma.

McBoyle et al. (12) reviewed 1,483 cases of invasive breast cancer and found only 22 cases (1.5%) that were more than 90% TCs. The mean size of the TC was 1.2 cm. Only 1 of 22 patients (4.5%) had a lymph node metastasis and that was a single node. All patients were living and well after a mean follow-up of 3.5 years.

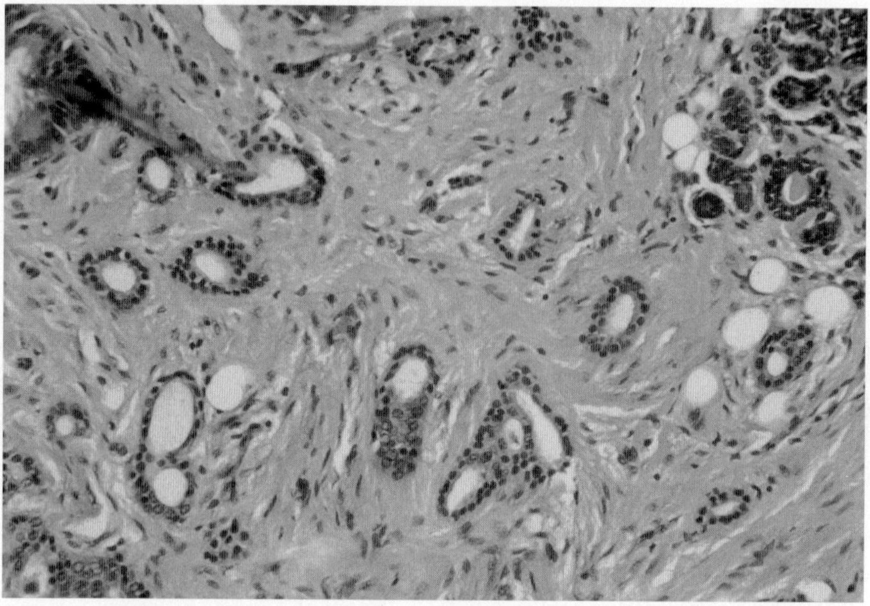

FIG. 8.4. Tubular carcinoma. Some of the invading ducts have bars across the lumen. All are open ducts, lined by a monolayer of cells with grade 1 nuclei.

The relatively small size of TCs and the association of TC with ordinary infiltrating ductal carcinoma of a larger size has been discussed by Peters et al. (13) and Cooper (14) who noted that, as the size of the carcinomas increases, so does the proportion of ordinary infiltrating ductal carcinomas, and that the higher grade ductal carcinoma is usually peripheral to the centrally located tubular component. These data, plus the increased incidence of TC found in screened cases, suggest that TC is an early indolent phase of ordinary invasive cancer of the breast. The authors emphasized the importance of distinguishing pure TC from the more aggressive infiltrating ductal carcinomas.

Tubular Carcinoma: Differential Diagnosis

From Benign Lesions

Even though TC has a good prognosis, overdiagnosis should be avoided. Differentiation from sclerosing adenosis (15–17), radial scar, and microglandular adenosis (18) may be difficult. Oberman and Fidler (5) noted that TC has an infiltrative border with a haphazard arrangement of ducts that are uniform in size throughout. The ductal lumina are always open, but there is occasional bridging. The myoepithelial layer is uniformly absent and a single layer of cells lines the lumina. Intraductal (or lobular) carcinoma *in situ* is often associated.

In distinction, sclerosing adenosis has a more circumscribed border with a nodular arrangement of ducts that are often attenuated in size and their lumina are often partially or completely obliterated. Multiple cell layers, frequently with a prominent myoepithelial layer, line the lumen. Intraductal epithelial bridging is absent, and DCIS or LCIS are associated only coincidentally. Sclerosing adenosis is usually 2 to 4 times the normal lobular size, retains the rounded lobular configuration, and is usually multiple. The ducts are distorted by the sclerotic process; some may be open and rounded, but the majority of ducts are slit-like or closed. The open ducts have a double cell layer, sometimes on each side, but others may show ductal and/or lobular hyperplasia. Atypical apocrine sclerosing lesions are similar to sclerosing adenosis, but they have large apocrine cells with atypical nuclei that feature large nucleoli in the epithelial component.

Microglandular adenosis may be larger than sclerosing adenosis. It is characterized by clear epithelial cells that do not have a myoepithelial layer; a basement membrane is present. Rosen (18) emphasized the pale-to-clear or vacuolated cytoplasm of the regularly shaped cuboidal cells of microglandular adenosis and emphasized that the glands appeared as neat, punched-out, and rounded structures. In contrast, the glands of TC, although open, are often oval or have angular contours, and the cytoplasm of the cells of TC are amphophilic or basophilic. McDivitt et al. (6) emphasized that in microglandular adenosis, the ducts may be open, the lumina may be prominent and rounded, and the cells lining these lumina may have apocrine snouts.

Radial scars have a starburst or daisy-like configuration, with a variety of ductal hyperplasias in the medium-sized ducts that extend radially from the center. The core has a dense fibroelastic stroma in which a very few small open ducts may be found. These ducts frequently have a double cell layer, but some seem to have a monolayer. Distinction from TC is based on the recognition of the presence of the ducts in the center of the radial scar, rather than by focusing on single ducts. TCs are larger than the core of a radial scar and have a stellate border.

From Ductal Carcinoma

Distinction of TCs from other invasive ductal carcinomas is important for prognostication. Stalsberg and Hartmann (19) reviewed 500 invasive carcinomas and classified them according to nuclear grade, mitotic activity, and tubularity, which they defined as the proportion of tumor cells adjacent to an open lumen. The authors found a continuum of cases with no sharp separation among the invasive carcinomas, but a group of 14 carcinomas with 70% or more tubularity, and nuclear and mitotic grades of 1 were not associated with lymph node metastasis or death from breast cancer.

Kader et al. (20) compared 171 cases of pure TC (90% or more TC) with 386 cases of mixed tubular/ductal carcinoma (75% to 90% TC) and reported 12.9%

and 23.9% lymph node metastases, respectively; however, TCs that were smaller than 2 cm and without either vascular or perineural invasion had a lymph node metastasis rate of 7%.

Papadatos et al. (21) compared 22 cases of pure TC (defined as 90% or more TC) with 9 cases of mixed tubular/well differentiated ductal carcinomas (defined as 75% to 90% TC) and reported metastasis to axillary lymph node in 1 of 22 cases of TC and 4 of 9 cases of mixed carcinomas. None of the carcinomas that was smaller than 1 cm had metastasized. Metaanalysis of 20 studies with 680 women showed 6.6% lymph node metastases among 244 women with TC and 25% nodal metastases among 149 women with mixed carcinomas.

In summary, pure TC, defined as a carcinoma with 90% small glands or tubules (which resemble ductules in nonneoplastic lobules, but which lack basement membranes and a myoepithelial layer) that infiltrate in a reactive stroma has a good prognosis, especially when it is less than 1 cm in diameter. As other elements of carcinoma with higher degrees of nuclear abnormality, mitotic rate and less ductal differentiation are added, and as the carcinomas grow in size, the prognosis is degraded.

CRIBRIFORM CARCINOMA

Page et al. (22) reviewed a group of 1,000 invasive breast cancers and found 51 invasive cribriform carcinomas, which were defined as invasive carcinomas with a cribriform pattern similar to that seen in the cribriform type of intraductal carcinoma (Fig. 8.5 and efigs. 8.5 to 8.8). Thirty-five cases were pure invasive cribriform carcinomas and 16 had cribriform elements admixed with less differentiated invasive ductal carcinoma. Twenty-eight of the 35 cases were associated with cribriform intraductal carcinoma, and the cells of both the invasive and *in situ* components were either low or intermediate in nuclear grade, in all cases. Sizes ranged from 1 to 14 cm (average 3.1 cm). Five of the patients had histologically positive nodes and seven had multifocal disease. Only one patient with purely infiltrating cribriform carcinoma died of breast cancer, and that patient had a higher grade contralateral carcinoma that caused death. The age range of the mixed cribriform/ductal carcinomas group was older and the size was also slightly larger, with an average of 4.2 cm. Nuclear grade was low, intermediate, or high in that group, and 6 of the 16 patients died of breast cancer, with all 6 deaths the result of the index carcinoma. Venable et al. (23) reported on 62 cases of infiltrating cribriform carcinoma, which represented 6.2% of all invasive carcinomas. Twelve of the 62 cases were pure cribriform carcinomas, 20 cases had a cribriform component of 50% or more of the infiltrating carcinoma, and the other 30 cases had less than a 50% cribriform component. Invasive cribriform carcinoma was associated with foci of TC in 15 cases and intraductal carcinoma was associated in 43 cases. During the follow-up period of 1 to 5 years, only two deaths from breast cancer were found and both of these were in the

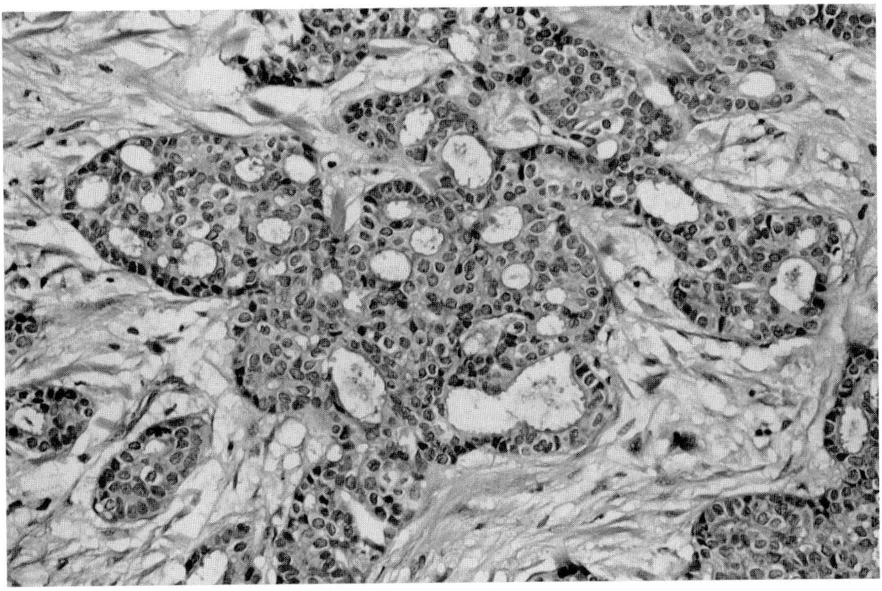

FIG. 8.5. Cribriform carcinoma. This is a well differentiated invasive carcinoma with a cribriform pattern more commonly seen in ductal carcinoma *in situ*.

cases in which the invasive cribriform component was less than one-half the cancer. Estrogen receptors were present in all of the pure and predominantly cribriform carcinomas, and 11 of the 16 assayed also expressed progesterone receptors. Marzullo et al. (24) described 5 additional cases of invasive cribriform carcinoma that had good outcomes.

INVASIVE PAPILLARY CARCINOMA

Intracystic papillary carcinoma with invasion of its capsule is discussed in Chapter 4. Invasive papillary carcinoma is relatively rare, accounting for less than 1% of invasive breast cancers. It is usually seen in postmenopausal women. The invasive component is characterized by a fibrovascular stalk, upon which tumor cells of nuclear grade 1 or grade 2 are found (Fig. 8.6 and efigs. 8.9 to 8.14). The tumors are usually small (2 to 3 cm in diameter) and circumscribed. Patients in the series reported by Fisher et al. (25) were frequently judged clinically to have enlarged axillary lymph nodes, but they showed a high degree of sinus histiocytosis and few metastases were found. Only 2 of 35 patients had four or more positive axillary lymph nodes, and there was evidence of treatment failure at 5 years in only 3 of 35 patients (8.5%) studied. This favorable prognosis was comparable to that observed in tubular, cribriform, and mucinous carcinomas and even better than the survival found for MC.

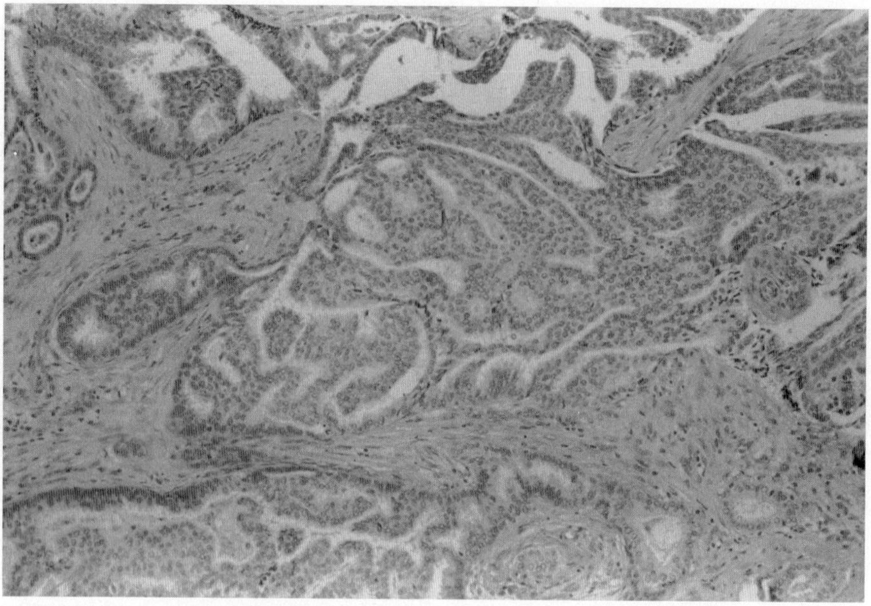

FIG. 8.6. Invasive papillary carcinoma. This invasive carcinoma forms a papillary structure as it invades through the desmoplastic stroma.

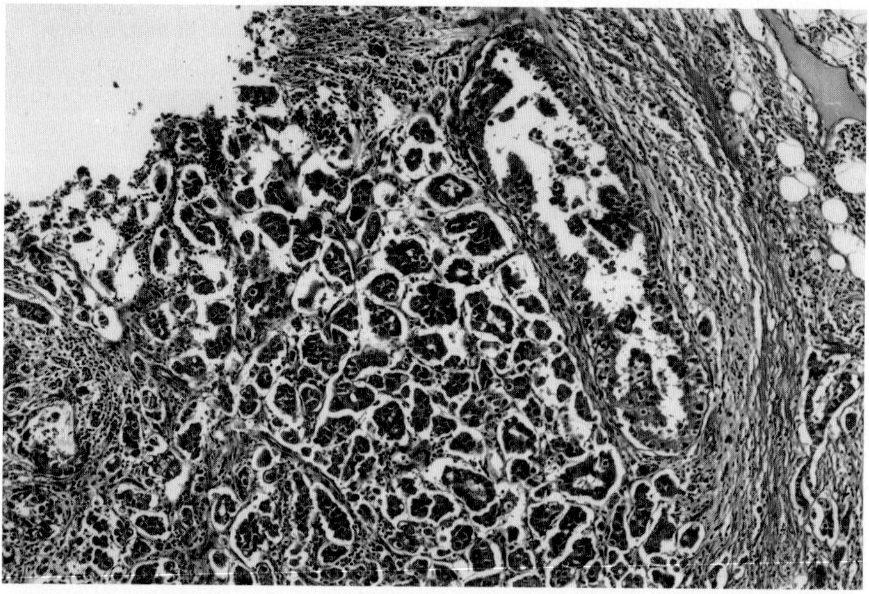

FIG. 8.7. Micropapillary carcinoma, *in situ* and invasive. The duct **to the right** has a micropapillary pattern of high grade ductal carcinoma *in situ.* **To the left**, there is an invasive micropapillary carcinoma with multiple groups in dilated spaces, which suggest lymphatics.

INVASIVE MICROPAPILLARY CARCINOMA

Invasive micropapillary carcinoma is also an unusual carcinoma, but, unlike papillary carcinoma, it has an aggressive behavior and a poor prognosis. Siriaunkgul and Tavassoli (26) described 9 cases that were characterized by the formation of micropapillae within clear spaces that were separated by fibrocollagenous stroma (Figs. 8.7 and 8.8 and efigs. 8.15 to 8.20). The pattern may be admixed with ordinary invasive ductal carcinoma. Middleton et al. (27) reported 14 cases of infiltrating micropapillary carcinoma in women who ranged in age from 37 to 58 years, with a mean of 50 years. Five (36%) were in stage II, 57% were in stage III, and one presented with stage IV disease. Psammoma bodies were found in 9 cases, 9 cases were grade II, and the other 5 cases were grade III carcinomas. Nine of 11 cases with follow-up had skin or chest wall recurrence, with an average time to recurrence of 24 months. Immunohistochemically, all cases stained positively for c-erbB-2, MIB-1 stained 30% to 60% of cells, and 75% of cells stained positively for p53.

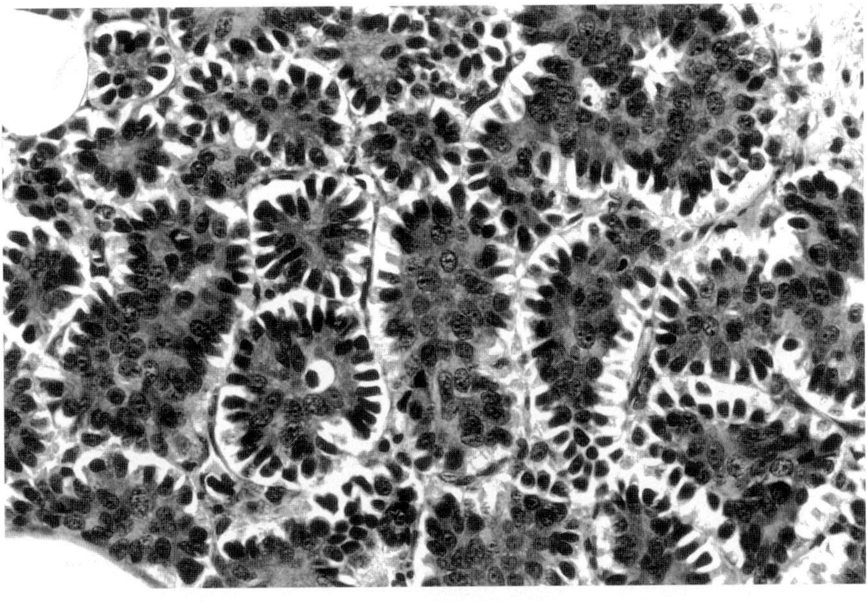

FIG. 8.8. Invasive micropapillary carcinoma. The dilated spaces contain structures that appear to be inverted micropapillary structures with cellular projections separating the group from the surrounding space.

MEDULLARY CARCINOMA

MC presents a paradox because it has the histology of a high-grade cancer, but it has a relatively favorable prognosis. MCs constitute approximately 5% to 8% of invasive mammary cancers. They are usually large (4 cm or more in diameter), grossly circumscribed, soft, gray-white, and have the fish-flesh appearance that is more often associated with lymphoma (Fig. 8.9 and efigs. 8.21 and 8.22), which they mimic both grossly and microscopically. Chalky streaks are not present, but hemorrhage and necrosis are often seen. Histologically, they are very poorly differentiated and grow in a simple sheet or synctium of cells without glands, ducts, papillae, or even trabeculae. A desmoplastic reaction is either absent or minimal, but there is a prominent lymphocytic infiltrate. At low magnification, they bear a distinct resemblance to large-cell lymphoma. MCs are composed of sheets of cells with abundant, delicate, and frequently basophilic cytoplasm, as distinct from the individual cells of lymphomas. The nuclei are large and vesicular with prominent nucleoli. Mitoses may be frequent (Figs. 8.10 and 8.11 and efigs. 8.23 to 8.27). The incidence of lymph node metastases from MC is about the same as it is with ordinary ductal cancers, but 5-year survival is significantly better in MC, even in the presence of lymph node metastases. This better prognosis has been attributed to the distinctive nature of the entity, its circumscription, and/or the extensive lymphoplasmocytic infiltrate, which is one of its chief diagnostic and prognostic characteristics.

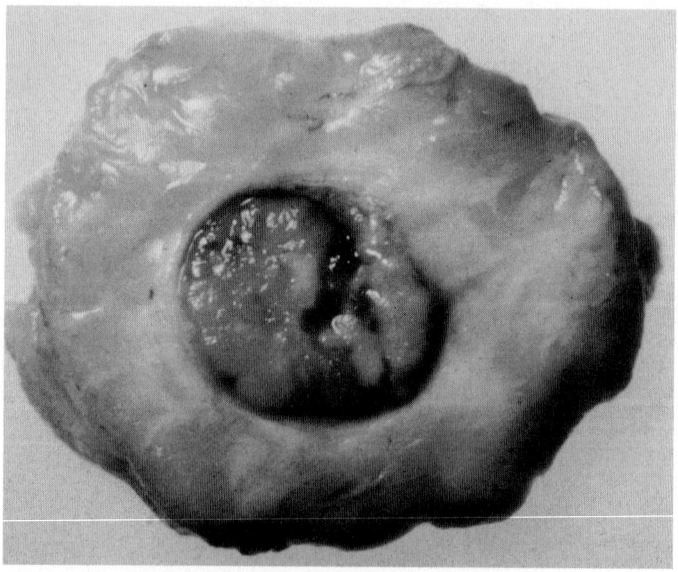

FIG. 8.9. Medullary carcinoma. The gross appearance is of a sharply circumscribed soft nodule that resembles a lymph node.

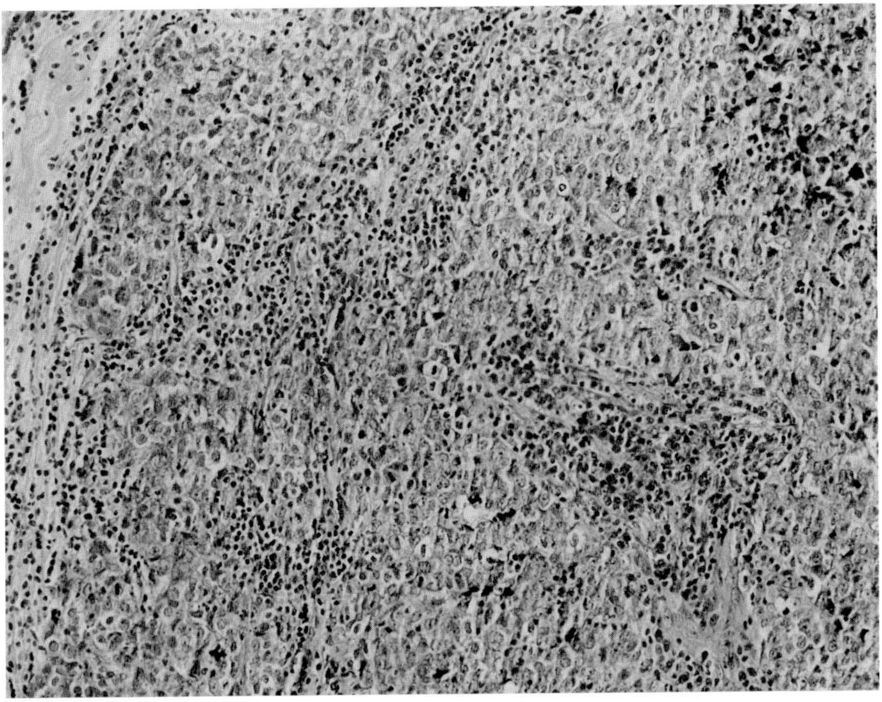

FIG. 8.10. Medullary carcinoma. The carcinoma is circumscribed. There is no desmoplastic reaction and the cells form no architectural features. A prominent lymphocytic infiltrate is present.

Moore and Foote (28) described MC in 1949 and noted its relatively favorable prognosis—a 5-year survival rate of 83%, even with a 43% incidence of axillary lymph node metastases. The critical importance of the lymphocytic infiltrate to the better prognosis was confirmed by Bloom and Field (29), who reported a 20-year survival rate of 74% for the entire group of patients with MC and a 20-year survival rate of 61% for patients with MC and axillary lymph node metastases.

There has been some question as to the strict definition of this group of carcinomas with such a favorable prognosis. Ridolfi et al. (30) addressed this problem in 1977. The authors considered typical MC to have a predominantly syncytial growth pattern (i.e., a solid growth of malignant epithelial cells without the formation of ducts, papillary structures, or other architectural features). MCs were grossly and microscopically circumscribed, there was no intraductal component, and nuclear grade was relatively low—that is, there was not much in the way of anaplasia or pleomorphism of the nuclei. Microglandular features were not present and, most importantly, there was a moderate to marked diffuse mononuclear infiltrate of inflammatory cells. An intraductal component was initially considered the basis for exclusion from the typical MC group, but analysis of this single feature showed that the presence of intraductal carcinoma was not inconsistent with the

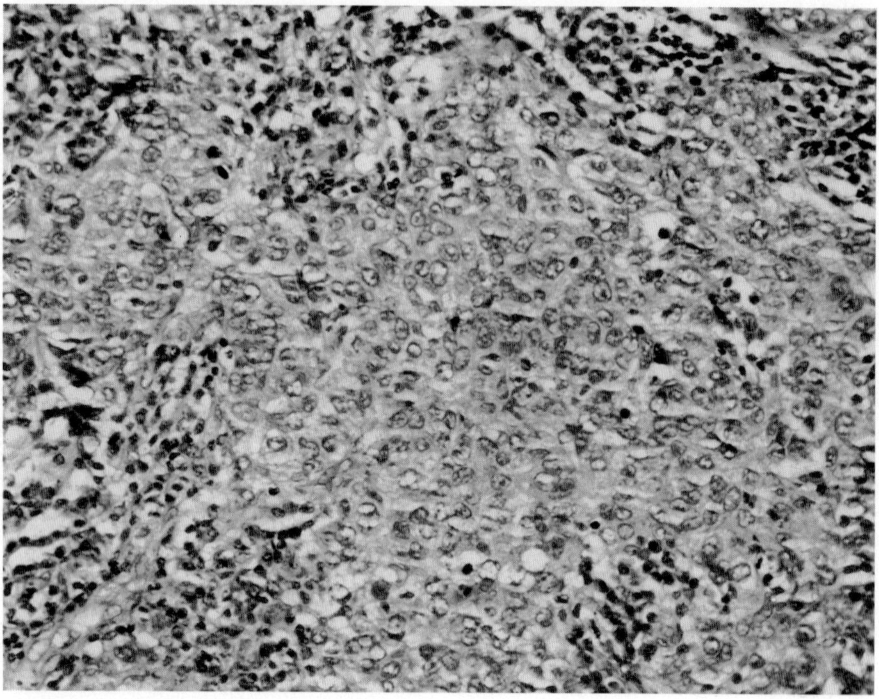

FIG. 8.11. Medullary carcinoma. At higher magnification, the cells are of nuclear grade 2 and form a synctium. The lymphocytic infiltrate is both within the groups of cells and at the periphery.

diagnosis of MC and that carcinomas excluded from the group, on the basis of this feature alone, behaved no differently from the MCs that did not have an intraductal component. Using this definition of MC, the authors found a significantly higher overall survival rate at 10 years (84%), even though there was a high frequency of axillary lymph node metastases. The more favorable prognosis applied, even when the nodal metastases were present. Smaller MCs had a better prognosis than larger ones, but the most important single prognostic feature within the group of MC was the density of the lymphoplasmocytic infiltrate. Patients who had a relatively sparse infiltrate had a diminished prognosis.

The authors described a group of atypical MCs that had some features of the typical MC, most often the syncytial growth pattern; however, atypical tumors had infiltrative margins, decreased mononuclear infiltrate, higher nuclear grade, and the presence of microglandular or ductular differentiation. The 10-year survival rate of patients with atypical MCs was significantly reduced to approximately 70%. Carcinomas that had a decreased amount of syncytial or solid growth pattern (i.e., less than 75% of the tumor with this histology) and the presence of three or more of the other atypical features were classified as non-medullary or ordinary infiltrating ductal carcinomas. The 10-year survival of the nonMCs was 63%. There was no significant difference between the survival curve of the atypical medullary and nonMCs, although there was a statistically significant difference between the survival curves of typical and atypical MCs. Wargotz and Silverberg (31) reported similar results. It is important to define MC strictly because it has a significantly better survival rate, even in the presence of axillary lymph node metastases.

Gaffey et al. (32) and Pedersen et al. (33–34) described the high level of interobserver variability in the histopathologic diagnosis of MC. Gaffey et al. (32) used six observers who employed the criteria set forth by Ridolfi et al. (30). Wargotz and Silverberg (31) found a consensus diagnosis of MC in only 70% of 53 previously diagnosed cases of MC. Their level of agreement was better than that found by Pedersen et al. (33), who compared the criteria proposed by the three classification schemes. Ridolfi et al. (30) required a syncytial growth pattern of greater than 75%, an intense infiltration of mononuclear inflammatory cells, microscopic circumscription, grade 2 or grade 3 nuclei, and no neoplastic glands or intraductal carcinoma. Wargotz and Silverberg (31) used similar criteria, but they did not utilize the presence or absence of intraductal carcinoma. As noted above, Ridolfi et al. (30) discarded the presence or absence of intraductal carcinoma as a criterion for exclusion from the MC group. Pedersen et al. (34) required only a syncytial growth pattern and an inflammatory infiltrate. It is of interest to note that the survival figures for all three of these studies are favorable, compared to those of most studies of comparable size invasive ductal carcinomas. Yazawa (35) found frequent expression of HLA-DR antigen in MCs of the breast and suggested that this might account for the favorable prognosis. Gaffey et al. (36) studied 52 MCs and found Epstein–Barr virus in none of them. The mononuclear infiltrate was composed predominantly of T cells that were CD3-positive in nearly all cases, CD3/CD4-positive in 36% of cases, and CD3-positive and CD4-negative in 64% of cases. Natural killer cells and histiocytes were virtually absent. The immunophenotyping of the lymphocytic infiltrate did not relate to the diagnosis of MC, the presence of axillary lymph node metastases, or to the overall surgical outcome.

Summary

MCs have an intense lymphoplasmocytic infiltrate, a rounded border, and minimal desmoplastic reaction. The cells grow in sheets (syncytia) of large uniform cells that do not form ducts or other architectural structures. Ductal carcinoma *in situ* (DCIS) may be present, but it is rarely observed. The prognosis of MC is better than that of ductal carcinoma, even with lymph node metastases.

MUCINOUS (COLLOID, GELATINOUS) CARCINOMA

Norris and Taylor (37) described 102 cases of mucinous carcinoma of the breast. These patients had approximately the same age distribution, clinical pre-

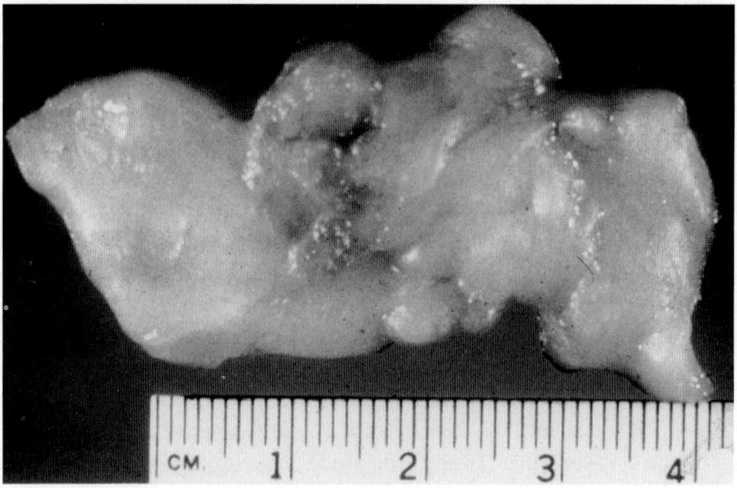

FIG. 8.12. Colloid or mucoid carcinoma. Grossly, the lesion is circumscribed and without architectural features. By palpation, it would be soft and sticky.

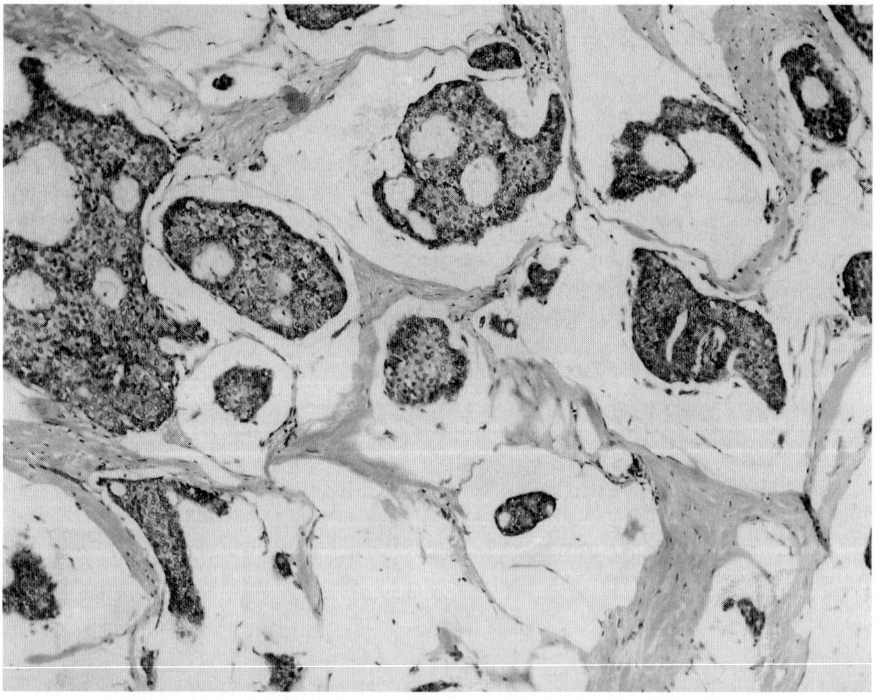

FIG. 8.13. Colloid or mucinous carcinoma. Microscopically, the groups of malignant cells float in pools of mucus. There is little or no stromal reaction to the mucus. The epithelial cells may be of a variety of nuclear and histologic grades.

sentation, and localization of the primary tumors as those with other types of carcinoma of the breast. Grossly mucinous carcinomas are circumscribed and soft to palpation, with a large amount of sticky mucinous substance (Fig. 8.12 and efig. 8.28). Microscopically, the bulk of the mass is mucin, in which groups of tumor cells appear to float. Groups of cancer cells form ducts, sheets, or cribriform groups and are of low or intermediate, but usually not high, nuclear grade. Despite the lakes of mucus, signet ring cells are unusual. There is little or no desmoplastic reaction in most of the tumor, but there may be some at the very periphery of the lesion, which demarcates the carcinoma from the surrounding mammary tissue (Fig. 8.13 and efigs. 8.29 and 8.30).

Norris and Taylor (37) separated the mucinous carcinomas into a large group of 62 patients who had tumors that were comprised entirely of mucinous carcinoma and a small group of 40 patients who had mucinous carcinoma that was combined with areas of infiltrating ductal carcinoma with a desmoplastic reaction (Fig. 8.14). Only 10% of the patients with pure mucinous carcinoma had recurrence or metastasis, but 42% of the patients with mucinous carcinoma, combined with infiltrating ductal carcinoma, had recurrence or metastasis after

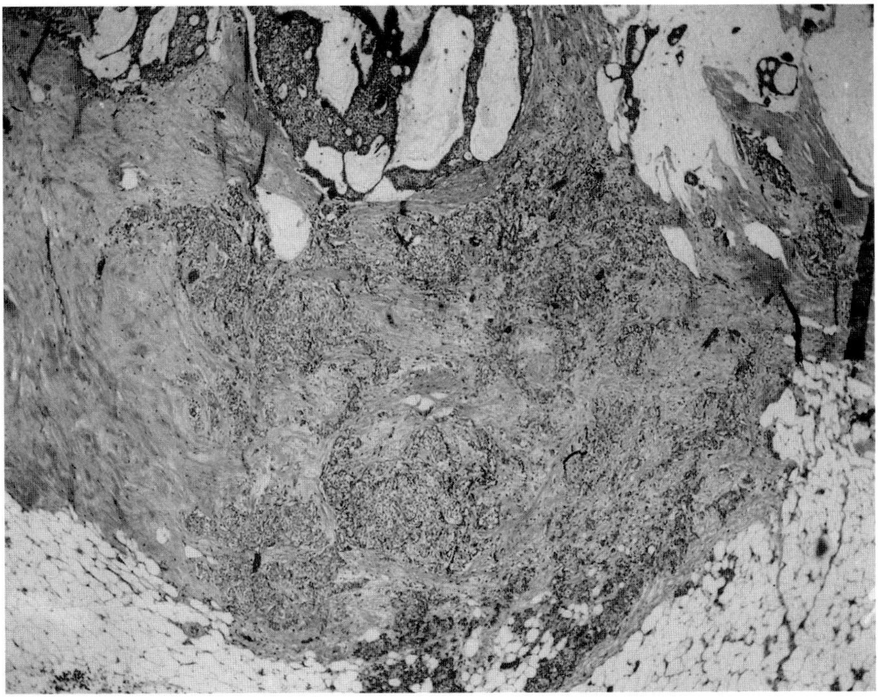

FIG. 8.14. Mixed ductal and colloid carcinoma. Groups of malignant cells float in pools of mucus (**upper**). Ductal structures invade a desmoplastic stroma (**lower**). This tumor has the prognosis of the ductal carcinoma.

surgery. After exclusion of noncancer deaths, the actuarial survival was 80% in the pure mucinous group and 62% in the mixed mucinous/ductal carcinomas. Only 1 of 27 patients in the pure mucinous group who was treated by radical mastectomy had axillary metastases; however, 15 of 32 patients in the mixed category were found to have axillary lymph node metastases. Five of the 6 patients with pure mucinous carcinoma who subsequently died of cancer had axillary lymphadenectomies, but only 2 of these patients had lymph node metastases. Among patients with either pure mucinous or mixed mucinous/infiltrating ductal carcinomas, those with carcinomas that were larger than 4 cm in diameter had a poorer survival rate than those with smaller tumors. In the pure mucinous carcinoma group, none of the 12 patients with tumors that were less than 2 cm in diameter died of cancer. Only 1 of 18 patients with a tumor that measured between 2 and 4 cm in diameter died of cancer. Of the 6 patients with pure mucinous carcinomas who died of breast cancer, 2 developed carcinoma in the contralateral breast and may have died of those second primaries. In 3 patients, the diagnosis was made on the basis of a single microscopic section, and the possibility of mixed histology could not be excluded. In 2 other patients, the tumors measured 12 and 15 cm in diameter. The authors stressed the distinction between pure colloid carcinoma, which has a good prognosis, and the colloid component in ordinary infiltrating ductal carcinoma, which does not have a major ameliorating effect on the prognosis. Clayton (38) confirmed these findings, as did Toikkanen and Kujari (39). Mucin that contains invasive ductal carcinoma (efig. 8.31) does not share this good prognosis.

Melamed et al. (40) found 113 cases of colloid carcinoma among 5,000 patients who had primary operable breast cancer. The age distribution and clinical presentation of the patients in this series were no different from those in other series of carcinomas of the breast. The carcinomas were divided into three categories. Fifty-one patients had pure colloid carcinomas; 78.4% of these patients were alive at 5 years. Forty-eight patients had a mixture of gelatinous and infiltrating ductal carcinoma; 62.5% of these patients were alive at 5 years. Eight patients had a slight colloid component in an invasive ductal carcinoma, and only 50% of these patients were alive at 5 years. Among patients who were treated by radical mastectomy, axillary lymph node metastases were present in 36% of the pure colloid group, 47% of the mixed group, and 63% of the slight colloid component group. The 5-year survival in patients who had no lymph node metastases was excellent in all three groups. A progressive decrease in survival was associated with an increase in the number of axillary lymph node metastases, but, even in patients with multiple lymph node metastases from pure mucinous carcinoma, the 5-year survival rate was 57%, compared with only 20% in the group in which colloid carcinoma was only a minor component. In general, pure gelatinous carcinomas tended to be smaller than those in which another component was present, but when correction was made for both tumor size and presence or absence of axillary lymph node metastases, there was still a better survival rate in the pure gelatinous carcinoma group.

Silverberg et al. (41) divided 42 cases into pure colloid and mixed colloid/infiltrating ductal carcinoma. Negative axillary lymph nodes were found in 71% of the pure group and in 42% of the mixed group. Death from cancer occurred within 5 years in 14% of those with the pure colloid carcinomas and in 30% of those in which another component was present. Rasmussen et al. (42) gave similar figures.

Anan et al. (43) studied 52 cases of pure mucinous carcinoma. The authors found comedo type extensive intraductal spread in 11% of cases, lymphatic invasion in 4% of cases, and lymph node metastases in 4% of cases, with no lymph node metastases from primaries that were smaller than 3 cm. Because of these features, the authors considered mucinous carcinoma favorable for breast conserving surgery, but presented no follow-up information.

Some cases of DCIS seem to contain (and eventually become surrounded) by mucus (efigs. 8.32 to 8.34).

Koenig and Tavassoli (44) reported on four cases of multicystic tumors that ranged in size from 0.8 to 19 cm. The cyst walls, in these tumors, were lined by tall columnar bland mucin-producing cells that were virtually identical to mucinous cystadenocarcinomas of the ovary or pancreas. Multiple areas of stromal invasion were found in association with foci of nonmucinous cells with eosinophilic squamoid cytoplasm. All four cases were negative for estrogen and progesterone receptors and for cytokeratin 20; however, cytokeratin 7 was expressed. One of 3 patients had axillary lymph node metastasis and all four patients were alive 11 to 22 months after diagnosis.

Summary

Mucinous (colloid) carcinomas are characterized by pools of mucus in which a variety of types and groups of carcinoma cells float. When the colloid pattern is mixed with that of invasive ductal carcinoma, the prognosis becomes that of ductal cancer. The better prognosis of colloid carcinoma is primarily related to its usual low stage. With lymph node metastases, its prognosis is that of ductal carcinoma with lymph node metastases.

The differential diagnosis of colloid carcinoma includes those carcinomas with only a partial mucoid component but also pools of mucus in which no carcinoma is evident. In 1986, Rosen (45) described six cases of mucocele-like lesions of the breast in which there appeared to be a ruptured cyst in which both mucinous material and benign epithelium had spilled out into the surrounding stroma (Figs. 8.15 and 8.16 and efigs. 8.35 to 8.39). The author likened this condition to mucocele of the salivary gland. All of the patients were well at the end of the follow-up period. The author cautioned against the overdiagnosis of colloid carcinoma unless malignant cells were evident and the overdiagnosis of colloid carcinoma on needle biopsy or fine needle aspiration.

Ro et al. (46) reported seven cases of mucocele-like tumors of the breast, all of which were associated with either atypical ductal hyperplasia or mucinous

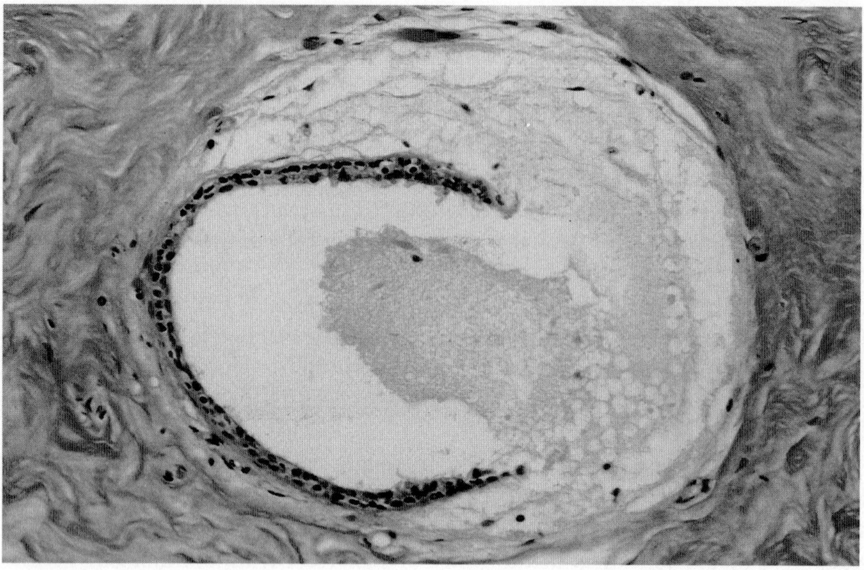

FIG. 8.15. Mucocele. This normal duct appears to have ruptured and spilled mucus into the periductal stroma.

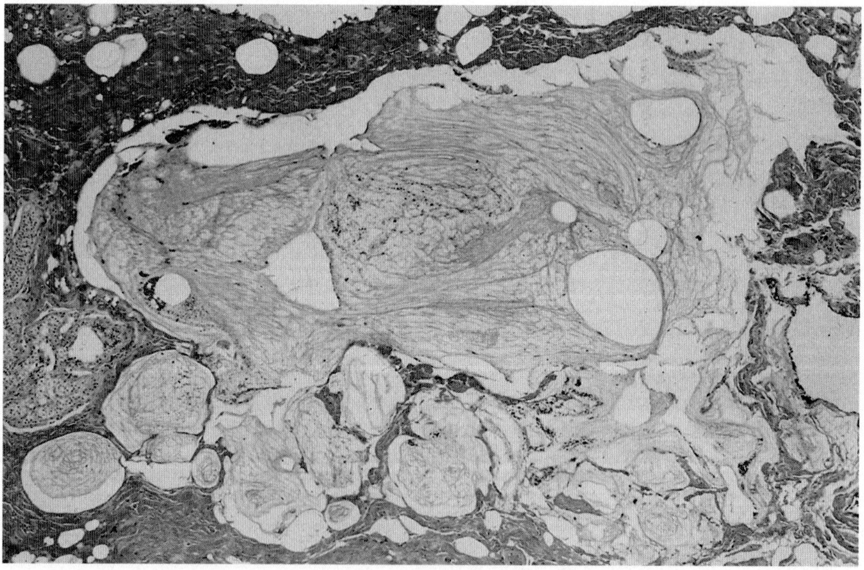

FIG. 8.16. Mucocele. An abundance of mucus appears in the nonreactive stroma. There are no groups of epithelial cells present, without which a diagnosis of carcinoma cannot be made.

carcinoma. All seven patients presented with palpable masses. The lesions were cystic, and pools of neutral or nonsulfated acid mucin contained microscopic foci of mucinous carcinoma or areas of atypical ductal hyperplasia in which there was abundant intraluminal mucus. The authors, however, suggested a conservative approach to the treatment of these individuals. These cases suggest that some mucinous carcinomas with malignant cells in the stroma may be "ruptured" ducts that have displaced DCIS in the stroma and that they may therefore not be truly invasive carcinomas. That may be true for some cases, but other cases appear to be truly invasive carcinomas that are surrounded by pools of mucus, fully capable of regional and distant metastasis. Unfortunately, there is no good way to distinguish between the two possibilities.

DUCTAL CARCINOMA VERSUS BETTER PROGNOSIS SUBTYPES

Tubular, cribriform, papillary, medullary, and colloid carcinomas are distinct clinicopathologic entities when pure. If there is an admixture of ductal carcinoma, there is erosion of the good prognosis that is proportional to the size of the ductal component. As the ductal component becomes dominant, prognosis is based on grade and stage rather than type.

INFILTRATING DUCTAL CARCINOMA

The majority of breast carcinomas fall into the category of invasive ductal carcinoma, due to their propensity to form small gland-like or ductal structures that bear some resemblance to the acini that are found in lobules of normal breast tissue. Some carcinomas do not form structures with lumens. Instead, they grow in sheets, cords, or trabeculae and are referred to as carcinoma NOS or as poorly differentiated infiltrating duct carcinomas. When the term "breast cancer" is not further defined, it means invasive ductal carcinoma. Eighty percent of invasive breast cancers are called ductal carcinoma, scirrhous carcinoma, carcinoma simplex, carcinoma NOS, or adenocarcinoma. Elements of the other subtypes of carcinomas may be present, but, in general, if the ductal component is predominant, it dictates the prognosis. This grouping of cases has the features of a "waste basket" because it is composed of those carcinomas that are not segregated as a distinct subtype. As a result, "ductal" does not reliably describe the appearance of the invasive carcinoma and a wide variety of histologies may be present. Ductal has practical merit in creating a large group in which prediction of clinical outcome is based on grade, stage, and the other prognostic factors (Chapter 9), rather than histology.

Classic infiltrating ductal carcinomas are grossly firm stellate tumors with chalky streaks (Fig. 8.17 and efig. 8.40). Microscopically, they are characterized by a growth of malignant cells of varied nuclear and cytoplasmic morphology that usually form small gland-like spaces (ducts), but the cancer cells may also grow wholly or partially in solid sheets, trabeculae, and they may have a small

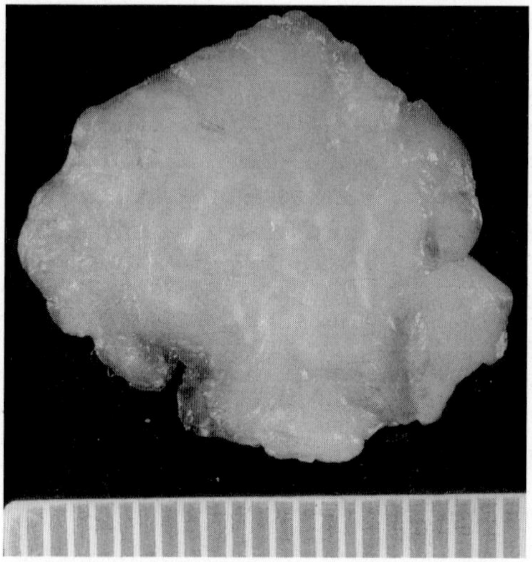

FIG. 8.17. Invasive ductal carcinoma. The sharply circumscribed angular tumor is characterized by chalky white streaks.

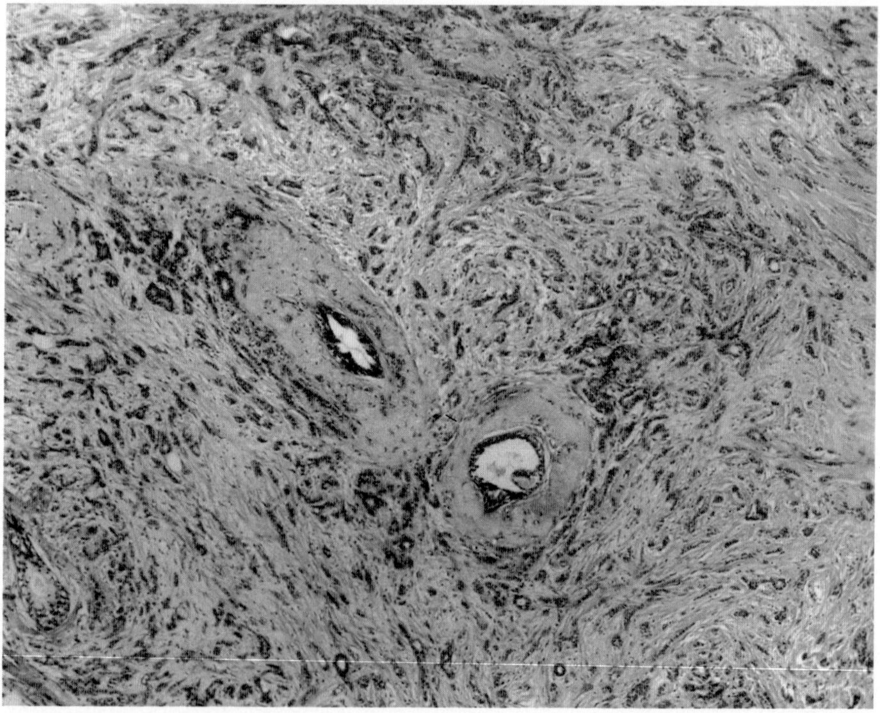

FIG. 8.18. Invasive ductal carcinoma. The ducts are rimmed by an elastotic stroma that presents grossly as white streaks. The desmoplastic stroma is infiltrated by ductal structures.

single file component or be complex structures that are composed of combinations of these elements. Although the focus here is appropriately on the epithelial elements, invasive ductal carcinomas also are characterized by a significant stromal desmoplastic reaction that is composed of fibroblasts, collagen, elastin, a variable number of inflammatory cells, and newly formed small and large blood vessels that often make up the bulk of the "tumor" mass, produces its hardness and stellate shape, and is responsible for many of the biologic features that are associated with the carcinoma (Figs. 8.18 to 8.21 and efigs. 8.41 to 8.49). Stromal elements are intimately involved in tumor growth. Angiogenesis is required for expansion beyond about 5 mm in size and the interaction of growth factors and their receptors among malignant cells and stromal cells plays a major role in carcinogenesis. E-cadherin is usually expressed by invasive ductal carcinoma (efig. 8.50).

Dabbs (47) found a good correlation between nuclear grade and S-phase fraction in 82 invasive ductal carcinoma cases. In 89% of the cases in which fresh tissue was used, sampling error was the greatest cause of discordant values, specimen quality was second, and tumor heterogeneity was third. A better cor-

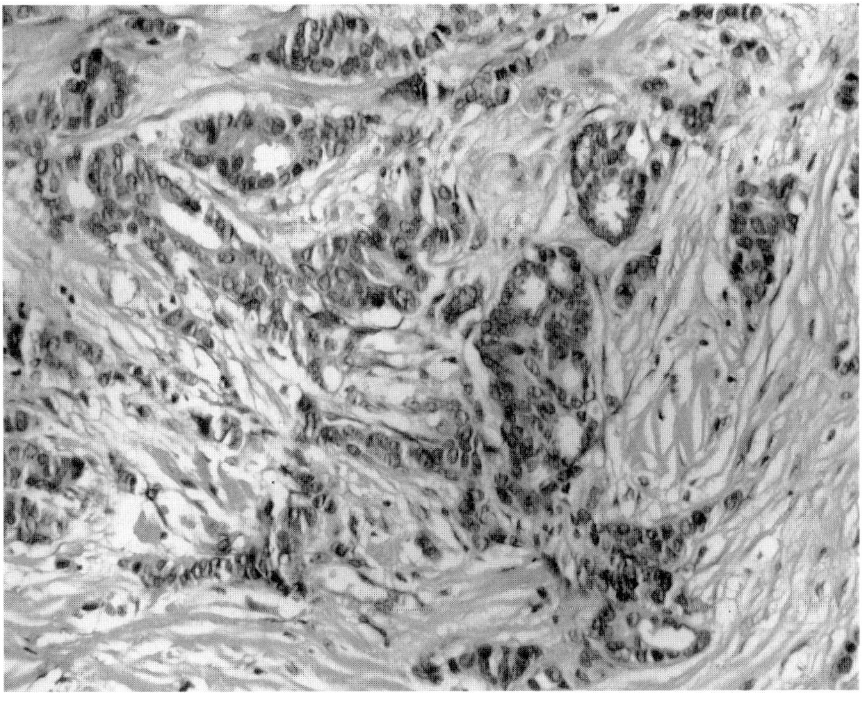

FIG. 8.19. Invasive ductal carcinoma. The desmoplastic stroma is infiltrated by complex ductal structures with low nuclear grade.

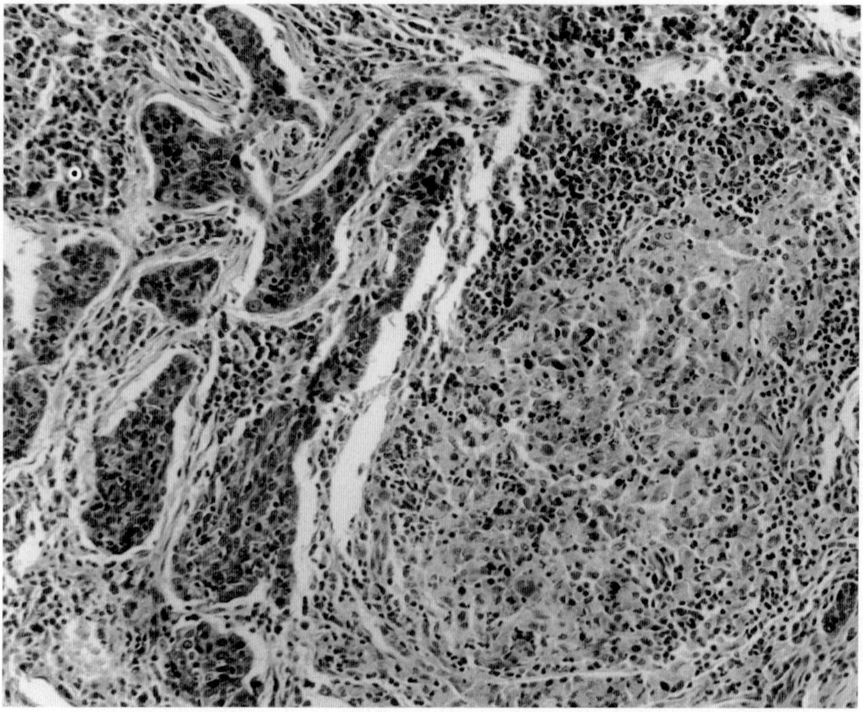

FIG. 8.20. Invasive ductal carcinoma. This desmoplastic and inflamed stroma is infiltrated by trabecular groups of cells with high nuclear grade.

relation was found when S-phase fraction was determined from the paraffin blocks. The author also found correlation of nuclear grade III carcinomas with c-erbB-2 staining. Twelve percent of carcinomas that were positive for c-erbB-2 were of nuclear grade 2. Clayton and Hopkins (48) found mitotic count a good predictor of both grade and prognosis in node-negative ductal carcinomas. Lampejo et al. (49) studied 215 cases of infiltrating ductal carcinoma in which there was also a DCIS component and found a correlation between poorly differentiated DCIS and grade III infiltrating carcinomas. In this study, the type of intraductal carcinoma correlated with disease-free survival and overall survival. The ultrastructural appearance of invasive ductal carcinoma is of a poorly differentiated adenocarcinoma, (efigs. 8.51 to 8.53).

Invasive carcinomas may have central necrosis and clear cytoplasm (efigs. 8.54 and 8.55).

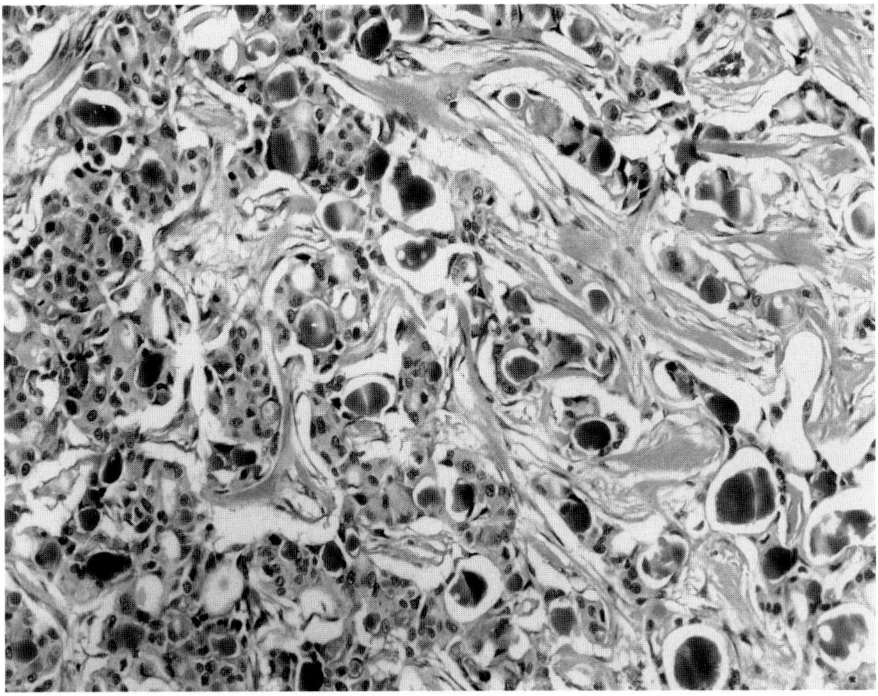

FIG. 8.21. Invasive ductal carcinoma. Mucus is present in the extracellular lumens that are formed by these invasive ducts. This is not mucoid or colloid carcinoma because it does not have pools of mucus.

INFILTRATING LOBULAR CARCINOMA

Infiltrating lobular carcinomas (ILCs) constitute 5% to 10% of invasive breast cancers. Their gross appearance is not as diagnostic as that of the more common infiltrating ductal carcinomas. ILC are not as firm, their borders are not as distinct, and they grossly resemble an inflammatory lesion (Fig. 8.22 and efig. 8.56). Microscopically, they are composed of small cells with hyperchromatic, usually bland, grade 1 nuclei and relatively small amounts of cytoplasm. Cancer cells frequently align themselves in single files, with molding of adjacent nuclei as they infiltrate between the bands of surrounding collagen, and they frequently stream around uninvolved ducts or lobules to form a target pattern. ILC may infiltrate as individual cells and occasionally form small trabeculae focally (Figs. 8.23 to 8.26 and efigs. 8.57 to 8.62).

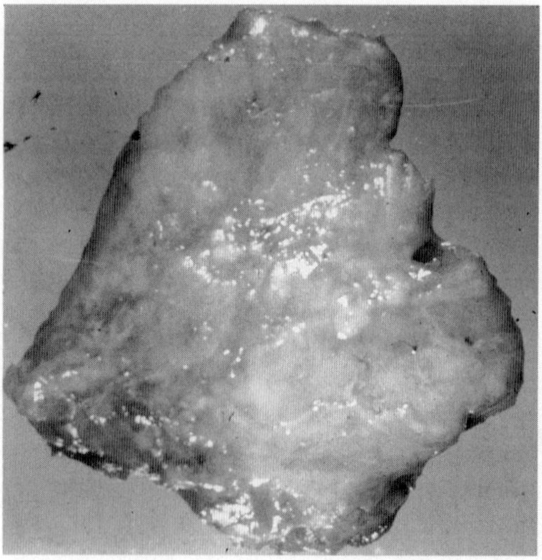

FIG. 8.22. Invasive lobular carcinoma. This carcinoma is not circumscribed and it lacks the white streaks characteristic of the ductal carcinoma.

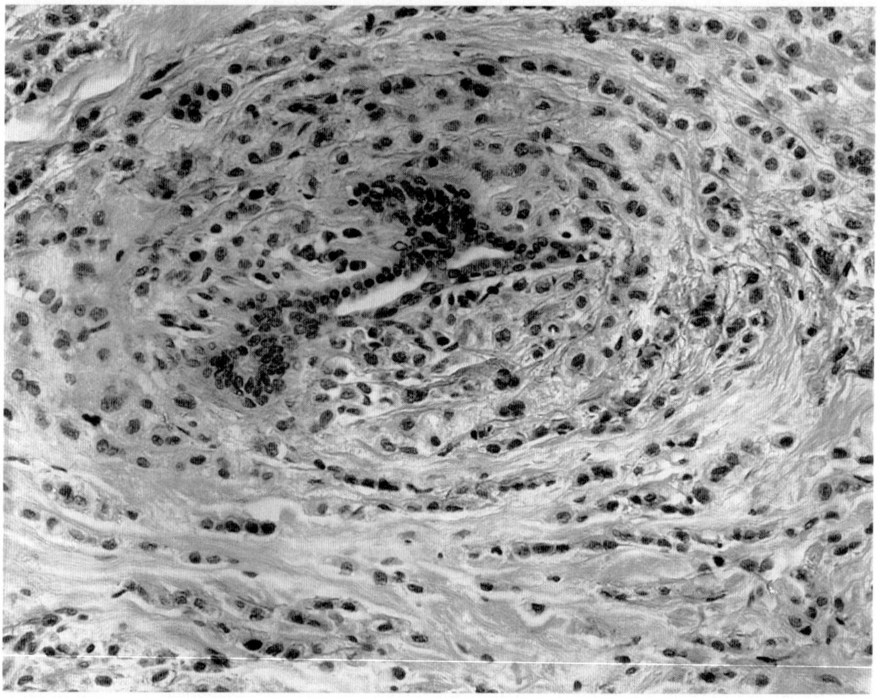

FIG. 8.23. Invasive lobular carcinoma. The small cells with grade 1 nuclei are arranged in single files and insinuate themselves in the stroma around a normal duct. No desmoplastic reaction is elicited.

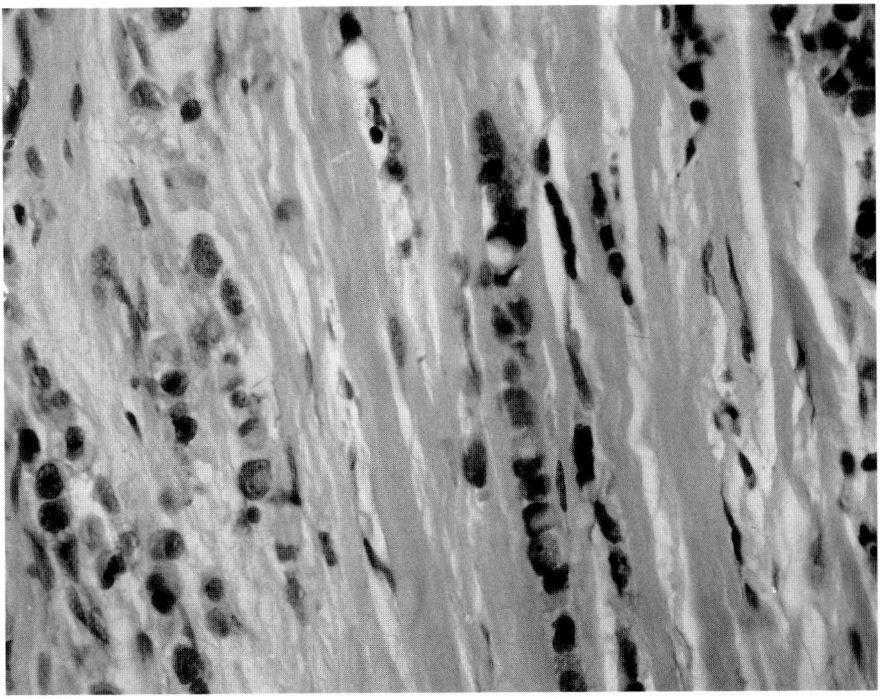

FIG. 8.24. Invasive lobular carcinoma. The single files of cells have round hyperchromatic nuclei without nucleoli or mitotic activity. Rare signet ring cells are present.

The term "lobular" refers to the type of invasive carcinoma that is most often associated with LCIS and its utility is discussed in Chapter 5. It does not imply that the cell of origin is fundamentally different between ductal and lobular carcinoma, but there is a significant difference in the interaction of malignant cells and stroma. ILC insinuates itself into the breast architecture, without eliciting the desmoplastic reaction that is characteristic of invasive ductal carcinoma. This feature is important for clinical presentation, tumor shape, and especially for delineation of margins. The adhesion molecule E-cadherin is reliably expressed by invasive ductal carcinoma and demonstrably absent from ILC. Desmoplasia and angiogenesis are less prominent in ILC. As a result, ILC "hides" among normal breast structures, thereby making it difficult to palpate a mass and define its limits. This allows ILC to grow to a larger size before detection. The higher stage may account for some of its relative aggressiveness and may overcome its "good" prognostic profile of estrogen and progesterone receptor positivity, absence of HER2/neu expression, diploid composition, and low S-phase. The tendency to follow and involve normal structures also may be an important factor in the apparently multifocal presentation, as invasive lobular carcinoma moves from its origin, along the collecting duct system, involving the lobules as

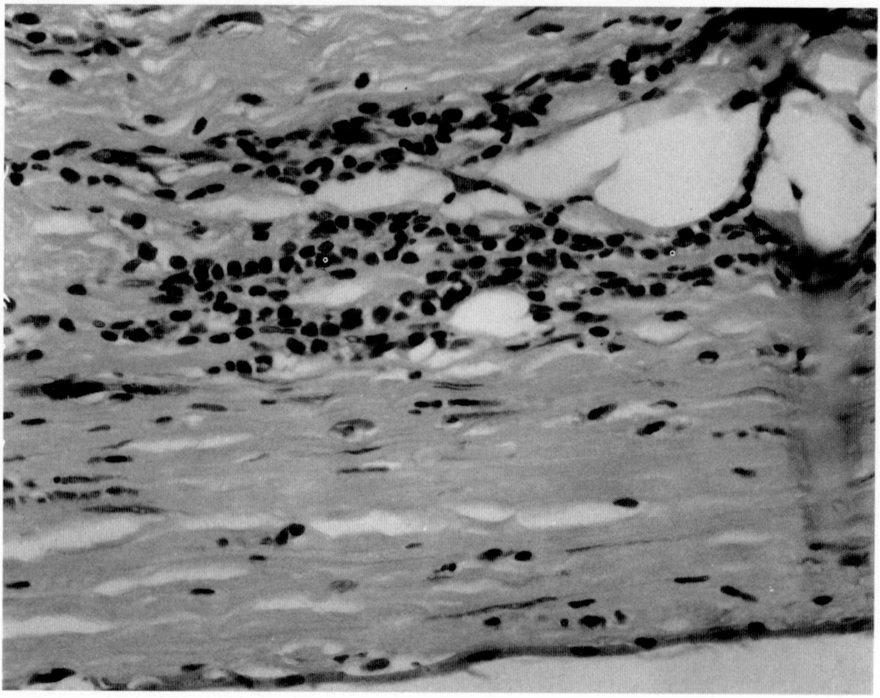

FIG. 8.25. Lymphocytes. Occasionally, lymphocytes may line up in single files and simulate invasive lobular carcinoma.

it goes. Nodules of invasive lobular carcinoma also may be limited in size by their inability to elicit angiogenesis in the stroma.

Ashikari et al. (50) reviewed 354 cases of infiltrating lobular carcinomas of the breast and found that 23% were bilateral, compared with only 15% of infiltrating ductal carcinomas. In comparison with infiltrating ductal carcinomas, infiltrating lobular carcinomas were more often fatal and were considered the most aggressive of all the invasive breast cancers. The overall 5-year survival of patients with infiltrating lobular carcinoma was 70% and the 10-year survival was 46%, compared with a 5-year survival of 73% and a10-year survival of 57% among patients with infiltrating ductal carcinomas.

Invasive lobular carcinoma is usually associated with LCIS, but Fechner (51) addressed the problem of diagnosing ILC in the absence of LCIS. The author used the classic pattern of ILC with single files and target, or bull's-eye formations of invasive single files of malignant cells in periductal stroma of normal ducts. Of 17 patients with invasive lobular carcinoma without LCIS, 7 patients developed contralateral breast carcinomas. Four of these 7 patients had infiltrating lobular carcinomas (2 patients with LCIS and 2 patients without LCIS), 1 patient had LCIS alone, 1 patient had comedocarcinoma, and 1 patient had infil-

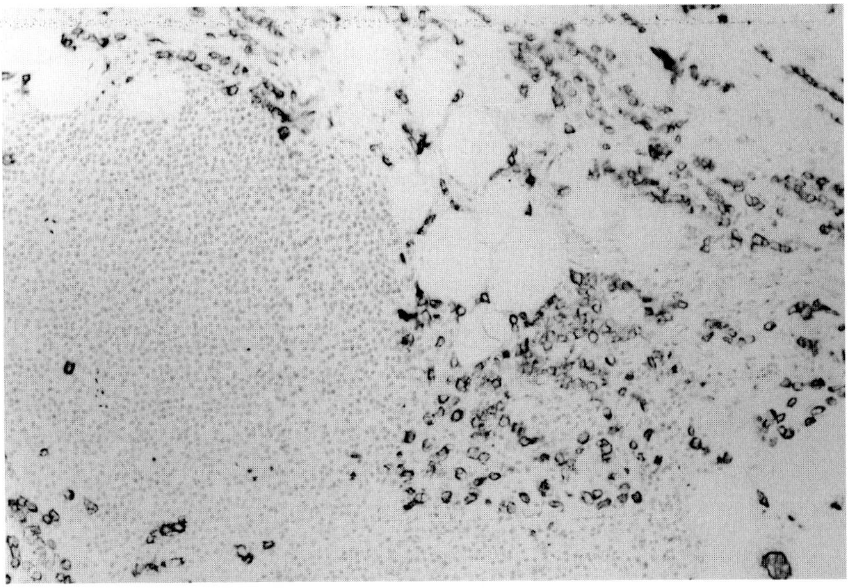

FIG. 8.26. Invasive lobular carcinoma. Keratin stain outlines the invasive lobular carcinoma cells and distinguishes them from the lymphoid nodule (**left**).

trating ductal carcinoma. Fechner (51) suggested that the high incidence of bilateral cancer observed in this series indicated the reliable identification of the entity of infiltrating lobular carcinoma in the absence of its accompanying carcinoma *in situ.*

Van Bogaert and Maldague (9) reported on 22 cases of infiltrating lobular carcinoma, including a variant pattern. Thirteen carcinomas had at least some of the classic single file pattern, and, in six cases, this was the predominant component. Nine cases were associated with LCIS, but, in nine other cases, there was a confluent or solid pattern with a high incidence of mucin-secreting cells in the primary tumor and in the axillary lymph node metastases. One of the cases was a signet ring carcinoma, which is discussed subsequently.

LCIS is a frequent accompaniment of infiltrating lobular carcinoma, occurring in about 50% of cases, and is helpful in identifying the variant cases, but is not required for the diagnosis of infiltrating lobular carcinoma. Its presence also is not an indication that the histology is lobular rather ductal invasive carcinoma, because LCIS may accompany infiltrating ductal carcinoma, and DCIS may (less commonly) accompany infiltrating lobular carcinoma.

Du Toit et al. (52) compared 171 patients with ILC with 342 patients with nonlobular invasive carcinomas and reported that the ILC patients survived longer, more often responded to endocrine treatment for systemic disease, and were more often bilateral, however, the patients also failed locally more often after conservative surgery and radiation. Sastre-Garau et al. (53) compared 726 cases of ILC with 249 cases of mixed lobular/ductal carcinomas and 10,061 cases of nonlobular invasive carcinoma and reported that ILC were larger, more often low grade, more frequently expressed estrogen receptor, were found in older patients, and were associated with fewer lymph node metastases. The authors found no difference in incidence of multicentricity, overall survival, locoregional control, disease-free interval, or rate of metastatic spread among the three groups when treated with conservative surgery and radiation.

Silverstein et al. (54) compared 161 patients with ILC with 1,138 patients with infiltrating ductal carcinoma. The authors found that the ILCs were more difficult to diagnose clinically and they were larger and more difficult to excise completely. Nevertheless, nodal positivity was 32% for ILC, compared with 37% for infiltrating ductal carcinomas. The 7-year breast cancer-specific survival rate was 83% for lobular carcinomas and only 77% for invasive ductal carcinomas. Patients who were treated with radiotherapy had a better disease-free survival rate and breast cancer-specific survival rate than patients with invasive ductal carcinoma who were treated with radiotherapy. The authors answer the question that is the title of their article, "Infiltrating lobular carcinoma: Is it different from infiltrating duct carcinoma?" by recommending that the lobular carcinoma subtype not be a major factor in determining therapy.

Variants of Lobular Carcinoma

Du Toit et al. (52) studied 171 cases of ILC and divided them into the following subtypes: classic, 30%; mixed, 46%; tubulolobular, 14%; solid, 6%; and alveolar, 4%. (Efigs. 8.61 and 8.62 present the solid/alveolar variant.) The 12-year actuarial survival was 100% for the tubulolobular subtype and 47% for the solid subtype. The other three subtypes were intermediate between these extremes. DiCostanzo et al. (55) compared the prognosis of 176 patients with the classic or single file pattern of infiltrating lobular carcinoma with 54 patients with variant invasive lobular carcinoma histology, including solid, alveolar, and mixed patterns. The classic invasive lobular carcinoma patients were younger and more likely to have microscopic multifocality and ductular extension of LCIS, but there was no significant difference in tumor size, axillary lymph node status, median survival, or time to recurrence between the classic and variant groups. When compared with a matched group of infiltrating ductal carcinomas, the stage I classic invasive lobular carcinoma patients had a higher disease-free survival rate than comparable patients with infiltrating ductal carcinoma. DiCostanzo (55) suggested that the unmodified term "infiltrating lobular carcinoma" should be restricted to those carcinomas that exhibit the classic single file microscopic architectural pattern in at least 85% of the invasive carcinomas.

SIGNET RING CELL CARCINOMA

Signet ring cell carcinoma (Fig. 8.27 and efigs. 8.63 to 8.66) was reported by Steinbrecher and Silverberg (56) as five cases of invasive mammary carcinomas that were characterized by the presence of numerous cells that contained large cytoplasmic mucinous vacuoles, which deformed the nucleus to produce the characteristic signet ring configuration. The large amounts of extracellular mucin seen in colloid carcinoma were not present. One of the five patients died of disease at 34 months, and another patient was living with metastases at 25 months. The other three patients were free of disease 3 to 8 months after diagnosis. The gross appearance of the signet ring cell carcinomas was like that of lobular carcinoma. Microscopically, the malignant cells grew in cords of infiltrating cells that were frequently single or in the single files that is seen in lobular carcinoma. PAS-positive, diastase-resistant material was present, as was mucicarminophilic material in the rounded structures that were apparently cytoplasmic vacuoles that pushed the nuclei aside in a signet ring configuration. Ultrastructurally, the tumor cells contained numerous intracellular lumina that gave the appearance of vacuoles on light microscopy. The incidence of signet ring cells was highest in infiltrating lobular carcinomas; signet ring cells were rarely seen in infiltrating ductal carcinomas and colloid carcinomas. LCIS was present in 3 of the 5 cases.

Merino and LiVolsi (57) reported on 24 cases of signet ring cell carcinoma of the breast. In each of the cases, infiltrating lobular carcinoma was recognized and,

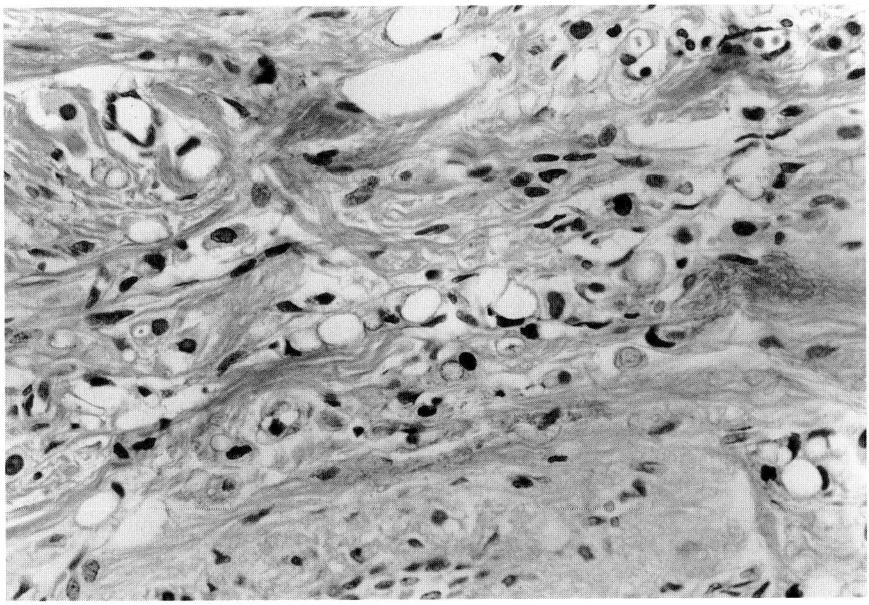

FIG. 8.27. Invasive lobular carcinoma, signet ring variant. The signet ring configuration of the cells is evident.

in 46% of the cases, LCIS also was present. Sixty percent of the patients were dead of disease at 7 years and, in four of the patients, there were metastases to the stomach, large and small bowel, and gallbladder. Five of the patients had hydronephrosis that was caused by metastatic signet ring cell carcinoma in the ureters. Eltorky et al. (58) described 11 cases of the signet ring cell variant of invasive lobular carcinoma, defined as lobular carcinoma in which more than 20% of the malignant cells appeared as signet ring cells. Ten of the 11 cases were positive for estrogen and progesterone receptors. The authors suggested that tamoxifen had a favorable effect on survival. Cormier et al. (59) reported gastric metastases, either alone or concurrent with other sites of metastases, in 14 of 31 cases of metastatic lobular carcinoma. Harris et al. (60) reviewed clinical and autopsy data on the pattern of metastasis from 76 cases of metastatic ductal carcinoma and 14 cases of metastatic lobular carcinoma. The authors reported that lung parenchymal metastases were more common in invasive ductal carcinoma; however, bone metastases, carcinomatous meningitis, and peritoneal and retroperitoneal metastases were more commonly found in the infiltrating lobular carcinomas.

Pleomorphic Variant of Invasive Lobular Carcinoma

Weidner and Semple (61) reviewed 16 cases of pleomorphic infiltrating lobular carcinoma, defined as classic infiltrating lobular carcinoma with a single file pattern in which the nuclei are of higher grade than in classic infiltrating lobular carcinoma (Fig. 8.28 and efigs. 8.67 to 8.69). The 16 patients with pleomorphic infiltrating lobular carcinoma all had nuclei of nuclear grade 2 or grade 3, whereas the cases of classic invasive lobular carcinomas had nuclei of grade 1 by the Bloom (62) criteria. Survival to recurrence was significantly worse for patients with pleomorphic infiltrating lobular carcinoma, as was recurrence in node-negative cases. Node-positive cases were 30 times more likely to experience recurrent disease than were node-positive cases of classic infiltrating lobular carcinomas. Eusebi et al. (63) reported ten cases of pleomorphic lobular carcinoma, defined as classic single cell infiltration in which the cells lacked the appropriate cytologic features. In these cases, many of the cells showed apocrine differentiation. Gross cystic disease fluid protein15 was expressed in LCIS, and six of the patients died within 42 months of diagnosis of this aggressive variant of lobular carcinoma.

Ladekari and Sorensen (64) studied 53 consecutively treated cases of invasive lobular carcinoma that had a median follow-up of 6.6 years. The prognostic indicators in this group were clinical stage of disease, mean nuclear volume, mitotic index, and nuclear index. These quantitative data support the view that the pleomorphic variant of invasive lobular carcinoma has a more aggressive course than the classic variant.

Middleton et al. (65) studied 38 cases of pleomorphic invasive lobular carcinoma. Six cases were in stage I, 19 cases were in stage II, 12 cases were in stage III, and 1 case was in stage IV. Twenty-nine percent of carcinomas had a signet ring cell component. Pleomorphic LCIS was present in 45% of cases. Estrogen receptor and HER2/neu were immunohistochemically stained in 81% of cases.

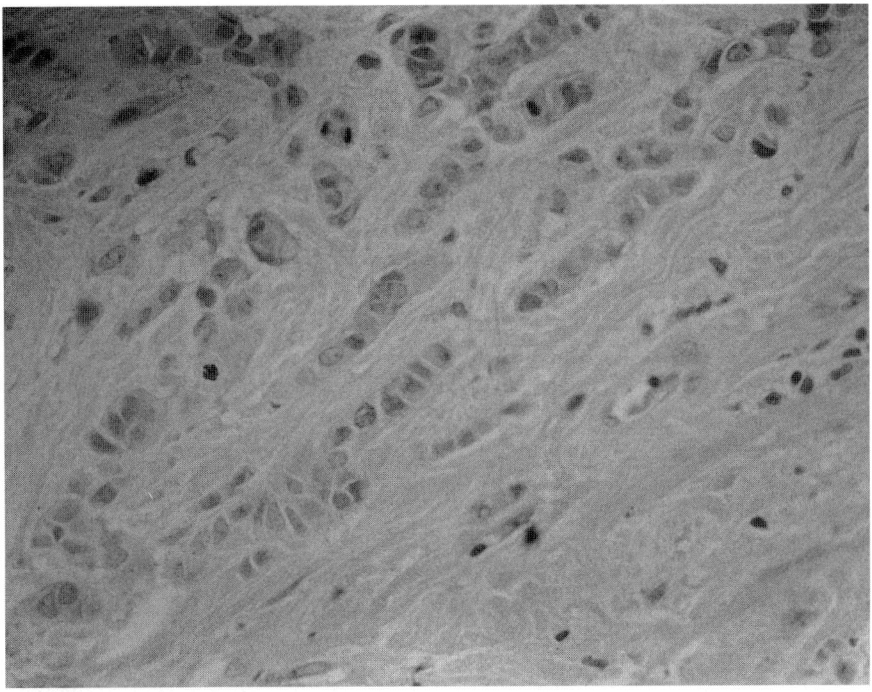

FIG. 8.28. Invasive pleomorphic lobular carcinoma. The single file pattern is maintained, but the nuclei are pleomorphic, some are large and angular, and mitotic figures are evident.

In follow-up over 1 to 15 years, nine patients died of disease, three patients were living with disease, and seven patients had no evidence of disease. Six patients had developed contralateral carcinomas.

Summary

Classic infiltrating lobular carcinoma is characterized by single files of relatively bland malignant cells that infiltrate between the collagen bands and around normal ducts in a target pattern. These cells also may infiltrate singly or take on a "signet ring" shape. Higher nuclear grade is indicative of a worse prognosis. The carcinomas are frequently multifocal and are usually associated with LCIS. A minor component of the single file pattern also may be seen as part of an infiltrating carcinoma that is dominated by an invasive ductal pattern.

TUBULOLOBULAR CARCINOMA

Fisher et al. (66) described 24 cases of tubulolobular invasive breast carcinoma as a variant of invasive lobular cancer with small tubules, as well as cords of neoplastic cells, in a configuration similar to that of classic invasive lobular carcinoma. This variant had a significantly better survival than classic invasive lobular carcinoma. Green et al. (67) compared 17 cases of tubulolobular carcinoma to 90 cases of pure TC and reported a higher incidence of multifocality (29% versus 20%) and axillary lymph node metastases (43% versus 12%) in the tubulolobular group. Multifocality was associated with lymph node metastases in both groups.

APOCRINE CARCINOMA

Apocrine metaplasia commonly accompanies cystic changes and is one of the features that helps to identify intraductal proliferations as benign in nature. There are, however, rare instances of apocrine carcinoma. Most of these are intraductal carcinomas (68,69) (Chapter 4), but Mossler et al. (70) reported six invasive apocrine carcinomas. The patients were all postmenopausal and had tumor masses that varied in size from 1 to 3.5 cm in diameter. All of the tumors were yellow or grayish stellate masses. In one case, carcinoma was fixed to the skin and pectoral muscle and, in three other cases, axillary lymph node metastases were present. Microscopically, the malignant cells were characterized by large active-appearing nuclei that had very low mitotic rates and little pleomorphism (Fig. 8.29 and efigs. 8.70 and 8.71). The cytoplasm was characterized by the presence of "apocrine snouts" and a granular eosinophilic cytoplasm that

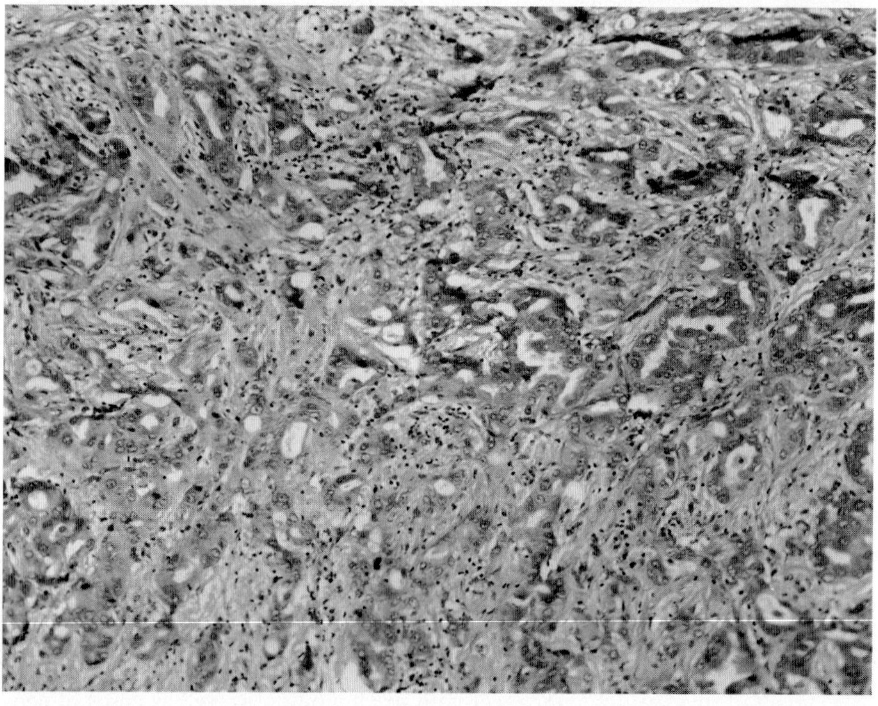

FIG. 8.29. Invasive apocrine carcinoma. The cytoplasm has a granular eosinophilia, but the overall pattern is that of invasive ductal carcinoma.

was documented by electron microscopy to be the result of numerous 400- to 600-nm osmiophilic membrane-bound vesicles that were concentrated along the luminal border of the cells. All of the tumors were well differentiated and tubular components were present as well. Follow-up information is not available on these cases, but the presence of lymph node metastases in 4 of the 6 patients indicates that they were at least moderately aggressive tumors.

Apocrine carcinomas also have been called "sweat gland carcinomas" because of their resemblance to axillary dermal appendage glands.

CLEAR CELL CARCINOMA: LIPID AND GLYCOGEN-RICH

Ramos and Taylor (71) found 13 lipid-rich carcinomas among 900 mammary carcinomas in adults. Grossly, they were poorly circumscribed and ranged in size from 1.5 to 4 cm. Histologically, they were invasive carcinomas, but the desmoplastic reaction that is characteristic of the usual ductal carcinoma was not present and they were associated with either DCIS or LCIS. The malignant cells were similar to those seen in secretory carcinoma, but they were distinguished by the presence of stainable neutral lipid in the cytoplasm (Figs. 8.30 and 8.31 and efigs. 8.72 and 8.73) and the demonstration of lipid droplets by electron

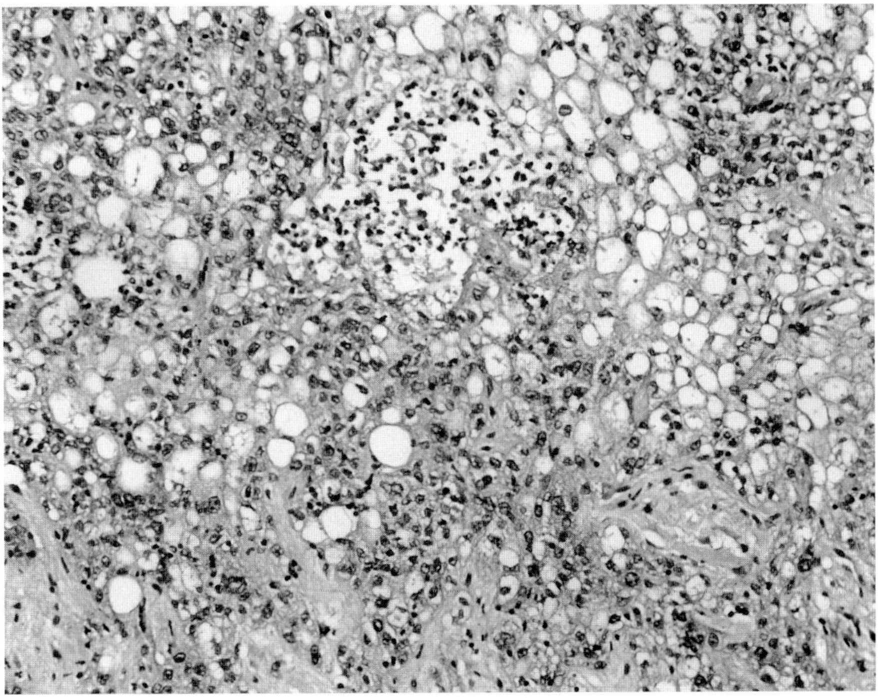

FIG. 8.30. Lipid rich carcinoma. The invasive carcinoma is characterized by cells with large vacuoles.

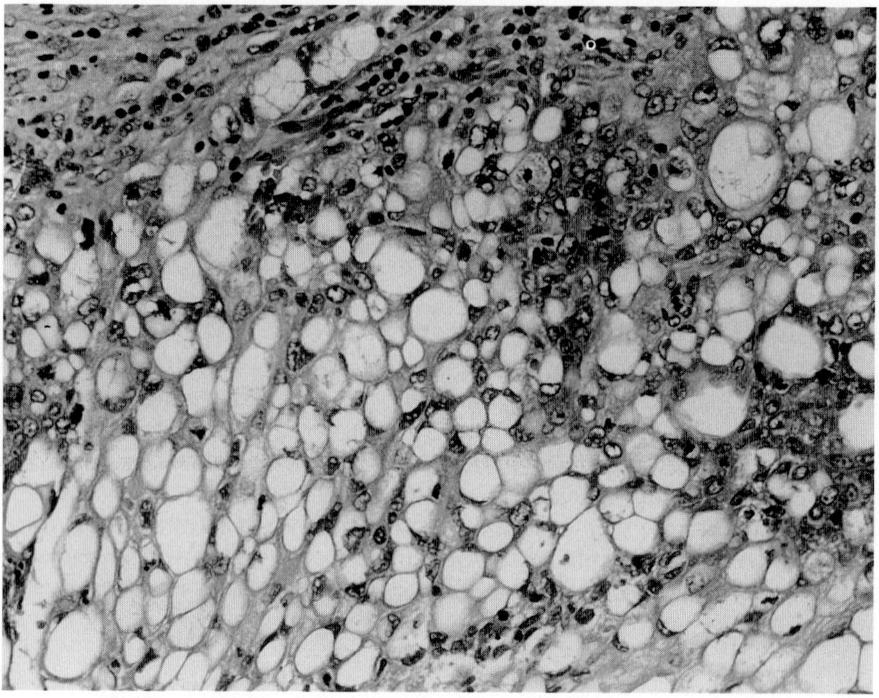

FIG. 8.31. Lipid rich carcinoma. At higher magnification, the nuclear anaplasia of the vacuolated cells is evident. Mucus stain is negative and oil-red-O is positive.

microscopy. In addition, needle-like crystals were observed in the mitochondria of these tumors. In 7 of the 13 patients, evidence of metastatic disease was evident within 2 years, and 5 patients died during this period. One patient died 6 years after treatment.

Varga (72) reported a similar case in which the lipid-rich cells were immunohistochemically stained for cytokeratin, vimentin, S-100 protein; the cells were focally stained for progesterone receptor and carcinoembryonic antigen (CEA). Toikkanen and Joensuu (73) described a glycogen-rich clear cell carcinoma of the breast with a similar appearance on H&E stain in which there was extensive PAS-positivity, with disappearance after digestion by diastase.

HISTIOCYTOID CARCINOMA

In 1973, Hood et al. (74) described 13 cases of breast cancer that were metastatic to the eyelid. Eight of these patients had metastases with a histiocytoid pattern, which puzzled pathologists and led them to suggest a variety of benign diagnoses. These eight tumors were composed of large individual cells that did not join together to form groups. Their nuclei were, in general, centrally placed and hyperchromatic. The cytoplasm was abundant and contained occasional large vacuoles and numerous small ones, which were positive by mucicarmine and PAS stain and contained hyaluronidase-resistant alcian blue-positive material in 3 of 8 cases. The authors stressed the histologic similarity of the metastases to the appearance of fat necrosis and lipid-laden macrophages and the peculiar location of the metastases. Walford and ten Velden (75) reported two cases of *in situ* and invasive histiocytoid carcinoma with features suggestive of an apocrine variant of lobular carcinoma. The histiocytoid variant is distinguishable from the lipid-rich carcinoma because it contains mucopolysaccharide in the cytoplasm of the cells and is negative on fat stain, whereas the reverse is true for the lipid-rich carcinoma.

CARCINOID (NEUROENDOCRINE) TUMORS OF THE BREAST

In 1977, Cubilla and Woodruff (76) reported eight cases of primary carcinoid of the breast. The gross appearance of the tumors was similar to that of other invasive carcinomas of the breast; however, microscopically, the tumors resembled carcinoids that were found elsewhere in the body (Figs. 8.32 to 8.36 and efigs. 8.74 to 8.80). Argyrophilic granules were noted in each case and, in all three cases in which electron microscopy was carried out, membrane-bound dense-core granules that measured approximately 250 nm in average diameter

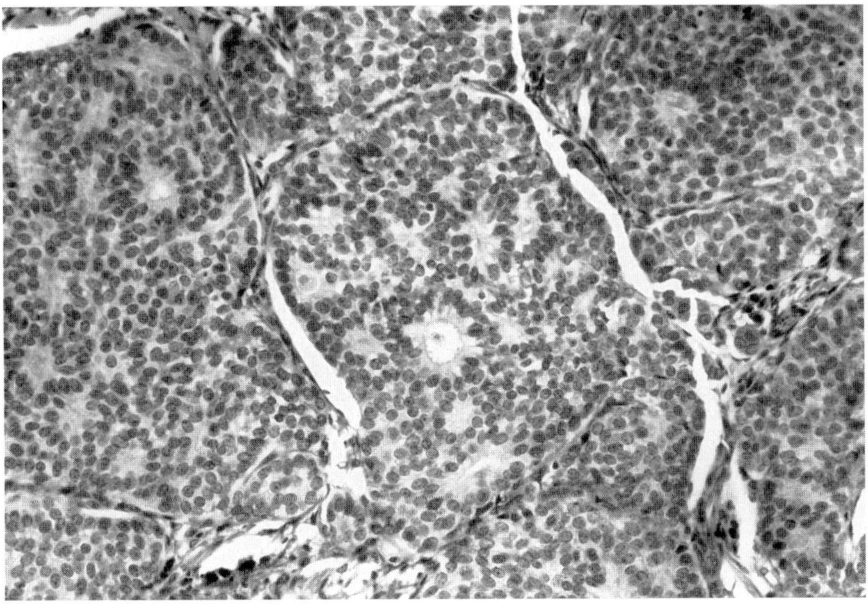

FIG. 8.32. Carcinoid. The small cells have regular round nuclei. Pseudorosettes are prominent.

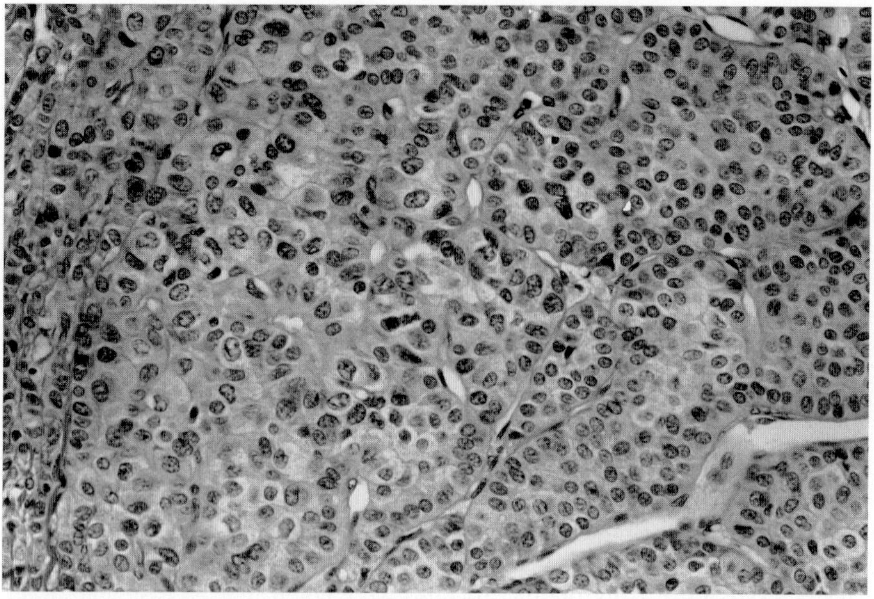

FIG. 8.33. Carcinoid. Ribbon and mosaic patterns are made up of cells with grade 2 nuclei.

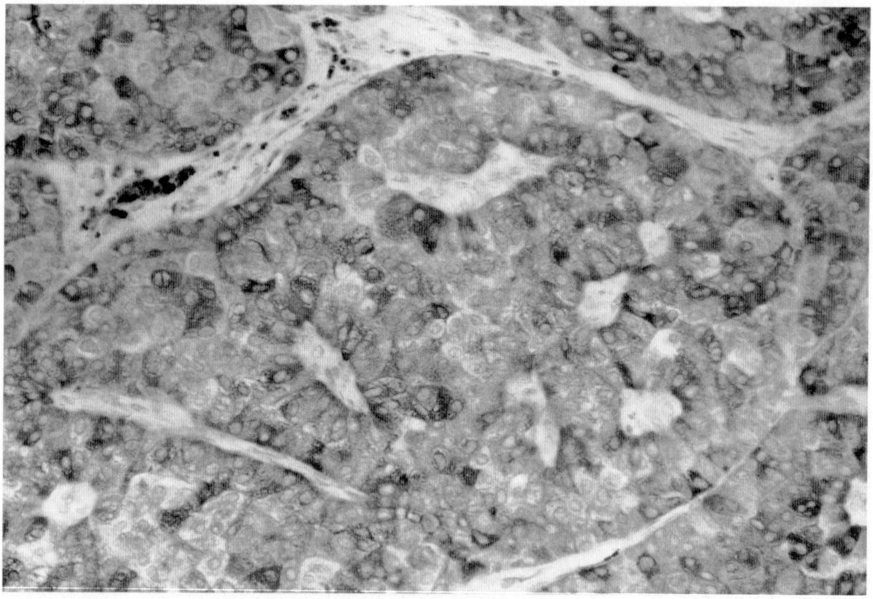

FIG. 8.34. Carcinoid. The immunostain is for chromogranin A.

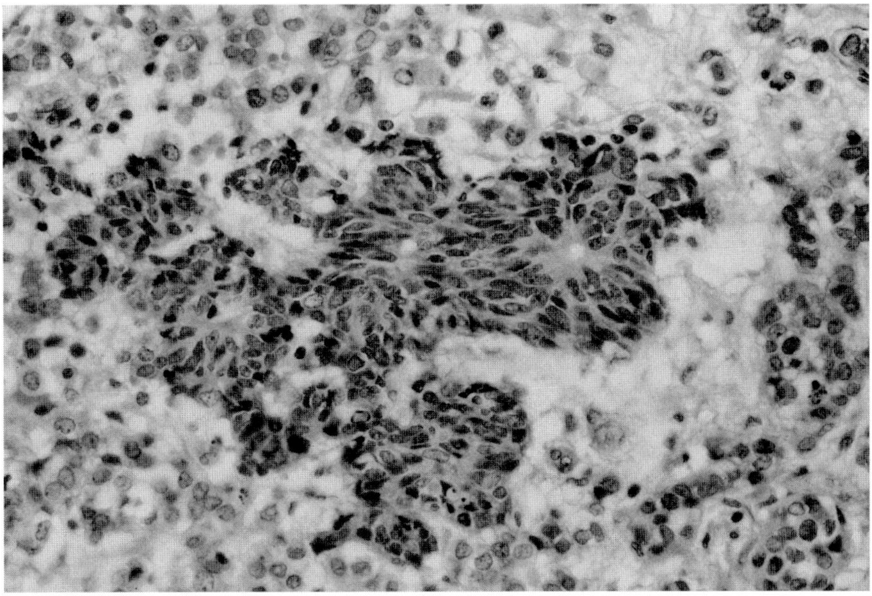

FIG. 8.35. Carcinoid. In this axillary metastasis from the neuroendocrine carcinoma of the breast (**preceding photomicrographs**), pseudorosettes are present, but the nuclei have taken on the features of a small cell carcinoma.

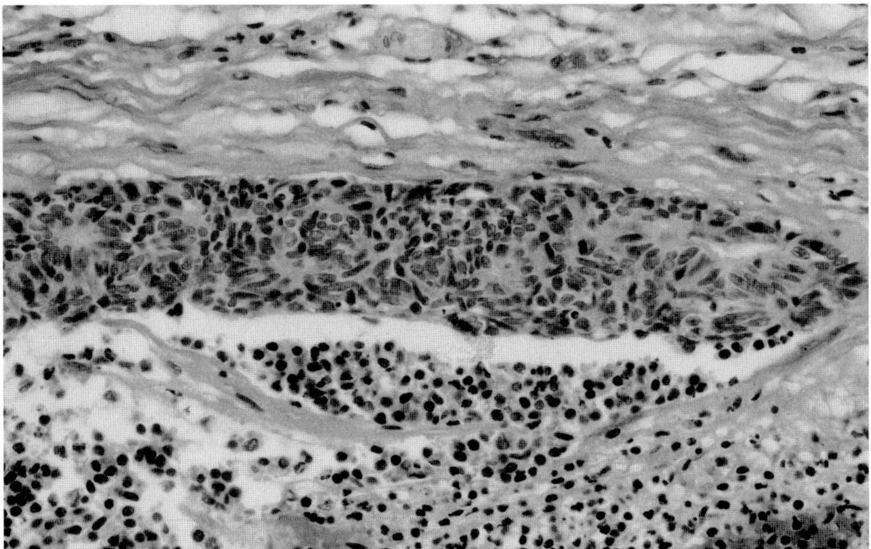

FIG. 8.36. Small cell carcinoma. This carcinoma has pseudorosettes, but dense hyperchromatic nuclei, numerous mitotic figures, and extensive necrosis.

were found and considered to be neurosecretory granules, confirming the carcinoid nature of the tumors that was suggested by their histologic appearance and argyrophilia. Bussolati et al. (77) found immunoreactivity for chromogranin A in one-half the argyrophilic breast carcinomas studied, but the behavior of the neuroendocrine tumors was not demonstrably different from that of infiltrating ductal carcinomas. Three of 4 patients who had tumors that measured 3 cm or larger died of widespread metastases, and a fourth patient was alive with disseminated disease. Patients with tumors that were smaller than 2 cm and who had negative axillary lymph nodes were living and free of disease after a relatively brief follow-up period. Intraductal carcinoma was present in three cases.

Subsequently, Taxy et al. (78) and Partanen and Syrjanen (79) found argyrophilia in ductal and lobular carcinomas, and colloid carcinomas were found to be especially argyrophilic.

Fetissof et al. (80) found argyrophilic cells in 7 of 46 infiltrating ductal carcinomas, 3 of 19 lobular carcinomas, and 7 of 20 colloid carcinomas. The authors did not find argyrophilic cells in any of 2 lactating adenomas, 19 dysplasias, or 12 fibroadenomas. Argyrophilia was noted in both the invasive and *in situ* components, as well as in axillary lymph node metastases. The authors also studied these tumors immunohistochemically for a number of hormones, but none were demonstrated. Electron microscopy on two tumors showed what appeared to be mucin-containing vacuoles in the cytoplasm. This finding, plus the frequent association of colloid carcinomas with argyrophilia, suggested that the cells might contain mucus rather than neurosecretory granules. Clayton et al. (81) studied 20 unselected breast carcinomas for argyrophilia and found it in 10 carcinomas. Immunoperoxidase localization of intracytoplasmic lactalbumin was present in 7 of the 10 cases, confirmed in 2 cases by ultrastructural immunoperoxidase staining. The structures that stained in this manner were membrane-bound, dense-core granules varying in size from 95 to 450 nm. The authors concluded that argyrophilia in breast cancers may be a result of the presence of lactational differentiation, rather than carcinoid differentiation. Sapino et al. (82) discussed immunostaining for neuroendocrine markers in breast cancer cells as a distinct morphologic phenotype of unknown clinical significance. The authors also found evidence that suggests that apocrine metaplasia was associated with the neuroendocrine phenotype (83).

Tumors that have the histology, immunohistochemical profile, ultrastructural appearance, and behavior of carcinoids are found in the breast. They usually have atypical features—mitotic figures, necrosis and/or nuclear anaplasia—and are aggressive carcinomas, with a propensity for regional and distant metastasis. Curiously, they usually express estrogen receptor protein.

Shin et al. (84) reported nine cases of small cell carcinoma of the breast that ranged in size from 1.3 to 5 cm in diameter. In four cases, small cell was found with a component of more usual invasive mammary carcinoma of ductal or lobular types, and *in situ* carcinoma was present in seven cases (efig. 8.36). Immunohistochemical staining revealed consistent staining for keratin and neuroendocrine markers in six cases. Five cases expressed estrogen and progesterone receptors and all cases were negative for HER2/neu and positive for bcl-2. Four of eight patients had axillary lymph nodes metastases, but all patients were alive 3 to 35 months after surgery; however, metastases had appeared in two cases.

METAPLASTIC CARCINOMA

A small number of carcinomas of the breast are associated with a sarcomatous element that is most often spindled in form and resembles fibrosarcoma; however, the histology of a high-grade sarcoma, chondrosarcoma, or osteosarcoma is present rarely. Numerous examples have been previously cited in which a carcinoma with the histology of an ordinary infiltrating ductal carcinoma is focally associated with another type of carcinoma, notably tubular, colloid, or medullary, and, in each of these instances, the presence of the infiltrating ductal carcinoma dictates the behavior of the lesion. So it is when the carcinoma is associated with a sarcomatous element. These are aggressive malignant tumors that metastasize to axillary lymph nodes (as carcinomas do and sarcomas do not) and metastasize to other organs (as do both carcinomas and sarcomas). The metastases may take the carcinomatous and/or sarcomatous form.

There is considerable discussion on the nature of mixed carcinomas and sarcomas of the breast, as there is for these tumors in other organs. It has been suggested that they arise independently or together or that the more common carcinoma differentiates as a sarcoma. McDivitt et al. (85) supported the view that the sarcomatous elements differentiated from the carcinoma cells. Although this view may not be correct (although I believe that it is), it focuses the attention of the observer on the carcinomatous component, which, all agree, determines the prognosis.

The review of the literature on metaplastic carcinomas by Harris and Persaud (86) noted 16 cases, of which 8 cases metastasized. Five of the 8 cases metastasized to axillary nodes. One metastasis showed both carcinoma and sarcoma; the other metastases showed only carcinoma. Grossly, metaplastic carcinomas tend to be large, and differentiation to cartilage or bone may be grossly evident. Oberman (87) noted relatively good survival in a group of 29 cases.

Matrix-producing Carcinoma

Wargotz and Norris (88) reported 26 metaplastic carcinomas that they distinguished as matrix-producing carcinomas. All of the tumors had obvious carcinoma that was moderately or poorly differentiated, with occasional foci of

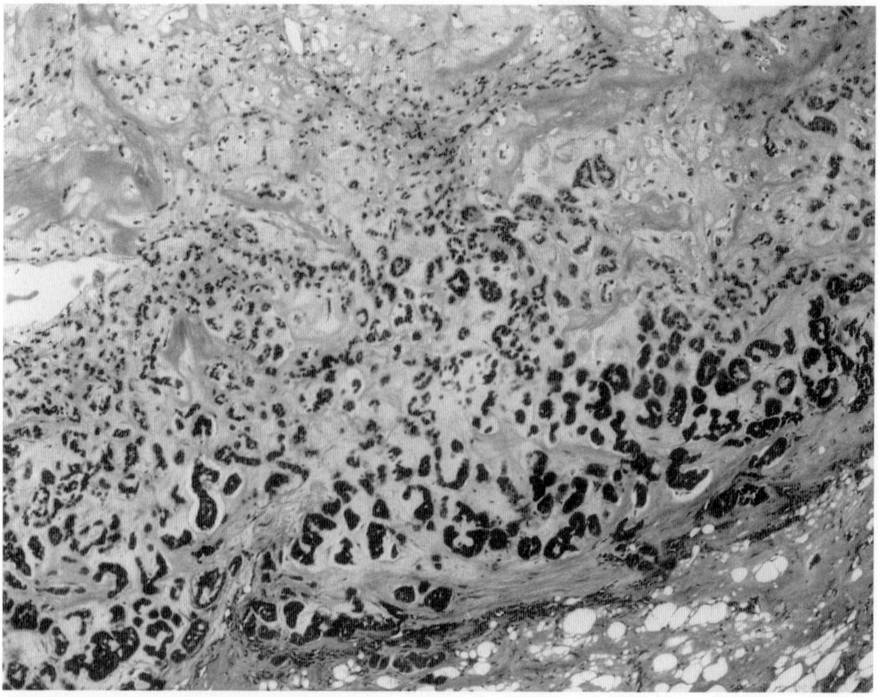

FIG. 8.37. Metaplastic carcinoma with chondroid matrix. The chondroid matrix is formed by the epithelioid groups of malignant cells.

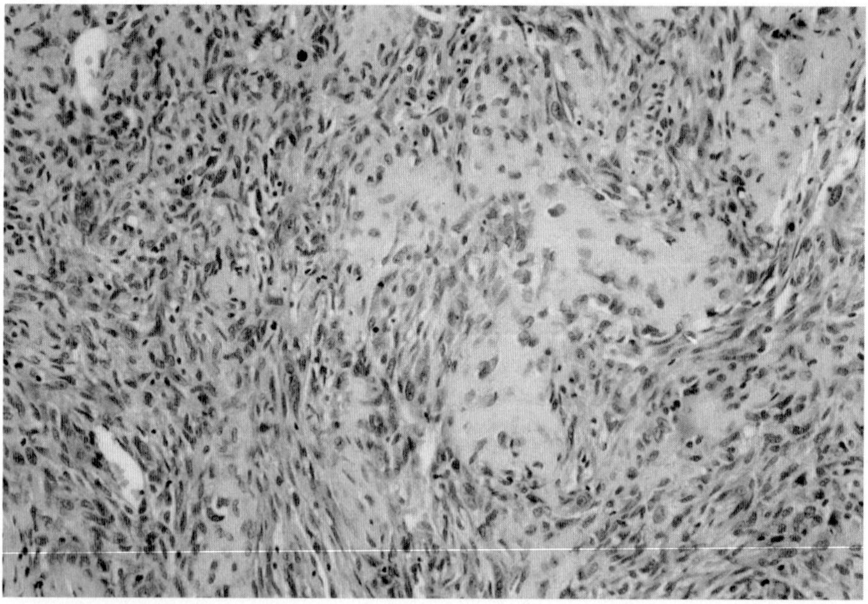

FIG. 8.38. Metaplastic carcinoma with osteoid matrix. These malignant cells form osteoid, giving an overall appearance similar to that of osteogenic sarcoma.

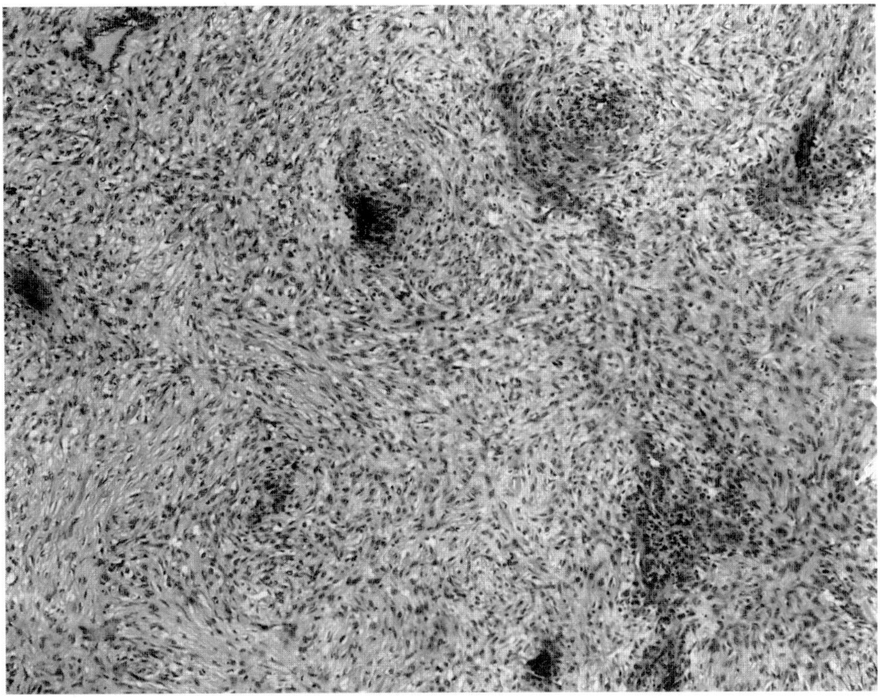

FIG. 8.39. Carcinosarcoma/carcinoma with spindled metaplasia. A malignant spindle neoplasm seems to spin out of the epithelial component.

squamous or apocrine metaplasia, growing in tubules, cords, or masses. Colloid carcinoma was the predominant type. In addition, all the tumors had cartilaginous (Fig. 8.37 and efigs. 8.81 to 8.84) or osteoid (Figs. 8.38 and 8.39 and efigs. 8.85 and 8.86) and lacked an intervening spindle cell element (Fig. 8.40). The tumors varied in size from 5 mm to 12 cm, with a mean diameter of 3.9 cm. The tumors that recurred and metastasized were larger and more cellular than those that did not metastasize. The presence of atypical cartilaginous metaplasia was the best predictor of recurrence and metastasis. Most of the recurrent tumors eventually metastasized, and the 5-year survival rate was 70% for patients treated by mastectomy (23 patients) and 50% for those treated by local excision.

Chieng et al. (89) reported on 32 cases of metaplastic carcinoma. Ten cases had a cartilaginous component; 2 cases, an osseous component; and 20 cases, an osteocartilaginous component. Lymph node metastases were found in 6 of 26 patients who underwent axillary adenectomy. Five-year survival was 60%, which was more favorable than a comparable group of invasive ductal carcinomas, after adjustment for size and nodal status.

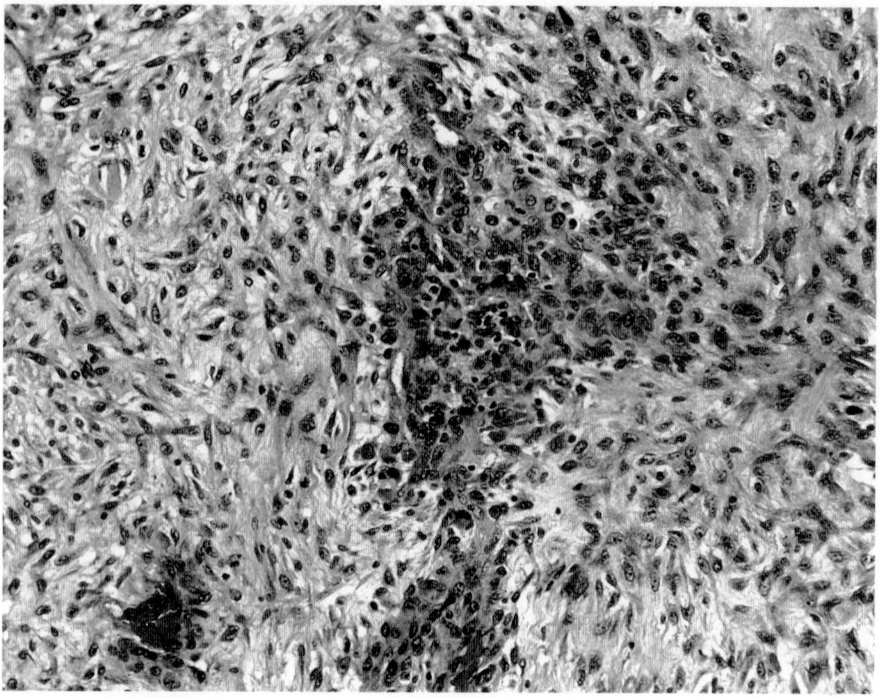

FIG. 8.40. Carcinosarcoma/carcinoma with spindle metaplasia. At higher magnification, the malignant epithelial group is not separated from the invasive malignant spindle cells.

CARCINOSARCOMA

In 1989, Wargotz and Norris (90) described 70 examples of carcinosarcoma of the breast, in which an infiltrating carcinoma was contiguous (or subtly merged) with a highly cellular mitotically active pleomorphic spindle cell stroma that appeared to be sarcomatous (Figs. 8.39 and 8.40). The spindle cell component comprised at least 50% of the neoplasm and was dominant in most cases. The cases in which chondrosarcoma or osteosarcoma was evident were considered matrix-producing carcinomas. Forty of the cases were studied by immunohistochemistry, which revealed immunoreactivity for keratin in the spindle component in 55% of cases. Virtually all of the cases were immunoreactive for vimentin and most of them stained for actin and S-100 protein. Electron microscopy revealed features of a sarcoma in the spindle cell element. The accumulative 5-year survival rate was 49%, which was worse than the survival rate that was observed for metaplastic carcinomas with matrix production. Axillary dissections were done on 50 of the cases, and 13 patients (26%) were found to have lymph node metastases, with carcinoma in 7 of those patients, sarcoma in 3 patients, and both carcinomatous and sarcomatous elements present in the axillary lymph node metastasis in 1 patient.

Spindle Cell Carcinoma

Gersell and Katzenstein (91) described six cases of spindle cell carcinoma of the breast in which there were transition areas from squamous cell carcinoma to the malignant spindle cells, which is seen in squamous cell carcinomas of the esophagus, upper respiratory tract, and lung. The squamous components were cystic and usually of high nuclear grade. Some of the areas contained benign-appearing squamous epithelium. The spindle cell component resembled that of a fibrosarcoma with foci of myxoid change. In one case, there was extensive intraductal carcinoma. Electron microscopy of the fibroblast-like cells of the tumor showed numerous tonofilaments, indicating epithelial differentiation. There was a prominent scirrhous reaction to the tumor and an extensive inflammatory reaction in one case. The authors stressed the importance of distinguishing this lesion from stromal sarcoma and cystosarcoma phyllodes. Four of the six patients underwent radical mastectomy, but none had metastases in the axillary lymph nodes. One patient had local recurrence after excisional biopsy, and one patient died of tumor, but the histology of the metastases from this lesion is not known. The association of one of the tumors with intraductal carcinoma is useful in the identification of the tumor as a primary lesion that originates in the ductal epithelium of the breast.

Wargotz et al. (92) reported 100 examples of spindle cell carcinoma of the breast, in which carcinoma was evident by light microscopy in 83 cases; however, carcinoma was only identified in the other 17 cases by immunoreactivity to keratin. In 98% of the cases, the spindle component was immunoreactive for keratin and also for vimentin, actin, and S-100 protein, suggesting to the authors that the spindle component had myoepithelial features. The 5-year survival rate for spindle cell carcinoma was 64%. Of 47 patients with axillary lymph node dissections, only 3 patients had positive nodes. Features that were predictive of recurrence and metastasis included size, cellularity, mitotic rate, and pleomorphism of the spindle cell component (Fig. 8.41 and efigs. 8.87 and 8.88).

Gobbi et al. (93) reported on a group of 30 cases of invasive ductal carcinomas with bland spindle cells that mimicked fibromatosis infiltrating the parenchyma at the periphery. The epithelial and some of the spindle cells were immunohistochemically stained for vimentin and one or more of the cytokeratins. Seven of 8 patients who were treated by local excision recurred, but only 1 of 10 patients who were treated by wide excision recurred. None metastasized regionally or systemically.

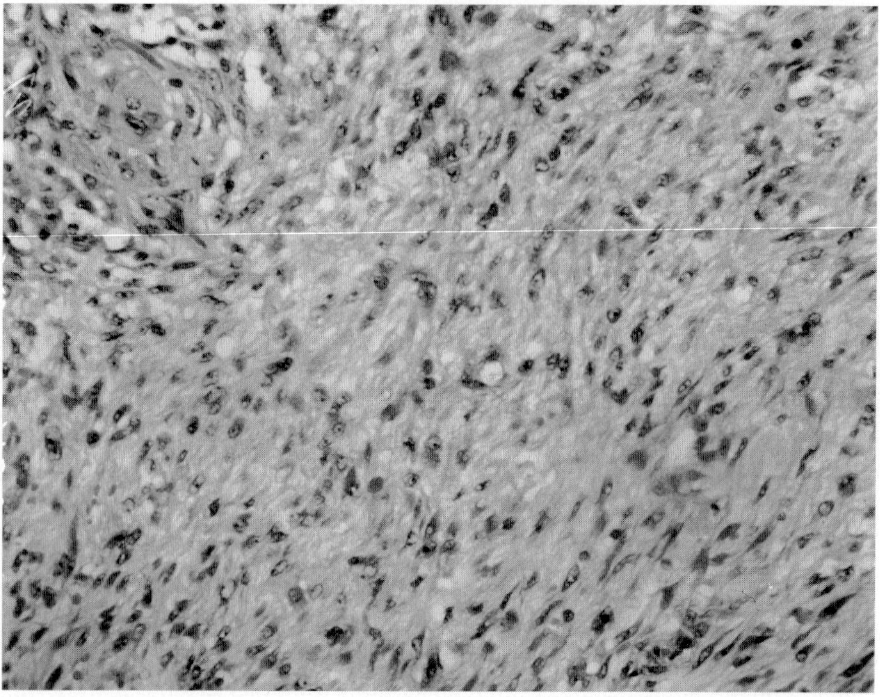

FIG. 8.41. Spindle cell carcinoma. This spindle cell malignant tumor has a high nuclear grade. Although no epithelial features are evident on H&E, immunostain is positive for keratin.

Mammary Carcinomas with Osteoclast-like Giant Cells

Agnantis and Rosen (94) described eight cases of mammary carcinoma with osteoclast-like giant cells. The tumors were not grossly distinctive, and the invasive component of the tumor was either of the ordinary infiltrating ductal variety, infiltrating lobular variety, or a combination of the two. There was a scirrhous reaction to the tumor and an inflammatory reaction in which osteoclast-like giant cells were abundant in six cases and focally present in two cases (Fig. 8.42 and efigs. 8.90 to 8.92). In the four patients with axillary lymph node metastases, giant cells were not present, but in two of the patients, visceral metastases contained osteoclast-like giant cells. Solid and pleomorphic forms of carcinoma were present in five cases and squamous or spindle forms were found in three cases. Osseous metaplasia was found focally in one case. Clinically, the carcinomas behaved like ductal carcinomas of the breast. Rosen (95) also called attention to the presence of giant cells, which are not of the osteoclast-like variety in benign breast biopsy specimens. They may simulate the presence of invasive cancer.

Wargotz and Norris (96) described 29 examples of metaplastic carcinoma with osteoclastic giant cells in the stroma. Histologically, they had a dominating

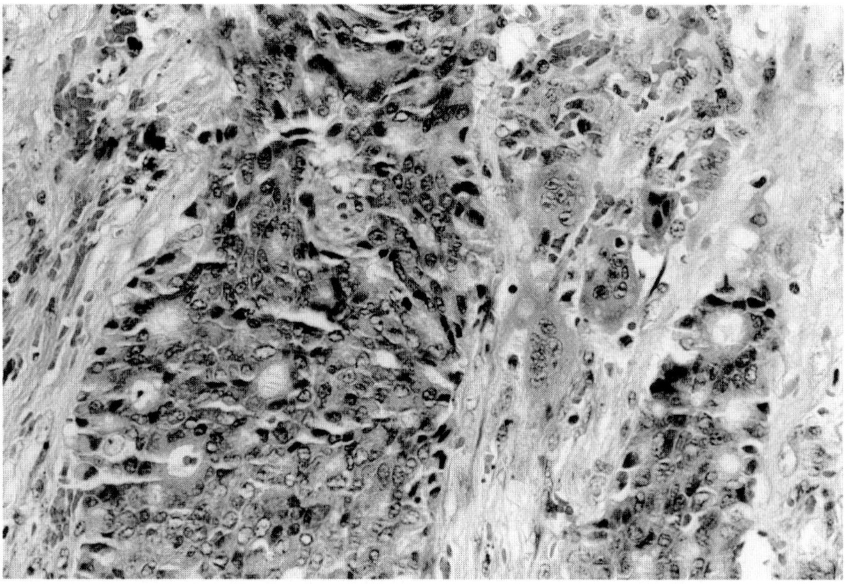

FIG. 8.42. Osteoclastic giant cells with invasive ductal carcinoma. Several multinucleated histiocytes with the appearance of osteoclasts are present in the stroma, adjacent to invasive carcinoma.

bland spindle or sarcomatous component, although obvious invasive carcinoma was present in 23 of the 29 cases. The osteoclastic giant cells were admixed within the cellular stroma and were immunoreactive for vimentin and actin, but not for keratin. The stromal component of the neoplasms was immunoreactive for keratin in 63% of cases and for epithelial membrane antigen in 33% of cases. It was also immunoreactive for actin and S-100 protein. Nineteen of the 29 cases had osseous or cartilaginous differentiation. The 5-year survival rate was 68%, which was similar to that of the cases in which there was matrix production. Two of 17 patients with axillary lymph node dissections had lymph node metastases. Eleven of the 29 patients developed distant metastases, most often to the lungs. Size predicted for metastatic disease, with metastases occurring in 7 of the 11 patients who had carcinomas that were greater than 6 cm, but in only 1 of 6 patients with tumors that were 2.9 cm or smaller. Circumscription was related to the lack of recurrence.

Metaplastic Carcinoma Versus Stromal Sarcoma

Large areas of metaplastic carcinoma may be indistinguishable from sarcoma, and therefore, when a diagnosis of nonphyllodes sarcoma of the breast is entertained, it is important to exclude carcinoma in sarcomatous form because of its propensity to metastasize to axillary lymph nodes. Immunohistochemistry with

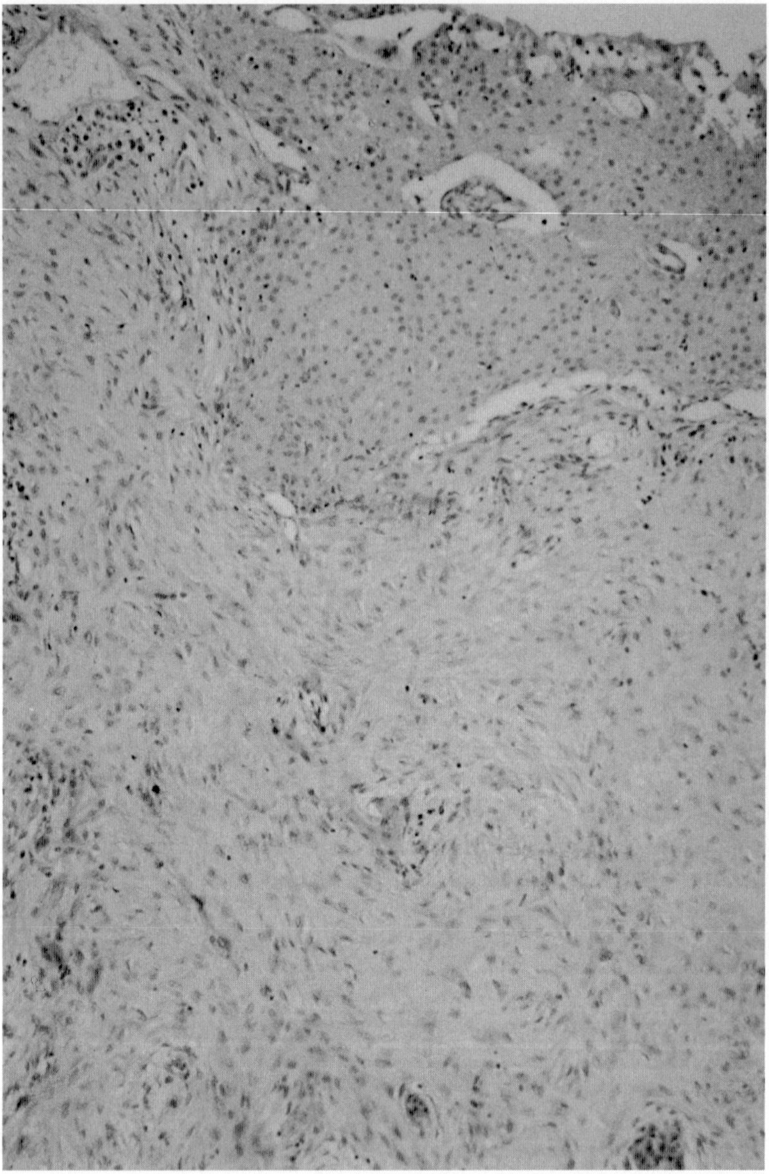

FIG. 8.43. Squamous cell carcinoma. A cystic space is lined by a thick keratinizing squamous cell carcinoma. The surrounding stroma is infiltrated by small nests of malignant squamous cells.

antibodies to keratins are usually useful in resolving this problem, if multiple histologic sections do not.

SQUAMOUS CELL CARCINOMA

Fisher et al. (97) described five cases of squamous cell carcinoma of the breast, which histologically had the characteristic appearance of squamous cell carcinoma that might have arisen in any of a number of organs. Three of the 5 cases had prominent cystic features, imparting a leaf-like or phyllode microscopic pattern (Fig. 8.43 and efigs. 8.92 to 8.98). None of the five patients had axillary lymph node metastases, but one of the patients died of systemic disease. Large bizarre malignant-appearing giant cells were present, as were some osteoclast-like multinucleated giant cells. The rarity of squamous cell carcinoma of the breast was noted by Toikkanen (98), who found only three examples among 4,000 breast cancer cases. Those three carcinomas were extremely aggressive, with a mean survival time of only 8.3 months. The author also noted the presence of necrosis and a cystic pattern. The mode of histogenesis of these tumors remains obscure, but they are considered to derive from the ductal epithelium, rather than from the skin. Eusebi et al. (99) described an acantholytic variant.

Wargotz and Norris (100) described 22 examples of pure ductal squamous cell carcinoma of the breast. The sizes ranged from 1.5 to 12 cm, with a mean of 3.9 cm. There was a tendency toward cyst formation. Microscopically, all were inva-

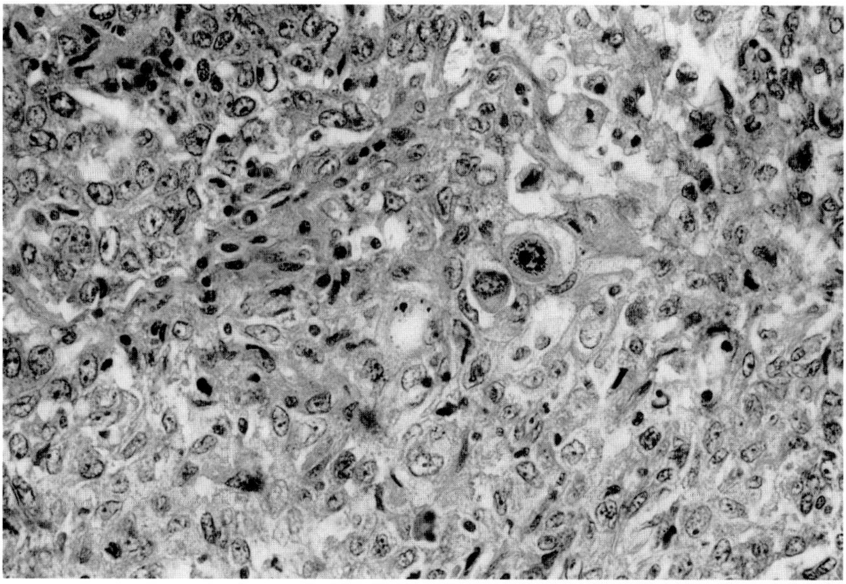

FIG. 8.44. Squamous cell carcinoma. This poorly differentiated malignant tumor has grade 3 nuclei. In the center, there are keratinized cells with large markedly hyperchromatic nuclei.

sive carcinomas with squamous cell differentiation (see fig. 8.44). Lymph node metastases were present in 2 of 19 women who had axillary dissections. The 5-year disease-free survival rate was 63%. No specific factor was predictive of local recurrence, but larger tumors tended to metastasize more often.

Mucoepidermoid Carcinoma

Fisher et al. (101) described five cases of low-grade mucoepidermoid carcinoma in which the squamous elements were associated with ductal elements that were similar to mucoepidermoid carcinomas of salivary glands (Figs. 8.45 and efigs. 8.99 and 8.100). The mucoid component contained PAS-positive material. Although the high-grade appearance of the squamous cell carcinoma was noted, the five patients with low-grade mucoepidermoid carcinomas did not have axillary lymph node metastases, and all were alive at the end of the follow-up period.

Adenosquamous Carcinoma

Van Hoeven et al. (102) described 32 cases of low-grade adenosquamous carcinoma. Origin from an intraductal papillary tumor was found in 12 cases, with three showing adenomyoepitheliomatous features. Squamous differentiation, as well as a glandular/ductal component, was present in all cases. The size range

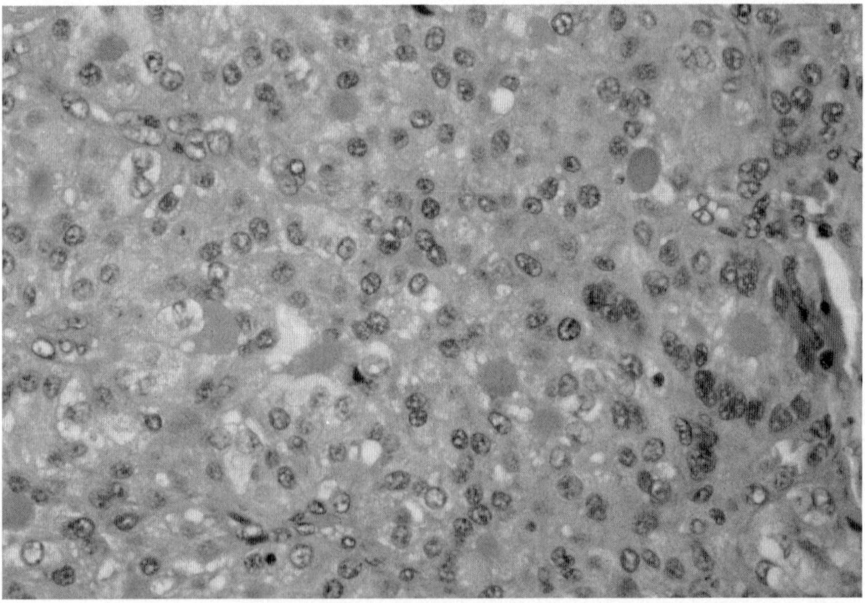

FIG. 8.45. Mucoepidermoid carcinoma. Duct-like structures with secretion are evident. Between them are intermediate cells characteristic of mucoepidermoid carcinoma.

was from 6 mm to 8.6 cm, with a mean of 2.8 cm. One of 12 patients with axillary adenectomy had a lymph node metastasis, and one patient with an 8-cm adenosqamous carcinoma had a metastatic deposit in the lung at the time of presentation. Twenty of 25 patients had no recurrence. One patient treated with local resection had a local recurrence that was fatal because of invasion of the thorax. Estrogen and progesterone receptors were negative in 13 of 15 cases. The authors suggested aggressive therapy for adenosquamous carcinomas that were 3-cm or greater in diameter, because of their aggressive local behavior.

REFERENCES

1. Haffty B, Perrotta P, Ward B, et al. Conservatively treated breast cancer: outcome by histologic subtype. *Breast J* 1997;3:7–14.
2. Stalsberg H, Thomas DB. Age distribution of histologic types of breast carcinoma. *Int J Cancer* 1993;54:1–7.
3. Rosen PP, Lesser ML, Senie RT, et al. Epidemiology of breast carcinoma. III. Relationship of family history to tumor type. *Cancer* 1982;50:171–179.
4. Somerville JE, Clarke LA, Biggart JD. c-erbB-2 overexpression and histological type of *in situ* and invasive breast carcinoma. *J Clin Pathol* 1992;45:16–20.
5. Oberman HA, Fidler WJ Jr. Tubular carcinoma of the breast. *Am J Surg Pathol* 1979;3:387–396.
6. McDivitt RW, Boyce W, Gersell D. Tubular carcinoma of the breast: clinical and pathological observations concerning 135 cases. *Am J Surg Pathol* 1982;6:401–411.
7. Taylor H, Norris HJ. Well differentiated carcinoma of the breast. *Cancer* 1970;25:687–692.
8. Lagios MD, Rose MR, Margolin FR. Tubular carcinoma of the breast: association with multicentricity, bilaterality, and family history of mammary carcinoma. *Am J Clin Pathol* 1980;73:25–30.
9. Van Bogaert L, Maldague P. Infiltrating lobular carcinoma of the female breast: deviations from the usual histopathologic appearance. *Cancer* 1980;45:979–984.
10. Parl FF, Richardson LD. The histologic and biologic spectrum of tubular carcinoma of the breast. *Hum Pathol* 1983;14:694–698.
11. Deos PH, Norris HJ. Well-differentiated (tubular) carcinoma of the breast: a clinicopathologic study of 145 pure and mixed cases. *Am J Clin Pathol* 1982;78:1–7.
12. McBoyle MF, Razek HA, Carter JL, et al. Tubular carcinoma of the breast: an institutional review. *Am Surg* 1997;63:639–644; discussion 644–635.
13. Peters GN, Wolff M, Haagensen CD. Tubular carcinoma of the breast: clinical pathologic correlations based on 100 cases. *Ann Surg* 1981;193:138–139.
14. Cooper HS. Tubular carcinoma of the breast. *Cancer* 1978;42:2334–2342.
15. Eusebi V. Nonencapsulated sclerosing lesion of the breast. *Am J Clin Pathol* 1980;73:456.
16. Taylor HB, Norris HJ. Epithelial invasion of nerves in benign disease of the breast. *Cancer* 1967;20: 2245–2249.
17. Tremblay G. Elastosis in benign sclerosing ductal proliferation of the female breast. *Am J Surg Pathol* 1977;1:155–160.
18. Rosen PP. Microglandular adenosis. A benign lesion simulating invasive mammary carcinoma. *Am J Surg Pathol* 1983;7:137.
19. Stalsberg H, Hartmann WH. The delimitation of tubular carcinoma of the breast. *Hum Pathol* 2000; 31:601–607.
20. Kader HA, Jackson J, Mates D, et al. Tubular carcinoma of the breast: a population-based study of nodal metastases at presentation and of patterns of relapse. *Breast J* 2001;7:8–13.
21. Papadatos G, Rangan AM, Psarianos T, et al. Probability of axillary node involvement in patients with tubular carcinoma of the breast. *Br J Surg* 2001;88:860–864.
22. Page DL, Dixon JM, Anderson TJ. Invasive cribriform carcinoma of the breast. *Histopathology* 1983;75:525.
23. Venable JG, Schwartz AM, Silverberg SG. Infiltrating cribriform carcinoma of the breast: a distinctive clinicopathologic entity. *Hum Pathol* 1990;21:333–338.
24. Marzullo F, Zito F, Marzullo A, et al. Infiltrating cribriform carcinoma of the breast: a clinico-pathologic and immunohistochemical study of 5 cases. *Eur J Gynaecol Oncol* 1996;17:228–231.

25. Fisher ER, Palekar AS, Redmond C, et al. Pathologic findings from the National Surgical Adjuvant Breast Project (protocol no. 4). VI. Invasive papillary cancer. *Am J Clin Pathol* 1980;73:313–322.
26. Siriaunkgul S, Tavassoli F. Invasive micropapillary carcinoma of the breast. *Mod Pathol* 1993;6: 660–662.
27. Middleton LP, Tressera F, Sobel ME, et al. Infiltrating micropapillary carcinoma of the breast. *Mod Pathol* 1999;12:499–504.
28. Moore OS, Foote FWJ. The relatively favorable prognosis of medullary carcinoma of the breast. *Cancer* 1949;2:635–642.
29. Bloom HJG, Field JR. Impact of tumor grade and host resistance on survival of women with breast cancer. *Cancer* 1971;28:1580–1589.
30. Ridolfi RL, Rosen PP, Port A, et al. Medullary carcinoma of the breast: a clinicopathologic study with 10 year follow-up. *Cancer* 1977;40:1365–1385.
31. Wargotz ES, Silverberg SG. Medullary carcinoma of the breast: a clinicopathologic study with appraisal of current diagnostic criteria. *Hum Pathol* 1988;19:1340–1346.
32. Gaffey MJ, Mills SE, Frierson HF Jr, et al. Medullary carcinoma of the breast: interobserver variability in histopathologic diagnosis. *Mod Pathol* 1995;8:31–38.
33. Pedersen L, Holck S, Schiodt T, et al. Inter- and intraobserver variability in the histopathological diagnosis of medullary carcinoma of the breast, and its prognostic implications. *Breast Cancer Res Treat* 1989;14:91–99.
34. Pedersen L, Zedeler K, Holck S, et al. Medullary carcinoma of the breast, proposal for a new simplified histopathological definition. *Brit J Cancer* 1991;63:591–595.
35. Yazawa T. Frequent expression of HLA-DR antigen in medullary carcinoma of the breast: a possible reason for its prominent lymphocytic infiltration and favorable prognosis. *Appl Immunohistochem* 1993;1:296.
36. Gaffey MJ, Frierson HF Jr, Mills SE, et al. Medullary carcinoma of the breast identification of lymphocyte subpopulations and their significance. *Mod Pathol* 1993;6:721–728.
37. Norris HJ, Taylor HB. Prognosis of mucinous gelatinous carcinoma of the breast. *Cancer* 1965;18: 879–885.
38. Clayton F. Pure mucinous carcinoma of the breast: morphologic features and prognostic correlates. *Hum Pathol* 1986;17:34–38.
39. Toikkanen S, Kujari H. Pure and mixed mucinous carcinomas of the breast: a clinicopathologic analysis of 61 cases with long-term follow-up. *Hum Pathol* 1989;20:758–764.
40. Melamed M, Robbins GF, Foote FW. Prognostic significance of gelatinous mammary carcinoma. *Cancer* 1961;14:699–704.
41. Silverberg SG, Kay S, Chitale AR, et al. Colloid carcinoma of the breast. *Am J Clin Pathol* 1971;55: 355–363.
42. Rasmussen BB, Rose C, Christensen. I Prognostic factors in primary mucinous breast carcinoma. *Am J Clin Pathol* 1987;87:155–160.
43. Anan K, Mitsuyama S, Tamae K, et al. Pathological features of mucinous carcinoma of the breast are favourable for breast-conserving therapy. *Eur J Surg Oncol* 2001;27:459–463.
44. Koenig C, Tavassoli FA. Mucinous cystadenocarcinoma of the breast. *Am J Surg Pathol* 1998;22: 698–703.
45. Rosen PP. Mucocele-like tumors of the breast. *Am J Surg Pathol* 1986;10:464–469.
46. Ro JY, Sneige N, Sahin AA, et al. Mucocelelike tumor of the breast associated with atypical ductal hyperplasia or mucinous carcinoma. A clinicopathologic study of seven cases. *Arch Pathol Lab Med* 1991;115:137–140.
47. Dabbs DJ. Ductal carcinoma of breast: nuclear grade as a predictor of S-phase fraction. *Hum Pathol* 1993;24:652–656.
48. Clayton F, Hopkins CL. Pathologic correlates of prognosis in lymph node-positive breast carcinomas. *Cancer* 1993;71:1780–1790.
49. Lampejo OT, Barnes DM, Smith P, et al. Evaluation of infiltrating ductal carcinomas with a DCIS component: correlation of the histologic type of the *in situ* component with grade of the infiltrating component. *Semin Diagn Pathol* 1994;11:215–222.
50. Ashikari R, Huvos AG, Urban JA, et al. Infiltrating lobular carcinoma of the breast. *Cancer* 1973;31: 110–116.
51. Fechner RE. Infiltrating lobular carcinoma without lobular carcinoma *in situ*. *Cancer* 1972;29: 1539–1545.

52. du Toit RS, Locker AP, Ellis IO, et al. Invasive lobular carcinomas of the breast—the prognosis of histopathological subtypes. *Br J Cancer* 1989;60:605–609.
53. Sastre-Garau X, Jouve M, Asselain B, et al. Infiltrating lobular carcinoma of the breast: clinicopathologic analysis of 975 cases with reference to data on conservative therapy and metastatic patterns. *Cancer* 1996;77:113–120.
54. Silverstein MJ, Lewinsky BS, Waisman JR, et al. Infiltrating lobular carcinoma: Is it different from infiltrating duct carcinoma? *Cancer* 1994;73:1673–1677.
55. DiCostanzo D, Rosen PP, et al. Prognosis in infiltrating lobular carcinoma: an analysis of "classical" and variant tumors. *Am J Surg Pathol* 1990;14:12–23.
56. Steinbrecher JS, Silberberg SG. Signet-ring cell carcinoma of the breast: the mucinous variant of infiltrating lobular carcinoma. *Cancer* 1976;37:828–840.
57. Merino MJ, Livolsi VA. Signet ring carcinoma of the female breast: a clinicopathologic analysis of 24 cases. *Cancer* 1981;48:1830–1837.
58. Eltorky M, Hall JC, Osborne PT, et al. Signet-ring cell variant of invasive lobular carcinoma of the breast. *Arch Pathol Lab Med* 1994;118:245–248.
59. Cormier WJ, Gaffey TA, Welch JM, et al. Linitis plastica caused by metastatic lobular carcinoma of the breast. *Gastrointest Endosc* 1980;38:130–135.
60. Harris M, Howell A, Chrissohou M, et al. A comparison of the metastatic pattern of infiltrating lobular carcinoma and infiltrating duct carcinoma of the breast. *Br J Cancer* 1984;50:23–30.
61. Weidner N, Semple JP. Pleomorphic variant of invasive lobular carcinoma of the breast. *Hum Pathol* 1992;23:1167–1171.
62. Bloom HJG, Richardson WW. Histological grading and prognosis in breast cancer: a study of 1409 cases of which 359 have been followed for 15 years. *Br J Cancer* 1957;11:359–377.
63. Eusebi V, Magalhaes F, Azzopardi JG. Pleomorphic lobular carcinoma of the breast: an aggressive tumor showing apocrine differentiation. *Hum Pathol* 1992;23:655–662.
64. Ladekari M, Sorensen FB. Prognostic, quantitative histopathologic variables in lobular carcinomas of the breast. *Cancer* 1993;72:2602–2611.
65. Middleton LP, Palacios DM, Bryant BR, et al. Pleomorphic lobular carcinoma: morphology, immunohistochemistry, and molecular analysis. *Am J Surg Pathol* 2000;24:1650–1656.
66. Fisher ER, Gregorio RM, Redmond C. Tubulolobular invasive breast cancer: a variant of lobular invasive cancer. *Hum Pathol* 1977;8:679–683.
67. Green I, McCormick B, Cranor M, et al. A comparative study of pure tubular and tubulolobular carcinoma of the breast. *Am J Surg Pathol* 1997;21:653–657.
68. Frable WJ, Kay S. Carcinoma of the breast—histologic and clinical features of apocrine tumors. *Cancer* 1968;21:756–763.
69. Tavassoli FA, Norris HJ. Intraductal apocrine carcinoma: a clinicopathologic study of 37 cases. *Mod Pathol* 1994;7:813–818.
70. Mossler JA, Barton TK, Brinkous AD, et al. Apocrine differentiation in human mammary carcinoma. *Cancer* 1980;46:2463–2471.
71. Ramos CV, Taylor HB. Lipid-rich carcinoma of the breast: a clinicopathologic analysis of 13 examples. *Cancer* 1974;33:812–819.
72. Varga Z, Robl C, Spycher M, et al. Metaplastic lipid-rich carcinoma of the breast. *Pathol Int* 1998; 48:912–916.
73. Toikkanen S, Joensuu K. Glycogen-rich clear cell carcinoma of the breast: a clinicopathologic and flow cytometric study. *Hum Pathol* 1991;22:81–83.
74. Hood CL, Fong RL, Zimmerman LE. Metastatic mammary carcinoma in the eyelid with histiocytoid appearance. *Cancer* 1973;31:793–800.
75. Walford N, ten Velden J. Histiocytoid breast carcinoma: an apocrine variant of lobular carcinoma. *Histopathology* 1989;14:515–522.
76. Cubilla AL, Woodruff JM. Primary carcinoid tumor of the breast: a report of eight patients. *Am J Surg Pathol* 1977;1:283–292.
77. Bussolati G, Papotti M, Sapino A, et al. Endocrine markers in argyrophilic carcinomas of the breast. *Am J Surg Pathol* 1987;11:248–256.
78. Taxy JB, Tischler AS, Insalaco SJ, et al. Carcinoid tumor of the breast: a variant of conventional breast cancer? *Hum Pathol* 1981;12:170–179.
79. Partanen S, Syrjanen K. Argyrophilic cells in carcinoma of the female breast. *Virchows Arch* 1981; 391:45–49.

80. Fetissof F, Duboid MP, Arbeille-Brassart B, et al. Argyrophylic cells in mammary carcinoma. *Hum Pathol* 1983;14:127–134.
81. Clayton F, Sibley RK, Ordonez NG, et al. Argyrophilic breast carcinomas: evidence of lactational differentiation. *Am J Surg Pathol* 1982;6:323–333.
82. Sapino A, Righi L, Cassoni P, et al. Expression of the neuroendocrine phenotype in carcinomas of the breast. *Semin Diagn Pathol* 2000;17:127–137.
83. Sapino A, Righi L, Cassoni P, et al. Expression of apocrine differentiation markers in neuroendocrine breast carcinomas of aged women. *Mod Pathol* 2001;14:768–776.
84. Shin SJ, DeLellis RA, Ying L, et al. Small cell carcinoma of the breast: a clinicopathologic and immunohistochemical study of nine patients. *Am J Surg Pathol* 2000;24:1231–1238.
85. McDivitt RW, Steward FW, Berg JW. *Atlas of tumor pathology*, fasc. 2, 2nd series. Washington: Armed Forces Institute of Pathology, 1968:22–48.
86. Harris M, Persaud V. Carcinosarcoma of the breast. *J Pathol* 1974;112:99–105.
87. Oberman HA. Metaplastic carcinoma of the breast: a clinicopathologic study of 29 cases. *Am J Surg Pathol* 1987;11:918–929.
88. Wargotz ES, Norris HJ. Metaplastic carcinomas of the breast. I. Matrix-producing carcinoma. *Hum Pathol* 1989;20:628–635.
89. Chieng C, Cranor M, Lesser ME, et al. Metaplastic carcinoma of the breast with osteocartilaginous heterologous elements. *Am J Surg Pathol* 1998;22:188–194.
90. Wargotz ES, Norris HJ. Metaplastic carcinomas of the breast. III. Carcinosarcoma. *Cancer* 1989;64: 1490–1499.
91. Gersell DJ, Katzenstein A. Spindle-cell carcinoma of the breast: a clinicopathologic and utlrastructural study. *Hum Pathol* 1981;12:550–561.
92. Wargotz ES, Deos PH, Norris HJ. Metaplastic carcinomas of the breast. II. Spindle cell carcinomas. *Hum Pathol* 1989;20:732–740.
93. Gobbi H, Simpson JF, Borowsky A, et al. Metaplastic breast tumors with a dominant fibromatosis-like phenotype have a high risk of local recurrence. *Cancer* 1999;85:2170–2182.
94. Agnantis NT, Rosen PP. Mammary carcinoma with osteoclast-like giant cells: a study of eight cases with follow-up data. *Am J Clin Pathol* 1979;72:383–389.
95. Rosen PP. Multinucleated mammary stromal giant cells: a benign lesion that stimulates invasive carcinoma. *Cancer* 1979;44:1305–1308.
96. Wargotz ES, Norris HJ. Metaplastic carcinoma of the breast. V. Metaplastic carcinoma with osteoclastic giant cells. *Hum Pathol* 1990;21:1142.
97. Fisher ER, Redmond C, Fisher B, et al. Pathologic findings from the National Surgical Adjuvant Breast Project. VIII. Relationship of chemotherapeutic responsiveness to tumor differentiation. *Cancer* 1983;51:181–191.
98. Toikkanen S. Primary squamous cell carcinoma of the breast. *Cancer* 1981;48:1629–1632.
99. Eusebi V, Lamovec J, Cattani MG, et al. Acantholytic variant of squamous-cell carcinoma of the breast. *Am J Surg Pathol* 1986;10:855–861.
100. Wargotz E, Norris H. Metaplastic carcinomas of the breast. IV. Squamous cell carcinoma of ductal origin. *Cancer* 1990;65:272–276.
101. Fisher E, Gragorio R, Palekar A, et al. Mucoepidermoid and squamous cell carcinoma of the breast with reference to squamous metaplasia and giant cell tumors. *Am J Surg Pathol* 1983;7:15–27.
102. Van Hoeven KH, Drudis T, Cranor ML, et al. Low-grade adenosquamous carcinoma of the breast. A clinicopathologic study of 32 cases with ultrastructural analysis. *Am J Surg Pathol* 1993;17: 248–258.

9

Prognosis and Systemic Therapy

After the diagnosis of invasive carcinoma has been histologically established, attention turns to determining the prognosis and determining the most effective form of therapy. Prognostic indicators are examined in four categories: patient characteristics, features of the primary tumor (T), regional spread or lymph node status (N), and evidence of distant spread (M). The summation of features is the TNM staging of the American Joint Commission on Cancer (AJCC), which is reproduced at the end of this chapter. Fitzgibbons et al. (1) ranked prognostic factors according to three categories: 1, proven to be important; 2, factors whose import remains to be established; and 3, not sufficiently studied to be of value. Category 1 included TNM, grade, type, mitotic figure counts, and steroid hormone receptors; category 2 included HER2/neu, proliferation, angiolymphatic invasion, and p53; and category 3 included ploidy, microvessel density, and other growth factors.

PATIENT CHARACTERISTICS

Several factors are known to contribute to differences in stage at the time of presentation. Patient demographics include age, race, family history with related germline abnormalities, and temporal association with lactation. These features were discussed in Chapter 2, but recall here that younger women have a worse prognosis than older women with the same histology. Nixon et al. (2) analyzed data on 1,398 breast cancer patients. The authors found that women who were younger than 35 years had a higher rate of recurrence and distant metastasis that was associated with higher histologic grade, lymphatic invasion, tumor necrosis, and negative estrogen receptor (ER) status.

In the United States, African-American women have been shown to present at a higher overall stage at a younger age (3). Hunter et al. (4) recently reported that approximately one-half of the difference could be accounted for by a combination of limited screening, especially by mammography, delay in diagnosis, and a higher nuclear grade.

Family history, particularly with the expression of the BRCA1 gene, may influence the course of the breast cancer. All of these features interact with the histology of the carcinoma. Crisp et al. (5) reported on 131 cases that were detected by screening. The authors found cancers that were of lower stage and grade than in 71 cases that were detected clinically during the same period. Women who are lactating, who are by definition, in a younger age group, present at a higher stage and therefore have a worse outcome. Breast cancer during pregnancy and lactation is known to be associated with higher stage at presentation. Hoover (6) reviewed the literature on this topic and concluded that 70% to 89% of pregnant or lactating women with breast cancer presented with axillary node metastases and the associated poor prognosis, although stage for stage, the prognosis was comparable for lactating and nonlactating women. Termination of the pregnancy was not found to improve the prognosis, although it was required for the administration of aggressive chemotherapy regimens. Korzeniowski and Dyba (7) reported on 1,885 patients with breast cancer and found that survival rates decreased with an increase in the number of pregnancies and deliveries.

Although many prognostic factors have been reported at 5- and 10-year survival rates, a study by Brinkley and Haylittle (8) found the death rate from breast cancer, in patients with a history of breast cancer more than 20 years before, to be 16 times that of women who had never had breast carcinoma.

FEATURES OF THE PRIMARY TUMOR

Prognostic features observed in the primary tumor include type (Chapter 8), size, grade, other nuclear features, histologic features, vascular invasion, proliferation, and expression of steroid hormone receptors and HER2/neu.

Size

After the histologic type is determined, perhaps the most important prognostic feature is the size of the primary carcinoma. Unfortunately, determination of tumor size is not a trivial exercise because breast cancers are 3-dimensional, usually stellate structures made of different components that elicit varying degrees of reaction and are resected as balls of partly fibrous and partly fatty tissue. Clinical size estimate is frequently exaggerated because of the inability to distinguish carcinoma from the surrounding normal breast tissue. Estimation of size by the radiologist is frequently underestimated, due to the merging of normal and malignant radiodensities. Gross examination for tumor size is usually a highly reliable determination of an invasive ductal carcinoma, but it may be a serious underestimation of an invasive lobular carcinoma. Histologic measurement is the most precise method for carcinomas that fit onto a single slide that measures 2 × 4 cm, but the size of larger tumors must be estimated from either the gross examination or the aggregation of size from adjacent blocks. Size of the invasive component is the determining prognostic factor, but *in situ* and invasive elements

TABLE 9.1. *Survival Rates of 1,411 Treated Breast Cancer Cases by Grade*

Grade	No. cases	5 yr	10 yr	15 yr	20 yr
1	363	81	62	49	41
2	640	50	37	31	26
3	408	35	25	21	21

From Bloom HJG, Field JR. Impact of tumor grade and host resistance on survival of women with breast cancer. *Cancer* 1971;28:1580–1589, with permission (12).

are usually intertwined in such a way that it is impossible to distinguish size for either component alone. In the 25% of cases in which the *in situ* and invasive carcinomas are separate, the size of the invasive component alone should be used for staging purposes (9). For staging, a transparent plastic ruler is an invaluable piece of equipment.

Grade

The most widely used grading system is that suggested by Bloom et al. (10–12). The authors identified three characteristics of carcinomas: (a) degree of cytoplasmic differentiation, as evident from the formation of ducts; (b) nuclear pleomorphism; and (c) nuclear hyperchromasia and mitotic activity. Tumors with scores of 3 to 5 were grade I, scores of 6 and 7 were grade II, and scores of 8 and 9 were grade III. Bloom and Richardson (11) found 5-, 10-, and 15-year survival rates for grade I of 75%, 47%, and 32%; for grade II of 53%, 27%, and 19%; and for grade III of 31%, 18%, and 10%. Bloom and Field (12) found similar data (Table 9.1). Wolff (13) confirmed these figures in treated patients, and Bloom et al. (14) confirmed the figures in untreated patients (Table 9.2). Elston and Ellis (15) further refined and defined the Bloom criteria for grading and reaffirmed their value in predicting survival rates of groups of cases of breast cancer (Table 9.3). The value of this modified grading system was confirmed by Clayton and Hopkins (16) in a series of 399 node-positive cases, but Theissig et al. (17) reported only 72% concurrence in grade among three observers.

Elston and Ellis (15) published the Nottingham modification of the Bloom and Richardson method, which involves estimation of the percentage of tubule formation, the degree of nuclear pleomorphism, and an accurate mitotic count, using a defined field area (Table 9.3). Tubules are assigned 1 to 3 points if they

TABLE 9.2. *Survival Rates of 86 Untreated Breast Cancer Cases by Grade*

Grade	No. cases	5 yr	10 yr	13 yr
1	23	30	16	13
2	32	30	4	—
3	31	0	—	—

From Bloom HJG (14).

TABLE 9.3. *Bloom Grade with Elston Amplification*

	Bloom	Elston
Tubules	1, 2, or 3	> 75%, 10–75%, < 10%
Pleomorphism	1, 2, or 3	Small and regular Large and varied
Hyperchromasia and mitotic figures	1, 2 or 3	9/10, 10–9, :20
Grade: 3, 4, or 5 = I; 6 or 7 = II; 8 or 9 = III		

form greater than 75%, 10 to 75%, or less than 10% of the tumor. Point 1 nuclei are small regular and uniform, point 2 nuclei are moderately increased in size and variability, and point 3 nuclei have marked variation. Mitotic counts are field size dependent and two Leitz and one Nikon fields are given as illustrations. The number of mitotic figures per 10 fields for 1 point is 0 to 11; 2 points, 6 to 22; and 3 points, greater than 11 to 23, depending on fields that range in size from 0.44 to 0.63 mm in diameter. Calibration for field size is needed to employ this counting method. Grade I carcinomas are 3 to 5 points; grade II, 6 or 7 points; and grade III, 8 or 9 points. Recurrence-free survival from grade I carcinomas at 5 and 10 years is 75% and 64%, respectively; grade II carcinomas, 50% and 40%, respectively; and grade III carcinomas, 40% and 38%, respectively. Studies by Dalton et al. (18–19) addressed pathologist disagreement on grade. The authors found good prognostication if total point count was used, but less relationship to outcome if only the three grades were given.

Fisher et al. (20) described a grading scheme that utilizes nuclear and histologic features. Grade I nuclei are defined as uniform and small, without evident nucleoli, and they resemble those of normal duct cells. Grade III nuclei are large, pleomorphic, and hyperchromatic. Grade II nuclei are uniform, medium in size, and contain nucleoli. Histologic differentiation is based on the presence or absence of ducts (tubules or adenocystic structures). Histologic grades are assigned as follows: Grade I has nuclear grade I and ducts; grade III has nuclear grade II or grade III, but no ducts; and grade II is nuclear grade II or grade III with duct formation or nuclear grade II without ducts. In the series by Fisher et al. (21), only 3% of cases were grade I, 30% were grade II, and 67% were grade III. Five-year disease-free survival was 95% in grade I, 75% in grade II, and 60% in grade III. Nuclear and histologic grades can be separately reported for the Fisher scheme, and nuclear grade correlates better with outcome (21) than histologic or combined grade. Table 9.4 compares the Bloom and Fisher schemes. Overall, survival was better in the series of Fisher et al. (20) than in the series of Bloom and Richardson (11). In Chapter 8, grades of the carcinomas are given in the figure legends. (See Figs. 9.1 to 9.3 and efigs. 9.1 to 9.6).

The Nottingham index incorporates tumor size, stage, and grade into a single number that is highly predictive of survival, but lymph node status must be known in order to calculate this index (Table 9.5) (22).

TABLE 9.4. *Comparison of Bloom and Fisher grading schemes*

Grade	Bloom	Fisher
1	75% survival Little to moderate nuclear or mitotic activity Extensive duct formation	95% survival Nuclear grade 1 Duct formation
2	47% survival Moderate nuclear pleomorphism, hyperchromasia, and mitotic activity Little or no duct formation	75% survival Nuclear grade 2 or 3 with duct formation or nuclear grade 1 with no duct formation
3	32% survival Marked nuclear pleomorphism, hyperchromasia, and mitotic activity Little or no duct formation	60% survival Nuclear grade 2 or 3 No duct formation

Henson et al. (23) reviewed 22,616 cases and found that grade and stage (size) were not independent of each other. As breast cancers increase in size, the grade also increases. Carcinomas smaller than 0.5 cm were predominantly in grade I and grade II, whereas those between 3 and 3.9 cm in diameter were predominantly grade III.

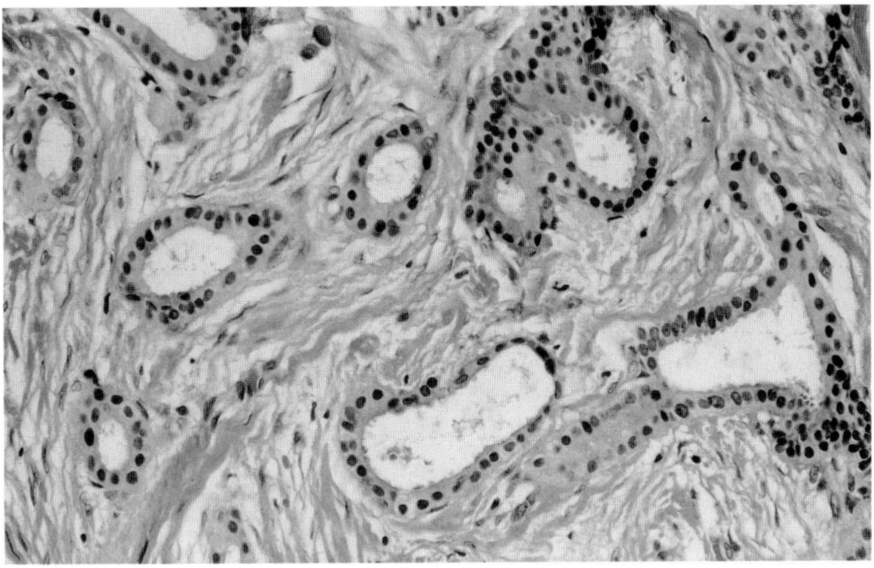

FIG. 9.1. Low grade invasive carcinoma. The nuclei are similar in size, small, round, and hyperchromatic. Mitotic figures are not present. All of the cancer cells form ductal structures.

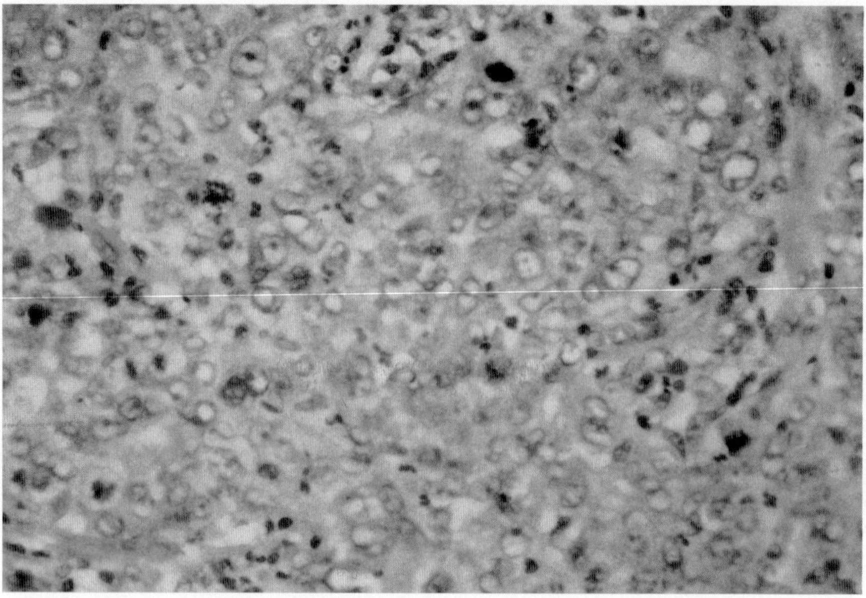

FIG. 9.2. Invasive carcinoma, high grade. The nuclei are irregular and pleomorphic and mitotic figures are present. No ducts are formed.

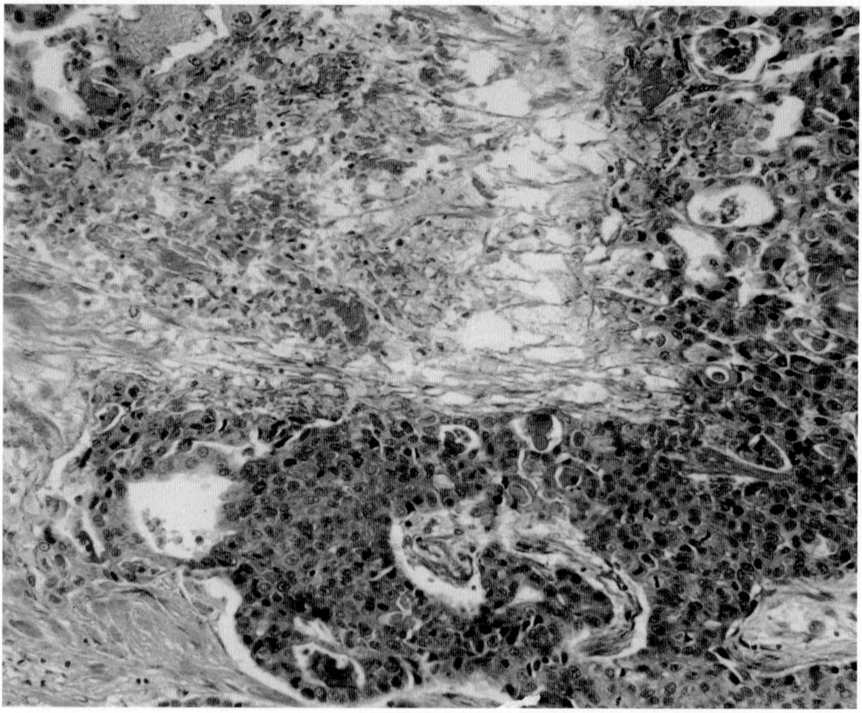

FIG. 9.3. Invasive carcinoma with tumor necrosis. A large field of tumor necrosis or apoptosis is evident in the center of this invasive carcinoma.

TABLE 9.5. *Nottingham prognostic index*

Index[a]	Annual mortality
<3.4	3%
3.5–5.3	7%
>5.3	30%

[a]Size –0.2 + lymph node stage (1–3) + grade (1–3).

Nuclear Features and Growth Rate

Subjective microscopic observations of nuclear morphology and mitotic counts can be supplemented with data derived by other techniques. The relative number of tumor cells in the S-phase (chromosomal replication) can be estimated from the thymidine-labeling index (TLI) by autoradiography of fresh tissue slides, or by staining and analysis with flow or static cytometry or by immunohistochemistry. McDivitt et al. (24) reported good correlation between S-phase estimates and S-phase measurements. Ploidy also may be estimated from flow cytometry. Meyer and Coplin (25) and Silvestrini et al. (26) documented a higher rate of relapse in node-negative patients with high S-phase values that were determined by TLI. Tubiani et al. (27) found TLI most predictive of survival in 128 breast cancer patients in stages I, II, and III. McDivitt et al. (24) studied ploidy, ER and progesterone receptor (PR) status, and TLI. The authors correlated these parameters with histologic parameters. Of 168 breast cancers, 45% were diploid, with a mean S-phase fraction (SPF) of 5.2%, compared with 10.3% for aneuploid carcinomas. ER-negative tumors had a higher SPF, but no higher incidence of aneuploidy. Necrosis in the invasive carcinoma, poor cytologic differentiation, aneuploidy, and high SPF correlated well, but neither ploidy nor SPF correlated with either tumor size or lymph node status. Dabbs (28) and Frierson (29) showed that ploidy and S-phase correlate well with nuclear and histologic grades that are derived from sections (Table 9.6).

Other authors have found aneuploidy to be a significant correlate of larger higher-stage breast cancers. Hedley et al. (30) documented this finding from

TABLE 9.6. *Flow cytometry data versus grade*

Grade[a]	No. cases	Aneuploid	S-phase fraction
1	8	0	0.6–4.8
2	21	29%	0.9–4.7
3	53	83%	5–26
Grade[b]	**No. cases**	**Aneuploid**	
1	30	40%	
2	48	70%	
3	40	83%	

[a]Dabbs et al. (28).
[b]Frierson et al. (29).

archival material in paraffin blocks by flow cytometry. Dressler et al. (31) reported on a study of 1,331 frozen samples of breast cancers for ER and PR, S-phase, and ploidy. Fifty-seven percent of the tumors were aneuploid, with a higher SPF (10.3%) than the diploid tumors (2.6%). Aneuploidy and high SPF correlated with ER and PR negativity, which has been shown elsewhere to correlate with poorer prognosis. High S-phase values in diploid, but not aneuploid, tumors correlated with positive axillary lymph nodes.

Data demonstrating that S-phase and, to a lesser extent, ploidy are important prognostic indicators that are independent of other prognostic information in node-negative cases are shown in Tables 9.6. Data concerning ploidy in node-negative and node-positive cases, and S-phase data in node-positive cases, are not as uniformly indicative of prognosis (32). Arnerlov et al. (33) and Arnerlov et al. (34) reported correlation between ploidy, S-phase, and the rate of tumor growth, as measured mammographically.

Other methods of estimating the rate of proliferation by cancer cells include immunostaining of nuclei for Ki-67 and proliferating cell nuclear antigen (PCNA), either of which may be semiquantitated by image analysis. Dervan et al. (35) showed correlation between estimates of cycling activity that were derived from immunostaining fresh frozen tissue for Ki-67 and from the immunostaining of paraffin-embedded material for PCNA. Isola et al. (36) found correlation between Ki-67 staining, S-phase, and mitotic counts. Other reports have shown (37–39) correlation of levels of proliferation antigens and prognosis. Measures of cell cycle activity, including p16, retinoblastoma, p53, cyclin D (40,41), and telomerase (42), also have been studied in breast cancer and have been found to correlate with prognosis.

Histologic Features

Fisher et al. (43) described the correlation of treatment failure with certain histologic characteristics of the carcinoma. A higher rate of treatment failure was associated with necrosis, an infiltrative border, and lymphatic or perineural invasion.

Several groups have attempted to establish a grading system by combining some of these characteristics. Fisher et al. (43) found correlations between prognosis and the degree of tumor differentiation, blood vessel invasion, patient age, and tumor size. Fisher et al. (21) found an increased responsiveness to chemotherapy in poorly differentiated carcinomas. Silverberg and Chitale (44) found a correlation in survival between relative amounts of intraductal and infiltrating ductal carcinomas. Among 14 patients in whom intraductal carcinoma was present in the absence of invasive cancer, there were no lymph node metastases, and the raw 5-year survival rate was 78.6%. Among 133 patients with carcinomas that were purely invasive, without an intraductal component, 58% had axillary lymph node metastases, and the 5-year survival rate was only 45%. There was a gradation between these two extremes that correlated with the percentage of the carcinoma that was invasive. Black et al. (45) found that the prognostically favorable features were nuclear grade, lymphocytic infiltration, perivenous groups of lymphocytes, and sinus histiocytosis in the lymph nodes.

Lane et al. (46) examined 241 cases of invasive carcinoma, excluding papillary and mucoid types. The authors divided the tumors into those that had a circumscribed contour from those that had an irregular or invasive contour. Tumors with a circumscribed contour were one-third larger, on average, than the irregular tumors. Eighty percent of the patients with circumscribed carcinomas were alive at 10 years, compared to only 38% of those with infiltrative contours. Kouchoukas et al. (47) found a similar difference in survival, depending on the type of margin. There was a significant difference in the incidence of axillary lymph node metastases when the more favorable carcinomas, which had pushing margins, were compared with the less favorable carcinomas, which had infiltrating margins; however, there was no difference in the survival rates between the two groups when they were corrected for stage.

Carter et al. (48) divided invasive ductal carcinomas into groups, depending on the nature of the border of the carcinoma and the presence or absence of necrosis within the tumor. The 10-year survival rate for patients with tumors that contained necrosis was only 35%, compared with 56% in those patients without evident necrosis. The necrotic tumor group had a 63% incidence of positive axillary lymph nodes, and the nonnecrotic tumors were associated with positive lymph nodes in only 42% of the cases. The survival rates of axillary node-positive patients were 19% with necrotic tumors and 43% for nonnecrotic tumors. Among 69 patients who were treated by radical mastectomy for necrotic tumors with an infiltrative margin, the incidence of axillary lymph node metastases was 75%. The survival rate in those patients with axillary lymph node metastases was 15%, and the overall 10-year survival rate was 29%. In 61 patients who were treated by radical mastectomy for circumscribed tumors without necrosis, 30% had axillary lymph node metastases. The survival rate at 10 years in those patients with axillary lymph node metastases was 44%, and the overall 10-year survival rate was 61%. Patients with nonnecrotic tumors with infiltrative margins and circumscribed tumors with necrosis present fell between these two extremes. When tumor size was analyzed according to border and necrosis, the 10-year survival rate of patients who had circumscribed nonnecrotic tumors did not decrease with the increase of the size of the primary carcinoma, but there was marked reduction in the 10-year survival rate with increasing size of the primary tumor in those tumors with necrosis and infiltrative borders (efigs. 9.7 to 9.9).

VASCULAR INVASION AND MICROVASCULAR DENSITY

Lymphatic or vascular invasion by carcinoma in the breast parenchyma is considered by some observers to be an excellent indicator of lymph node metastases (49,50), but Kister et al. (51) did not find it an important prognostic factor in the absence of lymph node metastases, and Gilchrist et al. (52) found so much variation among observers of this phenomenon that they doubted its reliability.

Immunohistochemical (IHC) staining for endothelial cells may help to clarify this observation. The clinical significance of vascular/lymphatic invasion in the breast remains unclear (Figs. 9.4 to 9.6 and efigs. 9.10 to 9.14). It is not considered in determining stage, but it correlates strongly with node status. Pinder et al. (53) investigated a consecutive series of 1,704 cases of primary operable invasive breast cancer for the presence of vascular/lymphatic invasion, as assessed on hematoxylin and eosin sections. The presence of vascular invasion, which was seen in 23% of the cases, correlated highly with lymph node metastases, tumor size, histologic grade, and tumor type. It also correlated highly with decreased survival and local recurrence of tumor.

Inflammatory breast cancer is T4d and is histologically diagnosed by finding carcinoma in dermal lymphatics. Ellis and Teitelbaum (54) distinguished breast cancers in which the overlying skin showed rubor and calor from those in which the dermal lymphatics were permeated by carcinoma. In most cases, the inflammatory clinical appearance was associated with permeation of the dermal lymphatics, but this is not always true. In the series by Meyer et al. (55), 20% of the patients with clinically inflamed skin had no dermal lymphatic involvement and 14% of those patients were alive at 5 years. Dermal lymphatic involvement, whether associated with clinical inflammation or not, was considered to be histologic evidence of inflammatory breast cancer (Fig. 9.6 and efig. 9. 15) (56–58). Dermal invasion is T4 (efig. 9.16).

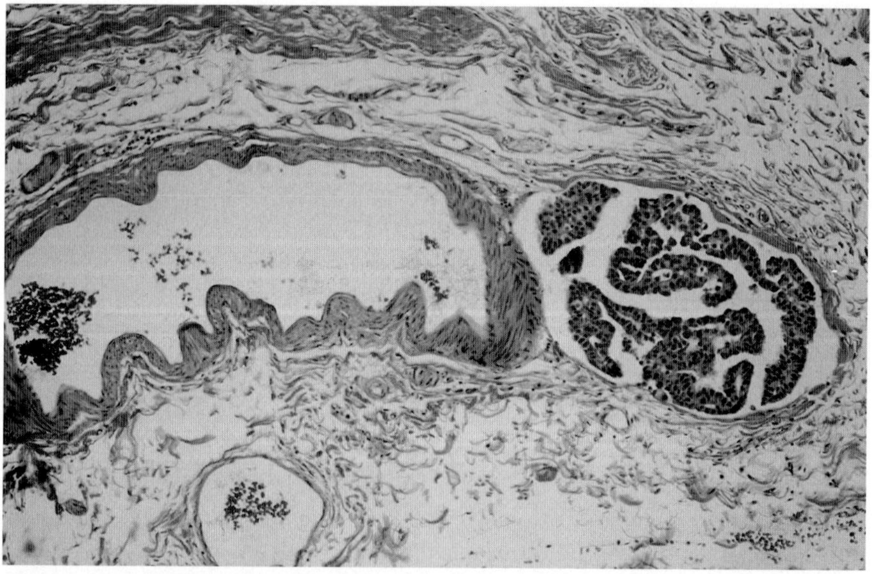

FIG. 9.4. Vascular invasion. The space adjacent to this small vein is identified as an angiolymphatic channel by the presence of endothelial cells. Location next to the vein suggests that it is a lymphatic. It is filled with metastatic carcinoma in a micropapillary configuration.

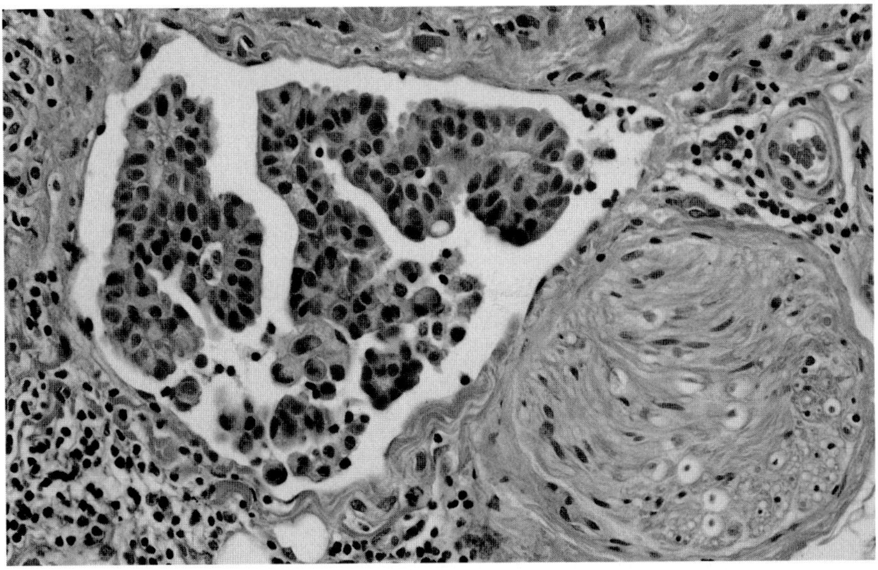

FIG. 9.5. Vascular invasion. This angiolymphatic space is lined by endothelial cells and is located next to a nerve. It is filled with carcinoma with a papillary configuration and low nuclear grade. In the breast stroma, the invasive carcinoma had a higher nuclear grade.

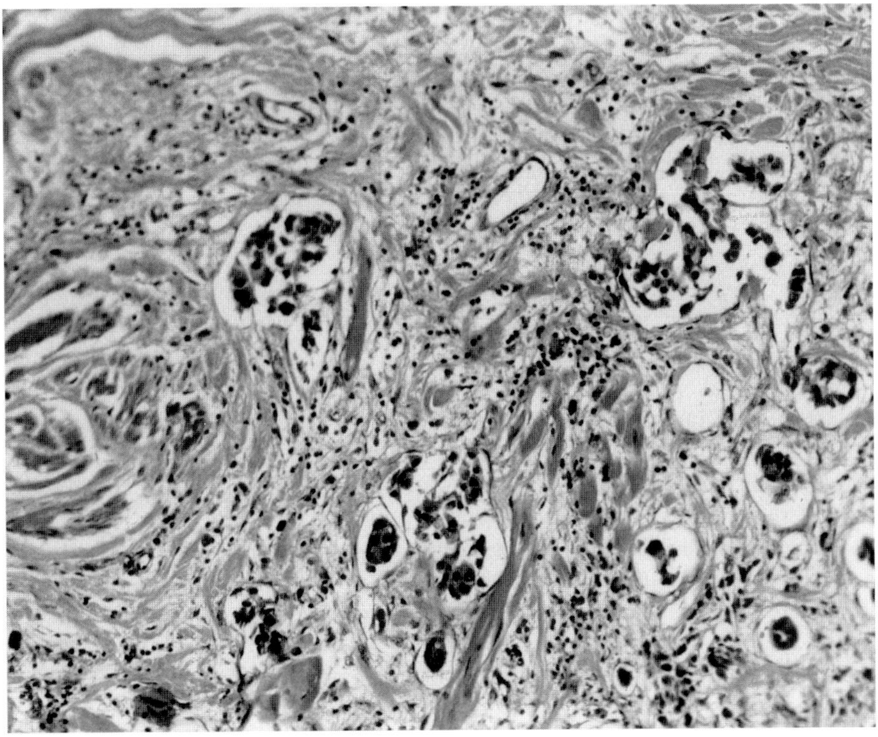

FIG. 9.6. Inflammatory carcinoma. Numerous groups of cancer cells fill and distend the lymphatics in the dermis of the nipple, identifiable by bands of smooth muscle. This finding is the histologic definition of inflammatory breast cancer.

Weidner et al. (59,60) described the relationship of microvascular density (MVD) with metastasis as a prognostic indicator. Using a prospective study of 165 consecutively resected breast cancers, the sections were stained with immunoperoxidase technique for factor VIII related antigen. Sections of the breast tumor that were stained with hematoxylin and eosin were used to select representative areas of the invasive component with a "hot spot"—the area in which the most active neovascularization had occurred. The number of microvessels per field at a magnification of 200 was counted. These findings were correlated with axillary lymph node status and overall and disease-free survival over an average follow-up of 51 months. All 17 patients with a microvessel density count greater than 100 relapsed during the period of observation. Five percent of the 30 patients with 33 or fewer microvessels relapsed. The 101 patients with intermediate numbers of blood vessels had an intermediate survival. Bosari et al. (61) described a similar study of 88 node-negative carcinomas and 32 node-positive carcinomas. The authors selected the three most vascular areas within a tumor and counted the microvessels within a microscopic field at a magnification of 200. The node-positive carcinomas had a significantly higher microvessel count than did the node-negative cases (99 versus 73). In the node-negative group, followed for 9 years, the patients with tumors having the higher microvessel density counts had a higher incidence of distant recurrence than did those with lower counts. A similar experience was found in the node-positive group. In this study, microvessel density associations with recurrence were independent of ploidy, S-phase, and other histologic parameters, with the exception of peritumoral vascular invasion. Other studies have not confirmed the prognostic utility of MVD, however (62,63).

Vascular endothelial growth factor (VEGF) is a major factor in neoangiogenesis that is related to proliferating cancer cells, and its expression by malignant cells is a predictor of both increased angiogenesis and poor prognosis (64–66).

Estrogen and Progesterone Receptors

Estrogen and progesterone play major roles in normal breast physiology, as discussed in Chapter 1. Battersby et al. (67) studied normal breast tissue and reported that progestins that occurred in the second part of the menstrual cycle were responsible for downregulating ERs. PRs did not vary in normal cycles, but increased with oral contraceptive use. ER and PR levels decrease as a function of the interval since last pregnancy. Expression of ER and PR in invasive carcinoma correlates positively with survival (Table 9.7) (68,69) and is an important indicator of the likelihood of response to hormonal manipulation. Estrogen inhibitors have been shown to decrease recurrence in both breasts when the index carcinoma is ER positive (70) and they have been shown to decrease the incidence of carcinoma in women at high risk for breast cancer (71).

Expression of ER also has been shown to correlate inversely with the rate of cellular reproduction (72). Ballare et al. (73) studied 14 PR-positive carcinomas and found that 69% of the cells that were synthesizing DNA were not expressing PR protein. Determination of the ER and PR levels in breast cancer has become part of the standard pathology work-up. The pathologist is in the best position to select material for ER and PR assays at the time of diagnosis of carcinoma. Although immunohistochemistry is now the most commonly employed methodology for steroid hormone receptor assay, the steroid-binding assay established the extensive correlation of numerical levels with response to therapy. An alternate method is enzyme immunoassay, which provides data that correlate well with steroid-binding assays, is less affected by endogenous steroids, and can be done on small samples, including needle aspirates.

Several monoclonal antibodies are available for the IHC evaluation of steroid hormone receptors on paraffin sections (74). McCarty et al. (75) reported that the correlation of IHC positivity to therapeutic response rates was comparable to those reported for biochemical assays when using fresh tissue or cells. Poulsen et al. (76), Andersen et al. (69), and Cheng et al. (77) addressed the problems of sensitivity of assays of fixed tissue and ways in which it may be enhanced, including the use of trypsin or pronase (Fig. 9.7 and efigs. 9.17 and 9.18).

Allred et al. reviewed the literature that compares ER analysis by IHC with the dextran-coated charcoal assay (DCCA) in 1990 (78) and again in 1998 (68). In 2,837 cases in which frozen sections were used for IHC, concordance ranged from 77% to 93%, with an average concordance of 86%. In 470 cases in which

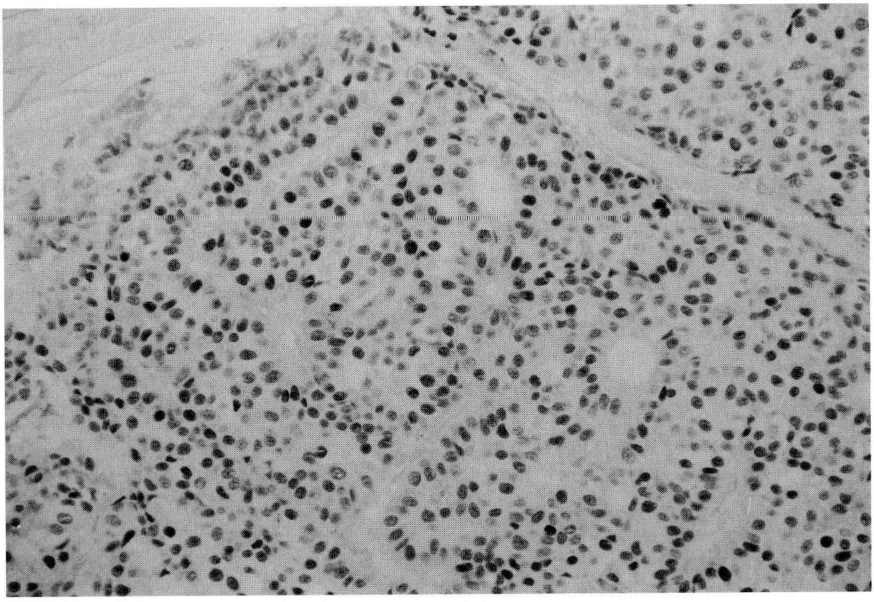

FIG. 9.7. Estrogen receptor expression. Immunostain for estrogen receptor demonstrates that the great majority of the nuclei are intensely stained with antibody to estrogen receptor protein. Staining is restricted to the nuclei.

paraffin sections were used for IHC, concordance ranged from 82% to 96%, with an average of 88%. On fine needle aspirated material from 423 cases, the range was 76% to 93%, with an average of 83%. About one-half of the discordant cases were ER-ICA-positive and DCCA-negative. At 3 years, disease-free survival of ER-ICA-positive cases was 76%, compared with 40% for ER-ICA-negative cases. Review of more recent data (68,79) shows good correlation among methods and that IHC staining is predictive of therapeutic response.

Pertschuk et al. (80) reported on ER-ICA and PR-ICA on frozen sections and found them to correlate well with DCCA ER and PR levels and with response to therapy in 600 cases. Colloid carcinoma was most likely to be ER/PR-positive and medullary carcinoma was least likely. The incidence of ER-ICA positivity increased with age. Five years after diagnosis, ER-ICA-positive cases had 74% disease-free survival, compared with 52% for ER-ICA-negative cases; PR-ICA-positive cases were 82% disease-free at 5 years, compared with 42% for PR-ICA-negative cases. PR-ICA was thus the better prognostic indicator.

In the report by Keshgegian and Cnaan (81), ER and PR positivity correlated with lower grade, lower S-phase, and a lower incidence of aneuploidy.

In 1993, Battifora et al. (82) reported that ER-ICA on paraffin sections had a concordance rate of 94% with DCCA and that the discordant cases were more accurately assayed by ER-ICA. Because of its greater ease of use and more universal applicability, Esteban et al. (83–86) and Taylor (87) reported that IHC had become the standard assay for steroid hormone receptors. Barnes and Millis (88) reviewed the history of methodology for assay of steroid hormone receptors in 1995 and concluded that immunohistochemistry had achieved dominance.

Leers and Nap (89) reported that diploid carcinomas had higher ER (81%) and PR (76%) levels than aneuploid carcinomas (47% for both). In nondiploid carcinomas, the diploid component had an ER of 66% and a PR of 62%, whereas the aneuploid component was 38% ER positive and 39% PR positive, which indicated a heterogeneous distribution of steroid hormone receptors in aneuploid carcinomas.

Several newer antibodies to ER have become available and, in general, are more "sensitive" because they stain more cells in more cases (90). It is not known how accurate each antibody is without outcome data that relates staining

TABLE 9.7. *Survival by estrogen receptor or progesterone receptor*

Status	5-yr survival
ER+	64%
ER–	24%
PR+	59%
PR–	40%

ER, estrogen receptor; PR, progesterone receptor.

to response to therapy, which may take years to accumulate. The studies reported by Rhodes et al. (91–93) indicate that reliability and reproducibility of immunostaining is good when there is strong expression of ER, but both decrease with a decreasing level of expression. False negative results, which indicate an inappropriately poor prognosis and deny the patient antiestrogen therapy, are more common and more worrisome than false positive results.

In our laboratory, positive and negative ER controls, as well as a positive antigenecity stain (factor VIII related antigen for the ubiquitous blood vessels), are done. Slides that contain invasive and *in situ* carcinoma and benign epithelium are chosen preferentially for immunostaining, and the score of all three components is reported. When there is no staining of any of the components and the factor VIII related antigen stain is negative, the procedure is repeated before a negative result is reported (efigs. 9.19 and 9.20).

Estrogen has been sequenced and found to have two forms, the classic alpha form that is assayed by most monoclonal antibodies and a beta form. Its gene is divided into 8 exons that encode a 65-kD protein with ligand-binding and DNA-binding domains. Activation by ligand leads to phosphorylation and dimerization to form a complex that activates transcription of target genes. ER beta is capable of heterodimerization with ER alpha, allowing for interactions between the two forms that may be of clinical significance (94).

HER2/neu

Slamon et al. (95) investigated the level of c-erbB-2–HER2/neu oncogene in 106 patients with primary breast cancer. The authors found a significant increase in the incidence of neu gene amplification in primary tumors of patients with metastatic carcinoma in more than three axillary lymph nodes, compared to the incidence of neu in carcinomas with negative or fewer than three positive axillary lymph nodes.

A second study (96) of 86 axillary node-positive patients who were followed for a median of 46 months showed amplification of the neu oncogene in 40% of cases, with a statistically significant correlation between the degree of gene amplification and mortality and shortened time to relapse. Gene rearrangement did not appear to be the mechanism of activation, because it was found in only 3 of the 189 tumors studied; in 2 of the 3 cases, neu was also amplified. Epidermal growth factor receptor oncogene was amplified in only 4 of the 189 cases.

Varley et al. (97) examined neu in tissue from 41 breast carcinomas. Amplification of neu sequences was observed in 7 of the 41 breast carcinomas, at a level of 5- to 40-fold. Rearrangements of the neu gene were not noted. Amplification of neu sequences was noted in the lymph node metastases from primary carcinomas with amplified neu sequences, but the levels of amplification were lower in the metastases than in the primary tumor. The authors also found a striking correlation between neu amplification and poor short-term prognosis. Even though the correlation between poor prognosis and neu amplification was strong, the authors noted no correlation between neu amplification and class, grade, estrogen status, menopausal status, or stage of disease. Slamon et al. (96) noted a correlation between neu amplification and positive ER, but not with PR status.

Van de Vijver et al. (98) detected amplification of the human neu oncogene in 16 of 95 invasive mammary carcinomas that were accompanied by overexpression of neu complementary mRNA. Van de Vijver et al. (99) compared IHC staining for neu protein with known gene copy numbers in 189 cases and found that staining correlated with gene amplification, but only 14% of the cases were stained, and positivity did not correlate with nodal status or disease-free survival. It did correlate with tumor size. Forty-two percent of 45 cases of comedocarcinoma were immunohistochemically stained when antibodies to neu protein were used, but none of the other types of ductal carcinoma *in situ* (DCIS) were stained.

Press et al. (100) reviewed the expression of HER2/neu in fetal and normal tissues and found high levels in fetal tissues and normal levels in cells of the gastrointestinal, respiratory, reproductive, and urinary tracts, as well as in the skin, breast, and placenta. HER2/neu was reported by Soomro et al. (101) in cases of ductal carcinoma, but not in cases of mucinous, medullary, tubular, cribriform, and papillary carcinoma (i.e., those types of breast cancer with a relatively good prognosis).

The association of HER2/neu amplification and/or overexpression with prognosis is varied across the literature. Press and Pike (102) matched 105 patients with recurrent breast cancer with 105 women who had no recurrence and they used immunohistochemistry to assess HER2/neu expression in archival tissue blocks. Overexpression was found in 41 of 105 relapse cases, but it was found in only 21 of 105 matched disease-free controls. Rilke et al. (103) studied 1,210 archival surgical specimens, with a follow-up for 19 years. Overexpression of the p185 protein that is encoded by HER2/neu showed a negative impact on survival in node-positive but not in node-negative cases. Toikkanen et al. (104) looked at another group of cases with a median follow-up of 30 years and found that HER2/neu expression predicted poor survival among node-positive cases. Tsuda et al. (105) studied 176 consecutive cases of breast cancer retrospectively and found that the copy number of c-erbB-2 strongly correlated with the histologic grade, number of mitotic figures, and degree of nuclear atypia, but its prognostic effect was absorbed within histologic grade when a multiple regression analysis was carried out. Battifora et al. (106) found correlation of decreased overall survival and decreased disease-free survival among 245 stage I and stage II neu-positive breast cancers that were studied by immunohistochemistry on paraffin-embedded tissue, but the decreased survival was found only in a group of low-stage low-nuclear grade patients. Allred et al. (107) also found poor survival in a subset of neu-positive node-negative cases with small ER-positive, predominantly invasive, carcinomas.

Parkes et al. (108) found no significant correlation between the overexpression of c-erbB-2, messenger RNA, and clinical behavior in 70 patients. Rosen et al. (109) reviewed IHC staining for HER2/neu in 440 node-negative cases with a median follow-up of 10 years and found no correlation with prognosis. The authors did find that only 10% of medullary carcinomas stained for HER2/neu, whereas one-half of the ductal and lobular carcinomas were stained. Clark and McGuire (110) studied 362 tumors from patients with both node-positive and node-negative breast cancer. Thirty-two percent of the node-negative patients and 31% of the node-positive patients had amplification of the HER2/neu oncogene. Amplification did not correlate with disease-free or overall survival. Pierce and Merino (111) studied 107 paraffin-embedded specimens by immunohistochemistry from a group of stage I or stage II breast cancers from randomized trial. Overexpression of c-erbB-2 did not predict for recurrent disease in this group.

Press et al. (112) suggested that the variation in the prognostic value of immunostaining for HER2/neu may be a consequence of different antibodies and techniques that are used in retrospective analyses. The authors surveyed 7 polyclonal and 21 monoclonal antibodies and found that the ability to detect overexpression of neu was extremely variable when paraffin-embedded sections were used. DiGiovanna and Stern (113) suggested that the variation in correlation with prognosis may be a result of variability in the activation of p185 and they described an antibody to a specifically activated tyrosine-phosphorylated form of p185.

Lehrer et al. (114) reported a correlation of HER2/neu protein levels with a significantly increased likelihood of a family history of breast cancer, but Borresen et al. (115), reviewing a larger series of cases, found no correlation between a positive history of breast cancer and c-erbB-2 amplification.

The ability of HER2/neu to predict for response to specific types of chemotherapy is more important than its prognostic value. Application of trastuzumab (Herceptin) therapy for human breast cancers that are characterized by the overexpression of p185 is now in clinical use, as is the IHC assay for neu to predict for response. Trastuzumab is a humanized monoclonal antibody to the extracellular domain of HER2/neu receptor, which inhibits growth of cancer cells that overexpress HER2/neu. Use of the antibody in ongoing, and planned clinical trials were reviewed by Perez and Hortobagyi (116) and McKeage and Perry (117).

Neu expression also may predict for response to chemotherapy, with the use of topoisomerase II inhibitors (doxorubicin and epirubicin). HER2/neu oncogene and topoisomerase II are located on adjacent loci, at 17q12-q21, and amplification of neu may indicate a similar amplification of topoisomerase II. Neu expression also has been shown to indicate a loss of response to tamoxifen therapy. At the present time, there remains considerable discussion of methodology for the HER2/neu assay, which most accurately predicts response to immunotherapy or chemotherapy. The utilization of an IHC assay for expression of p185, for determination of neu expression (Figs. 9.8 and 9.9 and efigs. 9.21 to 9.23) and of fluorescent *in situ* hybridization (FISH) technique, which deter-

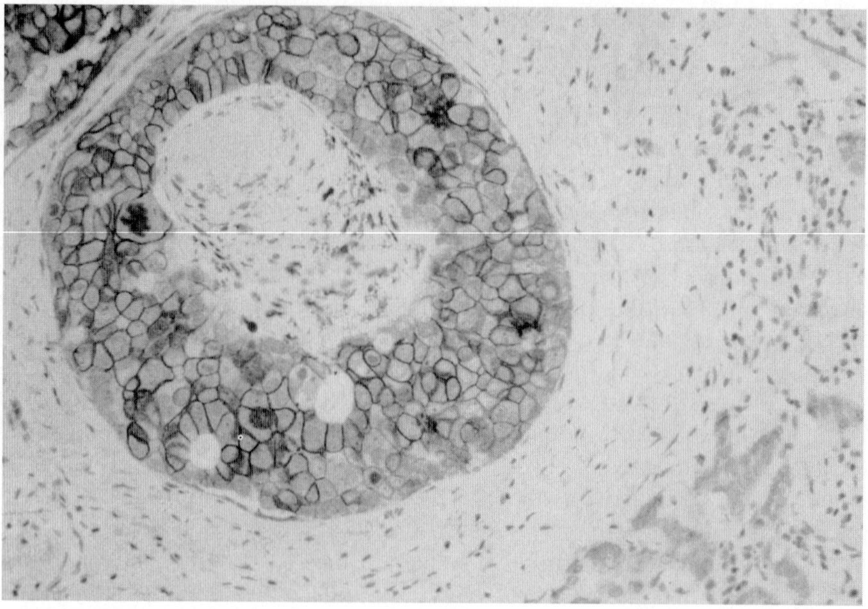

FIG. 9.8. HER2/neu immunoreactivity. Comedocarcinoma is immunohistochemically stained for HER2/neu in an entirely membranous pattern. Note that the ductal carcinoma *in situ* is stained, but the invasive component (**lower right**) is unstained.

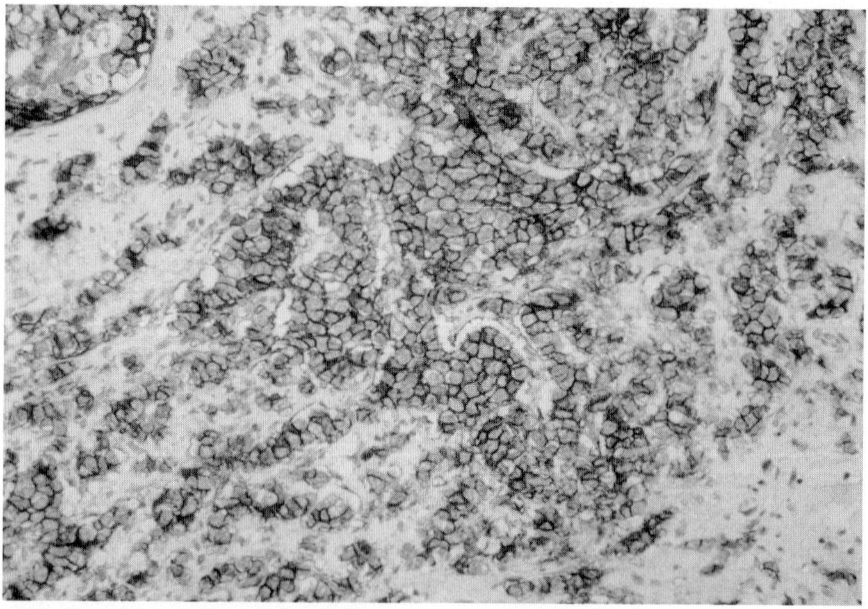

FIG. 9.9. HER2/neu expression. In this carcinoma, the invasive component is universally stained robustly in a membranous pattern.

mines amplification (efig. 9.24), or the most efficient combination of these two methods, has not yet been settled (118–123).

Lymph Node Status

Lymph node status is usually the prime determinant of stage in operable breast cancer, and evaluation of the histology of axillary lymph nodes is of critical importance in prognosis and in determining the need for adjuvant chemotherapy, at least in premenopausal women.

Fisher et al. (124) found that patients with three or fewer positive nodes had no significant decrease in survival, compared with those with negative nodes. This was confirmed in a large study that had an extended follow-up (21). Although differences between patients with three axillary lymph node metastases and those with four seemed difficult to accept conceptually, there appeared to be statistical justification for making this stepwise grouping to increase the number of cases in subsets of study groups. However, studies by Fisher et al. (124) showed a progressive linear decrease in survival with each increment in the number of positive nodes (Table 9.8).

Because the number of positive nodes correlates with survival, physicians who excise and examine nodes would be well advised to read the excellent article by Wilkinson and Hause (125) on the statistical probability of finding metastases of various sizes. The authors studied a geometric model to determine the probability of finding a metastasis in a lymph node section. The likelihood of success varied both with the size of the metastasis and the size of the node. When a single section is taken through the center of a lymph node, the probability of finding a peripherally located 2-mm metastasis in a 5-mm node is 73%; however, in a 10-mm lymph node, the probability is only 30% (Figs. 9.10 and 9.11 and efigs. 9.25 to 9.29). The authors suggested that nodes be cut into four or more pieces and embedded on nonfacing surfaces. When sectioned in this manner, the probability of finding a 2-mm metastasis in a 5-mm node is 100% and, in a 10-mm node, the probability is 82%. These probabilities indicate that small axillary lymph node metastases may be inapparent after what most pathologists would consider an intensive histologic examination. This level of uncertainty should figure into any discussion of staging data. Larger metastases (efigs. 9.30 and 9.31) are found much more readily.

TABLE 9.8. *Disease-free survival according to number of positive axillary lymph nodes*

No. positive nodes	5-yr survival
0	85%
1	64%
2	57%
3	57%
4	40%

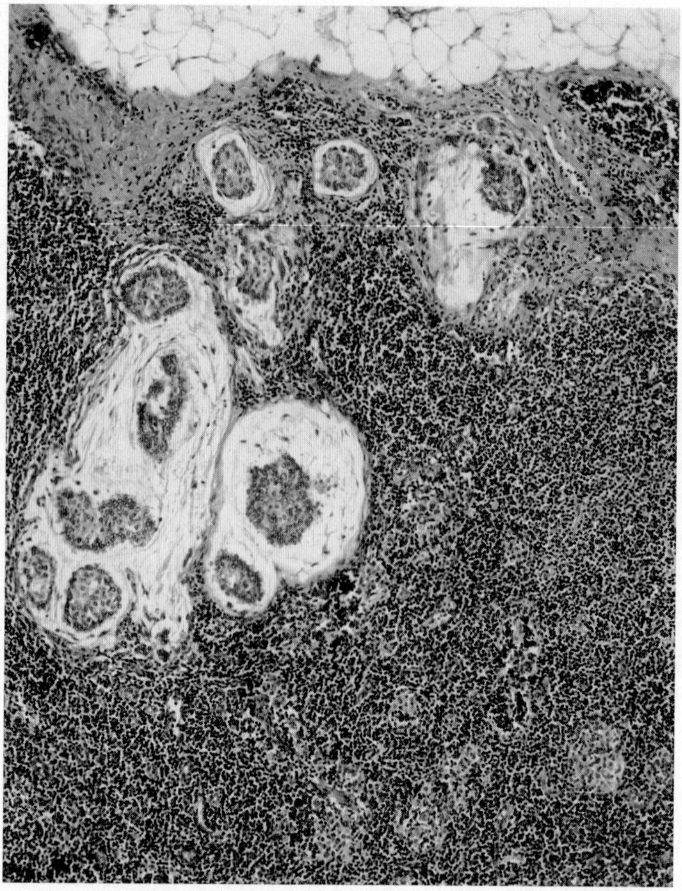

FIG. 9.10. Metastatic colloid carcinoma. Although unusual, metastases of colloid carcinoma may be found. This increase in stage diminishes the otherwise good prognosis of colloid carcinoma. In this photomicrograph, the micrometastases are less than 2 mm in diameter, but they are clearly evident from the pools of mucus that surround the groups of cancer cells.

Metastatic spread beyond the capsule into axillary connective tissue should be noted as pN1biii.

Trojani et al. (126) studied reportedly negative lymph nodes from mastectomy specimens with 10 years of follow-up, by staining immunohistochemically for epithelial markers—cytokeratin, epithelial membrane antigen (EMA), and human milk fat globulin. The authors found 14% of the cases to have micrometastases stained for each and every one of the epithelial markers. Among the patients with invasive ductal carcinoma, clinical recurrence was observed in 31% of those with micrometastases, but in only 8% of those without micrometastases.

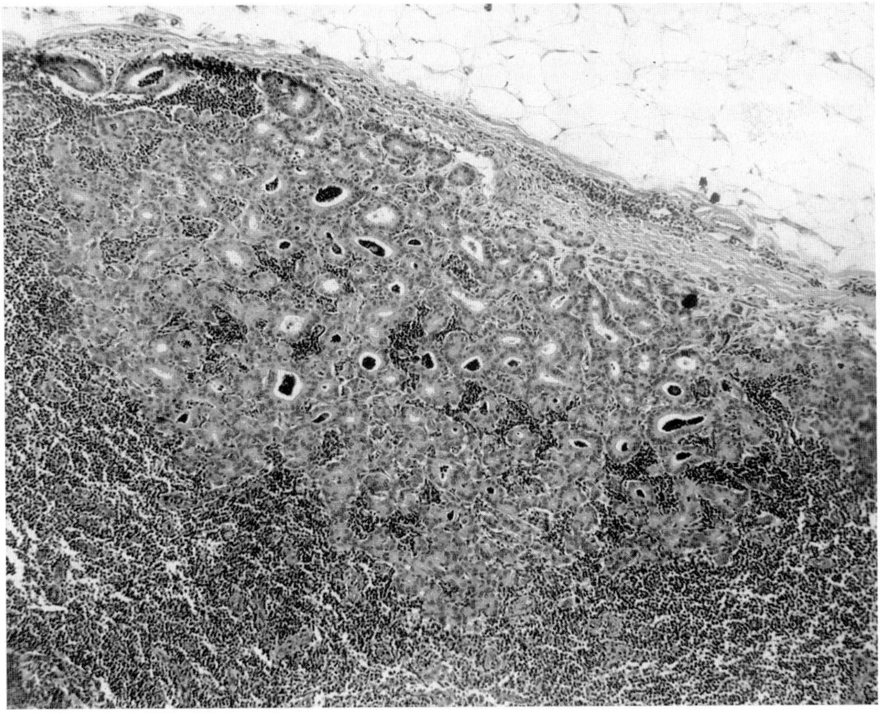

FIG. 9.11. Metastatic ductal carcinoma. This 1 mm micrometastasis is present in the peripheral sinus and adjacent sinusoid. No desmoplastic reaction is present.

In cases of invasive lobular carcinoma of the classic type, the problem is more difficult. Lachman et al. (127) reported on 8 of 12 patients with invasive lobular carcinoma and reportedly negative axillary lymph nodes. Three of the 8 patients were found to have micrometastases when immmunohistochemically stained for keratin (Figs. 9.12 to 9.15 and efigs. 9.33 to 9.37). The authors urged the use of keratin immunohistochemistry for the identification of metastases in cases of invasive lobular carcinoma.

Sentinel Lymph Nodes

The axilla contains lymph nodes that are associated with the lymphatic drainage from the breast and also the lymphatic drainage from the arm. It is important to determine the status of the lymph nodes that are associated with lymphatic drainage from the breast for accurate staging, but removal of lymph nodes that are primarily associated with the lymphatics of the arm may provide misleading information and cause morbidity in a high percentage of cases. The worst complication of axillary lymphadenectomy is lymphedema of the arm, but

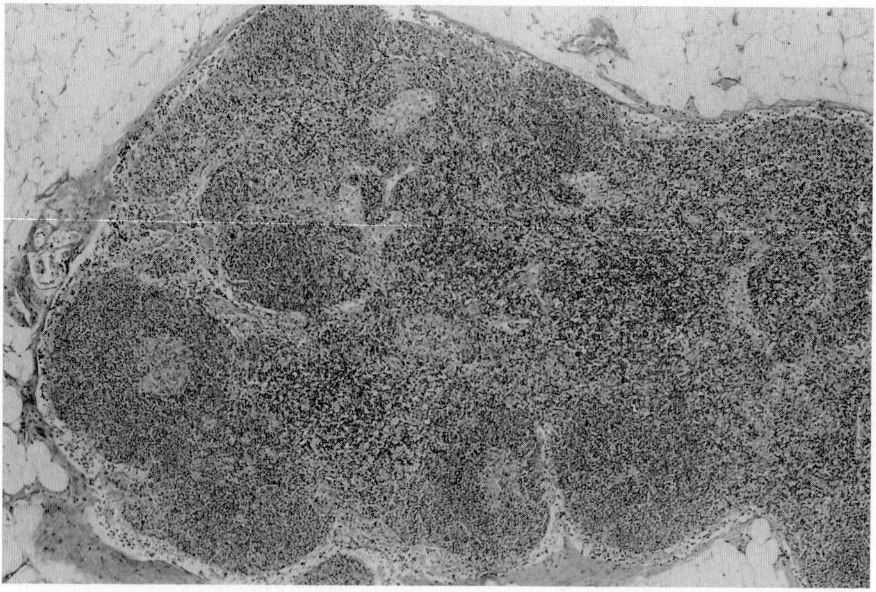

FIG. 9.12. Metastatic lobular carcinoma. The architecture of this lymph node appears to be intact and there is no evident mass lesion.

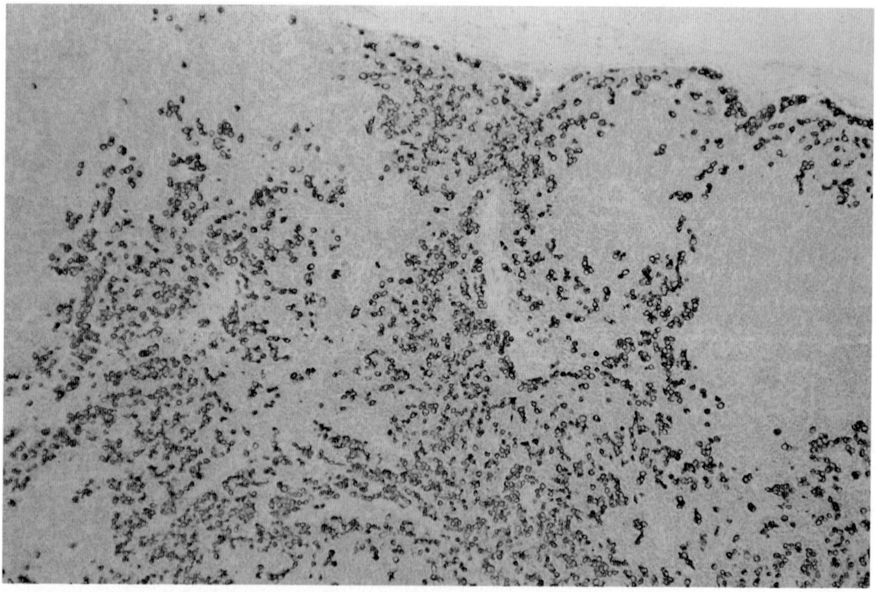

FIG. 9.13. Metastatic lobular carcinoma. Immunostain for keratin displays the large number of metastatic cells present in the peripheral sinus and sinusoids.

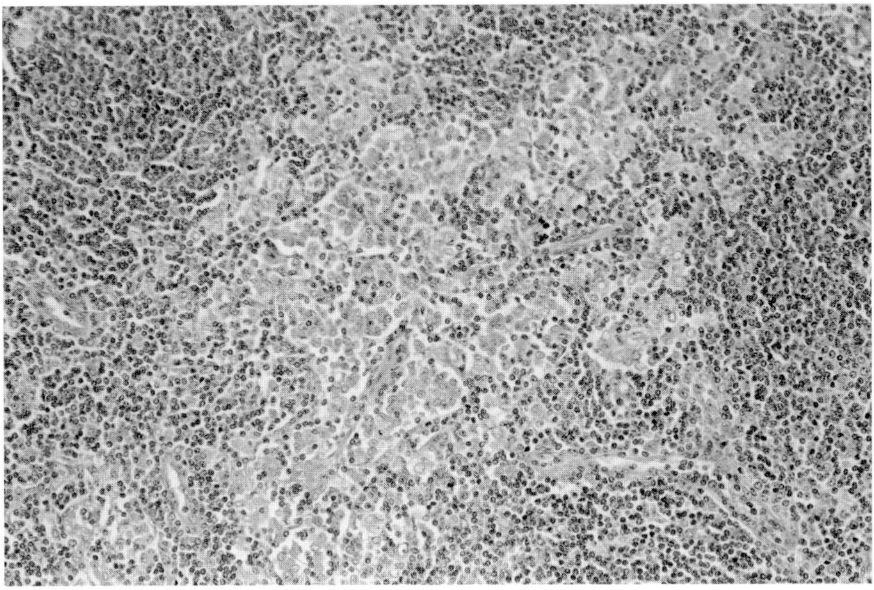

FIG. 9.14. Metastatic lobular carcinoma. This sinusoid is distended by cells that resemble the histiocytes seen in Fig. 9.16.

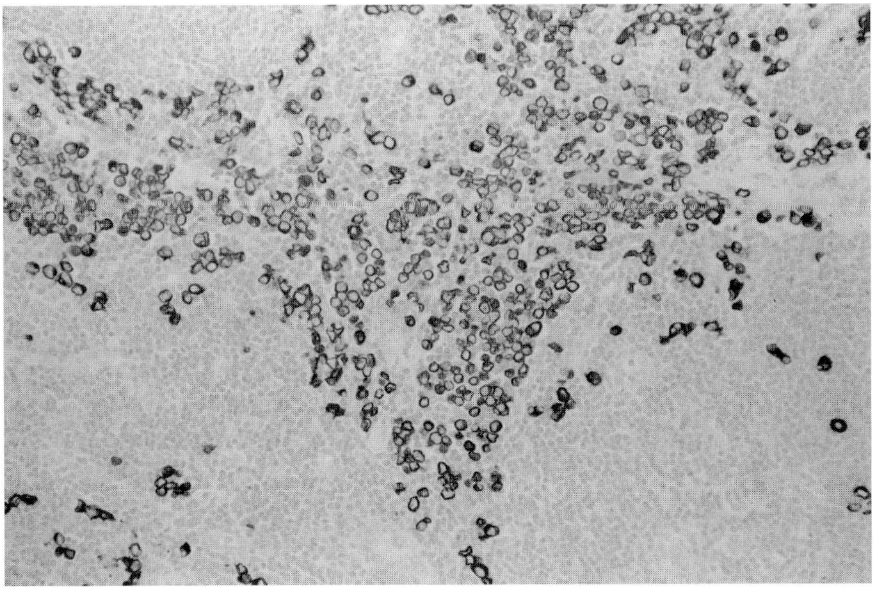

FIG. 9.15. Metastatic lobular carcinoma. This immunostain for keratin reveals the numerous metastatic cells of classic invasive lobular carcinoma.

limitation of movement by scar retraction and loss of sensitivity from sectioning of the long thoracic nerve may occur. As a result, it is necessary to remove the smallest number of lymph nodes required for accurate staging.

The sentinel lymph node technique was adapted from successful usage in patients with malignant melanoma. Radioactive material and a blue dye are injected into the breast, and the sentinel lymph nodes are localized with a Geiger counter as those that contain the largest amount of radioactive material. Identification of the sentinel lymph node is confirmed at the time of excision by tracking the blue dye.

Do sentinel lymph nodes accurately reflect the axillary nodal status? Do they accurately predict the prognosis for the purposes of therapy? The answer to the first question is a clear "yes," but data from follow-up are needed to answer the second question, and we are years away from that information. Weaver et al. (128) documented that surgeons are able to identify sentinel lymph nodes in 93% of cases, with at least one sentinel lymph node present beneath the hot spot in 98% of these cases. Sentinel lymph nodes were identified outside the axilla in internal mammary or supraclavicular locations in 8% of cases, with 3% of those lymph nodes positive for metastatic breast cancer. The observed accuracy in predicting the final axillary lymph node status was 97%, with a sensitivity of a positive node at 89% and specificity at 100%. The false negative rate was 11%, and the predictive value of a negative sentinel lymph node was 96%. Among 385 cases, 267 cases had negative sentinel lymph nodes and, of these, 14 had positive nonsentinel lymph nodes when the axillary dissection was completed. Among 104 patients with positive sentinel lymph nodes, 61 had negative nonsentinel lymph nodes at the completion of axillary dissection. Sentinel lymph nodes are therefore much more likely than nonsentinel nodes to contain a lymph node metastasis when there are lymph node metastases and are also highly indicative that the axilla is free of metastatic disease when the sentinel lymph node is negative.

With removal of a smaller number of lymph nodes, more intense scrutiny of each individual lymph node has been implied. Multiple sections and IHC stains for cytokeratin have been suggested as ancillary techniques for the identification of occult metastases, which are defined as those which cannot be found on the original H&E section. Note that the finding of micrometastases that are smaller than 2 mm in diameter was shown by Huvos et al. (129) to be of no prognostic significance and it is not used as an indication of node positivity in the staging scheme presented by the 5th Edition of the AJCC Cancer Staging Manual. Fisher et al. (130) found that 1.3 mm was a more predictive maximum size of micrometastasis. The 6th Edition of the AJCC Cancer Staging Manual uses 0.2 mm as the cutoff point. Weaver et al. (128) presented a study of multiple sections with cytokeratin staining on 214 node negative cases. In 18% of the false negative sentinel lymph node cases, there was evidence of occult metastasis and, in 1.4% of nonsentinel lymph nodes, occult metastases were found. All of the micrometastases were less than 1 mm in diameter, 90% were less than 0.5 mm, and 60% were less than 0.1 mm. Hansen et al. (131) showed that a single metastasis that was less than or equal to 2 mm in size and detected by immunohistochemistry had no impact on the 5-year disease-free survival or the overall 5-year survival, compared to lymph nodes that were negative. Disease-free survival was decreased by 25% in patients with axillary lymph node metastases that were larger than 2 mm in diameter.

Summary of this data indicates that sentinel lymph node procedures are of value and that they have a high level of reliability in predicting the presence or absence of lymph node metastases. The significance of micrometastases of whatever size and detected by H&E or by immunohistochemistry does not appear to have a strong impact on prognosis. In reporting axillary lymph nodes, sentinel and nonsentinel, the pathologist should give the size of the largest metastasis histologically found and describe how it was identified. The number of positive lymph nodes and total number of lymph nodes also should be provided. The 6th Edition of the AJCC Cancer Staging Manual recognizes the number of nodes with metastases, the size of the metastases, and the way in which the metastases were found (see Appendix, page 397).

Some observers have attempted to correlate reactive lymph node changes with a favorable response to the cancer (132). Sinus histiocytosis has been found by some authors (133,134) to correlate with a better prognosis, but others (135,136) have found no such effect.

AXILLARY PRESENTATION OF BREAST CANCER

Carcinoma may present as an axillary lymph node metastasis in the absence of an apparent breast primary tumor. This unusual situation presents a classic problem in surgical pathology—the search for the unknown primary tumor. The first step in the solution is to make certain that one is not dealing with the primary tumor itself, rather than a metastasis. Carcinoma may arise in mammary tissue that is sufficiently high in the axilla to approximate the location of lymph nodes. The identification of nodal architecture—specifically, the presence of a peripheral sinus—is therefore critical in determining that a metastasis is present.

The second step is to make sure that the lesion is malignant. Sinus histiocytosis may assume an epithelioid appearance and may mimic carcinoma (Fig 9.16 and efig. 9.38). Edlow and Carter (137) and Turner and Millis (138) have reported ectopic histologically benign breast lobules with apocrine metaplasia in axillary lymph nodes, in association with sclerosing adenosis (Figs. 9.17 to 9.20 and efigs. 9.39 to 9.41). Origin of carcinoma in heterotopic tissue such as this is a possibility, but it should be considered highly unlikely. Aggregates on nevus cells in the capsule of an axillary node should not be mistaken for cancer. These are usually in the capsule and not in the lymph node. They are positive for S-100 protein, but breast cancer cells also may stain for that antigen. Location and histology are the best guides to diagnosis (Figs. 9.21 and 9.22 and efigs. 9.42 and 9.43).

The third step is to rule out lymphoma, melanoma, or carcinoma that is metastatic from a known primary tumor by history, microscopy, stains, surface markers, immunohistochemistry, or a combination of these techniques. Melanoma or carci-

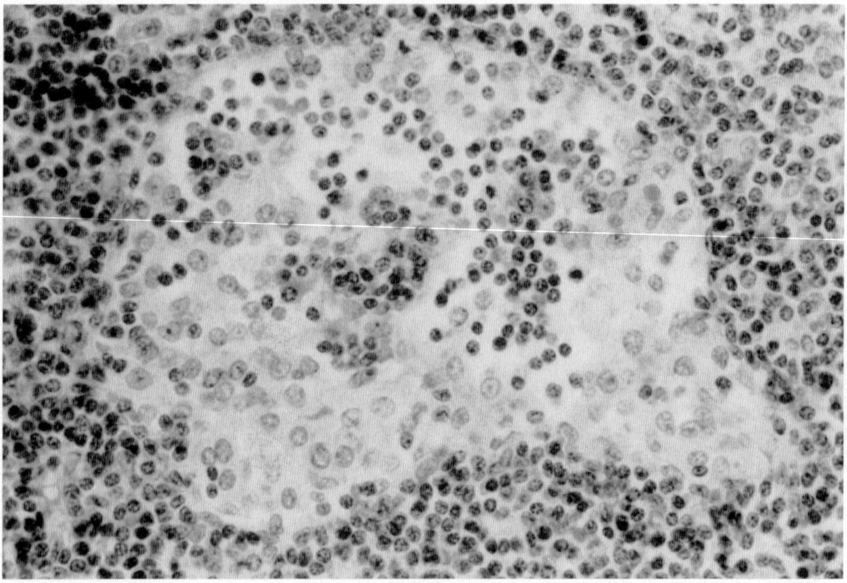

FIG. 9.16. Sinus histiocytes. The resemblance of these individual sinus histiocytes and their tendency to group together makes it difficult to distinguish them from bland nonduct forming carcinoma cells.

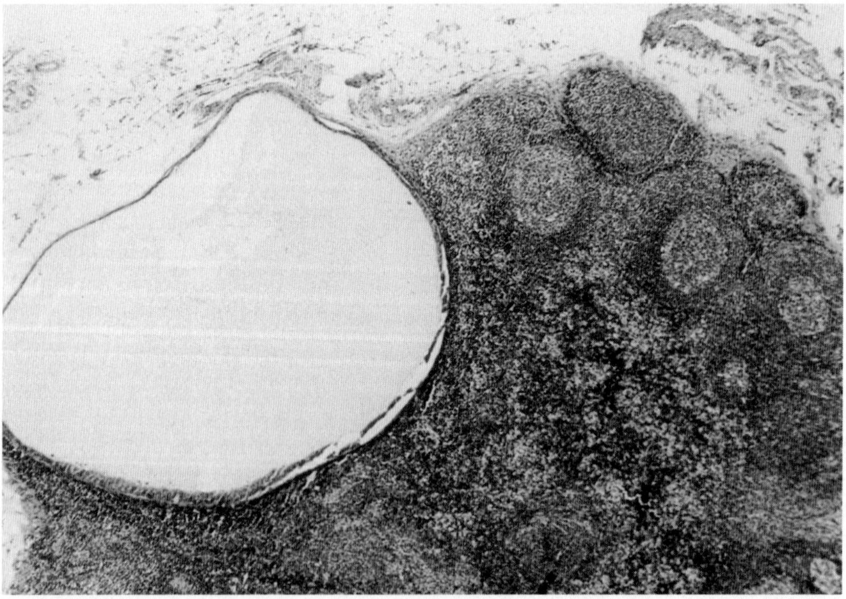

FIG. 9.17. Benign breast tissue in an axillary lymph node. A cystic space is present under the capsule of an axillary lymph node that was found in association with extensive sclerosing adenosis and fibrocystic change in the breast.

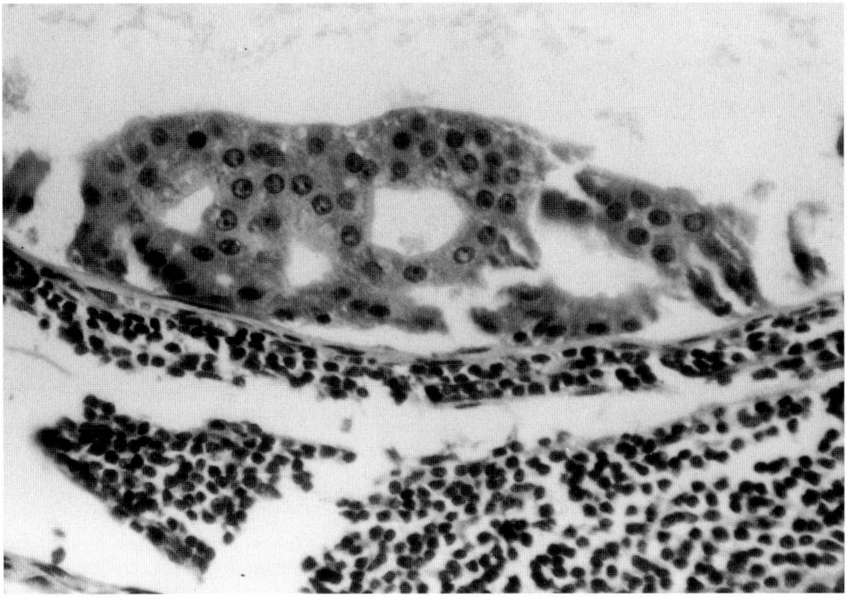

FIG. 9.18. Benign breast tissue in an axillary lymph node. The cyst shown in Fig. 9.17 is lined by this apocrine epithelium with a benign histologic appearance.

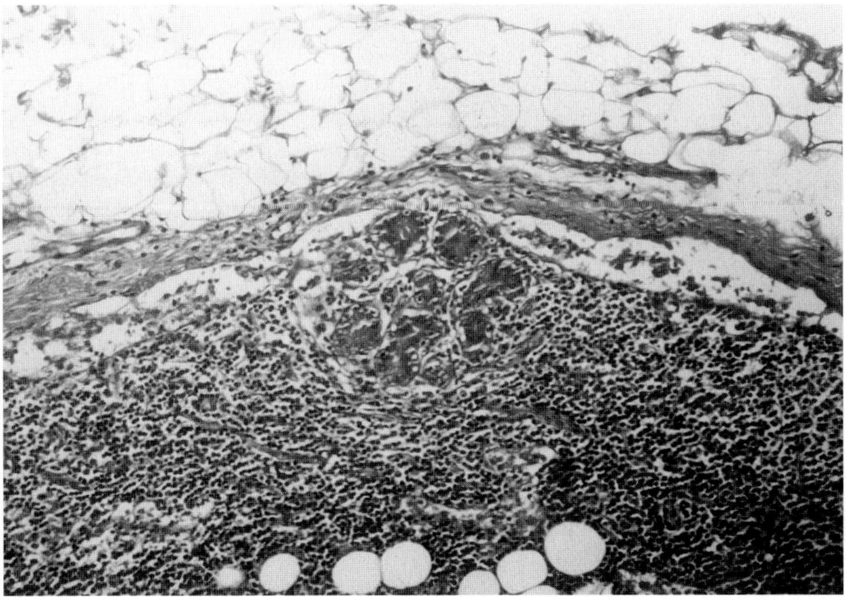

FIG. 9.19. Benign epithelium in an axillary lymph node. A demarcated lobule is evident under the capsule within the peripheral sinus of this lymph node.

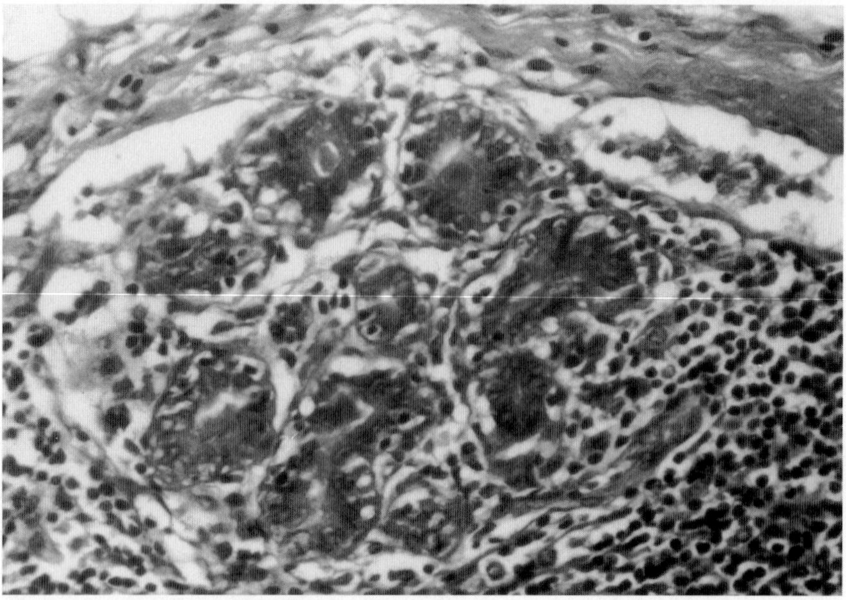

FIG. 9.20. Benign epithelium in an axillary lymph node. At higher magnification of the lobule shown in Fig. 9.19, the terminal ducts are composed of epithelial and myoepithelial cells and there appears to be intact encircling basement membrane. Secretion is present in the lumina of some of these ducts. Although epithelium was present in the lymph nodes, this patient did not have evidence of cancer in the breast and was clinically well years after the incidental removal of the lymph node.

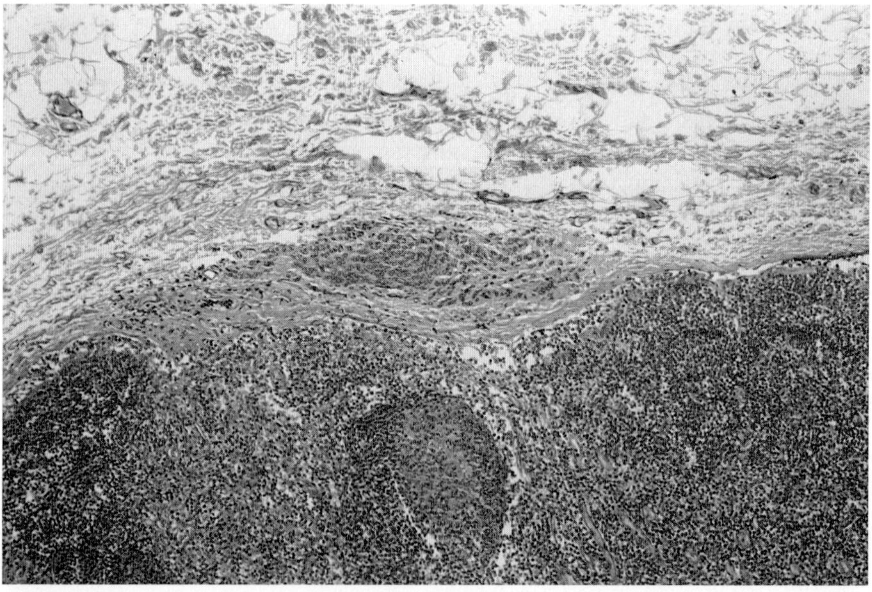

FIG. 9.21. Nevus cells in the capsule of an axillary lymph node. Within the capsule, but outside the peripheral sinus, there is a collection of large clear cells. This location is characteristic for nevus cells.

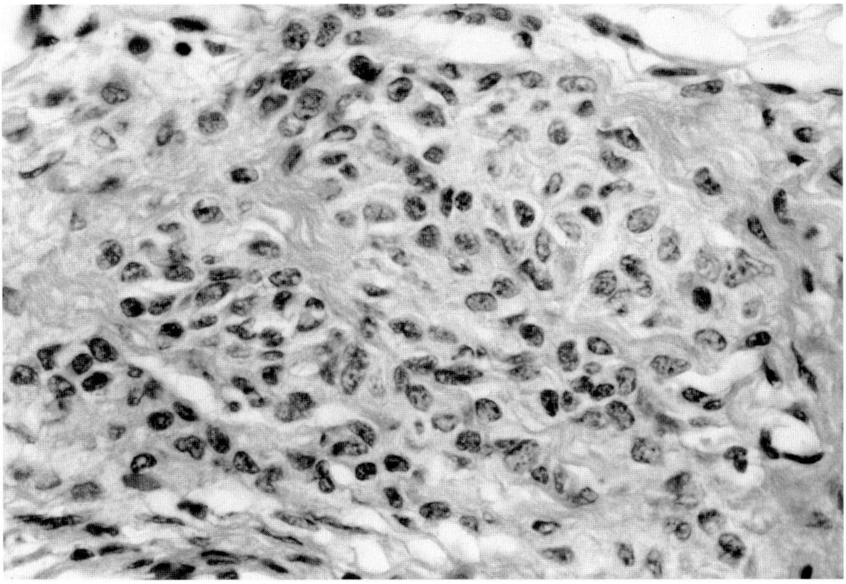

FIG. 9.22. Nevus cells in an axillary lymph node capsule. The benign nature of the nevus cells is evident. They are immunoreactive for S-100 protein, but not for keratin.

noma of the skin or skin appendages of the arm or chest may metastasize to the axilla, but this is usually known clinically (Figs. 9.23 to 9.26 and efigs. 9.44 to 9.47).

Metastatic carcinoma that is found in an axillary lymph node of a woman with a histologic appearance compatible with mammary carcinoma is strong circumstantial evidence that the breast contains the primary cancer, because the lymphatic drainage to the axilla is from the breast or the arm under ordinary circumstances. In the terminal stages of carcinomatosis, carcinoma from many primary sites—lung, gastrointestinal tract, or ovary—may metastasize to the axillary lymph nodes, but those primary tumors are almost always clinically evident. Metastasis from an occult abdominal primary tumor to an axillary lymph node is a rare event (see efigs. 9.48 and 9.49 for a renal cell carcinoma metastasis), although metastasis to a subclavicular lymph node, especially one that is on the left, is not.

Patel et al. (139) reported on 29 cases of carcinoma that presented in the axillary lymph nodes of women who had no clinically evident primary tumor. Workup failed to reveal an extramammary primary tumor in any of the women; mammography revealed a lesion in only 8 of 17 women. Mastectomy was done in all cases. Breast cancer was found in 16 patients (75% of the patients who had abnormal mammograms and in 44% of those with negative mammograms). The 16 patients in whom a breast primary tumor was found had 5- and 10-year recurrence-free survival rates of 25% and 5%, respectively, whereas the 13 patients in

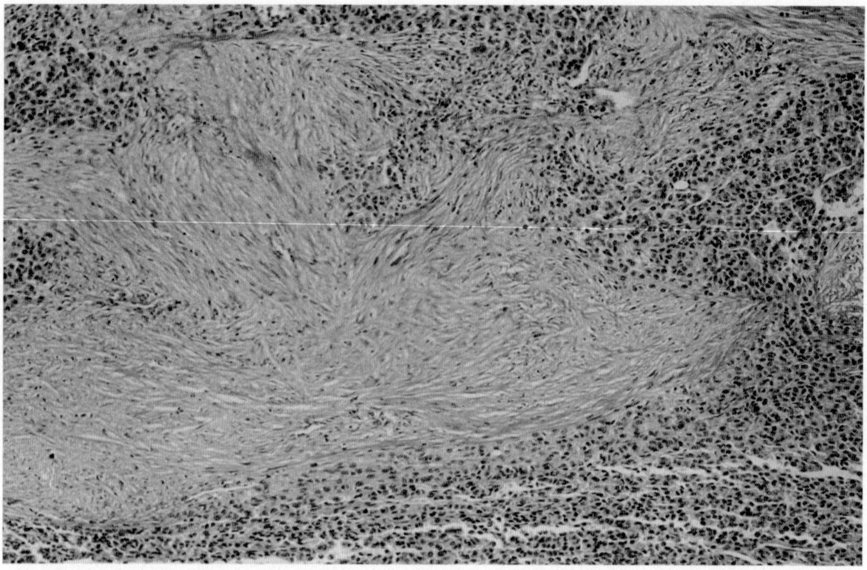

FIG. 9.23. Metastatic melanoma in an axillary lymph node. This patient had a classic variant of invasive lobular carcinoma of the breast and axillary lymph node dissection. The peculiar large scar with associated neoplastic cells was found within one of the nodes.

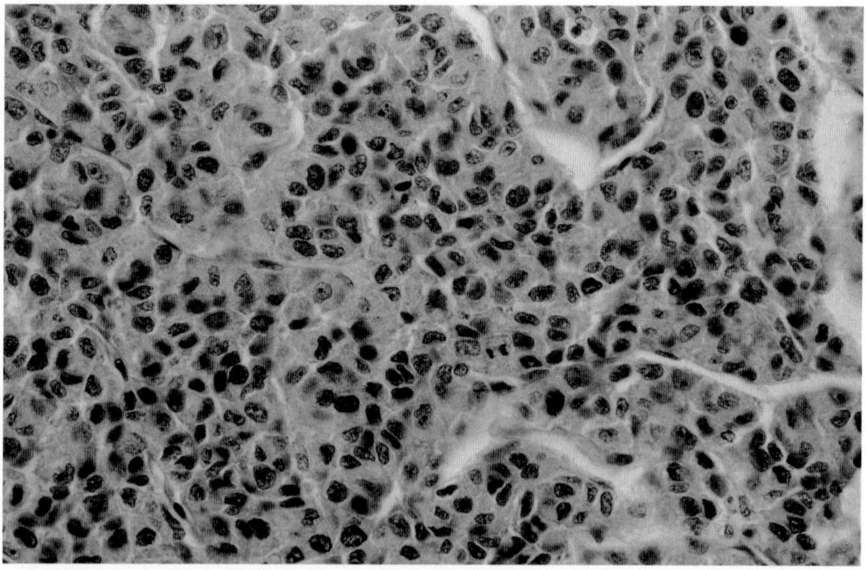

FIG. 9.24. Metastatic melanoma in an axillary lymph node. The cords of malignant cells shown in Fig. 9.23 are seen at higher magnification. They do not resemble lobular carcinoma. Immunostain for S-100 protein and HMB45 were positive and stain for keratin was negative.

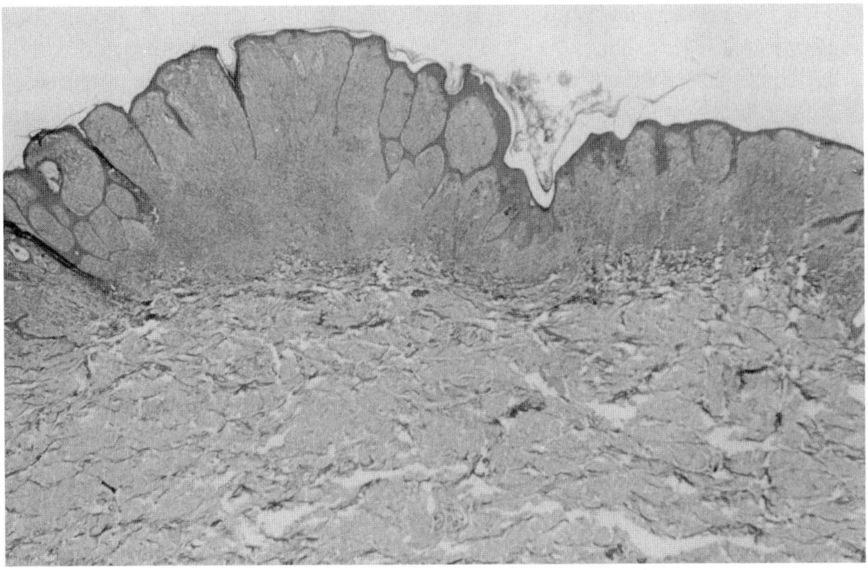

FIG. 9.25. Primary melanoma. In the patient whose lymph nodes are illustrated in Figs. 9.23 and 9.24, a history of melanoma of the skin of the back was elicited after immunohistochemical demonstration that the metastasis in the axillary lymph node was melanoma. This is the primary skin melanoma.

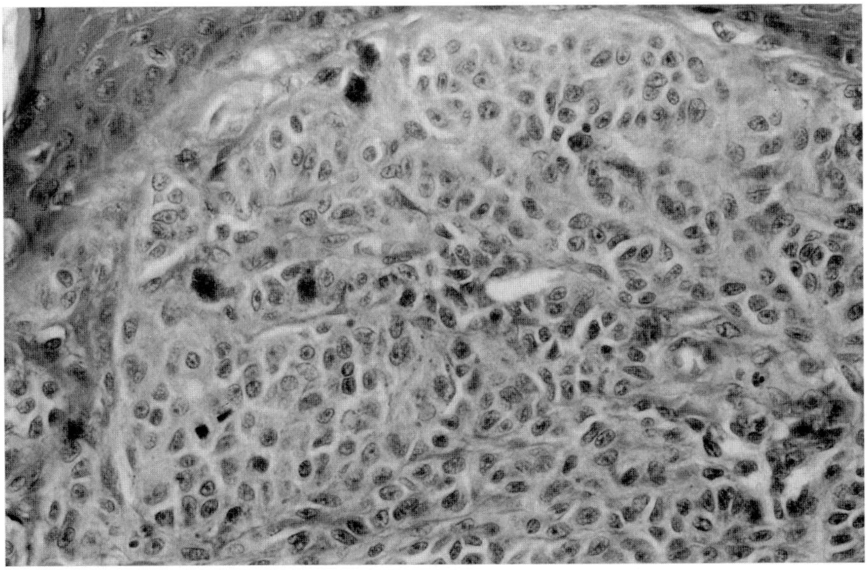

FIG. 9.26. Primary melanoma. At higher magnification, the malignant nature of the melanocytic cells and their resemblance to the metastasis are evident.

whom no breast primary tumor was found had 5- to 10-year recurrence-free survival rates of 30%. Survival related more to the number of positive nodes than to the finding of a breast primary tumor. No other primary tumor manifested itself during follow-up of these cases. The authors suggested that carcinoma in an axillary lymph node of a middle-aged woman should be considered metastatic from the breast, until proven otherwise, because of both the high likelihood of finding a breast primary tumor and the reasonably good likelihood of salvage by mastectomy (efigs 9.49 to 9.53). Rosen (140) reported eight such cases in which mastectomy revealed only noninvasive carcinoma, indicating that the carcinoma, especially the invasive component, may be quite small. All eight of those patients were free of disease 1 to 14 years after mastectomy. Rosen and Kimmel (141) reported on 48 occult breast carcinomas that presented as axillary lymph node metastases; the cases were followed for an average of 5 years. Only 24% of the cases had mammograms suggestive of or positive for malignancy, and 62% had ER-positive metastases. Primary cancer was found in the breast in 75% of cases, of which only 79% were invasive carcinomas. Of 27 invasive cancers, 22 were ductal, 2 cases each were lobular and medullary, and 1 case was a colloid carcinoma. The average size of the primary tumor was 1.5 cm, and 20 patients had four or more positive nodes. Sixty percent were disease-free at 5 years, comparing favorably with a matched group of stage II cases that presented with a breast lesion.

Ellerbroek et al. (142) reported on 42 cases of occult breast primary tumors that had 72% survival at 5 years. Only 2 cases were shown to have cancer in the breast, but, with radiotherapy as the primary treatment, the 5-year risk of local recurrence was 17%, compared with 57% for those who were not irradiated or treated by mastectomy. Metastasis from a contralateral carcinoma may occur, but it is usually late in the course of the disease. Although medullary and colloid carcinomas have the least desmoplastic reaction and therefore are more difficult to detect, most occult primary tumors are of the ordinary ductal carcinoma variety (143–146). Estimation of levels of ERs/PRs, lactalbumin, gross cystic disease fluid protein 15 (GCDFP-15), and other antigens may be helpful in confirming the origin of the carcinoma as mammary. Significantly elevated ER levels, especially if associated with elevated PR levels, indicate breast origin, although low levels of ER may be found in other primary tumors. Wick et al. (147) reported a 95% predictive index for antibodies to GCDFP-15 with immunohistochemistry. The other primary tumors that were positive with this antibody were salivary and sweat gland carcinomas and prostate cancer, which rarely metastasize to the axilla or breast and are usually known clinically. Lactalbumin had a 50% predictive index in the same study. Confirmation with the ancillary information that is provided by immunohistochemistry may be reassuring because it is always difficult to recommend mastectomy or radiotherapy without identification of a primary carcinoma in the breast. However, carcinoma in an axillary lymph node, with histology that is consistent with mammary origin, is still likely to be metastatic breast cancer if a careful search for another primary tumor is unproductive.

Occult breast primary tumors give rise to axillary lymph node metastases with much greater frequency than systemic metastases. Conversely, a breast carcinoma that is not apparent in either the breast or the axilla is rarely detected as a systemic metastasis.

Distant Metastasis

Distant metastasis is breast cancer that has reached beyond regional spread. Internal mammary nodes are considered an extension of regional spread, but they are of poorer prognostic significance. They are N3 nodes, which denote stage III. Breast cancer is one of the few cancers that often metastasizes to bone, which it may involve aggressively and without visceral involvement. Metastases are commonly found in lung, pleura, liver, brain, and ovary; however, other sites, including the GI tract and lower urinary tract, may be involved and no site is completely privileged from metastatic breast cancer.

The best indications that a metastasis is from the breast are a history of potentially metastasizing primary breast cancer and a comparison with the histologic appearance of the breast primary. ERs and PRs, although not entirely specific, are the best IHC markers of breast origin. Other markers, such as GCDFP-15, have been used, as discussed under the axillary presentation of breast cancer. An IHC profile may be used to rule out other primaries in the appropriate clinical setting.

Staging

After the diagnosis of invasive carcinoma has been histologically established, prognosis is primarily dictated by the staging criteria for breast cancer that was formulated by the American Joint Committee for Cancer Staging and End Results and the International Union Against Cancer, according to the TNM system, where T depicts tumor; N, regional lymph nodes; and M, distant metastasis. These factors can be evaluated by (a) clinical assessment before surgery; (b) surgical evaluation, based on biopsy specimens taken at limited surgery; or (c) pathologic assessment after resection. Pathologic evaluation is the most reliable. Fisher et al. (148) noted a 32% discrepancy between the clinical and histologic classification of lymph nodes, with a 24% clinical false positive rate and a 39% clinical false negative rate.

Rosen et al. (149) studied clinical and pathologic staging of the axillary lymph nodes of 203 patients who were treated by modified or radical mastectomy. The authors reported overall error rates of 33% and 38% for patients with T1 and T2 tumors, respectively. Forty-eight percent of the patients who were classified clinically as T2NO were pathologically T2N1 (false negative) and 41% of women who were staged clinically as T1N1 were really T1NO (false positive).

The currently recommended staging system for breast carcinoma was adopted, in 1997, by the AJCC and the International Union Against Cancer (UICC). The system was published in *Manual for Staging of Cancer* (150). A comparison of changes in the new 6th Edition is shown on page 397.

Staging is based on size and spread of the primary tumor (T), extent of regional axillary lymph node metastasis (N), and distant metastases (M). The most recent version focuses on subdividing the T1 and the N categories. TNM denotes clinical stage and pTNM refers to pathologic staging.

The classification is meant only for histologically confirmed carcinoma of the breast. The seven anatomic subsites that are identified in the female breast are the nipple, central subareolar region, four quadrants, and the axillary tail. The male breast is not subdivided. All other staging categories apply equally to carcinoma of the male breast.

If more than one carcinoma is present in a breast, the tumor with the highest T category is used for staging. Simultaneous bilateral breast cancers are staged separately.

Clinical staging is used when it is the only information available, but it is recognized that it is less accurate than pathologic staging. The size of the primary tumor is often overestimated clinically, and the clinical assessment of axillary lymph nodes is not accurate.

Staging Categories

The following TNM definitions and stage groupings for carcinoma of the breast are the same for the AJCC and the Union Internationale Contre le Cancer (UICC)/TNM projects. This staging system for carcinoma of the breast applies to infiltrating (including microinvasive) and *in situ* carcinomas. Microscopic confirmation of the diagnosis is mandatory, and the histologic type and grade of carcinoma should be recorded.

Anatomy

Primary Site. The mammary gland, situated on the anterior chest wall, is composed of glandular tissue within a dense fibroareolar stroma. The glandular tissue consists of approximately 20 lobes, each of which terminates in a separate excretory duct in the nipple.

Regional Lymph Nodes. The breast lymphatics drain by way of three major routes: axillary, transpectoral, and internal mammary. Intramammary lymph nodes are considered with, and coded as, axillary lymph nodes for staging purposes. Metastasis to any other lymph node is considered distant (M1), including supraclavicular, cervical, or contralateral internal mammary. The regional lymph nodes are:

1. Axillary (ipsilateral): interpectoral (Rotter's) nodes and lymph nodes along the axillary vein and its tributaries, which may be (but are not required to be) divided into the following levels:
    (a) Level I (low-axilla): lymph nodes that are lateral to the lateral border of the pectoralis minor muscle.

(b) Level II (mid-axilla): lymph nodes that are located between the medial and lateral borders of the pectoralis minor muscle and the interpectoral (Rotter's) lymph nodes.
(c) Level III (apical axilla): lymph nodes that are medial to the medial margin of the pectoralis minor muscle, including those designated as subclavicular, infraclavicular, or apical.

Note: Intramammary lymph nodes are coded as axillary lymph nodes.

2. Internal mammary (ipsilateral): lymph nodes that are located in the intercostal spaces, along the edge of the sternum in the endothoracic fascia.
   Any other lymph node metastasis is coded as a distant metastasis (M1), including supraclavicular, cervical, or contralateral internal mammary lymph nodes.

Metastatic Sites. All distant visceral sites are potential sites of metastasis. The four major sites of involvement are bone, lung, brain, and liver, but this widely metastasizing disease has been found in many other sites.

RULES FOR CLASSIFICATION

Clinical Staging

Clinical staging includes physical examination, with careful inspection and palpation of the skin, mammary gland, and lymph nodes (axillary, supraclavicular, and cervical), imaging, and pathologic examination of the breast *or* other tissues to establish the diagnosis of breast carcinoma. The extent of tissue that is examined pathologically for clinical staging is less than that required for pathologic staging (see section on pathologic staging). Appropriate operative findings are elements of clinical staging, including the size of the primary tumor and chest wall invasion, and the presence or absence of regional or distant metastasis.

Pathologic Staging

Pathologic staging includes all data used for clinical staging, surgical exploration, and resection, as well as pathologic examination of the primary carcinoma, including not less than excision of the primary carcinoma with no macroscopic tumor in any margin of resection by pathologic examination. A case can be classified pT for pathologic stage grouping, if there is only microscopic, but not macroscopic, involvement at the margin. If there is tumor in the margin of resection by macroscopic examination, it is coded TX because the extent of the primary tumor cannot be assessed. If there is no clinical evidence of axillary metastasis, resection of at least the low axillary lymph nodes (level I)—that is, those of the pectoralis minor muscle—should be performed for pathologic (pN) classification. Such a resection will ordinarily include six or more lymph nodes. Metastatic nodules in the fat adjacent to the mammary carcinoma within the breast, without evidence of residual lymph node tissue, are classified as regional lymph node metastases (N). Pathologic stage grouping includes any of the following combinations: pTpNpM, pTpNcM, or cTcNpM.

TNM CLASSICIFICATION

Primary Tumor

The clinical measurement that is used for classifying the primary tumor (T) is the one judged to be most accurate for that particular case (e.g., physical examination or imaging, such as a mammogram). The pathologic tumor size for classification (T) is a measurement of *only the invasive component.* For example, if there is a 4.0-cm intraductal component and a 0.3-cm invasive component, the tumor is classified T1a. The size of the primary tumor is measured for T classification before any tissue is removed for special studies, such as for ERs.

Microinvasion of Breast Carcinoma

Microinvasion is the extension of cancer cells beyond the basement membrane into the adjacent tissues, with no focus more than 0.1 cm in greatest dimension. When there are multiple foci of microinvasion, the size of only the largest focus is used to classify the microinvasion. (Do not use the sum of all the individual foci.) The presence of multiple foci of microinvasion should be noted, as is the case with multiple larger invasive carcinomas.

Multiple Simultaneous Ipsilateral Primary Carcinomas

The following guidelines are used when classifying multiple simultaneous ipsilateral primary (infiltrating, macroscopically measurable) carcinomas. These criteria do not apply to one macroscopic carcinoma that is associated with multiple separate microscopic foci.

1. Use the largest primary carcinoma to classify T.
2. Enter into the record that this is a case of multiple simultaneous ipsilateral primary carcinomas. Such cases should be analyzed separately.

Simultaneous Bilateral Breast Carcinomas

Each carcinoma is staged as a separate primary carcinoma in a separate organ.

Inflammatory Carcinoma

Inflammatory carcinoma is a clinicopathologic entity that is characterized by diffuse brawny induration of the skin of the breast with an erysipeloid edge, usually without an underlying palpable mass. Radiologically, there may be a detectable mass and characteristic thickening of the skin over the breast. This clinical presentation is due to tumor embolization of dermal lymphatics. The tumor of inflammatory carcinoma is classified T4d.

Paget's Disease of the Nipple

Paget's disease of the nipple, without an associated tumor mass (clinical) or invasive carcinoma (pathologic), is classified Tis. Paget's disease, with a demonstrable mass (clinical) or an invasive component (pathologic), is classified according to the size of the tumor mass or invasive component.

Skin of the Breast

Dimpling of the skin, nipple retraction, or any other skin change, except those described under T4b and T4d, may occur in T1, T2, or T3, without changing the classification.

Chest Wall

The chest wall includes ribs, intercostal muscles, and serratus anterior muscle, but not pectoral muscle.

DEFINITION OF TNM

Definitions for classifying the primary tumor (T) are the same for clinical and pathologic classification. The telescoping method of classification can be applied. If the measurement is made by physical examination, the examiner will use the major headings (T1, T2, or T3). If other measurements (such as mammographic or pathologic) are used, the telescoped subsets of T1 can be used.

Primary Tumor

TX Primary tumor (T) cannot be assessed
TO No evidence of primary tumor
Tis Carcinoma *in situ*: intraductal carcinoma, lobular carcinoma *in situ*, or Paget's disease of the nipple, with no tumor
T1 Tumor 2 cm or less in greatest dimension
- T1mic Microinvasion of 0.1 cm or less in greatest dimension
- T1a Tumor is more than 0.1 cm, but not more than 0.5 cm in greatest dimension
- T1b Tumor is more than 0.5 cm, but not more than 1 cm in greatest dimension
- T1c Tumor is more than 1 cm, but not more than 2 cm in greatest dimcnsion

T2 Tumor is more than 2 cm, but not more than 5 cm in greatest dimension
T3 Tumor is more than 5 cm in greatest dimension
T4 Tumor can be any size, with direct extension to (a) chest wall or (b) skin, only as described below
- T4a Extension to chest wall
- T4b Edema (including peau d'orange) or ulceration of the skin of the breast or satellite skin nodules that are confined to the same breast
- T4c Both (T4a and T4b)
- T4d Inflammatory carcinoma (see definition of inflammatory carcinoma in the introduction)

Note: Paget's disease that is associated with a tumor is classified according to the size of the tumor

Regional Lymph Nodes

NX Regional lymph nodes (N) cannot be assessed (e.g., previously removed)
N0 No regional lymph node metastasis
N1 Metastasis to movable ipsilateral axillary lymph node(s)
N2 Metastasis to ipsilateral axillary lymph node(s) fixed to one another or to other structures
N3 Metastasis to ipsilateral internal mammary lymph node(s)

Pathologic Classification

pNX Regional lymph nodes cannot be assessed (e.g., previously removed or not removed for pathologic study)
pN0 No regional lymph node metastasis
pN1 Metastasis to movable ipsilateral axillary lymph node(s)
- pN1a Only micrometastasis (none larger than 0.2 cm)
- pN1b Metastasis to lymph node(s), any nodes that are larger than 0.2 cm
- pN1bi Metastasis in 1 to 3 lymph nodes, any nodes that are more than 0.2 cm and all nodes that are less than 2 cm in greatest dimension
- pN1bii Metastasis to 4 or more lymph nodes, any more than 0.2 cm and all less than 2 cm in greatest dimension
- pN1biii Extension of tumor beyond the capsule of a lymph node metastasis that is less than 2 cm in greatest dimension
- pN1biv Metastasis to a lymph node that is 2 cm or more in greatest dimension

pN2 Metastasis to ipsilateral lymph nodes that are fixed to one another or to other structures
pN3 Metastasis to ipsilateral internal mammary lymph node(s)

Distant Metastasis

MX Distant metastasis (M) cannot be assessed
M0 No distant metastasis
M1 Distant metastasis [includes metastasis to ipsilateral supraclavicular lymph node(s)]

Stage Grouping

Stage 0	TIS	N0	M0
Stage I	T1*	N0	M0
Stage IIA	T0	N1	M0
	T1*	N1**	M0
	T2	N0	M0
STAGE IIB	T2	N1	M0
	T3	N0	M0
STAGE IIIA	T0	N2	M0
	T1*	N2	M0
	T2	N2	M0
	T3	N1	M0
	T3	N2	M0
STAGE IIIB	T4	Any N	M0
	Any T	N3	M0
STAGE IV	Any T	Any N	M1

* *Note*: T1 includes pT1mic

***Note*: The prognosis of patients with N1a is similar to that of patients with pNO (see page 397 for a comparison of stages in the 5th and 6th Editions of the AJCC Cancer Staging Manual.)

REFERENCES

1. Fitzgibbons P, Page D, Weaver D, et al. Prognostic factors in breast cancer: College of American Pathologists consensus statement 1999. *Arch Pathol Lab Med* 2000;124:966–78.
2. Nixon AJ, Schnitt SJ, Geiman R, et al. Relationship of tumor grade to other pathologic features and to treatment of patients with early stage breast carcinoma treated with breast-conserving therapy. *Cancer* 1996;78:1426–1431.
3. Elmore JG, Moceri VM, Carter D, et al. Breast carcinoma tumor characteristics in black and white women. *Cancer* 1998; 83:2509–2515.
4. Hunter C, Redmond C, et al. Breast cancer: factors associated with stage at diagnosis in black and white women. *J Natl Cancer Inst* 1993;85:1129–1137.
5. Crisp W, Higgs M, et al. Screening for breast cancer detects tumors at an earlier biological stage. *Br J Surg* 1993;80:863–865.
6. Hoover HC Jr. Breast cancer during pregnancy and lactation. *Surg Clin North Am* 1990;70:1151–1163.
7. Korzeniowski S, Dyba T. Reproductive history and prognosis in patients with operable breast cancer. *Cancer* 1994;74:1591–1594.
8. Brinkley D, Haylittle JL. The curability of breast cancer. *Lancet* 1975;2:95–97.
9. Seidman JD, Schnaper LA, Aisner SC. Relationship of the size of the invasive component of the primary breast carcinoma to axillary lymph node metastasis. *Cancer* 1995;75:65–71.

10. Bloom HJG. Prognosis in carcinoma of the breast. *Br J Cancer* 1950;4:259–288.
11. Bloom HJG, Richardson WW. Histological grading and prognosis in breast cancer: a study of 1409 cases of which 359 have been followed for 15 years. *Br J Cancer* 1957;11:359–377.
12. Bloom HJG, Field JR. Impact of tumor grade and host resistance on survival of women with breast cancer. *Cancer* 1971;28:1580–1589.
13. Wolff B. Histological grading in carcinoma of the breast. *Br J Cancer* 1966;20:36–40.
14. Bloom HJG, Richardson WW, Harries EJ. Natural history of untreated breast cancer (1805–1933): comparison of untreated and treated cases according to histological grade of malignancy. *Br Med J* 1962;2:213–221.
15. Elston C, Ellis I. Pathological prognostic factors in breast cancer. I. The value of histological grade in breast cancer: experience from a large study with long-term followup. *Histopathology* 1991;19: 403–410.
16. Clayton F, Hopkins CL. Pathologic correlates of prognosis in lymph node-positive breast carcinomas. *Cancer* 1993;71:1780–1790.
17. Theissig F, Kunze K, Haroske G, et al. Histologic grading of breast cancer. Interobserver reproducibility and prognostic significance. *Pathol Res Pract* 1990;186:732–736.
18. Dalton LW, Page DL, Dupont WD. Histologic grading of breast carcinoma: a reproducibility study. *Cancer* 1994;73:2765–2770.
19. Dalton LW, Pinder SE, Elston CE, et al. Histologic grading of breast cancer: linkage of patient outcome with level of pathologist agreement. *Mod Pathol* 2000;13:730–735.
20. Fisher ER, Redmond C, Fisher B. Histologic grading of breast cancer. *Pathol Ann* 1980;15:239–251.
21. Fisher ER, Costantino J, Fisher B, et al. Pathologic findings from the National Surgical Adjuvant Breast Project (protocol 4): discriminants for 15-year survival. *Cancer* 1993;71:2141–2150.
22. Galea MH, Blamey RW, Elston CE, et al. The Nottingham Prognostic Index in primary breast cancer. *Breast Cancer Res Treat* 1992;22:207–219.
23. Henson DE, Ries L, Freedman LS, et al. Relationship among outcome, stage of disease, and histologic grade for 22,616 cases of breast cancer: the basis for a prognostic index. *Cancer* 1991;68:2142–2149.
24. McDivitt R, Stone K, et al. A proposed classification of breast cancer based upon kinetic information derived from a comparison of 168 operable breast cancers. *Cancer* 1986;57:269–276.
25. Meyer JS, Coplin MD. Thymidine labeling index, flow cytometric S-phase measurement, and DNA index in human tumors: comparisons and correlations. *Am J Clin Pathol* 1988;89:586–595.
26. Silvestrini R, Daidone MG, Gasparini G. Cell kinetics as a prognostic marker in node-negative breast cancer. *Cancer* 1985;56:192–1987.
27. Tubiani M, Pejovic MJ, Reymond A. Kinetic parameters and the course of the disease in breast cancer. *Cancer* 1981;47:937–943.
28. Dabbs DJ. Ductal carcinoma of breast: nuclear grade as a predictor of S-phase fraction. *Hum Pathol* 1993;24:652–656.
29. Frierson HFJ. Grade and flow cytometric analysis of ploidy for infiltrating ductal carcinomas. *Hum Pathol* 1993;24:24–29.
30. Hedley DW, Friedlander ML, Taylor IW, et al. Method for analysis of cellular DNA content of paraffin-embedded pathologic material using flow cytometry. *J Histochem Cytochem* 1983;31:1333–1335.
31. Dressler LG, Seamer LC, Owens MA, et al. DNA flow cytometry and prognostic factors in 1,331 frozen breast cancer specimens. *Cancer* 1988;61:420–427.
32. Fisher B, Gunduz N, Constantino J, et al. DNA flow cytometric analysis of primary operable breast cancer: relation of ploidy and S-phase fraction to outcome of patients in NSABP B-04. *Cancer* 1994; 68:1465–1475.
33. Arnerlov C, Emdin SO, Lundgren B, et al. Breast carcinoma growth rate described by mammographic doubling time and S-phase fraction: correlation to clinical and histopathologic factors in a screened population. *Cancer* 1992;70:1928–1934.
34. Arnerlov C, Emdin SO, Lundgren B, et al. Mammographic growth rate, DNA ploidy, and S-phase fraction analysis in breast carcinoma: a prognostic evaluation in a screened population. *Cancer* 1992;70:1935–1942.
35. Dervan PA, Magee HM, Buckley C, et al. Proliferating cell nuclear antigen counts in formalin-fixed paraffin-embedded tissue correlate with Ki-67 in fresh tissue. *Am J Clin Pathol* 1992;97:S21–S28.
36. Isola JJ, Helin HJ, Helle MJ, et al. Evaluation of cell proliferation in breast carcioma: Comparison of Ki-67 immunohistochemical study, DNA flow cytometric analysis, and mitotic count. *Cancer* 1990;65:1180–1184.

37. Frierson HFJ, Gaffey MJ, Zukerberg LR, et al. Immunohistochemical detection and gene amplification of cyclin D1 in mammary infiltrating ductal carcinoma. *Mod Pathol* 1996;9:725–730.
38. Leonardi E, Girlando S, Serio G, et al. PCNA and Ki 67 expression in breast carcinoma: correlation with clinical and biological variables. *J Clin Pathol* 1992;45:416–419.
39. Barbareschi M, Girlando S, Mauri FM, et al. Quantitative growth fraction evaluation with MiB1 and Ki67 antibodies in breast carcinomas. *Am J Clin Pathol* 1994;102:171–175.
40. Geradts J, Ingram CD. Abnormal expression of cell cycle regulatory proteins in ductal and lobular carcinomas of the breast. *Mod Pathol* 2000;13:945–53.
41. Landberg G. Multiparameter analyses of cell cycle regulatory proteins in human breast cancer: a key to definition of separate pathways in tumorigenesis. *Adv Cancer Res* 2002;84:35–56.
42. Landberg G, Nielsen NH, Nilsson P, et al. Telomerase activity is associated with cell cycle deregulation in human breast cancer. *Cancer Res* 1997;57:549–554.
43. Fisher ER, Gregario RM, Fisher B. The pathology of invasive breast cancer. *Cancer* 1975;36:1–85.
44. Silverberg SG, Chitale AR. Assessment of significance of proportions of intraductal and infiltrating tumor growth in ductal carcinoma of the breast. *Cancer* 1973;32:830–837.
45. Black MM, Barclay THC, Hankey BF. Prognosis in breast cancer utilizing histologic characteristics of the primary tumor. *Cancer* 1975;36:2048–2055.
46. Lane N, Goskel H, Salerno RW, et al. Clinicopathologic analysis of the surgical curability of breast cancers: a minimum ten-year study of a personal series. *Ann Surg* 1961;153:483–498.
47. Kouchoukas NT, Ackerman LV, Butcher HR. Prediction of axillary nodal metastases from the morphology of 10 mammary carcinomas: guide to operative therapy. *Cancer* 1967;20:948.
48. Carter D, Pipkin RD, Shepard RH, et al. Relationship of necrosis and tumor border to lymph node metastases and 10-year survival in carcinoma of the breast. *Am J Surg Pathol* 1978;2:39.
49. Nime FA, Rosen PP, Thaler HT, et al. The prognostic significance of tumor emboli in extramammary lymphatics in patients with mammary carcinoma. *Am J Surg Pathol* 1977;1:25–30.
50. Weigand RA, Isenberg WM, Russo J, et al. Blood vessel invasion and axillary lymph node involvement as prognostic indicators for human breast cancer. *Cancer* 1982;50:962–969.
51. Kister SJ, Sommers SC, Haagensen CD, et al. Reevaluation of blood vessel invasion as a prognostic factor in carcinoma of the breast. *Cancer* 1966;19:1213.
52. Gilchrist KW, Gould VF, Hirschl S, et al. Interobserver variation in the identification of breast carcinoma in intramammary lymphatics. *Hum Pathol* 1982;13:170–172.
53. Pinder S, Ellis I, Galea M, et al. Pathological prognostic factors in breast cancer. III. Vascular invasion. *Histopathology* 1994;24:41–47.
54. Ellis DL, Teitelbaum SL. Inflammatory carcinoma of the breast: a pathologic definition. *Cancer* 1974;33:1045–1047.
55. Meyer AC, Dockerty MD, Harrington SW. Inflammatory carcinoma of the breast. *Surg Gynecol Obstet* 1948;87:417–424.
56. Lucas FV and Perez-Mesa C. Inflammatory carcinoma of the breast. *Cancer* 1978;41:1595–1605.
57. Pollak EW, Getzen LC. Inflammatory carcinoma of the breast. *Am J Surg Pathol* 1978;136:722–725.
58. Saltzstein SL. Clinically occult inflammatory carcinoma of the breast. *Cancer* 1975;34:382–388.
59. Weidner N, Semple JP, Welch WR, et al. Tumor angiogenesis and metastasis. Correlation in invasive breast carcinoma. *N Engl J Med* 1991;324:1–8.
60. Weidner N, Folkman J, Pozza F, et al. Tumor angiogenesis: a new significant and independent prognostic indicator in early-stage breast cancer. *J Natl Cancer Inst* 1992;84:1875–1887.
61. Bosari S, Lee A, DeLellis R, et al. Microvessel quantitation and prognosis in invasive breast carcinoma. *Hum Pathol* 1992;23:755–761.
62. Kaldjian E, Jin L, Lloyd R. Immunohistochemical analysis of breast carcinomas: correlation of estrogen and progesterone receptors, proliferative activity, tumor vascularity and lymph node metastasis. *Mod Pathol* 1992;5:14–21.
63. Sneige N, Singletary E, Sahin A. Multiparameter analysis of potential prognostic factors in node negative breast cancer patients. *Mod Pathol* 1992;5:18.
64. De Paola F, Granato AM, Scarpi E, et al. Vascular endothelial growth factor and prognosis in patients with node- negative breast cancer. *Int J Cancer* 2002;98:228–233.
65. Gasparini G. Prognostic value of vascular endothelial growth factor in breast cancer. *Oncologist* 2000;5:37–44.
66. Guidi AJ, Schnitt SJ, Fischer L, et al. Vascular permeability factor (vascular endothelial growth factor) expression and angiogenesis in patients with ductal carcinoma *in situ* of the breast. *Cancer* 1997;80:1945–53.

67. Battersby S, Robertson BJ, Anderson TJ, et al. Influence of menstrual cycle, parity and oral contraceptive use on steroid hormone receptors in normal breast. *Br J Cancer* 1992;65:601–607.
68. Allred DC, Harvey JM, Berardo M, et al. Prognostic and predictive factors in breast cancer by immunohistochemical analysis. *Mod Pathol* 1998;11:155–168.
69. Andersen J, Poulsen HS. Immunohistochemical estrogen receptor determination in paraffin-embedded tissue: prediction of response to hormonal treatment in advanced breast cancer. *Cancer* 1989;64:1901–1908.
70. Li CI, Malone KE, Weiss NS, et al. Tamoxifen therapy for primary breast cancer and risk of contralateral breast cancer. *J Natl Cancer Inst* 2001;93:1008–1013.
71. Vogel VG. Reducing the risk of breast cancer with tamoxifen in women at increased risk. *J Clin Oncol* 2001;19:87S–92S.
72. Munoz de Toro MM, Maffini MV, Kass L, et al. Proliferative activity and steroid hormone receptor status in male breast carcinoma. *J Steroid Biochem Mol Biol* 1998;67:333–339.
73. Ballare C, Bravo AI, Sorin I, et al. The expression of progesterone receptors coincides with an arrest of DNA synthesis in human breast cancer. *Cancer* 1991;67:1352–1358.
74. Tesch M, Shawwa A, Henderson R. Immunohistochemical determination of estrogen and progesterone receptor status in breast cancer. *Am J Clin Pathol* 1993;99:8–12.
75. McCarty KSJ, Miller LS, Cox EB, et al. Estrogen receptor analyses: correlation of biochemical and immunochemical methods using monoclonal antireceptor antibodies. *Arch Pathol Lab Med* 1985;109:716–721.
76. Poulsen HS, Ozello L, King WJ, et al. The use of monoclonal antibodies to estrogen receptors (ER) for immunoperoxidase detection of ER in paraffin sections of human breast cancer tissue. *J Histochem Cytochem* 1985;33:87–92.
77. Cheng L, Binder SW, Fu YS, et al. Demonstration of estrogen receptors by monoclonal antibody in formalin-fixed breast tumors. *Lab Invest* 1988;58:346–353.
78. Allred DC, Bustamante MA, Daniel CO, et al. Immunocytochemical analysis of estrogen receptors in human breast carcinomas: evaluation of 130 cases and review of the literature regarding concordance with biochemical assay and clinical relevance. *Arch Surg* 1990;125:107–134.
79. Elledge RM, Green S, Pugh R, et al. Estrogen receptor (ER) and progesterone receptor (PgR), by ligand-binding assay compared with ER, PgR and pS2, by immunohistochemistry in predicting response to tamoxifen in metastatic breast cancer: a Southwest Oncology Group Study. *Int J Cancer* 2000;89:111–117.
80. Pertschuk LP, Feldman JG, Kim Y-D, et al. Estrogen receptor immunohistochemistry in paraffin embedded tissues with ER1D5 predicts breast cancer endocrine response more accurately than H222Spg in frozen tissue and ligand-binding assays. *Cancer* 1996;77:2514–2519.
81. Keshgegian AA, Cnaan A. Proliferation markers in breast carcinoma: mitotic figure count, S-phase fraction, proliferating cell nuclear antigen, Ki-67, and MIB-1. *Am J Clin Pathol* 1995;104:42–49.
82. Battifora H, Mehta P, Ahn C, et al. Estrogen receptor immunohistochemical assay in paraffin-embedded tissue: a better gold standard? *Appl Immunohistochem* 1993;1:39–45.
83. Esteban JM, Battifora H, Warsi Z, et al. Quantification of estrogen receptors on paraffin-embedded tumors by image analysis. *Mod Pathol* 1991;4:53–57.
84. Esteban J, Dandalaft P, Mehta P, et al. Improvement on the quantification of estrogen and progesterone receptors on paraffin-embedded tumors by image analysis. *Am J Clin Pathol* 1993;99:32–38.
85. Esteban JM, Ahn C, Mehta P, et al. Biologic significance of quantitative estrogen receptor immunohistochemical assay by image analysis in breast cancer. *Am J Clin Pathol* 1994;102:158–162.
86. Esteban JM, Ahn C, Battifora H, et al. Predictive value of estrogen receptors evaluated by quantitative immunohistochemical analysis in breast cancer. *Am J Clin Pathol* 1994;102[Suppl]:S9–S12.
87. Taylor CR Paraffin section immunocytochemistry for estrogen receptor: the time has come. *Cancer* 1996;77:2419–2422.
88. Barnes DM, Millis RR. Oestrogen receptors: the history, the relevance and the methods of evaluation. In: Kirkham N, Lemoine NR, eds. *Progress in pathology*. 1995:89–114.
89. Leers MP, Nap M. Steroid receptor heterogeneity in relation to DNA index in breast cancer: a multiparameter flow cytometric approach on paraffin-embedded tumor samples. *Breast J* 2001;7:249–259.
90. Allred DC, Harvey JM, Berardo M, et al. Prognostic and predictive factors in breast cancer by immunohistochemical analysis. *Mod Pathol* 1998;11:155–168.
91. Rhodes A, Jasani B, Barnes DM, et al. Reliability of immunohistochemical demonstration of oestrogen receptors in routine practice: interlaboratory variance in the sensitivity of detection and evaluation of scoring systems. *J Clin Pathol* 2000;53:125–130.

92. Rhodes A, Jasani B, Balaton AJ, et al. Immunohistochemical demonstration of oestrogen and progesterone receptors: correlation of standards achieved on in house tumours with that achieved on external quality assessment material in over 150 laboratories from 26 countries. *J Clin Pathol* 2000; 53:292–301.
93. Rhodes A, Jasani B, Balaton AJ, et al. Study of interlaboratory reliability and reproducibility of estrogen and progesterone receptor assays in Europe. Documentation of poor reliability and identification of insufficient microwave antigen retrieval time as a major contributory element of unreliable assays. *Am J Clin Pathol* 2001;115:44–58.
94. Walker RA. Oestrogen receptor and its potential role in breast cancer development. *J Pathol* 1999; 188:229–30.
95. Slamon DJ, deKernion JB, Verma IM, et al. Expression of cellular oncogenes in human malignancies. *Science* 1984;224:256–262.
96. Slamon DJ, Clark GM, Wong SG, et al. Human breast cancer: correlation of relapse and survival with amplification of the HER-2/neu oncogene. *Science* 1987;235:177–182.
97. Varley JM, Swallow JE, Brammar WJ, et al. Alterations to either c-erbB-2 (neu) or c-myc proto-oncogenes in breast carcinomas correlate with poor short-term prognosis. *Oncogene* 1987;1:423–430.
98. Van de Vijver M, van de Bersselaar R, Devilee P, et al. Amplification of the neu (c-erbB-2) oncogene in human mammary tumors is relatively frequent and is often accompanied by amplification of the linked c-erbA oncogene. *Mol Cell Biol* 1987;7:2019–2023.
99. Van de Vijver MJ, Peterse JL, Mooi WJ, et al. Neu-protein overexpression in breast cancer. Association with comedo-type ductal carcinoma *in situ* and limited prognostic value in stage II breast cancer. *N Engl J Med* 1988;319:1239–1245.
100. Press M, Cordon-Cardo C, Slamon D. Expression of the Her2/neu oncogene in human adult and fetal tissues. *Oncogene* 1990;5:953–962.
101. Soomro S, Shousha S, Taylor P, et al. c-erbB-2 expression in different histological types of invasive breast carcinoma. *J Clin Pathol* 1991;44:211–214.
102. Press M, Pike MEA. HER2/neu expression in node negative breast cancer direct tissue quantitation by computerized image analysis and association of overexpression with increased risk of recurrent disease. *Cancer Res* 1993:53:4960–4970.
103. Rilke F, Colnaghi M, Cascinelli N, et al. Prognostic significance of Her2/neu expression in breast cancer and its relationship to other prognostic factors. *Int J Cancer* 1991;49:44–49.
104. Toikkanen S, Helin H, Isola J, et al. Prognostic significance of HER2 oncoprotein expression in breast cancer: a 30-year follow up. *J Clin Oncol* 1992;10:1044–1048.
105. Tsuda H, Hirohashi S, Shimosato Y, et al. Correlation between histologic grade of malignancy and copy number of c-erbB-2 gene in breast carcinoma: a retrospective analysis of 176 cases. *Cancer* 1990;65:1794–1800.
106. Battifora H, Gaffey M, Esteban J, et al. Immunohistochemical assay of neu/c-erb-2 oncogene product in paraffin-embedded tissues in early breast cancer: retrospective follow-up study of 245 stage I and II cases. *Mod Pathol* 1991;4:466–474.
107. Allred DC, Clark GM, Molina R. Overexpression of HER-2/neu and its relationship with other prognostic factors change during the progression of *in situ* to invasive breast cancer. *Hum Pathol* 1992; 23:974–979.
108. Parkes HC, Lillycrop K, Howell A, et al. c-erB2 mRNA expression in human breast tumours: comparison with c-erB2 DNA amplification and correlation with prognosis. *Br J Cancer* 1990;61:39–45.
109. Rosen PP, Lesser ML, Arroyo CD, et al. Immunohistochemical detection of HER2/neu in patients with axillary lymph node negative breast carcinoma: a study of epidemiologic risk factors, histologic features, and prognosis. *Cancer* 1995;75:1320–1326.
110. Clark G, McGuire W. Follow-up study of HER2/neu amplification in primary breast cancer. *Cancer Res* 1991;51:944–948.
111. Pierce L, Merino MEA. Is C-ERB b-2 a predictor of recurrence in early breast cancer? *J Radiat Oncol Biol Phys* 1994;28:395–403.
112. Press M, Hung G, Godolphin W, et al. Sensitivity of HER2/neu antibodies in archival tissue samples: a potential source of error in immunohistochemical studies of oncogene expression. *Cancer Res* 1994;54:2771–2777.
113. DiGiovanna M, Stern D. Activation state-specific monoclonal antibody detects tyrosine phosphorylated p185 neu/erb B-2 in a subset of human breast tumors overexpressing this receptor. *Cancer Res* 1995;55:1946–1955.
114. Lehrer S, Lee P, Tartter P, et al. Tumour HER2 protein in breast cancer and family history. *Lancet* 1993;341:1420–1421.

115. Borresen A-L, Ottestad L, Gaustad A, et al. Amplification and protein over-expression of the neu/HER2/c-erB-2 protooncogene in human breast carcinomas: relationship to loss of gene sequences on chromosome 17, family history and prognosis. *Br J Cancer* 1990;62:585–590.
116. Perez EA, Hortobagyi GN. Ongoing and planned adjuvant trials with trastuzumab. *Semin Oncol* 2000;27:26–32; discussion 92–100.
117. McKeage K, Perry CM. Trastuzumab: a review of its use in the treatment of metastatic breast cancer overexpressing HER2. *Drugs* 2002;62:209–243.
118. Ridolfi RL, Jamehdor MR, Arber JM. HER-2/neu testing in breast carcinoma: a combined immunohistochemical and fluorescence *in situ* hybridization approach (in process citation). *Mod Pathol* 2000;13:866–873.
119. Couturier J, Vincent-Salomon A, Nicolas A, et al. Strong correlation between results of fluorescent *in situ* hybridization and immunohistochemistry for the assessment of the ERBB2 (HER-2/neu) gene status in breast carcinoma. *Mod Pathol* 2000;13:1238–1243.
120. Jacobs TW, Gown AM, Yaziji H, et al. Comparison of fluorescence *in situ* hybridization and immunohistochemistry for the evaluation of HER-2/neu in breast cancer. *J Clin Oncol* 1999;17:1974–1982.
121. Lehr HA, Jacobs TW, Yaziji H, et al. Quantitative evaluation of HER-2/neu status in breast cancer by fluorescence *in situ* hybridization and by immunohistochemistry with image analysis. *Am J Clin Pathol* 2001;115:814–822.
122. Ridolfi RL, Jamehdor MR, Arber JM. HER-2/neu testing in breast carcinoma: a combined immunohistochemical and fluorescence *in situ* hybridization approach. *Mod Pathol* 2000;13:866–873.
123. Pauletti G, Dandekar S, Rong H, et al. Assessment of methods for tissue-based detection of the HER-2/neu alteration in human breast cancer: a direct comparison of fluorescence *in situ* hybridization and immunohistochemistry. *J Clin Oncol* 2000;18:3651–3664.
124. Fisher B, Bauer, M, Wickerham L, et al. Relation of number of positive axillary nodes to the prognosis of patients with primary breast cancer: an NSABP update. *Cancer* 1983;52:1551–1557.
125. Wilkinson EJ, Hause S. Probability in lymph node sectioning. *Cancer* 1974;33:1269.
126. Trojani M, de Mascarel I, Bonichon F, et al. Detection by immunohistochemistry and prognostic significance. *Br J Cancer* 1987;55:303–306.
127. Lachman MF, Ricci A Jr, Pedersen CA, et al. Detection of occult metastatic lobular carcinoma in axillary lymph nodes using anticytokeratin monoclonal antibodies. *Conn Med* 1992;56:65–68.
128. Weaver DL, Krag DN, Ashikaga T, et al. Pathologic analysis of sentinel and nonsentinel lymph nodes in breast carcinoma: a multicenter study. *Cancer* 2000;88:1099–1107.
129. Huvos AG, Hutter RV, Berg JW. Significance of axillary macrometastases and micrometastases in mammary cancer. *Ann Surg* 1971;173:44–46.
130. Fisher ER, Swamidoss S, Lee CH, et al. Detection and significance of occult axillary node metastases in patients with invasive breast cancer. *Cancer* 1978;42:2025–2031.
131. Hansen N, Grube B, Te W, et al. Clinical significance of axillary micrometastases in breast cancer: How small is too small? *Proc ASCO* 2001:24a.
132. Berg JW, Hutter RVP. Breast cancer. *Cancer* 1995;75:257–269.
133. Silverberg SG, Chitale AR, Hind AD, et al. Sinus histiocytosis and mammary carcinoma: study of 366 radical mastectomies and an historical review. *Cancer* 1970;26:1177.
134. Wernicke M. Quantitative morphologic assessment of immunoreactivity in regional lymph nodes of patients with carcinoma of the breast. *Surg Gynecol Obstet* 1975;140:919.
135. Kister SJ. Nuclear grade and sinus histiocytosis in cancer of the breast. *Cancer* 1969;23:570–575.
136. Tsakraklides V, Olson P, Kersey JH, et al. Prognostic significance of the regional lymph node histology in cancer of the breast. *Cancer* 1974;34:1259.
137. Edlow D, Carter D. Heterotopic epithelium in axillary lymph nodes: report of a case and review of the literature. *Am J Clin Pathol* 1973;59:666–668.
138. Turner DR, Millis RR. Breast tissue inclusions in axillary lymph nodes. *Histopathology* 1980;4:631–636.
139. Patel J, Nemoto T, Rosner D, et al. Axillary lymph node metastasis from an occult breast cancer. *Cancer* 1981;47:2923–2927.
140. Rosen PP. Axillary lymph node metastases in patients with occult noninvasive breast carcinoma. *Cancer* 1980;46:1298–1306.
141. Rosen PP, Kimmel M. Occult breast carcinoma presenting with axillary lymph node metastases: a follow-up study of 48 patients. *Hum Pathol* 1990;21:518–523.

142. Ellerbroek N, Holmes F, Singletary E, et al. Treatment of patients with isolated axillary nodal metastases from an occult primary carcinoma consistent with breast origin. *Cancer* 1990;66:1461–1467.
143. Fitts WT, Steiner GC, Enterline HT. Prognosis of occult carcinoma of the breast. *Surg Gynecol Obstet* 1963;106:460–463.
144. Grundfest S, Steiger E, Sebek B. Axillary adenopathy: use of estrogen receptor proteins as an aid in diagnosis. *Arch Surg* 1978;113:1108–1109.
145. Haupt HM, Rosen PP, Kinne DW. Breast carcinoma presenting with axillary lymph node metastases: an analysis of specific histologic features. *Am J Surg Pathol* 1985;9:165–175.
146. Westbrook KC, Gallager HS. Carcinoma presenting as an axillary metastasis. *Am J Surg* 1971;122: 607–612.
147. Wick MR, Lillemoe TJ, Copland GT, et al. Gross cystic disease fluid protein-15 as a marker for breast cancer: immunohistochemical analysis of 690 human neoplasms and comparison with alpha-lactalbumin. *Hum Pathol* 1989;20:281–287.
148. Fisher B, Wolmark N, Bauer M, et al. The accuracy of clinical nodal staging and of limited axillary dissection as a determinant of histologic nodal status in carcinoma of the breast. *Surg Gynecol Obstet* 1981;152:765–772.
149. Rosen PP, Fracchia AA, Urban JA, et al. "Residual" mammary carcinoma following simulated partial mastectomy. *Cancer* 1975;35:739–747.
150. CANCER AJCC. *American Joint Committee on Cancer staging manual*, 5th ed. Philadelphia: Lippincott-Raven Publishers, 1997:171–179.

10

Stromal Lesions

Although attention is usually focused on the epithelial changes of the breast, most clinically detectable abnormalities are the result of mammary stromal changes. Clinical examination or mammography does not differentiate normal tissue from cancer cells, but these procedures detect the hardness and radiodensity of the desmoplastic reaction to cancer cell growth. In many biopsies of benign breast tissue, the clinically suspicious abnormality is an irregular pattern of stromal density in the presence or absence of a variety of epithelial changes.

Before puberty, adipose tissue is the predominant component of breast stroma, but in adolescence, the stromal balance shifts to dense fibrovascular tissue, rich in collagen, with an admixture of smaller amounts of adipose tissue. After menopause, the balance returns to a predominance of adipose tissue, as it gradually replaces the fibrous tissue. It is therefore easier to screen postmenopausal women clinically and radiographically for the desmoplastic reaction that is associated with carcinoma, but uneven replacement of the fibrous stroma by fat may produce nodular densities or ridges that mimic cancer and often precipitate biopsy.

Intralobular stroma responds rapidly to growth factor stimulation and, during the reproductive years, it is apparently hormone-dependent, with dramatic changes during the menstrual cycle; however, interlobular stroma remains relatively constant. During lactation, intralobular stroma is thinned to the point where it is microscopically inapparent, but at other stages, it becomes dense and cellular (Chapter 1). Fibrous mastopathy is characterized by an unusually dense, relatively acellular, fibrous interlobular stroma.

GYNECOMASTIA AND JUVENILE HYPERTROPHY

Marked stromal density with periductal fibroblastic proliferation that is associated with a proliferating epithelial component occurs in the juvenile breast of young women as juvenile or virginal hypertrophy and in young men as gynecomastia. Gynecomastia occurs in about 10% of young men at the onset of puberty, but it persists in fewer than 5% for more than 1 year. It may occur in later years and is found often in men who are on estrogen therapy for carcinoma of the prostate. Clinically, it presents as a disk-like density of varying size, and surgical specimens are usually sharply circumscribed and densely fibrous (Fig. 10.1 and efig. 10.1). Microscopically, stromal cellular proliferation is limited to periductal areas, and there is an accompanying much less cellular increase in interlobular stroma (Fig. 10.2 and efig. 10.2). A peculiar epithelial proliferation is present in the lining cells of ducts (Fig.10.3). In young men, lobules are rarely present, but they may be found in older men who have taken estrogen for long periods of time (1). Juvenile hypertrophy in young women is grossly less circumscribed, but it is microscopically similar and associated with more interlobular stroma and more numerous lobules.

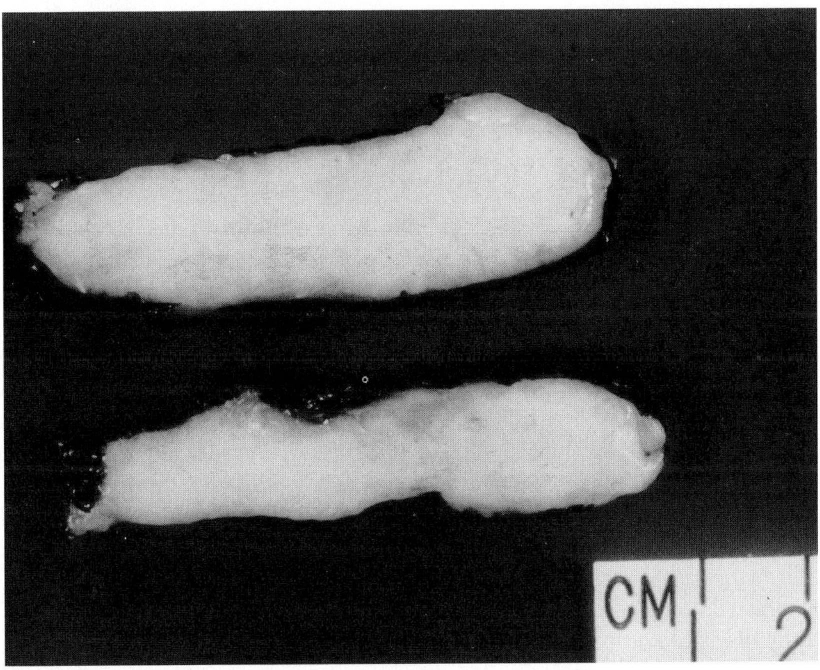

FIG. 10.1. Gynecomastia. The disk-like configuration of the fibrotic breast tissue is characteristic.

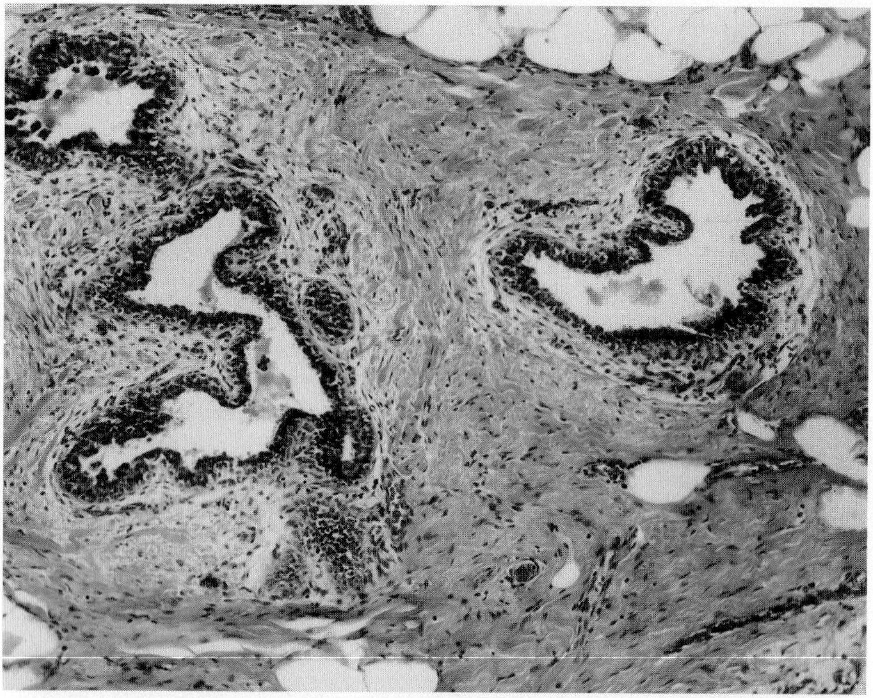

FIG. 10.2. Gynecomastia. There is a proliferation of the ducts and periductal stroma with a dense interlobular stroma that shows changes reminiscent of pseudoangiomatous stromal hyperplasia. No lobules are present.

FIBROADENOMA

Fibroadenoma (FA), the most common benign tumor of the breast, usually occurs in young adult women and presents as a dense circumscribed hypoechoic mass (Fig. 10.4 and efigs. 10.3 and 10.4). It is frequently examined by fine needle aspiration, which may be a source of potential false positive reports.

Histologically, FA can be seen as a proliferation of the fibroblasts of the intralobular stroma of adjacent lobules that coalesce to form a tumor mass. Each lobular unit is sharply demarcated by the relatively constant intervening interlobular stroma. Early in the natural history of FA, intralobular fibroblasts are numerous and they may produce a myxoid matrix or, rarely, contain an admixture of adipose tissue or smooth muscle (2). At low magnification, the basophilia of the proliferating lobular stroma contrasts with the eosinophilia of the interlobular stroma to reassure the pathologist that a benign lesion is present (Figs. 10.5 and 10.6 and efigs. 10.5 to 10.11). In the obsolescent phase, each area of intralobular stroma becomes less cellular, and the fibroblasts differentiate to produce denser collagen to leave a virtually noncellular nodule of collagenized matrix around a central terminal duct. In the postmenopausal woman, this lobular stroma may occasionally calcify or even focally ossify and present mammographically as a dense mass with clustered calcifications that are suggestive of carcinoma (Fig. 10.6).

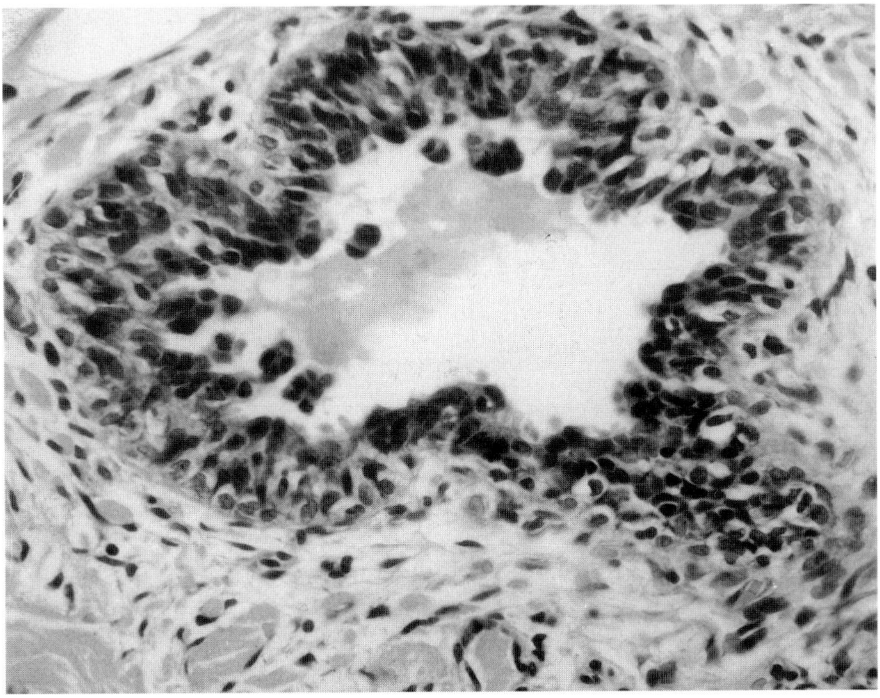

FIG. 10.3. Gynecomastia. A peculiar micropapillary proliferation of epithelial cells is present. Myoepithelium is prominent and there is a cellular periductal stroma. Changes similar to this are seen in juvenile hypertrophy of the female breast.

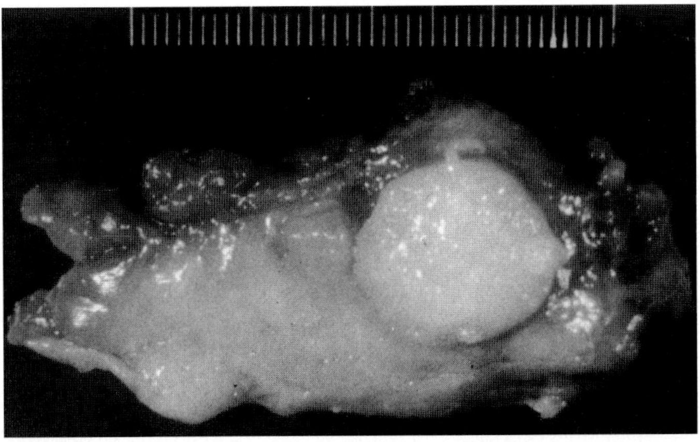

FIG. 10.4. Fibroadenoma. This sharply circumscribed nodule is firm to palpation. Smaller nodules at the 3 and 6 o'clock positions are present within the larger lesion.

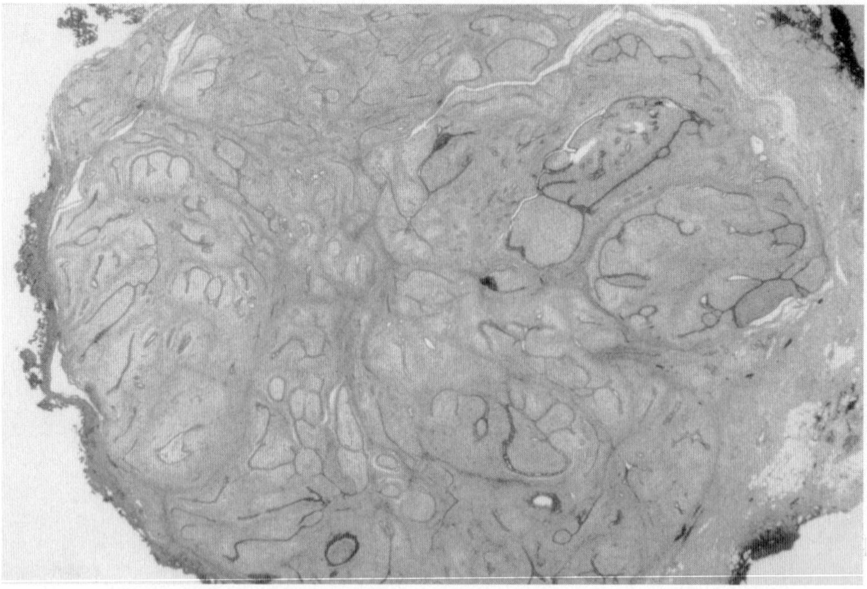

FIG. 10.5. Fibroadenoma. At low magnification, the nodularity is the result of proliferation of the stroma of multiple adjacent lobules that aggregate to form the larger mass. The terminal ducts are elongated in a stag-horn configuration. Acini are absent.

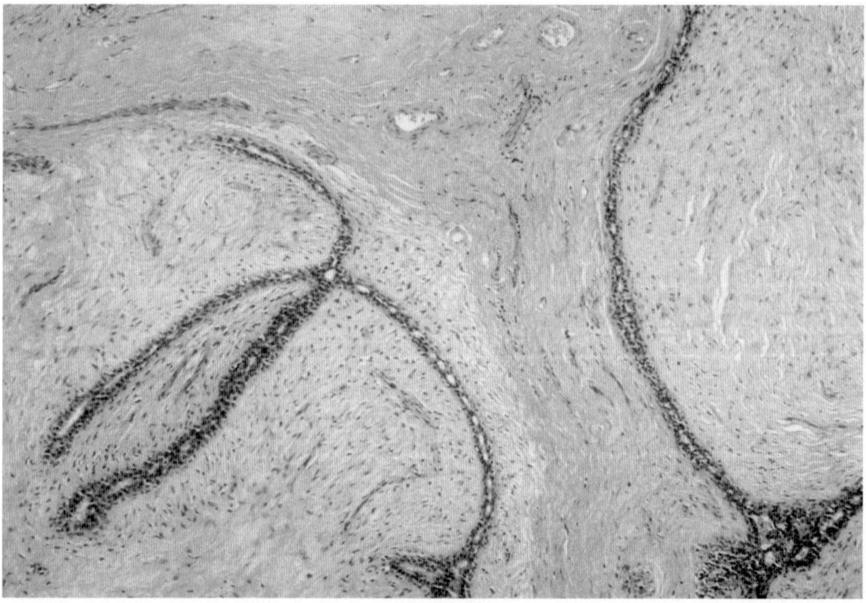

FIG. 10.6. Fibroadenoma. Clear separation of lobules is evident. Lobular stroma is proliferative, but interlobular stroma is not.

Both epithelium and stromal fibroblasts proliferate in FA, suggesting an interaction between the two tissue components. Sawhney et al. (3) found stromal mitotic figures to be concentrically related to epithelium and concluded that stromal growth was a result of stimulation by epithelial cells. The authors suggested that this was a feature of benign glandular/stromal neoplasms and that dependency of stromal fibroblasts on mitogenic stimulation by growth factors decreased as there was progression to stromal malignancy (cystosarcoma phyllodes). Epithelium in FA may show the full range of proliferative changes, described in the sections on intraductal and lobular lesions, with the same significance (4–6), although true ductal atypia is unusual and frank malignant change is quite rare. Kuijper et al. (7) studied 396 FAs and found carcinoma *in situ* in eight cases (five ductal and three lobular). No invasive carcinoma was found.

FAs are divided into pericanalicular and intracanalicular types, depending on stromal or epithelial predominance, but this has no known clinical significance. Histologically, FAs are characterized by the presence of elongated slit-like or staghorn ducts with proliferating lobular stroma that is capped by epithelium that projects into potential spaces (intracanalicular pattern) or proliferating lobular stromal fibroblasts in the periductal (pericanalicular) zone, with less proliferative activity in the intervening stroma.

The so-called juvenile FA (8) is one with proliferation of both epithelial and stromal components (efigs. 10.12 and 10.13). While usually seen in younger women, it has a broad age range and does not convey any elevated risk of recurrence or progression to malignancy.

Ansah-Boateng and Tavassoli (1) reported FAs and cystosarcoma phyllodes in men who had lobular differentiation in the breast tissues. The authors considered lobular development to be rare in men, unless there was a prolonged duration or intense elevation of estrogen stimulation beyond that which normally produced gynecomastia.

Acinar structures are usually not prominent in FA, but they may be retained and may contribute to the formation of histologically complex lesions, with combinations of intracanalicular and pericanalicular FA, sclerosing adenosis, and blunt duct adenosis that have varying degrees of epithelial proliferative activity in any or all of the components. No satisfactory nomenclature describes all of these localized glandular/stromal lesions.

Complex Fibroadenoma

Dupont et al. (9) studied 1,835 patients who had FAs, with follow-up, and reported that complex FAs, which were FAs with cysts (efigs. 10.14 to 10.16), sclerosing adenosis (efigs. 10.17 and 10.18), epithelial calcifications, or papillary apocrine changes had a 3.10 relative risk of developing invasive carcinoma, compared to a 3.88 relative risk for women with benign proliferative disease in the parenchyma adjacent to the FA. Complex FA, in patients with a family history of breast cancer, had a 3.72 relative risk of invasive carcinoma, compared to

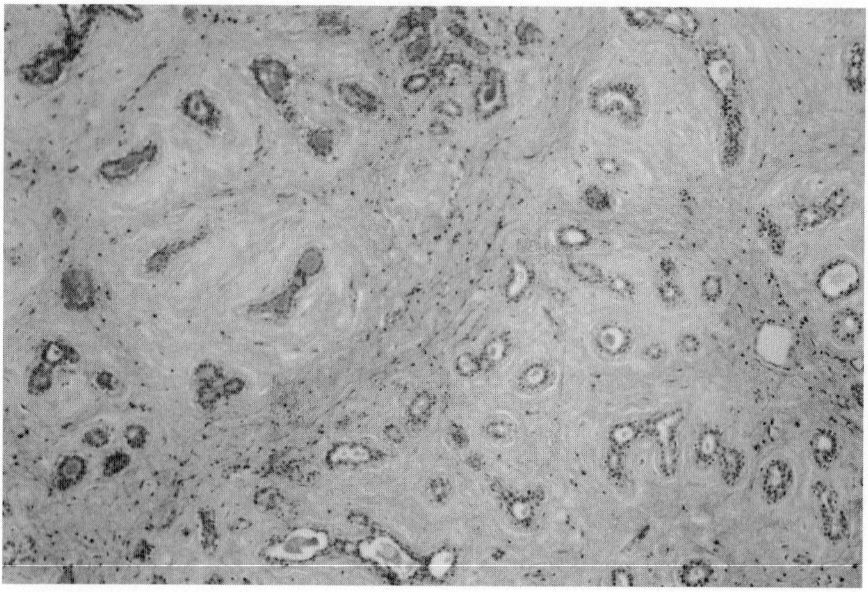

FIG. 10.7. Tubular adenoma. This proliferative lesion is part fibroadenoma (**left**), but has distended acinar structures characteristic of tubular adenoma (**right**).

women with a family history of breast cancer without FA. Noncomplex FA without family history was not associated with elevated risk of breast cancer.

Tubular Adenoma

Rosen and Oberman (10) used the term "tubular adenoma" to describe a glandular/stromal tumor that grossly and superficially resembled an FA, except that lobular units with dilated acini persisted (Fig. 10.7 and efigs. 10.19 to 10.21).

Fibroadenoma Versus Phyllodes Tumor

FAs may be large, single or multiple, and bilateral. They occur during adolescence or later, may attain great size, and are treated by observation or by simple excision without the likelihood of recurrence, unless multiple. The degree of cellularity in the stroma characteristically varies. Although the great majority of stromal/glandular lesions are benign, there are malignant counterparts (cystosarcoma phyllodes), and distinguishing the benign lesions from the malignant lesions is a classic problem for the surgical pathologist.

Much confusion has resulted from the use of the terms giant FA and benign cystosarcoma phyllodes (11–12), which indicates how difficult it may be to distinguish these entities. The extremes are readily distinguishable both grossly and histologically, but there is a difficult borderline group (Fig. 10.8 and efig.

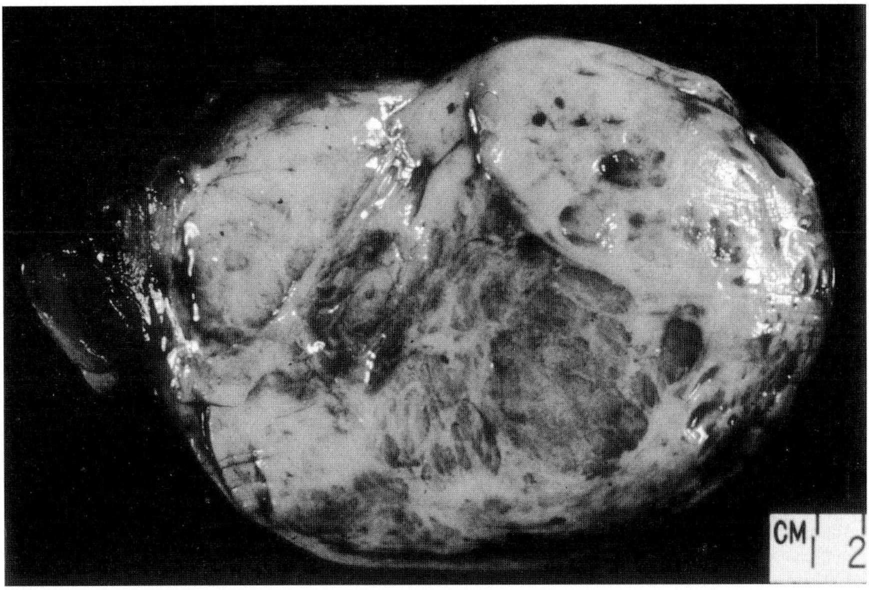

FIG. 10.8. Cellular fibroadenoma. The gross appearance is of a circumscribed nodular lesion that is fleshy and irregular.

10.22). Lesions with moderate (clearly benign) stromal cellularity may attain great size, and the term giant FA is appropriately applied to these cases. Tumors with a gross cystic structure, frond-like proliferation of epithelial and stromal elements within the cyst, and a markedly cellular, but not anaplastic or mitotically active fibroblastic component, were designated "phyllodes tumor" by Azzopardi (13) to avoid the oxymoron "benign cystosarcoma" for these borderline tumors. One of the histologic changes that indicates the progression from FA toward a more serious lesion is the disappearance of the contrast between basophilic lobular and eosinophilic interlobular stroma. Phyllodes tumors and cystosarcomas have an overall basophilic appearance, as fibroblasts between lobules become more proliferative, which has been termed stromal overgrowth. In the extreme, there is a monomorphous proliferation of fibroblasts from the basement membranes of one lobular unit to the basement membranes of the next. Figures 10.9 to 10.11 and efigs. 10.23 to 10.36 display the range of stromal proliferation in the intermediate lesions.

For lesions with borderline histology, there is an increased risk of local recurrence, but local excision is the indicated initial treatment for FA, phyllodes tumors, and cystosarcoma phyllodes. Recurrence of any glandular/stromal lesion should be viewed with concern, and both the initial and recurrent lesions should be examined carefully for evidence of an increase in stromal cellularity and anaplasia. However, metastasis from a phyllodes tumor is unlikely. Wide exci-

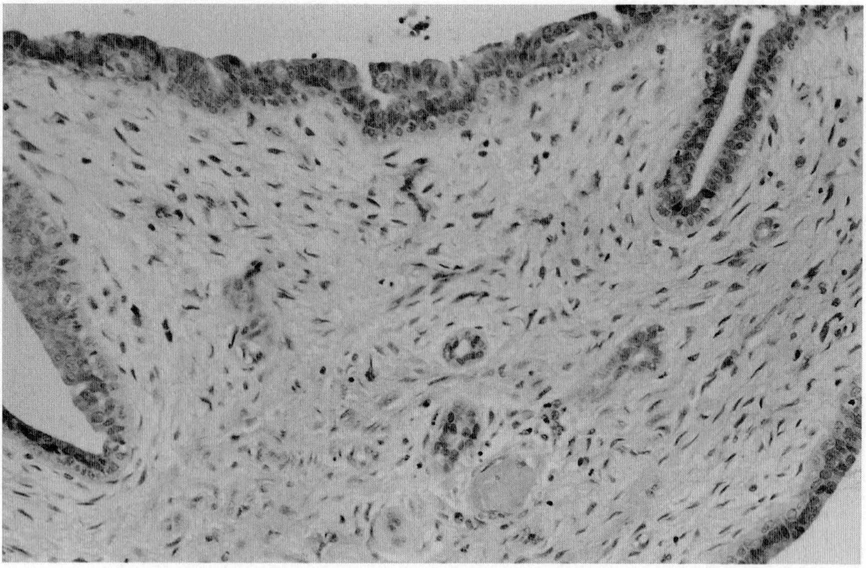

FIG. 10.9. Cellular fibroadenoma. Part of the proliferative lesion pushes out into a prominent frond-like pattern. The density of fibroblasts is increased.

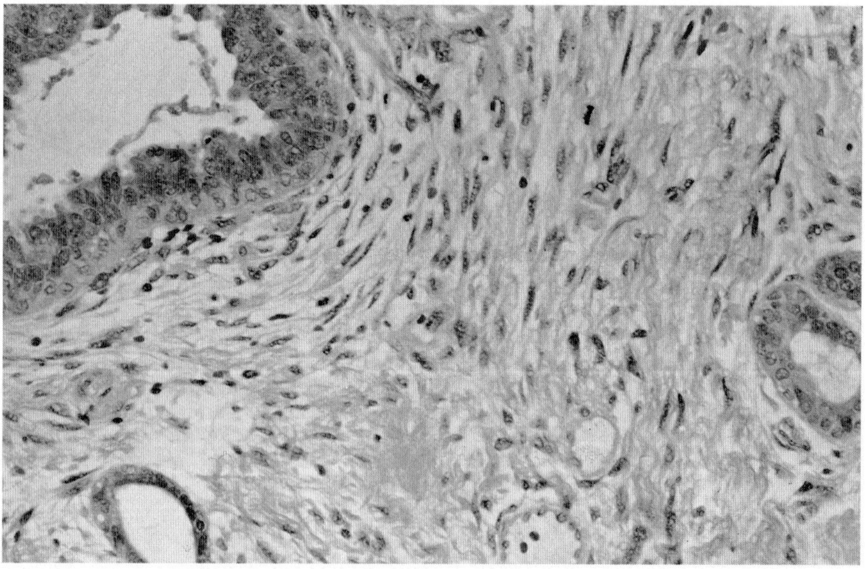

FIG. 10.10. Cellular fibroadenoma. The density of fibroblasts is increased, but the nuclei are not enlarged or anaplastic. A single mitotic figure is evident.

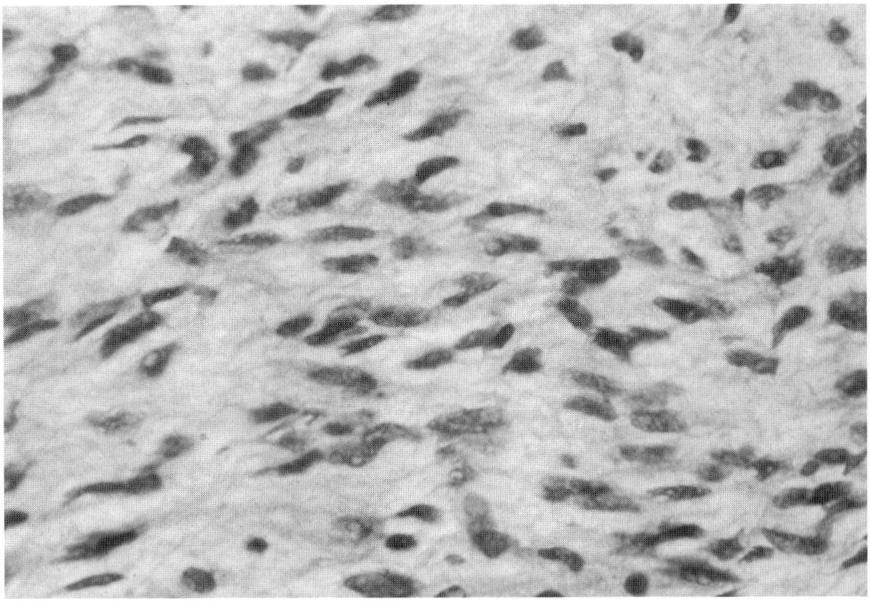

FIG. 10.11. Cellular fibroadenoma. The fibroblasts show no anaplasia or pleomorphism; however, their density is increased.

sion to prevent further recurrence and possible further progression in degree of malignancy is indicated.

Do cystosarcomas arise from FA? FA is quite common, and cellular FA is almost always seen in women in their childbearing years; cystosarcomas are rare and are often seen in postmenopausal women. The two lesions are both fibroepithelial, and cystosarcoma may contain histologically benign areas that are indistinguishable from those seen in FA. Progression of FA to sarcoma may occur, but it must be a rare event. A strong clinical case has been made for the *de novo* origin of true cystosarcomas.

El-Naggar et al. (14) studied 42 spindle cell-containing neoplasms of the breast by flow cytometry. The authors found that all 18 of the FAs, regardless of size, were diploid; phyllodes tumors were either diploid or aneuploid, with a striking correlation of survival with diploid status; and 7 stromal sarcomas were all aneuploid. Noguchi et al. (15) analyzed the clonality of 10 FAs and 5 phyllodes tumors by polymerase chain reaction (PCR) for restriction fragment polymorphisms of X-linked phosphoglycerokinase and differential methylation of this gene. The authors found the epithelial component of FA and phyllodes tumor and the stromal component of FA to be polyclonal and the stromal component of the phyllodes tumors to be monoclonal, thereby distinguishing the phyllodes lesions as neoplastic and the FA as hyperplastic, rather than as truly neoplastic.

No single criterion distinguishes FA from phyllodes tumor and no single criterion distinguishes phyllodes tumor from malignant cystosarcoma phyllodes. All are predominantly stromal neoplasms in which there is also proliferation of epithelium. Stromal histology determines the diagnosis. It should be stressed that there is often significant variation in stromal histology within a single lesion, which necessitates examination of multiple blocks to find the most cellular areas. It is not unusual to find areas indistinguishable from FA in a fully malignant cystosarcoma. Because of this, all lesions with the characteristic gross appearance of a phyllodes tumor or a leaf-like pattern of proliferative tissue, which extends into cystic spaces, cellular FA, and recurrent FA, should be examined thoroughly.

CYSTOSARCOMA PHYLLODES

Cystosarcoma phyllodes (CP) is the malignant glandular/stromal lesion, with the stromal element representing the malignancy with the ability to locally recur, invade and, rarely, to metastasize, and the epithelial component necessary for the

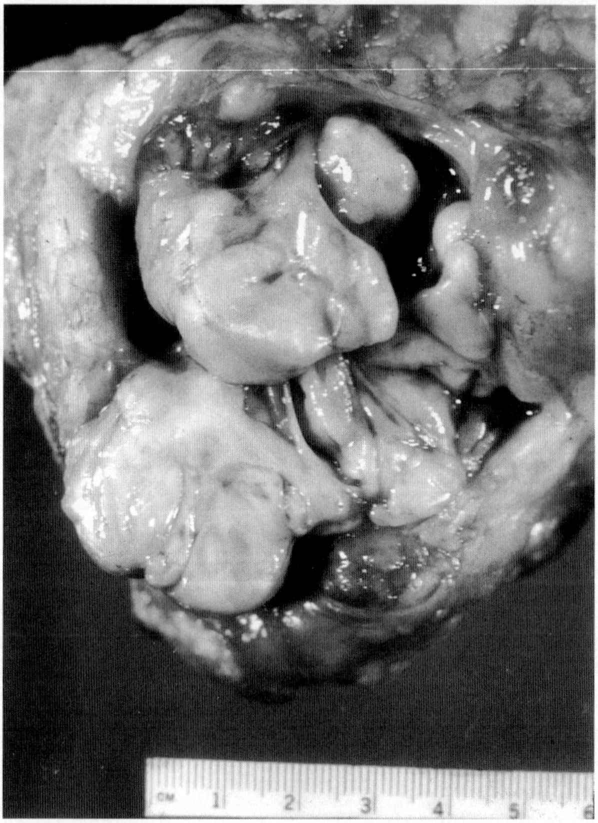

FIG. 10.12. Cystosarcoma phyllodes. Grossly, the outside border is circumscribed and the lesion is cystic with frond-like proliferation of fleshy structures into the cysts.

diagnosis, but not histologically malignant or capable of metastasis. CP presents as a large mass in women older, on average, than those with FA, although there is considerable overlap. Dusenbery and Frable (16) found little value in fine needle aspirations of CP, as one-half were diagnosed as carcinomas and there were also false negatives. Many CPs have a large, extremely active, and atypical epithelial component. Rarely, intraductal and even invasive ductal carcinomas have been found in association with cystosarcoma stroma.

Grossly, CP are large, usually cystic, and they have foci of hemorrhagic necrosis (Fig. 10.12 and efig. 10.37). The proliferating stromal cells have the appearance of fibroblasts and resemble low-grade or high-grade fibrosarcomas that have considerable variation in cellularity, pleomorphism, mitotic rate, and anaplasia (Figs. 10.13 to 10.22 and efigs. 10.38 to efig. 10.44).

Stromal overgrowth is prominent and it is an important diagnostic feature, but the degree of malignancy is primarily determined by the appearance of the proliferating fibroblasts. Size and invasion of the chest wall are useful observations and usually correlate with histology.

Malignant fibrous histiocytoma, osteosarcoma, chondrosarcoma, and liposarcoma may be seen as the malignant stromal component (Figs. 10.23 and 10.24 and

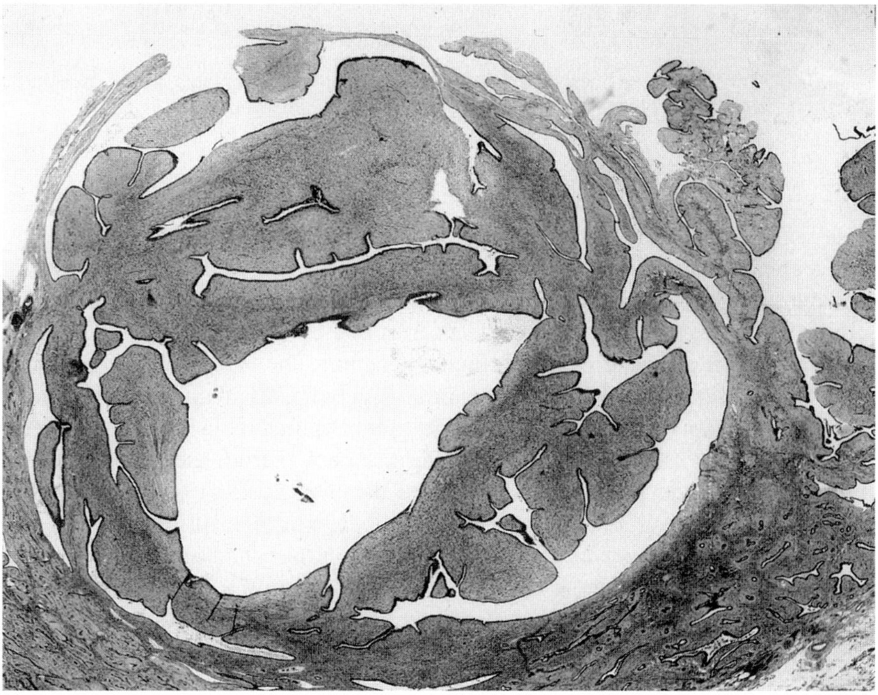

FIG. 10.13. Cystosarcoma phyllodes. At low magnification, palm-like fronds extend into the cystic space.

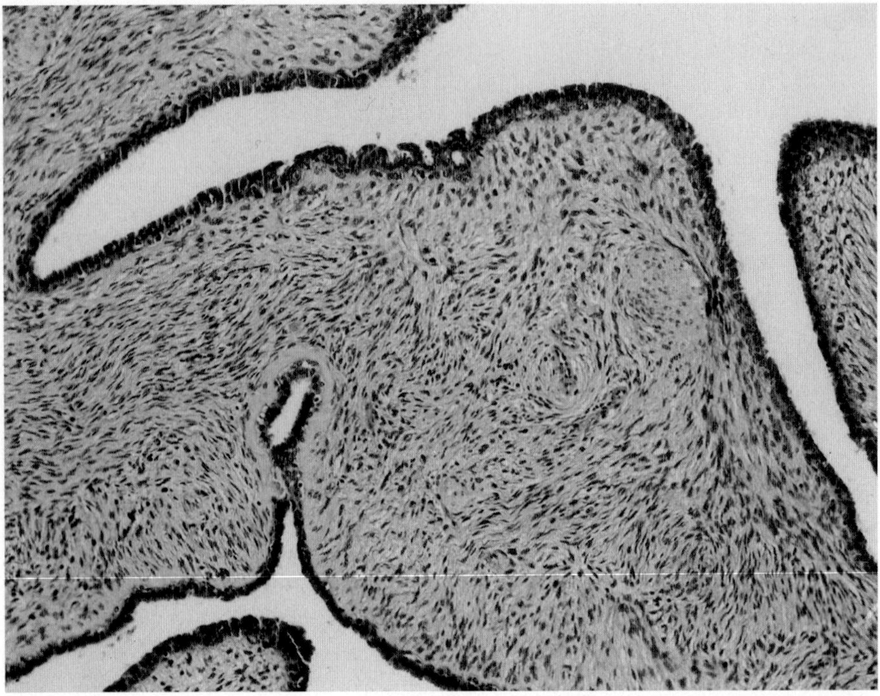

FIG. 10.14. Cystosarcoma phyllodes. The frond-like proliferation contains a high density of fibroblasts, but pleomorphism, anaplasia, and mitotic figures are not present.

efigs. 10.45 to 10.48). Powell and Rosen (17) reported 14 cases of CP with adipose tissue differentiation that ranged from mature adipose tissue in a histologically benign CP to high-grade pleomorphic liposarcoma in a malignant CP. Hemorrhage and necrosis were common features of the higher-grade lesions (18–21).

Norris and Taylor (22) reported on a series of 94 patients with CP and related their pathologic characteristics to clinical behavior. The features that best correlated with clinical behavior were size, mitotic activity, an infiltrative border, and cytologic atypism of the stromal cells. The authors pointed out that no single feature was wholly reliable in distinguishing the benign from the malignant cystosarcomas. Fifteen percent of the tumors that had pushing or circumscribed margins recurred, and 38% of those in which there was an infiltrating or invasive margin recurred. There was one fatal neoplasm in the 39 patients with pushing margins and nine fatal tumors in 26 patients with infiltrating or invasive margins. Only 2 of 30 patients with minimal cellular atypism died of tumor, and 13 of 53 patients with moderate or large amounts of cellular atypism died of tumors. No patient with a cystosarcoma that was smaller than 4 cm in diameter or with fewer than 3 mitotic figures per 10 high-power fields in the areas of greatest mitotic activity died because of tumor. However, 2 of 18 patients with tumors that were

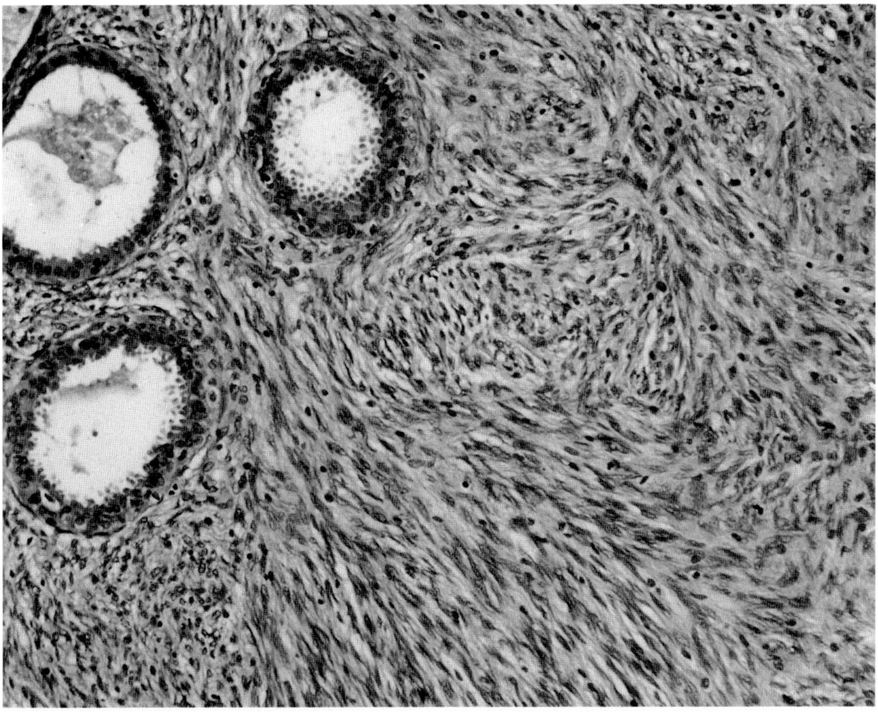

FIG. 10.15. Cystosarcoma phyllodes. The marked hypercellularity of the fibroblasts, which extend to the basement membrane around the ducts, is evident.

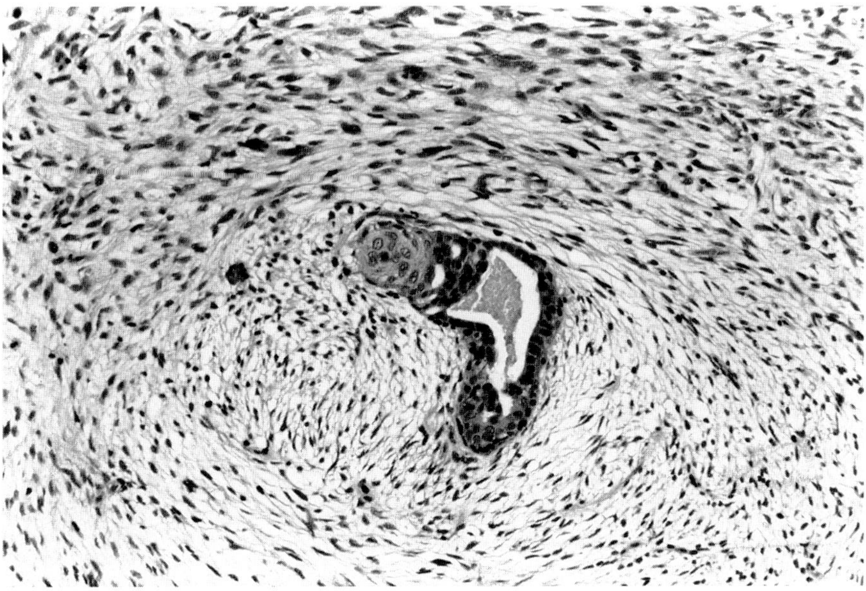

FIG. 10.16. Cystosarcoma phyllodes. The periductal stroma is markedly hypercellular with a mitotic figure present. There is virtually no difference between the periductal stroma and the interlobular stroma, which is as cellular. This is termed stromal overgrowth.

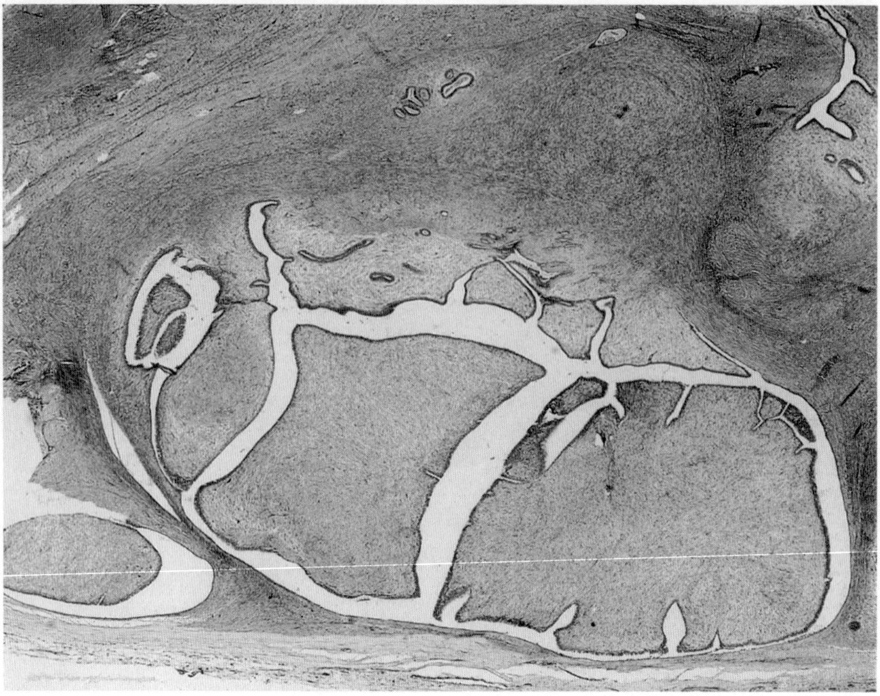

FIG. 10.17. Tumor with phyllodes pattern and marked variation in the cellularity of the stromal growth. In the pericystic area, there is moderate cellularity with a striking increase at the periphery.

smaller than 3.9 cm had recurrence and 4 of 23 patients with tumors that showed little mitotic activity had local recurrence.

Metastases from cystosarcoma to axillary lymph nodes were quite rare. In only one patient was this occurrence documented histologically, although axillary lymph node enlargement was not uncommon. Fifteen of the 94 patients died of CP. The longest survival after initial therapy among the fatal cases was 5.7 years, and recurrence was evident within 24 months in all but 3 cases. The lung was the most common site of metastasis, with pulmonary deposits in 12 of the 15 fatal cases, but the lesion may metastasize to other sites as well.

Hajdu et al. (23) summarized the clinicopathologic correlations of patients with recurrent CP according to the original histology. Twenty-eight (18%) of 150 women with previously benign CP developed recurrence. In these patients, the histologic appearance of the recurrence was of a higher grade than in the original. The majority of the recurrent benign cystosarcomas recurred more than 1.5 years after the primary surgery, whereas the time to recurrence in 4 (8%) of the 49 patients with originally malignant cystosarcoma was less. Only 1 of the 28 patients with recurrent "benign" cystosarcoma died of disseminated disease, but 2 of the 4 patients who had recurrent malignant cystosarcoma died with dissem-

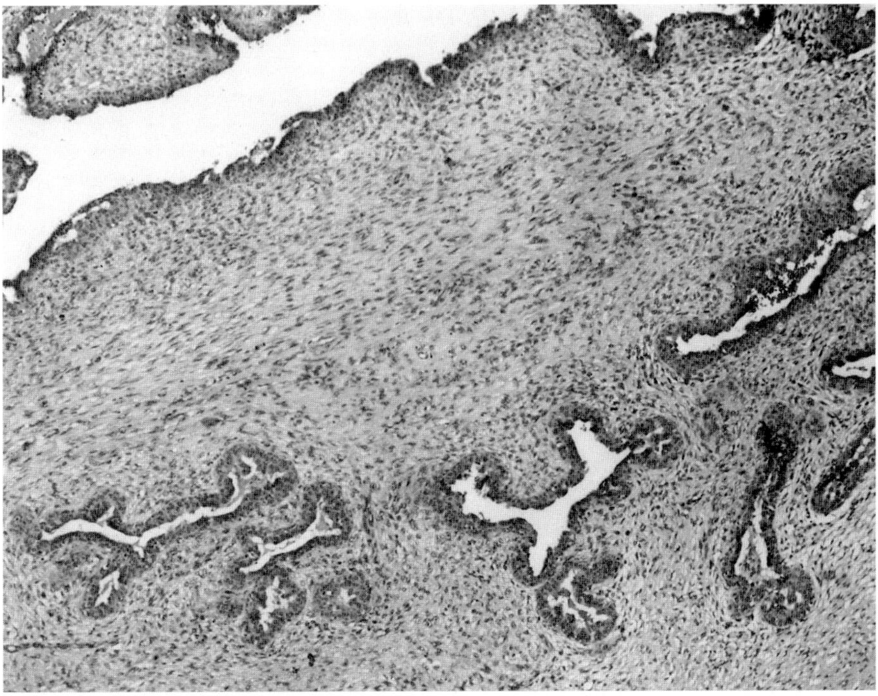

FIG. 10.18. Malignant cystosarcoma phyllodes. The fibroblastic density is increased in this area. Extension to the basement membrane of all epithelial structures is evident.

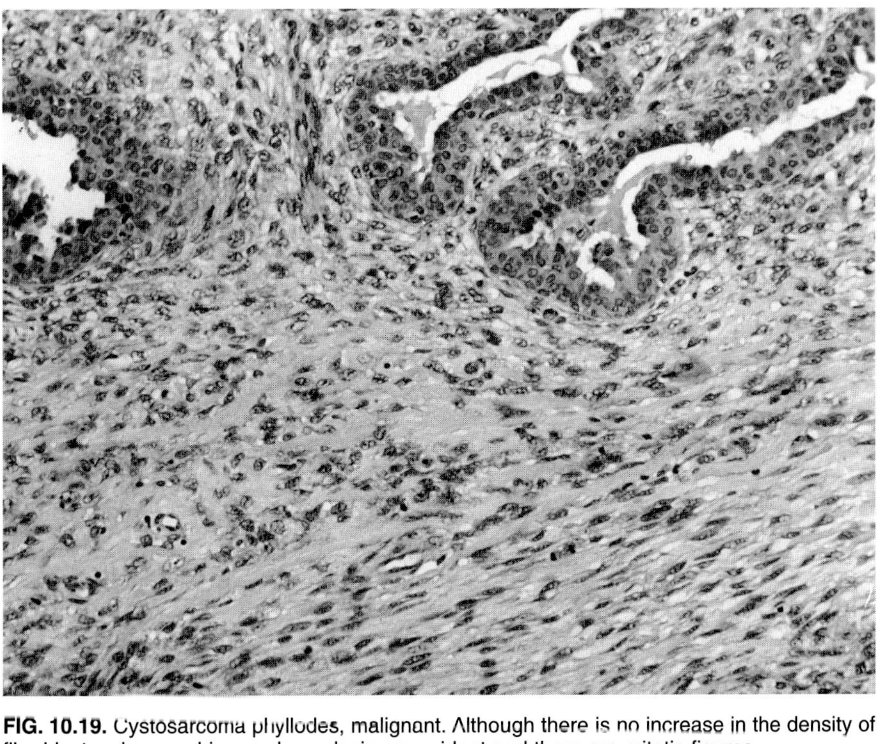

FIG. 10.19. Cystosarcoma phyllodes, malignant. Although there is no increase in the density of fibroblasts, pleomorphism and anaplasia are evident and there are mitotic figures.

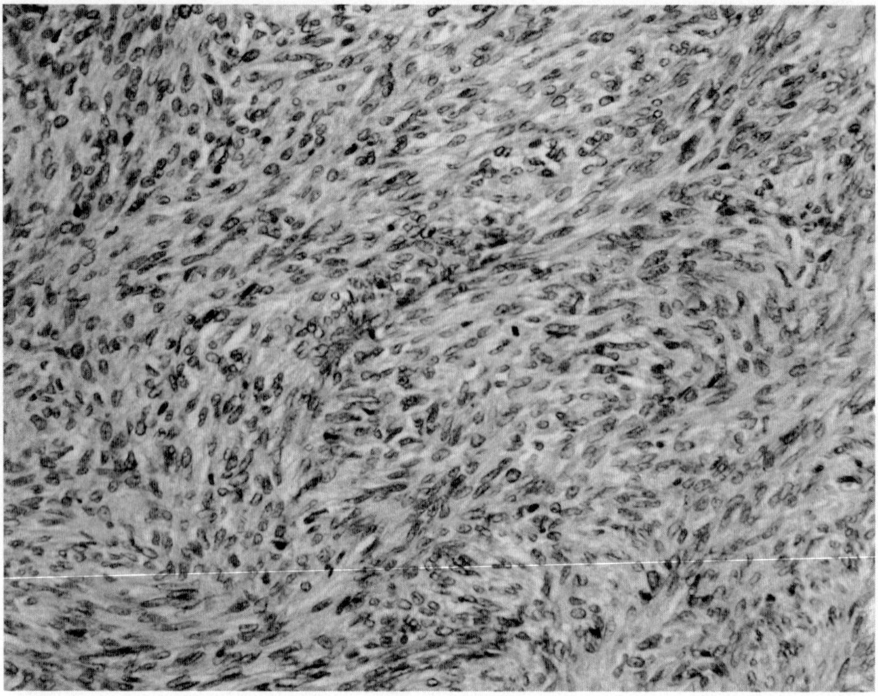

FIG. 10.20. Cystosarcoma phyllodes, malignant. The anaplasia and pleomorphism of the nuclei is part of this swirling pattern, similar to what might be seen in a malignant fibrous histiocytoma. The stromal component is dominant and is the malignant part of the tumor. Often an epithelial component can be found only after extensive sectioning. Differential diagnosis is stromal sarcoma, which is also treated by wide local excision.

inated disease 6 and 12 months, respectively, after their first surgery. In general, all recurrences were slightly more cellular than the original tumors, and intracystic extension of the tumor was common. Adequate surgical removal of cystosarcomas is needed to prevent recurrence.

Pietruska and Barnes (24) reported a retrospective analysis of 42 patients with CP. They divided cystosarcomas into benign, borderline, and malignant lesions. The benign lesions had 0 to 4 mitoses per 10 high-power fields, predominantly pushing margins, and slight to moderate stromal atypia. Borderline lesions had 5 to 9 mitoses per 10 high-power fields, moderate atypia, and either pushing or infiltrating margins. The malignant cystosarcomas had 10 or more mitoses per 10 high-power fields, predominantly infiltrating margins, and moderate to marked degrees of cytologic atypia. The epithelial component in this group was hyperplastic in one-third of cases, normal in one-third of cases, metaplastic in three cases, and atypical in two cases. In one case, there was a carcinoma associated with the malignant stroma. The authors associated an atrophic or normal epithelium with malignant cystosarcomas and a hyperplastic epithelium with the

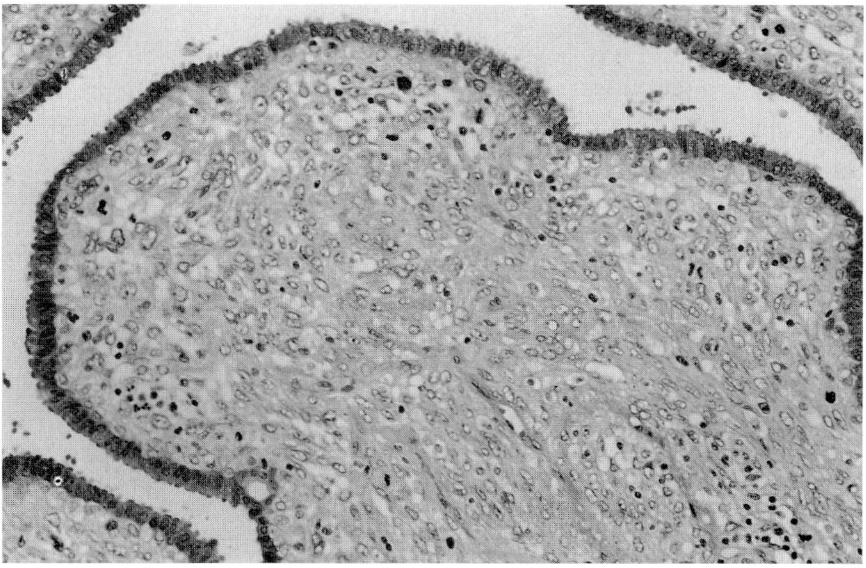

FIG. 10.21. Cystosarcoma phyllodes, malignant. The frond-like configuration is formed by proliferating stromal cells with numerous mitotic figures. A hyperplastic, but orderly, epithelium covers this frond-like structure.

more benign phyllodes tumors, but this is not universally observed. Local recurrence was noted in six patients from all three categories. One borderline tumor recurred 14 times and eventually proved fatal, as a result of contiguous pulmonary involvement. None of the tumors that were designated benign cystosarcoma developed systemic metastases. Three of the 19 women with malignant cystosarcomas died of metastatic disease, and another woman was alive 6 months after surgery, with metastases to both the lungs and the brain.

Reinfuss et al. (25) reviewed 55 cases of CP and confirmed the findings related above. Hawkins et al. (26) studied 33 cases and stressed the importance of stromal overgrowth as a criterion for predicting metastases from CP, in addition to the features previously noted. Stromal overgrowth was found in those CPs that most closely resembled sarcomas with little epithelial proliferation. From a literature review, the authors reported a 72% metastatic rate when stromal overgrowth was present. Local recurrence of a CP with stromal overgrowth was reported to be an especially ominous sign.

In summary, high-grade malignant tumors are readily recognized histologically. They are likely to recur locally, and about one-third of them may metastasize predominantly to the lung. The relatively benign group of phyllodes tumors has a significant risk of local recurrence, with the chance of progression in the recurrence; however, this local recurrence rarely invades the chest wall and thoracic cavity. Occasionally, what appears to be a benign lesion recurs locally as a malignant cystosarcoma, with the implication that it is then capable of metasta-

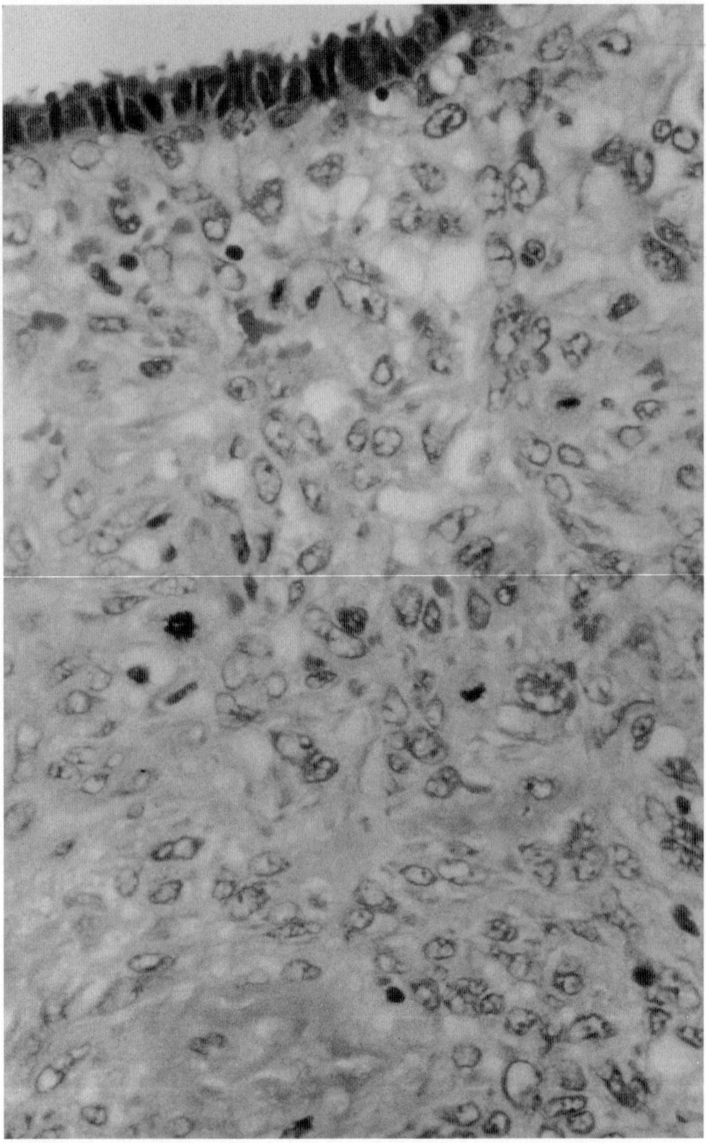

FIG. 10.22. Cystosarcoma phyllodes, malignant. Anaplastic and mitotically active nuclei of the fibroblasts, which extend to the basement membrane, under the proliferative, but benign, epithelium is depicted.

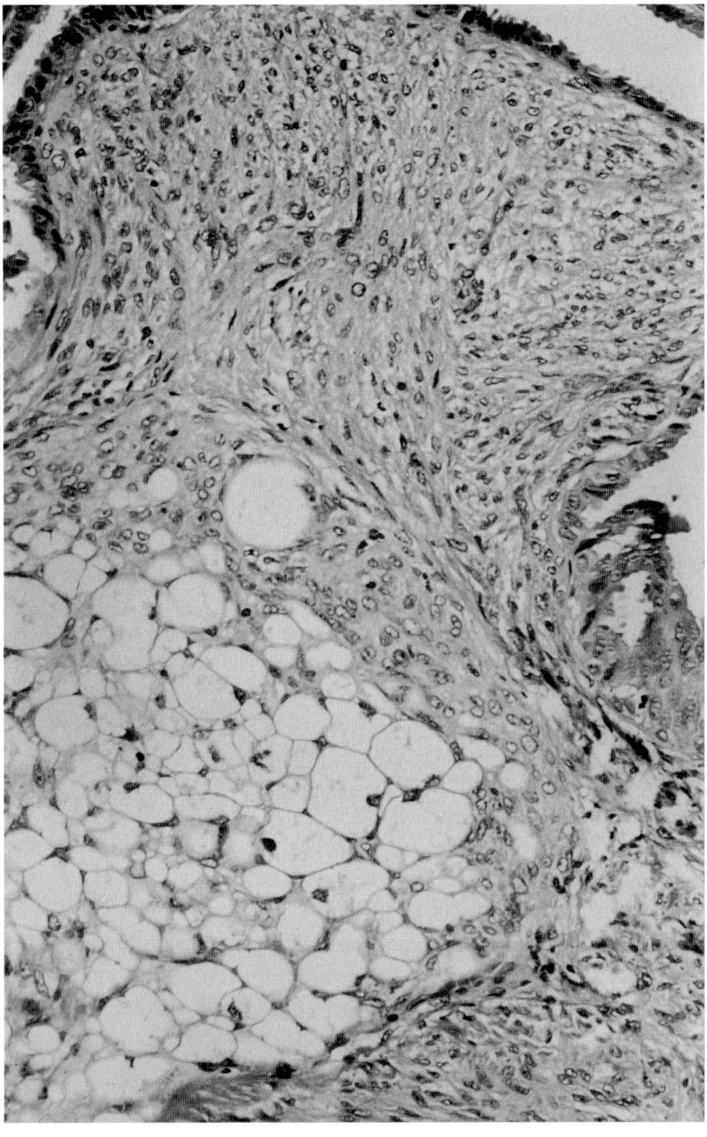

FIG. 10.23. Cystosarcoma phyllodes with liposarcoma as the malignant component. The frond-like phyllodes pattern is produced by fibroblastic and lipoblastic components. Benign epithelium covers the surface.

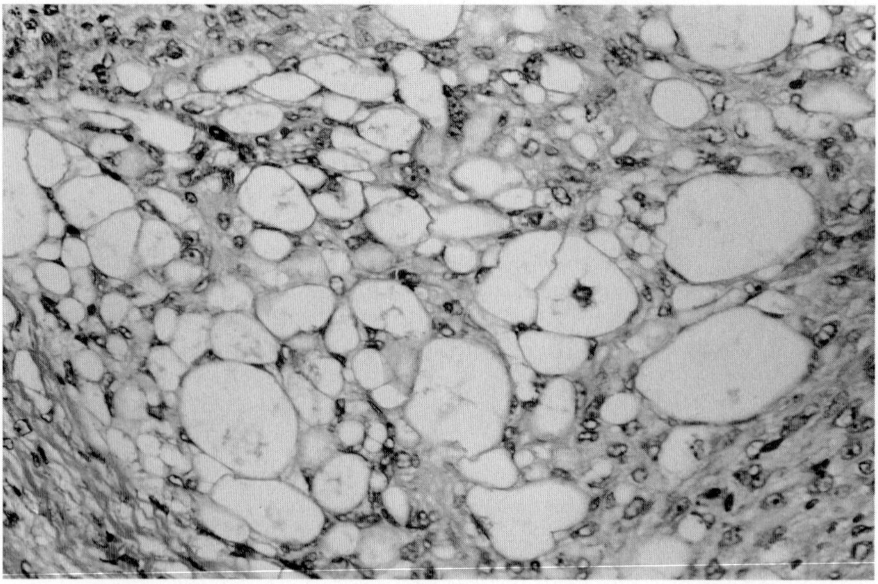

FIG. 10.24. Cystosarcoma phyllodes with liposarcoma. Moderately differentiated lipoblasts proliferate in this area. Distinction between liposarcoma of the breast and cystosarcoma with liposarcomatous component depends upon the finding of a benign epithelial component, which may be inapparent in most of the sections.

sis. A borderline group exists in which it is difficult to predict which of these two courses is the more likely (8,27,28). Adequate local excision is urged by all authors. The size and invasive nature of CP dictate the extent of the excision that is required, with larger or infiltrative lesions frequently treated by mastectomy. Axillary lymph node metastasis is unlikely, however, and radical mastectomy probably should not be recommended. Biopsy of enlarged axillary lymph nodes might prove useful in detecting the extremely unusual case of an axillary lymph node metastasis from cystosarcoma, but if lymph node metastasis is present, one should reexamine the case to make sure that the lesion is not a metaplastic carcinoma that mimics a CP. Immunohistochemical staining for keratin by malignant spindle cells indicates carcinoma.

STROMAL SARCOMA

Malignant CP may show extreme histologic variation within the lesion, and the epithelial component may be so inapparent as to suggest stromal sarcoma. In small biopsy specimens, or even in larger ones, the pathologist may be misled into a sarcoma diagnosis when an epithelial component is not found. It is best to withhold final diagnosis on a stromal malignancy until the complete excision, which is the treatment of choice for CP or sarcoma, has been fully evaluated.

There is no sarcoma that is unique to the stroma of the breast, but the mammary gland may rarely be the primary site of virtually any of the sarcomas that occur elsewhere in soft tissue (29–35). As in soft tissues, the most commonly observed pattern is the so-called malignant fibrous histiocytoma. The assessment of stromal breast lesions is based on the principles of soft tissue pathology that has been described in other texts (efigs. 10.49 and 10.50).

DIFFERENTIAL DIAGNOSIS

It is important to distinguish sarcoma from metaplastic carcinoma because of the more aggressive nature and likelihood of lymph node metastases in the latter. Immunostaining with keratin antibodies is useful in making this distinction (Fig. 10.25 and efigs. 10.51 to 10.53). Christensen et al. (36) reported on 100 cases of sarcomatoid tumors of the breast that were seen in Denmark between 1977 and 1987. Twenty-six cases were reported as sarcoma, but, on immunohistochemical study, 23 of the 26 cases were keratin-positive and therefore they were considered metaplastic carcinomas (Chapter 8). The CP cases and the three keratin-negative cases had a 21% local recurrence rate with no metastases, whereas the metaplastic carcinomas had a 50% metastatic rate with no local recurrences.

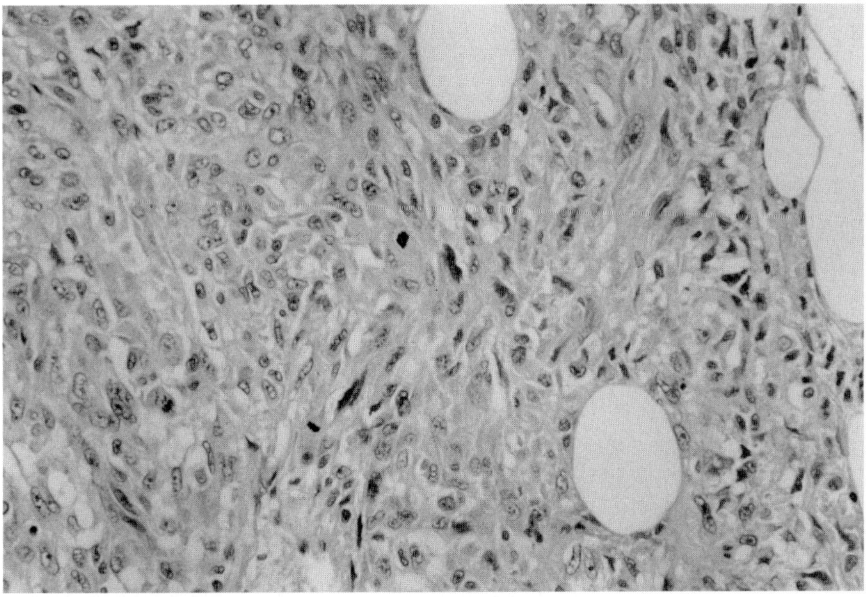

FIG. 10.25. Spindle cell carcinoma. This spindle cell epithelioid malignancy must be distinguished from malignant cystosarcoma phyllodes and stromal sarcoma for purposes of treatment. Immunohistochemical identification as an epithelial neoplasm is frequently useful.

Stromal changes, which may mimic sarcoma, are those seen after irradiation of benign stroma (efigs. 10.54 and 10.55) and radiation and/or chemotherapy changes in the carcinoma (efigs. 10.56 to 10.59).

BENIGN STROMAL TUMORS OTHER THAN FIBROADENOMA

Hamartoma

Linell et al. (37) described 15 cases of distinct tumor-like lesions of the breast that have a distinct mammographic appearance and can be easily shelled out at surgery. Grossly, hamartomas are variably sized well-circumscribed masses that have a smooth surface. Microscopically, they are made up of normal glandular structures, with both lobules and ducts distributed within a prominent, but not proliferative, fibrous stroma. Adipose tissue also is described as being part of the circumscribed mass (Figs. 10.26 and 10.27 and efigs. 10.60 and 10.61). Jones et al. (38) described 17 breast hamartomas with histologic features, including circumscribed fibrocystic disease, adenolipoma, FA with fat, and FA with lobules. Heterologous elements were found, which included cartilage and smooth muscle. Charpin et al. (39) found 41 hamartomas among 5,834 breast biopsies. Mammography showed sharply circumscribed densities that were separated from adjacent normal breast by a thin radiolucent zone. Grossly, hamartomas were well-delimited, white, pink, and fleshy with yellow islands of fatty tissue. Histologically,

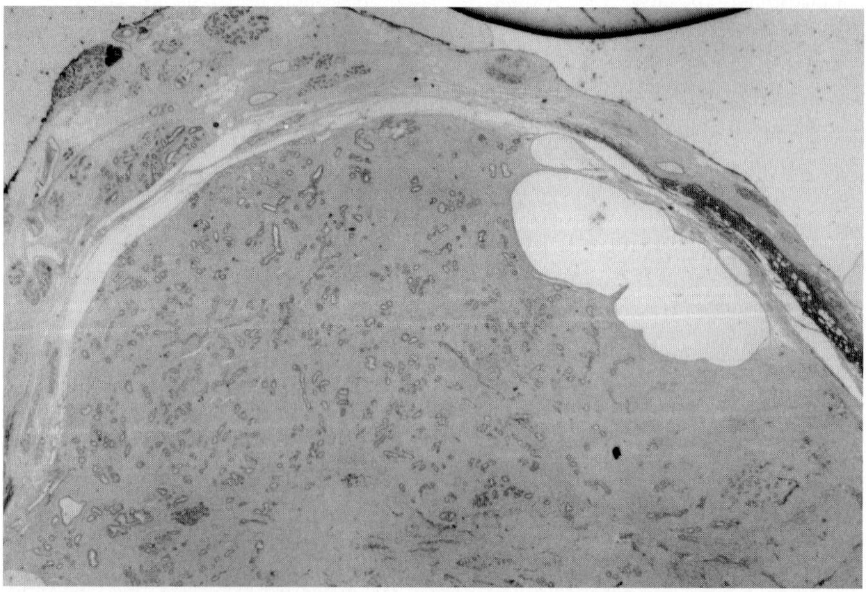

FIG. 10.26. Hamartoma. This sharply circumscribed lesion contains numerous lobules with acini, as well as adipose tissue.

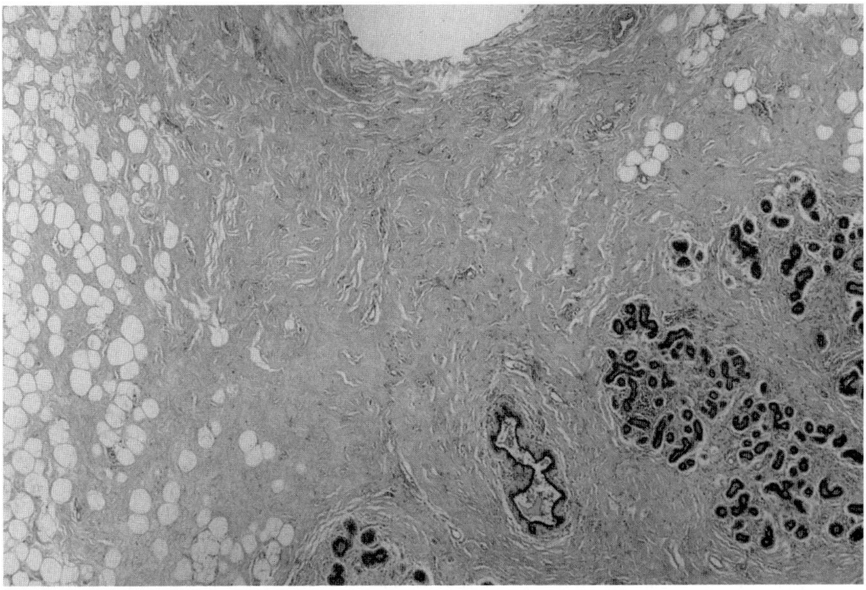

FIG. 10.27. Hamartoma. The lobular elements with ducts and acinar structures are embedded in a fibrous stroma with features of pseudoangiomatous stromal hyperplasia that contains a major element of adipose tissue.

hamartomas exhibited pushing borders with pseudoencapsulation and they consisted of stromal components with prominent fibrohyalin that were associated with islands of adipose tissue. The incorporated epithelial structures showed variable features of benign breast disease. Daya et al. (40) reported on 25 cases of breast hamartoma in patients who ranged in age from 18 to 89 years (mean age 45 years). Grossly, they were oval well-circumscribed masses that ranged in size from 1 to 7 cm, with a mean of 3.9 cm. Microscopically, the hamartomas had a stroma with varying amounts of fibroconnective and adipose tissue. A consistent and important diagnostic feature was the presence of both lobules and ducts, which distinguished hamartoma from FA, from which lobular structures are often absent.

FIBROMATOSIS

Fibromatosis occurs in the breast, but it is rare, and, in mammary tissue, it lacks the aggressive behavior that is characteristic of desmoid tumors in other sites that are related to the shoulder girdle. Histologically, it has dense bundles of collagen with a modest fibroblastic proliferation (Figs. 10.28 and 10.29 and efigs. 10.62 to 10.65). Gump et al. (41) reported on 13 cases of mammary fibromatosis, with recurrence in 3 of them, but no recurrence when negative resection margins were achieved. Pettinato et al. (42) found intracytoplasmic inclusion bodies with features of actin filaments by electron microscopy and immunohis-

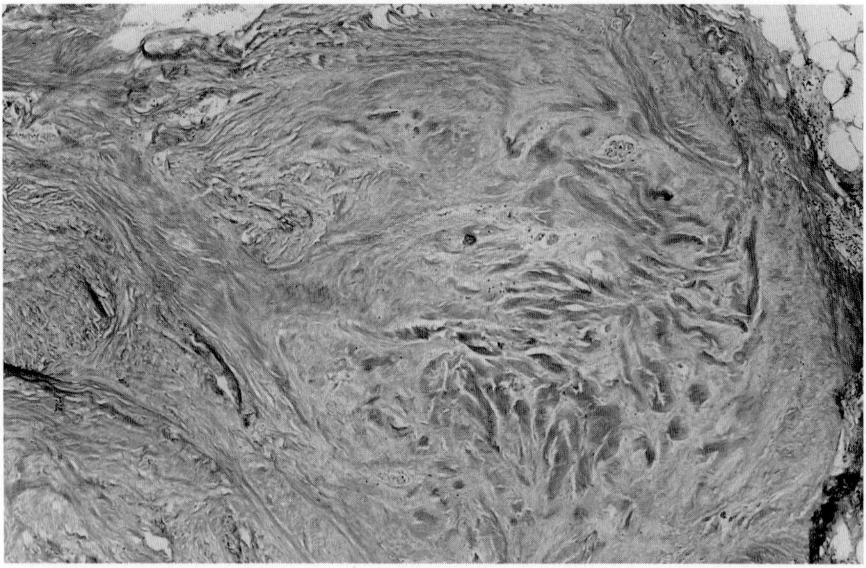

FIG. 10.28. Fibromatosis. This circumscribed dense 1.5 cm nodule was located in the breast parenchyma and simulated the gross appearance of a carcinoma. Although deeply placed, it is small and does not invade the chest wall or even much of the breast stroma.

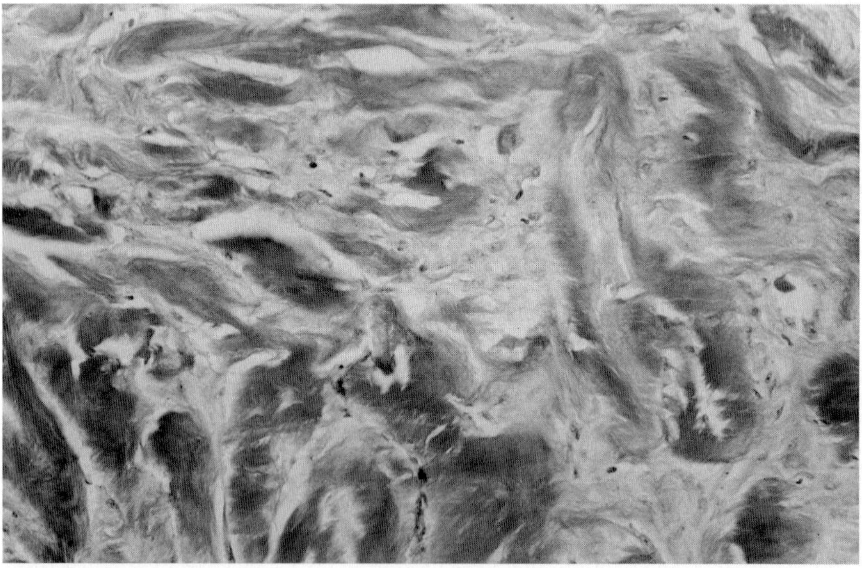

FIG. 10.29. Fibromatosis. The dense collagen bands characteristic of hypertrophic scar or extraabdominal desmoid are evident. Proliferation of fibroblasts is limited.

tochemistry that were similar to those seen in infantile digital fibrosis in two cases of mammary fibromatosis. Rasbridge et al. (43) found no evidence of estrogen receptors in six cases of mammary fibromatosis. Devouassoux-Shisheboran et al. (44) studied 33 cases of fibromatosis of the breast and found that none of them were immunohistochemically stained for estrogen, progesterone or androgen receptor. The authors did report that fibromatoses in women of childbearing years were more cellular and mitotically active, with a higher level of atypia than fibromatoses in older women.

MYOFIBROMA

Wargotz et al. (45) described 16 cases of benign mammary stromal tumors, which ultrastructurally had features of myofibroblasts. Eleven of the cases were in men and five cases were in women; the average age was 63 years. Grossly, they were circumscribed nodules, 1 to 4 cm in diameter. Microscopically, they had broad bands of hyalinized collagen and a haphazard arrangement of short spindle cell fascicles (Figs. 10.30 to 10.33 and efigs. 10.66 to 10.68). Desmin immunoreactivity was evident. None of the tumors recurred or metastasized, but two tumors were treated by mastectomy, indicating their histologic similarity to malignancy.

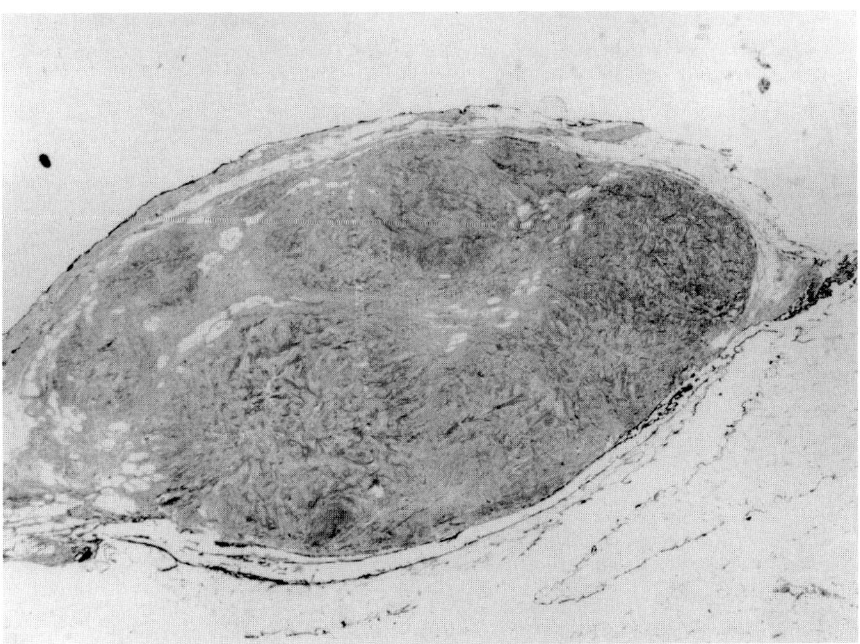

FIG. 10.30. Myofibroma. Grossly sharply circumscribed 1.5 cm nodule.

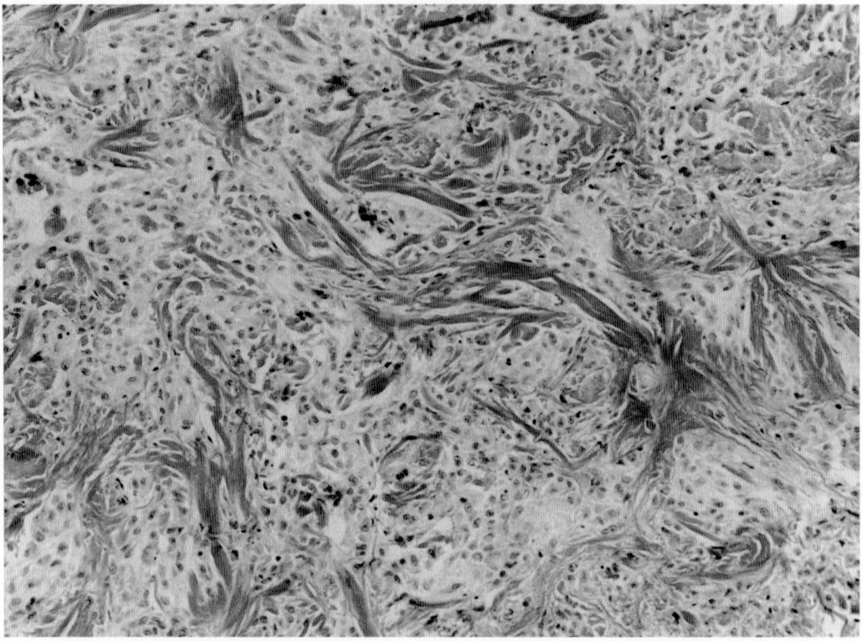

FIG. 10.31. Myofibroma. Broad bands of hyalinized collagen associated with a haphazard arrangement of short spindle cell fascicles.

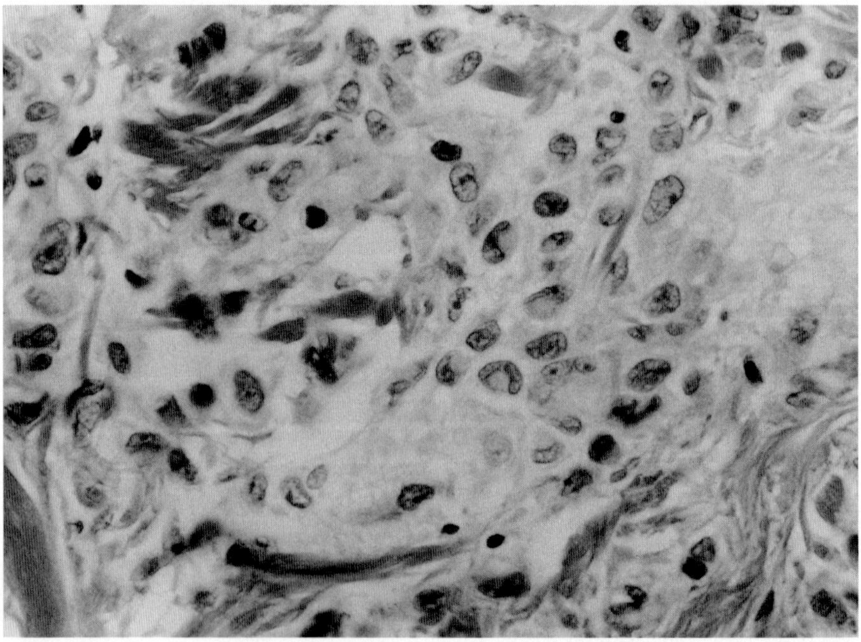

FIG. 10.32. Myofibroma. The individual spindle and histiocyte-like cells have active, but amitotic, nuclei.

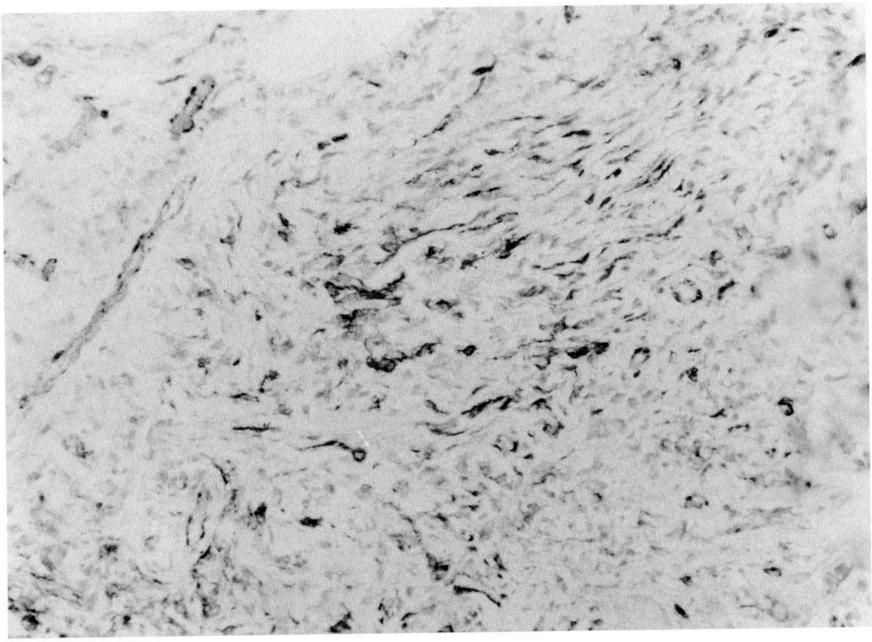

FIG. 10.33. Myofibroma. Desmin immunoreactivity is present.

LEIOMYOMA

Leiomyoma in the breast was described recently by Diaz-Arias et al. (46) and Kotsuma et al. (47). Grossly, microscopically, immunohistochemically, and ultrastructurally, mammary leiomyomas are the same as leiomyomas that are seen elsewhere.

Other benign stromal neoplasms have been reported as rarities in the breast.

VASCULAR LESIONS

Benign Vascular Tumors

Other than perilobular hemangiomas, which are incidentally found, and small cavernous angiomas in and around lobules (Fig. 10.34 and efigs. 10.69 and 10.70), benign vascular tumors rarely occur in the breast.

Rosen et al. (48) described five cases of venous hemangiomas that did involve the mammary parenchyma, but they were comprised of venous channels that were surrounded by smooth muscle layers. The venous channels appeared to be quite disorderly and varied in size (Fig. 10.35 and efigs. 10.71 to 10.74). The lesions were well circumscribed, but they varied in size from 1.0 to 5.3 cm in diameter. The five lesions occurred in women from ages 24 to 59 years. The

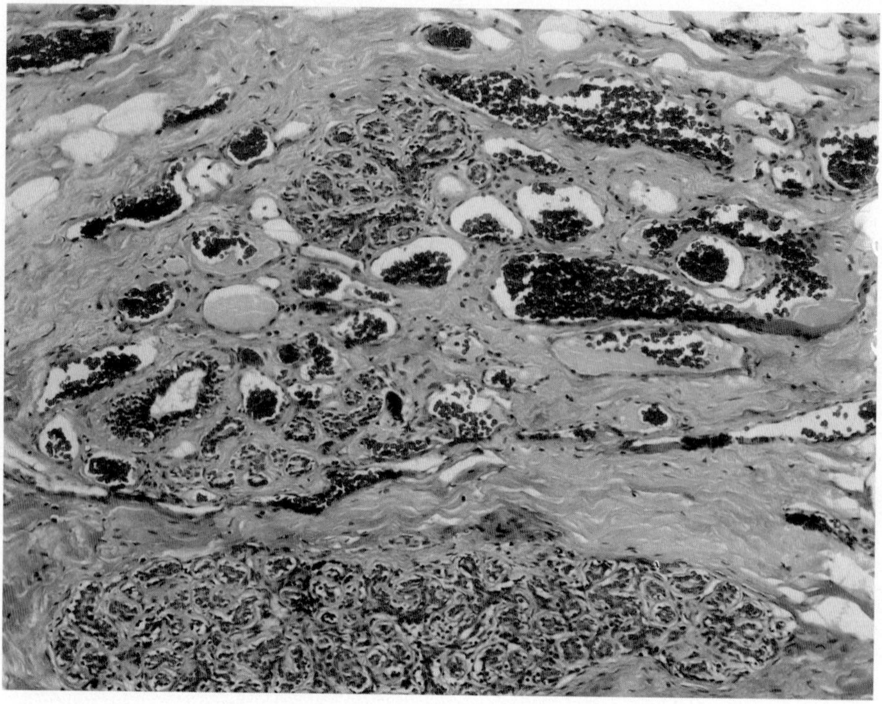

FIG. 10.34. Perilobular hemangioma. Dilated venous sized vascular channels that do not inter-anastamose and which lack a prominent endothelial lining surround this lobule.

lesions of four patients were locally excised, and one patient was treated by a mastectomy. All five patients were free of disease at the time of the report.

Jozefczyk and Rosen (49) also described 25 cases of hemangiomas. Eleven of the cases were so-called perilobular hemangiomas, which were grossly inapparent and measured less than 2 mm in size. In 5 of the 11 cases, there was some nuclear hyperchromasia or focal anastomoses of the vascular channels. Despite these areas of atypia, all of the patients were disease-free up to 10 years after excision. Perhaps this can be attributed to the very small size of the lesions. There were 14 clinically or grossly apparent hemangiomas, which varied in size from 3 mm to 2.1 cm, in greatest dimension. Eight of the hemangiomas also had cytologic atypia, but all of the patients were disease-free up to 5 years after the excision. In general, the hemangiomas, regardless of size, were quite well circumscribed and lobulated. They were composed of dilated nonanastomosing channels. Many of these had a prominent spindle cell cuff. There was some focal atypia of the nuclei, but there was no striking proliferative change within the endothelial cell population. The authors pointed out that in over one-half of the cases, large nonneoplastic feeding vessels were demonstrated in the vicinity of hemangiomas of the breast. (The same is true for other lesions of the breast,

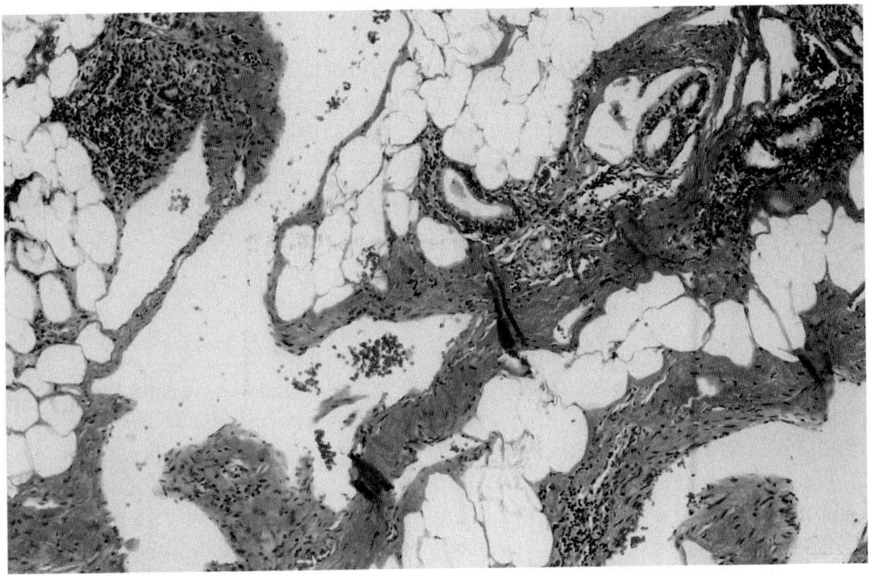

FIG. 10.35. Venous hemangioma. Large dilated vascular channels surround and cut up this lobule. The vascular channels do not interanastomose. The endothelial lining is inapparent.

including carcinomas.) Size is a relatively important criterion in distinguishing hemangiomas from angiosarcomas. Few lesions that are larger than 2 cm in diameter qualify as hemangiomas, and there are few angiosarcomas that are smaller than 2 cm in diameter. Nevertheless, the histologic appearance is of greater importance than is size.

Rosen (50) also described three cases of a lesion that he termed angiomatosis of the breast. All of these lesions were quite large, measuring approximately 9 cm in diameter. One lesion was congenital and had recurred twice over 39 years. In the other two patients, there was no recurrence 3 years after local excision or 2.2 years after mastectomy. These vascular lesions were comprised of dilated vascular and lymphatic channels that surrounded whole lobular units; however, the lesions did not invade the lobules in the same way as did angiosarcomas. The vascular channels were nonanastomosing, lined by a flat, relatively nonproliferative endothelium, and not surrounded by smooth muscle (efigs. 10.75 and 10.76). Morrow et al. (51) described a diffuse cystic angiomatosis of the breast that measured 11 cm in diameter. It was excised and it recurred in approximately 2 years, during gestation, as a 15-cm mass. Total mastectomy was carried out in order to remove the huge lesion. Follow-up after mastectomy, at approximately 1 year, was uneventful.

Rosen also described a variety of vascular lesions that occurred in the subcutis near the breast, but which did not involve the breast itself (52). These should be regarded as soft tissue vascular tumors (efigs. 10.77 to 10.80).

PSEUDOANGIOMATOUS STROMAL HYPERPLASIA

Vuitch et al. (53) described a pseudoangiomatous hyperplasia of the breast that is most often seen in areas with fibroadenosis. It is basically an artifact with separation of the fibrous stroma to form spaces that, despite their superficial appearance, are not vascular, a fact that can be verified by immunohistochemical staining for factor VIII related antigen (Figs. 10.36 to 10.38 and efigs. 10.81 and 10.82) (54).

Angiosarcoma

Angiosarcomas present clinically as mass lesions and may become quite large. When superficial, the masses have the warmth that is associated with large vascular masses. When studied by ultrasound, they produce the characteristics of turbulent blood flow. Microscopically, they involve breast parenchyma, evident by the presence of entrapped ducts and lobules, and they are characterized by interanastomosing channels that are lined by endothelial cells. The deceptively benign end of the histologic spectrum is characterized by plump numerous endothelial cells. High-grade angiosarcomas may present their lowest grade areas at their periphery, where biopsy is most frequent and where differentiation from a benign vascular tumor most difficult. The high-grade angiosarcomas may

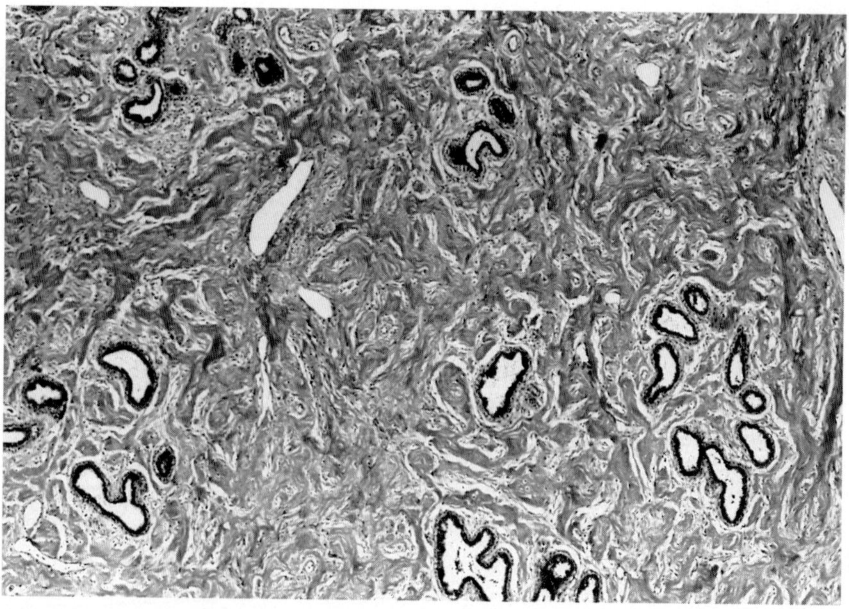

FIG. 10.36. Pseudoangiomatous stromal hyperplasia. The interlobular stroma is separated by what appear to be interanastomosing vascular channels.

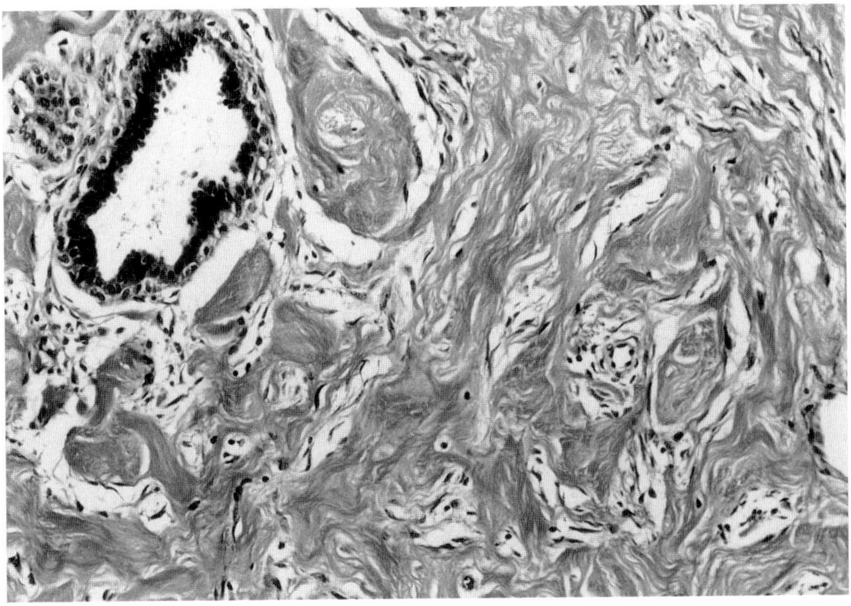

FIG. 10.37. Pseudoangiomatous stromal hyperplasia. Dense bundles of collagen are separated by spaces that contain spindled-shaped cells.

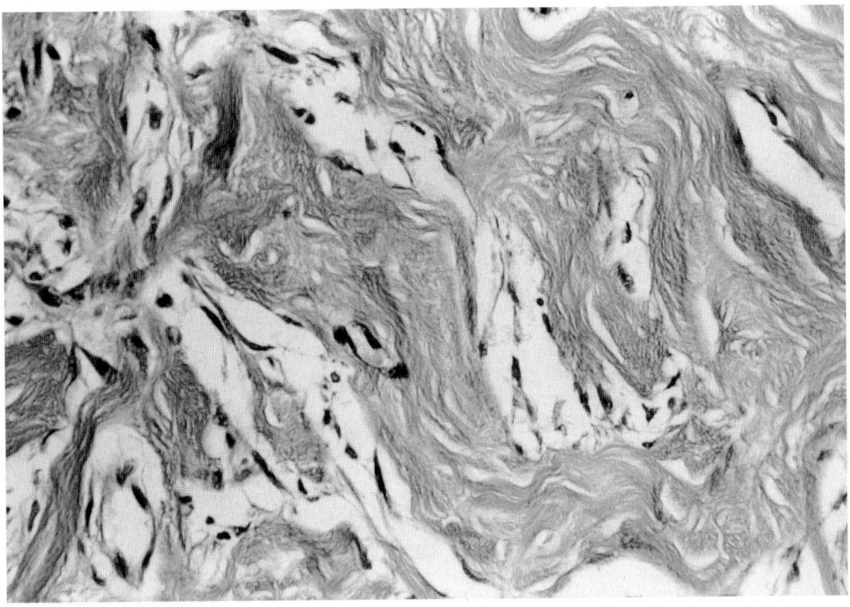

FIG. 10.38. Pseudoangiomatous stromal hyperplasia. At higher magnification, the spaces with spindle cells resemble dilated capillaries, but, immunohistochemically, these are fibroblasts that do not express endothelial markers.

appear as solid masses of anaplastic cells. Identification of the cells as endothelial is aided with immunohistochemical staining for factor VIII related antigen, CD34, and *Ulex europaeus* (Figs. 10.39 to 10.45 and efigs. 10.83 to 10.92).

In 1980, Chen et al. (55) reviewed the world literature on the subject and found that 87 cases of angiosarcoma of the breast had been recorded since its first documentation. The 3-year survival rate of reported cases was 38%, but the disease-free survival rate at 3 years was only 14%. Only 5 of the 87 cases with a 5-year survival were free of disease. The mean age at presentation was 35 years, with a range of 14 to 82 years. Most of the patients presented with a painless mass in the breast, although 11 patients presented with diffuse enlargement of the breast. The vascular nature of the lesion was evident clinically in 30 patients, but, in 32 of the 87 cases, the malignant nature of the lesion was not recognized in the initial biopsy. It was frequently confused with hemangioma, hematoma, or lymphangioma. In 18 patients, there was bilateral breast involvement. Most of the patients died of dissemination of the angiosarcoma, with metastasis to the lung, skin, bone, liver, brain, and ovary. Involvement of axillary lymph nodes was rare, however, and the treatment advised was simple mastectomy. The authors described the histology as being frequently well-differentiated and deceptively benign. Their differential diagnosis from angiosarcoma is generally limited to that of the perilobular hemangioma, which is microscopic in

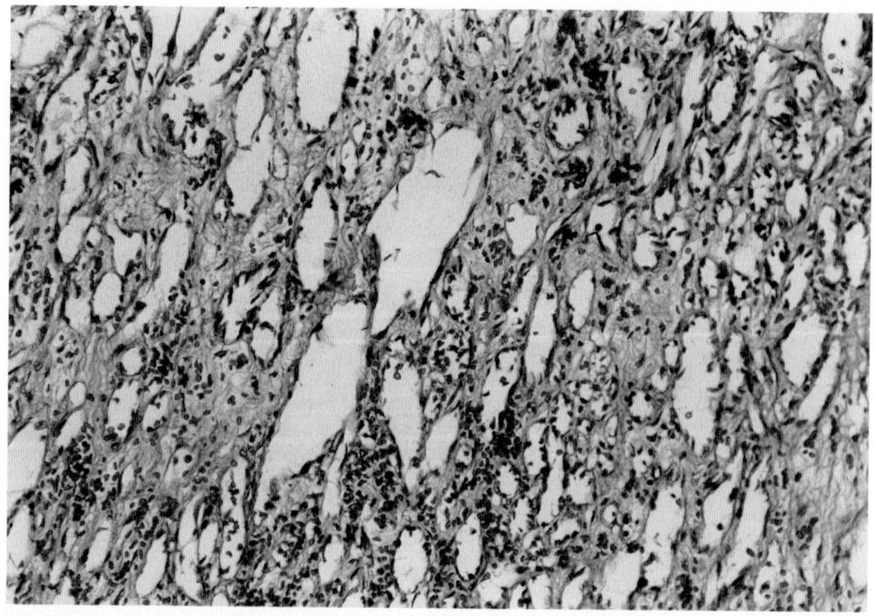

FIG. 10.39. Well differentiated angiosarcoma. Numerous dilated and anastomosing thin walled vascular channels are lined by endothelial cells. This deceptively bland appearance is often found at the periphery of an angiosarcoma and may lead to underdiagnosis.

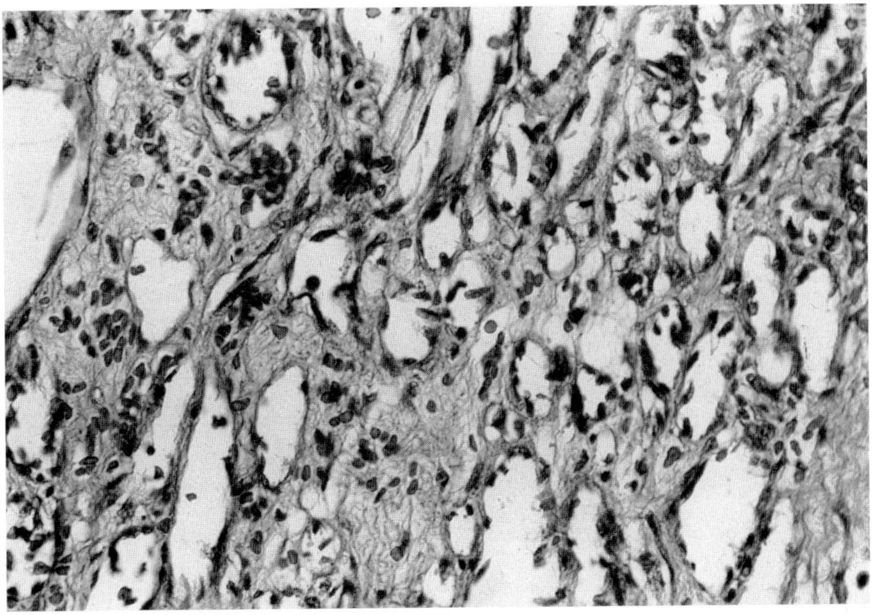

FIG. 10.40. Well differentiated angiosarcoma. At higher magnification, the prominence of the endothelial cells and their nuclei is evident. Occasionally, nuclei are plump and hyperchromatic.

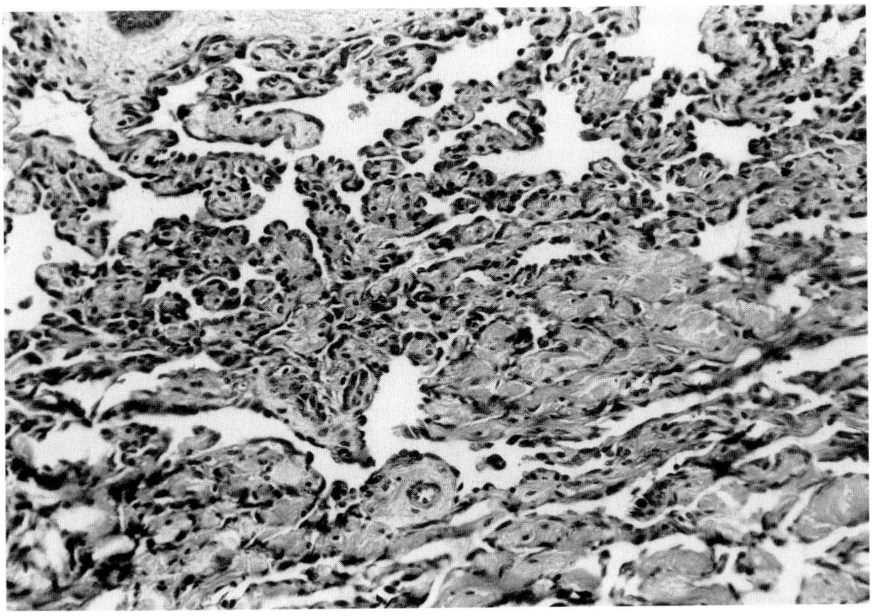

FIG. 10.41. Well differentiated angiosarcoma. Proliferation of endothelial cells is more prominent, and interanastomosis of the vascular channels is a prominent feature of these thin walled vessels.

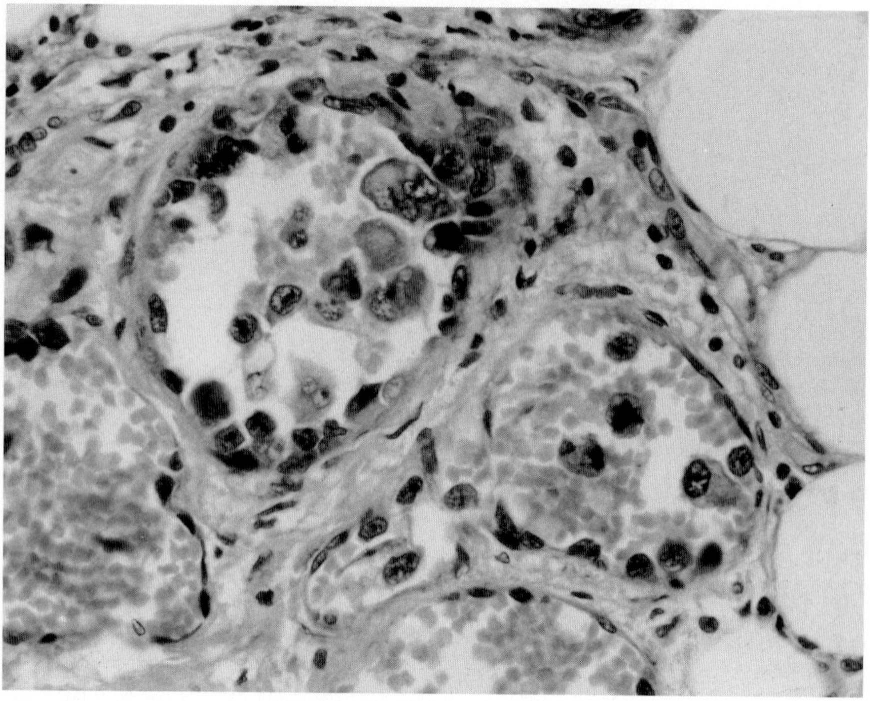

FIG. 10.42. Angiosarcoma. These dilated thin-walled vessels are lined by anaplastic endothelial cells that are indicative of malignancy.

size. The authors suggested that nuclear hyperchromatism of tumor cells, intraluminal tufting, and infiltration of fat and breast tissue indicated the sarcomatous nature of the vascular lesion. They did not distinguish various grades of angiosarcoma in their discussion.

Donnell et al. (56) described the pathologic features of 40 cases of angiosarcoma of the breast and related the histologic appearance of these lesions to the clinical course. The authors divided angiosarcomas into grades 1, 2, and 3. In all groups, the breast parenchyma was involved by a grossly evident vascular tumor that varied in size from 2 to 11 cm, with an average of 5.3 cm. In all groups, the lesion invaded breast parenchyma, was characterized by interanastomosing vascular channels, and contained endothelial cells with large hyperchromatic nuclei. In the grade 1 lesions, endothelial tufting was minimal. Papillary formations and solid and spindle cell foci were absent. The average size of the grade 1 lesions was 4.4 cm in diameter. Ten of the 13 patients with histologic grade 1 lesions were alive and free of disease, after an average follow-up of nearly 6 years. Seven patients had grade 2 lesions. These lesions were characterized by endothelial tufting and some papillary formations, solid and spindle cell foci, and occasional mitoses that were usually present in the papillary areas. The average size

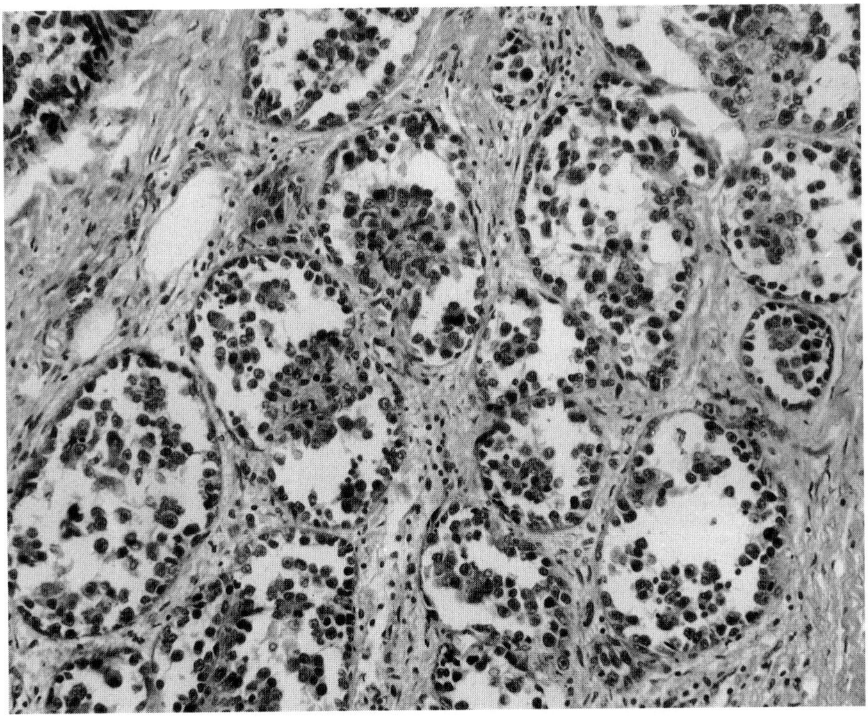

FIG. 10.43. The thin-walled vascular spaces are filled with cells proliferating in a micropapillary and "tufted" pattern of high grade angiosarcoma.

of these lesions was 4.5 cm in diameter, and the survival was comparable to that of patients with grade 1 lesions. Twenty of the 40 cases fell into the group 3 category. Histologically, grade 3 lesions had prominent endothelial tufting with papillary formations, solid and spindle cell foci, numerous mitoses, blood lakes, and necrosis. Fourteen of the 16 patients on whom follow-up was available had died of the disease. The overall 3-year disease-free survival rate of all groups was 41%, and, at 5 years, the figure was 33%. The authors pointed out that simple mastectomy was the treatment of choice and that actinomycin D had been effective as a chemotherapeutic adjuvant. Differential diagnosis offered for angiosarcoma included perilobular hemangiomas, hemangiomas that involved the soft tissue in the area (but not the breast parenchyma), and hemangiopericytoma. Three other cases included a juvenile hemangioendothelioma and two vascular anomalies. None of the benign lesions recurred.

Merino et al. (57) described 15 angiosarcomas of the breast with the histologic appearance stratified into well-differentiated (Figs. 10.24 to 10.26), moderately differentiated (Fig. 10.27), and poorly differentiated (Figs. 10.28 to 10.30) angiosarcoma. As in the study by Donnell et al. (56), the results showed that the histologic patterns of the tumors correlated closely with prognosis. The size of

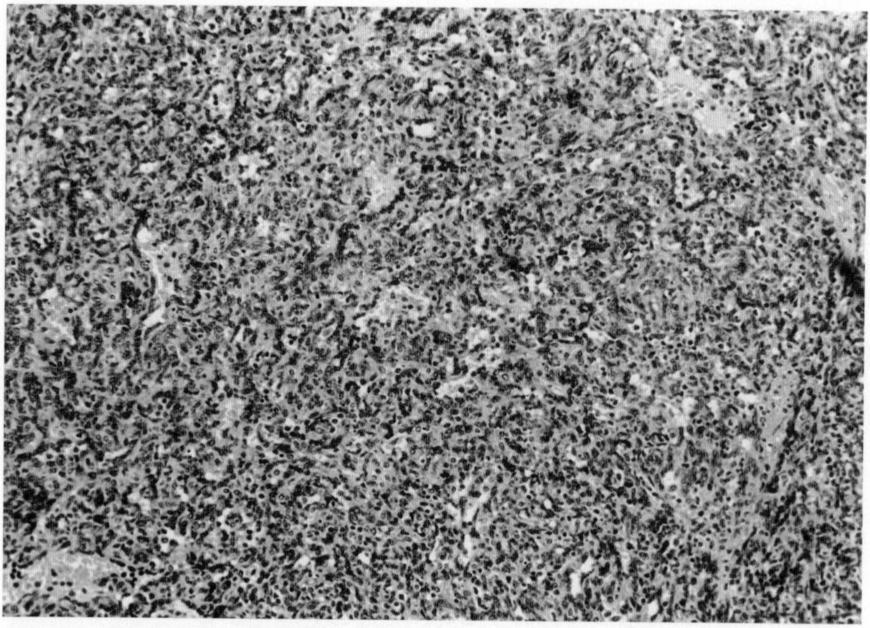

FIG.10.44. Poorly differentiated angiosarcoma. This is a solid proliferation of cells, which are obviously malignant, but cellularity is so high that the vascular channels are inapparent. Immunostaining for factor VIII related antigen and CD34 are diagnostic. Solid angiosarcoma has a grave prognosis.

the lesions studied ranged from 2 to 9 cm, and, in 11 of the 15 cases, the tumors were smaller than 5 cm. No correlation between size and prognosis was found. The smallest primary angiosarcoma to metastasize was 2 cm in greatest diameter. All lesions were of macroscopic size and all of them clearly infiltrated the breast parenchyma. All lesions were composed of anastomosing and intercommunicating vascular channels that were lined by plump endothelial cells. The well-differentiated lesions were characterized by well-formed vascular spaces that were lined by one or two layers of endothelial cells; there was no hemorrhage, necrosis, pleomorphism, or anaplasia. Mitoses were rare and were normal in all instances. Occasionally, the vascular spaces showed some areas of endothelial tufting and thrombosis, with evidence of organization of the thrombi by fibroblastic cells. Four of the five patients with well-differentiated lesions remained free of disease for as long as 24 years. The moderately differentiated angiosarcomas were composed predominantly of areas like those seen in well-differentiated angiosarcomas, but there were foci of solid tumor that comprised less than 20% of the total tumor masses present in patchy fashion throughout the neoplasm. Three of these four patients died of disease in less than 4 years. The poorly differentiated angiosarcomas were composed predominantly of solid

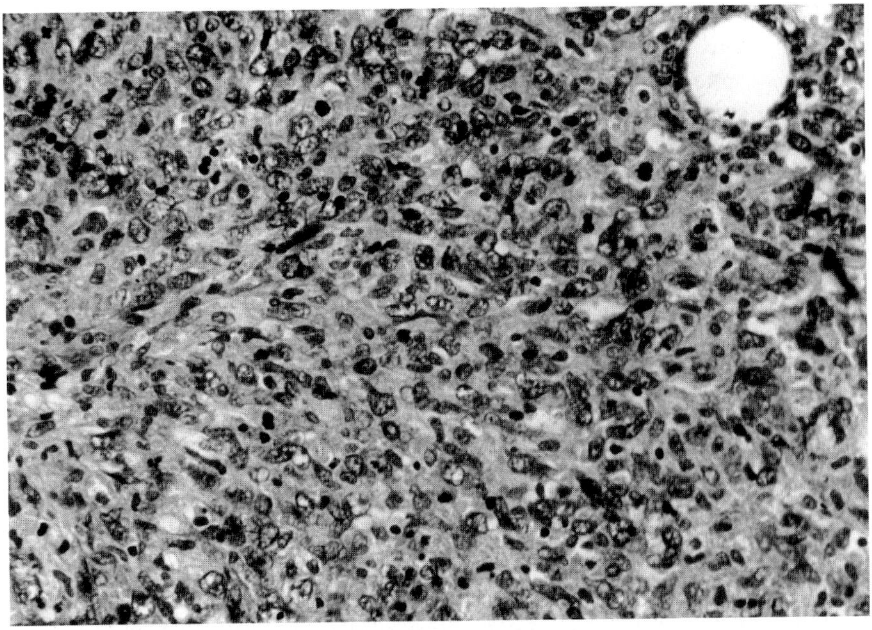

FIG. 10.45. Angiosarcoma. Obviously high grade sarcoma with minimal differentiation. There is immunohistochemical staining for CD34, but not for factor VIII related antigen. Electron microscopy may show minimal differentiation. It is rare for an angiosarcoma to be composed entirely of solid areas like this one. There are usually better differentiated areas that allow classification of this malignancy.

tumor, with few areas in which well-formed vascular spaces were evident. These tumors exhibited extensive areas of hemorrhage, necrosis, and marked cellular pleomorphism, with numerous mitotic figures. Within the solid areas, several of the tumors had a histologic appearance that resembled a malignant fibrous histiocytoma or a carcinoma. One tumor had giant cells with numerous bizarre nuclei. Three of the six patients who had poorly differentiated angiosarcoma were dead of disease within a short interval. The vascular nature of the neoplasms was demonstrated by staining with an immunoperoxidase technique for factor VIII related antigen. The endothelial cells that lined the vascular spaces, as well as the cells that made up the solid areas in the poorly differentiated tumors, stained for this antigen. Weibel–Palade bodies were identified on ultrastructural examination of two of these lesions. Both Donnell et al. (56) and Merino et al. (57) distinguished the histologic low-grade and high-grade angiosarcomas histologically, but the middle group was not as clearly defined. The intermediate group described by Donnell et al. (56) was quite similar in clinical behavior to that of the low-grade or well-differentiated angiosarcomas, whereas the intermediate group described by Merino et al. (57) was more similar to that of the poorly differentiated or high-grade angiosarcomas. Both studies showed that a vascular tumor of open anastomosing vascular channels, with little endothelial cell proliferation, has a relatively good prognosis and that solid areas of a tumor are of grave prognostic significance. Both studies also showed that even the relatively bland histologic appearance of the well-differentiated or low-grade angiosarcoma should not be underestimated, for patients with such tumors are likely to have local recurrence, if adequate treatment is not promptly instituted (58). Although the long-term survival from this rare lesion is still not good, stratification of the cases, according to histologic appearance, does provide some relief for the well-differentiated cases from the grim prognosis that has been assigned to this group as a whole.

Rosen et al. (59) updated their previous study of angiosarcoma in both follow-up and number of patients to 63. Twenty-five (40%) of the 63 patients had low-grade, type I (grade 1) lesions, with disease-free 5-year survival of 76% and a median length of disease-free survival of more than 15 years. Twenty-five (41%) of the patients had high-grade, type III (grade 3) angiosarcomas, with a disease-free 5-year survival of only 15% and a median disease-free interval of only 15 months. The higher-grade lesions metastasized widely to liver and lungs, but they also showed a curious predilection for spread to bones, skin, and contralateral breast. The intermediate category, which comprised only 19% of the 63 patients, was similar in behavior to the lower-grade angiosarcomas, with a 5-year disease-free survival of 70% and a median disease-free survival of more than 12 years. These type II angiosarcomas are similar to the type I (grade 1) angiosarcomas that were described by Donnell et al. (56); however, the former contains microscopic foci of more solid neoplastic endothelial cells. The high-grade angiosarcomas (type III or grade 3) have prominent overtly sarcomatous areas with areas of spindle cell sarcoma, as well as nuclear anaplasia, mitotic figures, necrosis, and hemorrhage.

Alles and Bosslet (60) reported on the immunohistochemical profile of angiosarcomas. The authors found that about one-half of the solid areas were negative for both factor VIII related antigen and *U. europaeus* I agglutinin. The papillary and slit-like patterns were positive for both markers in 85% of cases and all of the well-differentiated angiosarcomas stained with one or both of these markers. The authors described another antibody (BMA120), which stained all patterns of angiosarcoma.

Rosen et al. (59) noted the presence of type I patterns at the periphery, which is the likely site of a small biopsy specimen in many of the type III high-grade lesions.

Differential Diagnosis of Vascular Lesions in the Breast

Several vascular lesions of the breast have now been described, largely as a result of the efforts of Rosen et al. (48–50,52,54,61). In approaching this differential diagnosis, the pathologist should recall that two-thirds of vascular tumors of the breast are malignant and that angiosarcoma, even of high grade, may appear deceptively benign, especially at its periphery. Complete excision and extensive sampling of vascular lesions of the breast are to be encouraged before a definitive diagnosis is rendered. Nevertheless, fully one-third of mammary vascular lesions are benign.

Benign vascular tumors may involve the soft tissue in the vicinity of the breast; however, these tumors are extraparenchymal and are therefore evaluated as one would evaluate the histology of a soft tissue vascular lesion. Rosen (52) described three angiolipomas, three cavernous hemangiomas, one juvenile hemangioma, one venous hemangioma, and one papillary endothelial hyperplasia. Keys to the recognition of these tumors are (a) the absence of mammary gland involvement and (b) the histologic similarity to benign vascular lesions that is seen in other tissues.

Stewart–Treves Lesion

In 1948, Stewart and Treves (62) described six cases in which lymphangiosarcoma developed in lymphedematous arms after radical mastectomy for carcinoma of the breast. Stewart–Treves lesions are found clinically in the dermis and subcutis of lymphadenomatous extremities and they present as raised 2- to 3-mm nodules that have the blush of a capillary lesion. They do not present as a mass. Microscopically, dilated vascular channels are lined by plump to frankly anaplastic endothelial cells that form a lining to papillary tufts to solid masses (Figs. 10.46 to 10.48 and efigs. 10.93 to 10.97 and 10.101). Since then, over 100 cases of lymphangiosarcoma that arose in lymphedematous extremities have

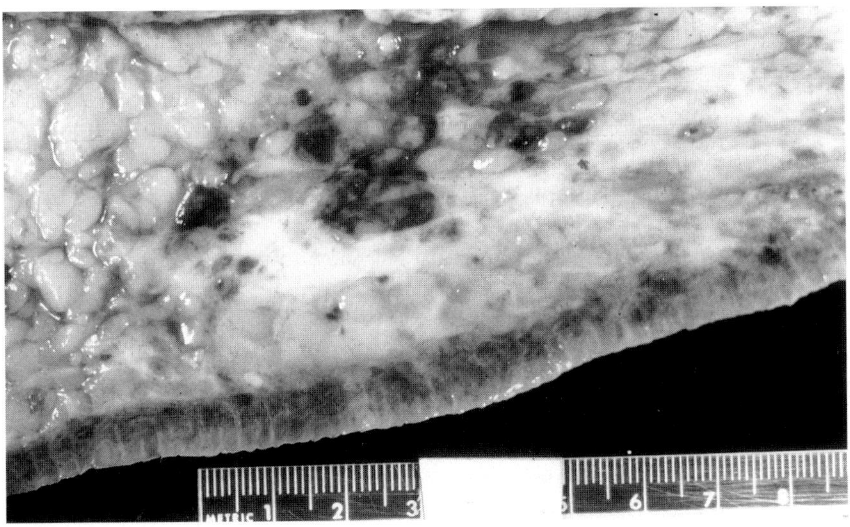

FIG. 10.46. Stewart–Treves lesion. The skin and subcutis are distended by numerous violatious nodules in the dermis and subcutis.

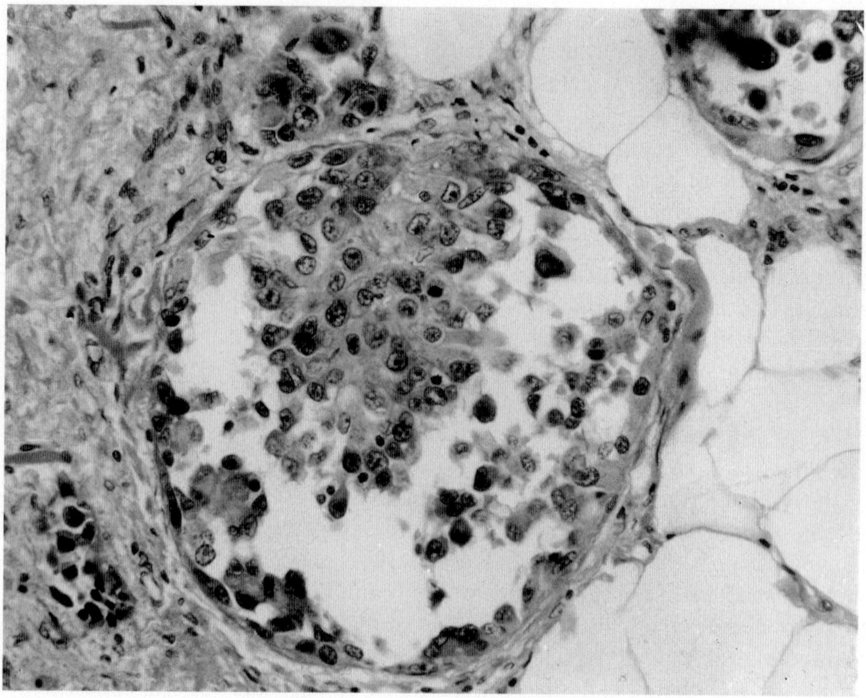

FIG. 10.47. Stewart–Treves lesion. Moderately differentiated angiosarcoma with dilated thin-walled vascular spaces that are filled with tufts of anaplastic endothelial cells.

been reported. In most of these cases, radical mastectomy was the factor that initiated the lymphedema (63–70), but the lesion has been reported following lymphedema with other tumors (71) and in patients with lymphedema in whom no tumor was previously present (72,73). Nemoto et al. (68) described the pathogenesis of the lesion. The authors found that a "hemangioma" developed clinically as a red spongy lesion in the skin and subcutaneous tissue and then in the deeper structures of the lymphedematous extremity; it subsequently enlarged and developed into a hemangiosarcoma. The view that the lesion is truly a sarcoma was challenged. Salm (74) described three such cases and suggested that they represented a peculiar retrograde metastasis of mammary carcinoma into the dilated and hemorrhagic vascular channels. Several electron microscopic studies were performed to determine if the lesion was of endothelial or epithelial origin. Unfortunately, these tumors are so poorly differentiated that it is difficult to distinguish primitive endothelial cells from primitive carcinoma cells on ultrastructural information alone.

Miettinen et al. (67) described two cases that were studied by electron microscopy that showed prominent pinocytotic vesicles and cell-to-cell junctions

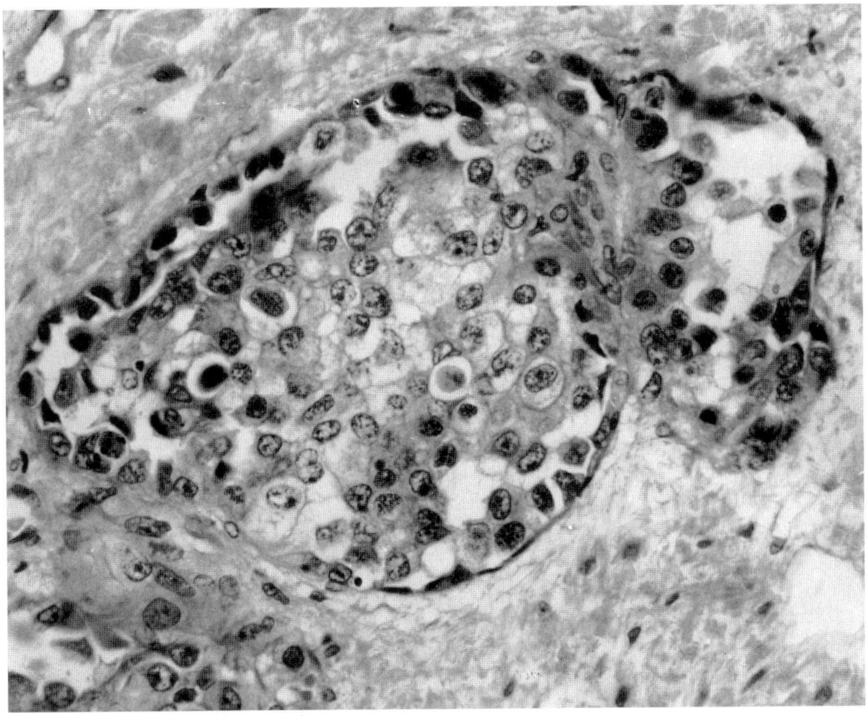

FIG. 10.48. Stewart–Treves lesion. This dilated thin-walled vascular space is filled with an epithelioid proliferation of anaplastic malignant cells. Immunostaining for CD34 and factor VIII related antigen is positive, but negative for epithelial markers.

but no other evidence of differentiation and no Weibel–Palade bodies. The authors then went on to stain the tumors immunohistochemically, using markers for keratin, vimentin, factor VIII related antigen, and *U. europaeus* lectin antibodies. Both tumors stained for factor VIII related antigen and *U. europaeus* lectin and were negative for keratin, demonstrating that the two cases were angiosarcomas.

Capo et al. (75) confirmed the finding of immunohistochemical staining for endothelial markers. The possibility that retrograde carcinomatous metastases may occur in a lymphedematous extremity cannot be excluded, but it appears that the Stewart–Treves lesion, as described (62), is an angiosarcoma, although it may be more of a hemangiosarcoma than a lymphangiosarcoma. Clinically, the lesions arise in the lymphedematous extremity, usually 10 years or more after the original treatment for breast cancer and they spread rapidly throughout the area of lymphedema. They also have a great propensity to disseminate widely, and 5-year survival is a rarity.

Post Irradiation Angiosarcoma

There is a growing number of case reports of angiosarcomas that arise in the bed of conservatively excised carcinomas that are treated with radiation (Chapter 2). Some of the angiosarcomas have appeared very rapidly after the completion of radiotherapy, but the localization of angiosarcoma to the irradiated site makes it difficult to escape the conclusion that they are induced by the radiation.

Grossly, the angiosarcomas appear as reddish spots, most commonly in the dermis, but they also may involve the conserved breast, either secondarily or primarily. The angiosarcomas vary considerably in size and they are frequently multiple. Histologically, angiosarcomas are characterized by the presence of dilated interanastomosing vascular channels lined by plump and frequently anaplastic endothelial cells (efigs. 10.98 to 10.100). These channels may combine or collapse to form a solid mass in which the differential diagnosis from recurrent carcinoma may be problematic without the use of immunohistochemistry. Angiosarcomas are immunohistochemically stained for factor VIII related antigen and CD34. Progesterone receptor has been reported as being expressed, but estrogen receptor has not. Carcinomas are distinguished by their expression of keratins. Macias-Martinez et al. (76) described an epithelioid variant of angiosarcoma.

Strobbe et al. (77) reported on 21 patients with angiosarcoma that was associated with breast conserving therapy; the patients were diagnosed in the Netherlands between 1987 and 1995. The median interval between radiation and the appearance of angiosarcoma was 74 months, with a range of 29 to 106 months. Detection of skin changes, followed by incisional biopsy, provided the diagnosis in all cases. Overall 2-year survival was 72% and disease-free survival at 2-years was 35%. After initial complete surgical resection, 2-year overall survival was 86%, compared to no survival after incomplete excision. The estimated incidence of angiosarcoma after breast conserving therapy, including radiation, was 0.16%.

Marchal et al. (78) described 9 cases of angiosarcoma among 20,000 patients who were treated with radiation in 11 centers over a period of 20 years. The median latency period between treatment of the breast carcinoma and diagnosis of angiosarcoma was approximately 74 months, with a range of 57 to 108 months. Mastectomy was the primary modality of therapy for the angiosarcoma. The median survival was 15.5 months, with only 1 of 9 patients alive, without progressive disease, at 32 months after salvage mastectomy. The authors reported the prevalence of angiosarcoma as 5 cases per 10,000, which was not different from the prevalence of primary breast angiosarcoma that occurred in nonirradiated breast. However, Cozen et al. (79) found a 59-fold risk of development of upper extremity angiosarcoma after treatment for breast cancer. There was an 11.6-fold risk of angiosarcoma of the chest and breast after treatment for breast cancer. Other sarcomas of the chest and breast had an overall risk of 3.3.

Pendlebury et al. (80) reported that the conserved breast was a likely site of development of sarcoma after a median latency period of 5.5 years. In their review, the authors found that the most frequent sarcoma was osteosarcoma of the scapula. The overall frequency of radiation-induced sarcoma at 10 years of follow-up was 0.2%.

Fineberg and Rosen (81) described three patients with cutaneous angiosarcoma and four patients with atypical vascular lesions after breast conserving surgery, axillary lymph node dissection, and radiation therapy for breast carcinoma. The three angiosarcomas, located mainly in the dermis, were multifocal or diffuse and of high grade, with solid cellular foci. These tumors developed at 3.5, 3.7, and 5.25 years after radiotherapy. Patients with atypical vascular lesions had not developed angiosarcoma or recurrent mammary carcinoma.

METASTASES TO THE BREAST

Metastases from carcinomas and sarcomas of the breast are all too common, but it is rare to find metastases from another primary tumor to the breast. When they occur, the primary tumor is known in nearly all cases. DiBonito et al. (82) reported on 12 cases of metastases to the breast that were studied at autopsy. The authors found that cutaneous melanoma was the most common and the most difficult to diagnose in the absence of a known primary tumor. The authors also found metastases from carcinomas of the ovary, kidney, stomach, lung, and pancreas. Laifer et al. (83) reviewed the literature on metastases to the breast from ovarian epithelial tumors. Metastases to the breast from the prostate were considered to be a diagnostic problem (84); however, such metastasis rarely occurs and it can usually be diagnosed accurately with the aid of immunohistochemical staining for prostate-specific antigen.

LYMPHOMA

Primary lymphomas of the breast are rarely seen and, when they are, their clinical presentation is as a mass lesion that is indistinguishable from other breast masses clinically. Primary lymphomas are distinguished from secondary lymphomas on the basis of the site of first diagnosis. Breast lymphomas are considered primary only if the lymphoma is restricted to the breast and axillary lymph nodes at the time of diagnosis. Two types were reported by Bobrow et al. (85) in their review of the literature: (a) an unusual Burkitt-type lymphoma seen in younger women as a rapidly progressive malignancy, often presenting bilaterally during lactation and (b) the more commonly seen, slowly progressive B-cell lymphoma, presenting unilaterally in older women (Figs. 10.49 and 10.50 and efigs. 10.102 and 10.103). (Efig. 10.104 is an angiotropic malignant lymphoma diagnosed in breast tissues incidental to a benign lesion.) The authors also reported one case of a true histiocytic lymphoma.

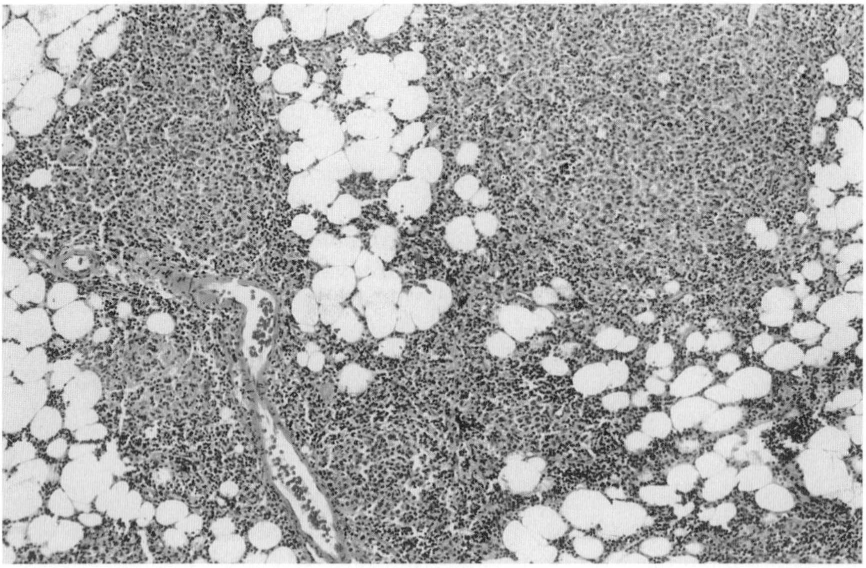

FIG. 10.49. Malignant lymphoma. The lymphoma infiltrates the stroma of the breast and surrounding epithelial and vascular structures.

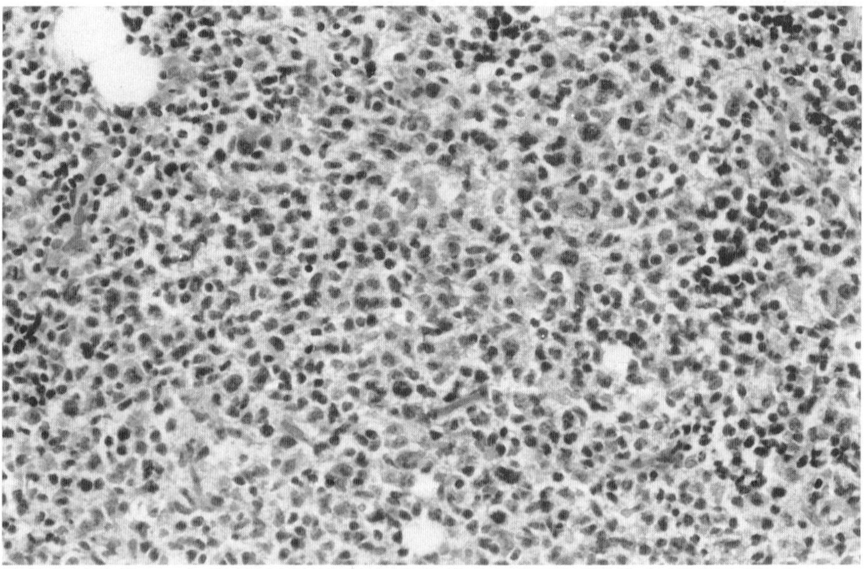

FIG. 10.50. Lymphoma. The cells are small noncleaved lymphocytes that are shown to be a B-cell phenotype. Differential diagnosis includes pseudolymphoma (to be ruled out with studies for clonality), secondary lymphoma (to be excluded by history and clinical studies), and invasive lobular carcinoma (to be ruled out by immunostains for epithelial markers).

There is a difference in the composition of cases reported in the various series of this rare lesion. Mattia et al. (86) reported on nine cases of primary lymphoma, all of which were B-cell lymphomas. Four cases had features of having arisen in mucosa-associated lymphoid tissue (MALT), evident as lymphoepithelial lesions. Three cases were free of disease, but one case progressed to immunoblastic lymphoma and was fatal. Three of four follicular lymphomas were fatal, and a small noncleaved-cell lymphoma was fatal at 31 months. Twenty-two systemic lymphomas also involved the breast; only one of them was of T-cell differentiation. Aozasa et al. (87) reported 19 cases from Japan in which the most common type of primary breast lymphoma was a diffuse large-cell type, with MALT lymphomas accounting for most of the rest. Jeon et al. (88) reported on 152 cases from Japan, all of which were B-cell lymphomas. Most of the B-cell lymphomas were of intermediate to high grade; none of them were MALT lymphomas. Arber et al. (89) reported on 41 primary breast lymphomas that had a high incidence of B-cell phenotype of intermediate to high grade, which was also found in the 20 lymphomas that secondarily involved the breast. The authors were unable to differentiate primary from secondary lymphomas in their studies. Cohen and Brooks (90) reported on 16 primary lymphomas and 18 secondary lymphomas, with a predominance of diffuse large-cell lymphoma. All were B-cell type, except for one T-cell lymphoma. Lymphoepithelial lesions and vascular invasion were found in both primary and secondary lymphomas. Topalovski et al. (91) reported on 22 cases of breast lymphomas, with diffuse large B-cell morphology the most common type. Primary and secondary lymphomas were seen with equal frequency.

Windrum et al. (92) described a mantle cell lymphoma of the breast. Kuper-Hummel et al. (93) reported on a 65-year-old woman who had a 4.5-cm., high-grade MALT-lymphoma that was apparently localized to the breast and treated with radiotherapy. Subsequently, gastric bleeding was shown on biopsy to be due to MALT-lymphoma that was associated with *Helicobacter pylori*. Chemotherapy was given with initial complete response, but it was followed in 6 months by recurrence of lymphoma and death from congestive heart failure. Brogi and Harris (94) recently reviewed the breast lymphoma literature and reported that most were large B-cell lymphomas. The relative incidence of maltomas varied from none to 44% of breast lymphomas in different series, but the consensus was that they had indolent behavior and good prognosis.

FAT NECROSIS

Necrosis of fat in the breast stroma is usually the result of trauma of either an incidental type or the result of a surgical procedure. The release of fat into the tissues elicits an intense macrophage and foreign body reaction that results in granulation tissue formation and eventually scar formation, sometimes with calcification. It may present as a mass (efigs. 10.105 and 10.106) and is histologically seen as reactive foamy macrophages (efig. 10.107).

REACTION TO SILICONE IMPLANTS

Mammary prosthetic implants consist of an envelope, usually composed of silicone elastomer, which contains gel silicone (95). (Silicon is an element that may be combined chemically with oxygen to form a gel, which is used to fill the envelope, or an elastomer, which is used to form the envelope of an implant. It can also be made in a polymer form, which is rigid and has been used in orthopedic prostheses.) The envelope may contain other materials, and the silicone gel may be replaced by saline. Baker et al. (96,97), Barker et al. (98), Bergman and van der Ende (99), and Rudolph et al. (100) reported that silicone gel "bled" through the intact silicone elastomer envelope into the adjacent tissue. The scar, foreign body reaction, and macrophage accumulation around the implant are components of the capsule (efigs. 10.108 to 10.110).

Huang et al. (101) suggested that the "squeeze" technique for breaking up the scar that forms in the capsule around the envelope of the implant might enhance the migration of silicone gel into the tissues. Baker et al. (97), Winding et al. (102), and several other authors (103–106) reported the presence of silicone in tissue around the implant. The authors reported a rough correlation between the amount of silicone present and the reaction in the form of myofibroblasts in the breast tissue. Migration of silicone gel into the tissues is probably enhanced, if the envelope of the implant grossly ruptures. Kasper (107) reported the tissue

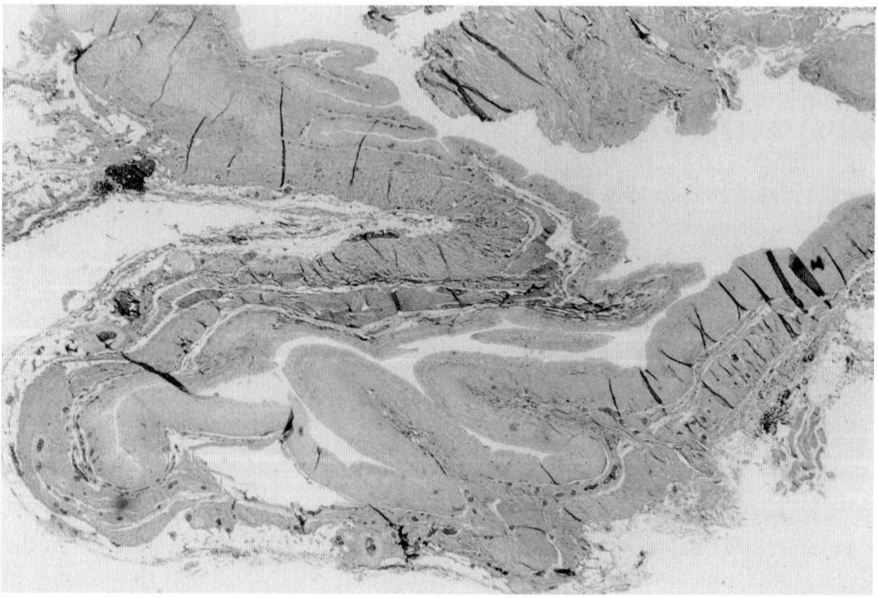

FIG. 10.51. Reaction to silicone implant. The cystic space is surrounded by a striking reaction with three separate zones—central bursal reaction, dense scar and foamy histiocytes. The dense fibrous scar is the most constant and prominent feature.

reaction to implants with a variety of materials in the silicone elastomer envelope. In one case of a silicone envelope that was filled with saline, there was a dense scar at the periphery of the capsule that was indistinguishable from the scar found when silicone gel was in the implant, indicating that the elastomer could provoke scar formation without the presence of gel silicone. Polyurethane also has been used in the envelope of some implants and is found in the dense scar of the tissue capsule that forms adjacent to the implant as a geometric-shaped birefringent material. In some cases, myofibroblasts form a bursal or synovium-like lining of the capsule immediately adjacent to the envelope (108,109). Squamous cell carcinoma at the interface with the envelope has been described by Kitchen et al. (110).

The histologic changes in the capsule are seen in a zonal distribution (Figs. 10.51 to 10.54 and efigs. 10.111 to efig10.117) (111). There is a dense scar and often synovialization immediately adjacent to the envelope of the implant. The scar may contain multinucleated giant cell granulomas in association with foreign material. If the material is refractile and birefringent, it may be polyurethane or some other component of the envelope. Silicone is refractile, but not birefringent. It can be seen off Kohler illumination. Silicone gel has been reported in the scar, but it is seen more often in foamy macrophages that are located outside of the scar in the surrounding breast tissue (Figs. 10.42 and 10.43). Corrin (112) and Hausner et al. (113) have reported silicone gel in axillary lymph nodes in patients with implants.

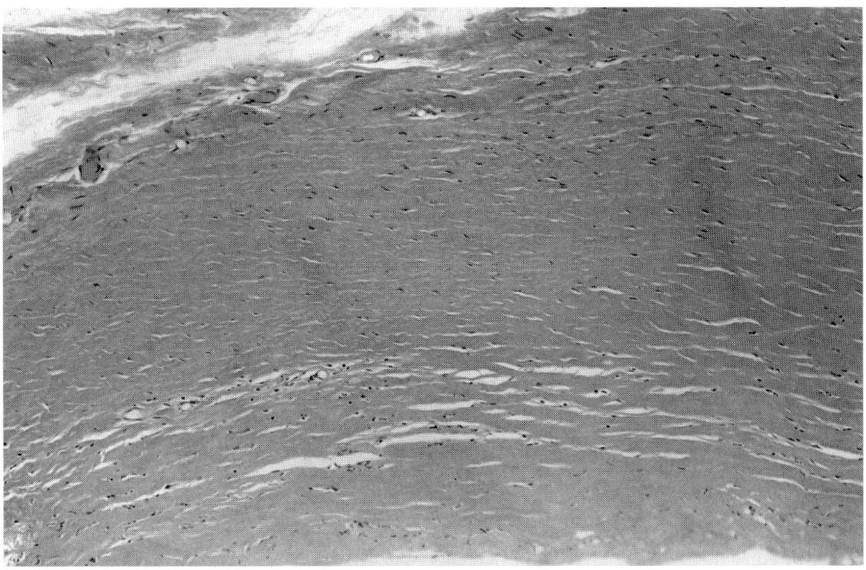

FIG. 10.52. Reaction to silicone implant. Much of the scar around the implant has dense collagen bands, basket-weave configuration, and lack of cellularity, which are similar to a pleural plaque.

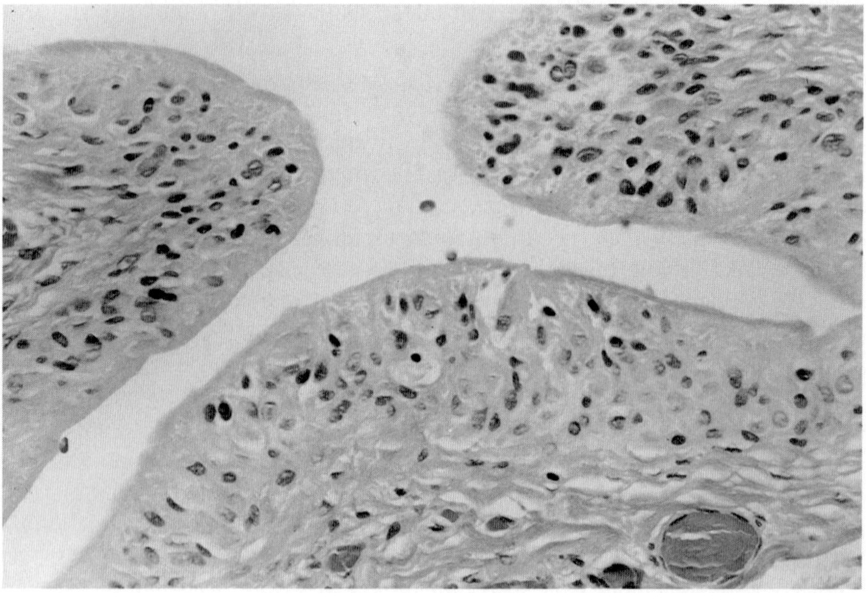

FIG. 10.53. Reaction to silicone implant. On the surface of the scar, toward the implant, myofibroblasts align themselves to produce a synovial or bursal appearance. Rarely, these develop an epithelioid appearance, which is suggestive of carcinoma. This bursal-like change is found in approximately 25% of capsules. Its cause is not known.

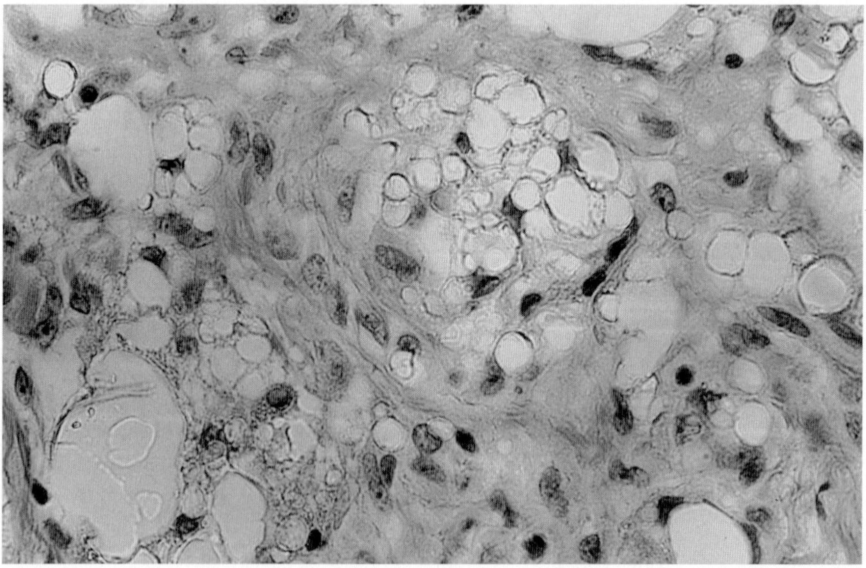

FIG. 10.54. Reaction to silicone implant. When there is abundant silicone in the surrounding tissues, it is ingested by numerous macrophages. The silicone is not birefringent, but refractile, and it is evident at the edge of the vacuoles within the macrophages.

REFERENCES

1. Ansah-Boateng Y, Tavassoli FA. Fibroadenoma and cystosarcoma phyllodes of the male breast. *Mod Pathol* 1992;5:114–116.
2. Cheatle C. Hyperplasia of epithelial and connective tissues in the breast: its relation to fibroadenoma and other conditions. *Br J Surg* 1923;10:436–455.
3. Sawhney N, Garrahan N, Douglas-Jones AG, et al. Epithelial-stromal interactions in tumors: a morphologic study of fibroepithelial tumors of the breast. *Cancer* 1992;70:2115–2120.
4. Anthony S-Y, Leong MB, Meredith DJ. Tubular carcinoma developing within a recurring cytosarcoma phylloides of the breast. *Cancer* 1980;46:1863–1867.
5. Fondo EY, Rosen PP, Fracchia AA, et al. The problem of carcinoma developing in a fibroadenoma: recent experience at Memorial Hospital. *Cancer* 1979;43:563–567.
6. McDivitt RW, Stewart FW, Farrow JH. Breast carcinoma arising in solitary fibroadenomas. *Surg Gynecol Obstet* 1967;125:572–576.
7. Kuijper A, Mommers EC, van der Wall E, et al. Histopathology of fibroadenoma of the breast. *Am J Clin Pathol* 2001;115:736–742.
8. Reddick RL, Shin TK, Sawhney D, et al. Stromal proliferations of the breast: an ultrastructural and immunohistochemical evaluation of cystosarcoma phylloides, juvenile fibroadenoma, and fibroadenoma. *Hum Pathol* 1987;18:45–49.
9. Dupont WD, Page DL, Parl FF, et al. Long-term risk of breast cancer in women with fibroadenoma. *N Engl J Med* 1994;331:10–15.
10. Rosen PP, Oberman HA. *Atlas of tumor pathology*, 3rd series. Washington: Armed Forces Institute of Pathology, 1993.
11. Rix DB, Tredwell JJ, Howard AP. Cystosarcoma phylloides (cellular intracanilicular fibroadenoma)—clinicopathologic relationship. *Can J Surg* 1971;14:31–37.
12. Trives N, Sunderland DA. Cystosarcoma phylloides—a benign and malignant tumor: a clinicopathologic study of 77 cases. *Cancer* 1951;4:1286–1332.
13. Azzopardi J. Problems in breast pathology. Philadelphia: WB Saunders, 1979.
14. El-Naggar A, Ro JY, McLemore D, et al. DNA content and proliferative activity of cystosarcoma phyllodes of the breast: potential prognostic significance. *Am J Clin Path* 1990;93:480–485.
15. Noguchi S, Motomura K, Inaji H, et al. Clonal analysis of fibroadenoma and phyllodes tumor of the breast. *Cancer Res* 1993;53:4071–4074.
16. Dusenbery D, Frable J. Fine needle aspiration of phyllodes tumor. Potential diagnostic pitfalls. *Acta Cytol* 1992;36:215–221.
17. Powell CM, Rosen PP. Adipose differentiation in cystosarcoma phylloses: a study of 14 cases. *Am J Surg Pathol* 1994;18:720–727.
18. Blichert-Taft M. Clinical course of cystosarcoma phylloides related to histologic appearance. *Surg Gynecol Obstet* 1975;140:929.
19. Fernandez BB, Hernandez FJ, Spindler W. Metastatic cystosarcoma phylloides: a light and E-M study. *Cancer* 1976;37:1737–1746.
20. McDivitt RW, Urban JA, Farrow JH. Cystosarcoma phylloides. *Johns Hopkins Med J* 1967;120:33–45.
21. Toker C. Cystosarcoma phylloides—an ultrastructural study. *Cancer* 1968;21:1171.
22. Norris HJ, Taylor HB. Relationship of histologic features to behavior of cystosarcoma phylloides: analysis of 94 cases. *Cancer* 1967;20:2090–2099.
23. Hajdu SI, Espinosa MH, Robbins GF. Recurrent cystosarcoma phyllodes: a clinicopathologic study of 32 cases. *Cancer* 1976;38:1402–1406.
24. Pietruska M, Barnes J. Cystosarcoma phyllodes: a clinicopathologic study of 42 cases. *Cancer* 1978;41:1974–1983.
25. Reinfuss M, Mitus J, Smolak K, et al. Malignant phyllodes tumours of the breast. A clinical and pathological analysis of 55 cases. *Eur J Cancer* 1993;29A:1252–1256.
26. Hawkins R, Schofield J, Fisher C, et al. The clinical and histologic criteria that predict metastases from cystosarcoma phyllodes. *Cancer* 1992;69:141–147.
27. Ward RM, Evans LH. Cystosarcoma phylloides: a clinicopathologic study of 26 cases. *Cancer* 1986;58:2282–2289.
28. Yeh IT, Francis DJ, Orenstein JM, et al. Ultrastructure of cystosarcoma phyllodes and fibroadenoma. A comparative study. *Am J Clin Pathol* 1985;84:131–136.
29. Austin RM, Dupree WB. Liposarcoma of the breast: a clinicopathologi study of 20 cases. *Hum Pathol* 1986;17:906–913.

30. Barnes L, Peitruska M. Sarcomas of the breast: a clinicopathologic analysis of 10 cases. *Cancer* 1977;40:1577–1585.
31. Berg JW, DeCosse JJ, Fracchia AA, et al. Stromal sarcomas of the breast. *Cancer* 1962;15:418.
32. Mittall KR, Gerald W, True L. Hemangiopericytoma of breast: report of a case with ultrastructural and immunohistochemical findings. *Hum Pathol* 1986;17:1181–1183.
33. Mufarrij AA, Feiner HD. Breast sarcoma with giant cells and osteoid. A case report and review of the literature. *Am J Surg Pathol* 1987;11:225–230.
34. Norris HJ, Taylor HB. Sarcomas and related mesenchymal tumors of the breast. *Cancer* 1968;22: 22–28.
35. Tavassoli FA, Weiss S. Hemangiopericytoma of the breast. *Am J Surg Pathol* 1982;5:745–752.
36. Christensen L, Schiodt T, Blichert-Toft M. Sarcomatoid tumors of the breast in Denmark from 1977 to 1987. A clinicopathologic and immunohistochemical study. *Eur J Cancer* 1993;29A:1824–1831.
37. Linell F, Ostberg G, Soderstrom J, et al. Breast hamartomas. An important entity in mammary pathology. *Virchows Arch* 1979;383:253–264.
38. Jones MW, Norris HJ, Wargotz ES. Hamartomas of the breast. *Surg Gynecol Obstet* 1991;173: 54–56.
39. Charpin C, Mathoulin MP, Andrac L, et al. Reappraisal of breast hamartomas. A morphological study of 41 cases. *Pathol Res Pract* 1994;190:362–71.
40. Daya D, Trus T, D'Souza TJ, et al. Hamartoma of the breast, an underrecognized breast lesion: a clinicopathologic and radiographic study of 25 cases. *Am J Clin Pathol* 1995;103:685–689.
41. Gump FE, Sternschein MJ, Wolff M. Fibromatosis of the breast. *Surg Gynecol Obstet* 1981;153: 57–60.
42. Pettinato G, Manivel JC, Gould EW, et al. Inclusion body fibromatosis of the breast: two cases with immunohistochemical and ultrastructural findings. *Am J Clin Pathol* 1994;101:714–718.
43. Rasbridge S, Gillett CE, Millis RR. Oestrogen and progesterone receptor expression in mammary fibromatosis. *J Clin Pathol* 1993;46:349–351.
44. Devouassoux-Shisheboran M, Schammel MD, Man YG, et al. Fibromatosis of the breast: age-correlated morphofunctional features of 33 cases. *Arch Pathol Lab Med* 2000;124:276–280.
45. Wargotz E, Weiss S, Norris H. Myofibroblastoma of the breast: 16 cases of a distinctive benign mesenchymal tumor. *Am J Surg Pathol* 1987;11:493–502.
46. Diaz-Arias A, Hurt M, Loy T, et al. Leiomyoma of the breast. *Hum Pathol* 1989;20:396–399.
47. Kotsuma Y, Wakasa K, Yayoi E, et al. A case of leiomyoma of the breast. *Breast Cancer* 2001;8: 166–169.
48. Rosen PP, Jozefczyk MA, Boram IH. Vascular tumors of the breast. IV. The venous hemangioma. *Am J Surg Pathol* 1985;9:659–665.
49. Jozefczyk MA, Rosen PP. Vascular tumors of the breast. II. Perilobular hemangiomas and hemangiomas. *Am J Surg Pathol* 1985;9:491–503.
50. Rosen PP. Vascular tumors of the breast. III. Angiomatosis. *Am J Surg Pathol* 1985;9:652–658.
51. Morrow M, Berger D, Thelmo W. Diffuse cystic angiomatosis of the breast. *Cancer* 1988;62: 2392–2396.
52. Rosen PP. Vascular tumors of the breast. V. Nonparenchymal hemangiomas of mammary subcutaneous tissue. *Am J Surg Pathol* 1985;9:723–729.
53. Vuitch MF, Rosen PP, Erlandson RA. Pseudoangiomatous hyperplasia of mammary stroma. *Hum Pathol* 1986;17:185–191.
54. Powell CM, Cranor ML, Rosen PP. Pseudoangiomatous stromal hyperplasia (PASH): a mammary stromal tumor with myofibroblastic differentiation. *Am J Surg Pathol* 1995;19:270–277.
55. Chen KT, Kirkegaard DD, Bocian JJ. Angiosarcoma of the breast. *Cancer* 1980;46:368–371.
56. Donnell RM, Rosen PP, Lieberman PH, et al. Angiosarcoma and other vascular tumors of the breast. *Am J Surg Pathol* 1981;5:629–642.
57. Merino MJ, Carter D, Berman M. Angiosarcoma of the breast. *Am J Surg Pathol* 1983;7:53–60.
58. Antman KH, Corson J, Greenberger J, et al. Multimodality therapy in the management of angiosarcoma of the breast. *Cancer* 1982;50:2000–2003.
59. Rosen PP, Kimmel M, Ernsberger D. Mammary angiosarcoma: the prognostic significance of tumor differentiation. *Cancer* 1988;62:2145–2152.
60. Alles JU, Bosslet K. Immunocytochemistry of angiosarcomas: a study of 19 cases with special emphasis on the application of endothelial cell specific markers to routinely prepared tissues. *Am J Clin Pathol* 1988;89:463–471.
61. Rosen PP, Rudolfi RL. The perilobular hemangioma: a benign microscopic vascular lesion of the breast. *Am J Clin Pathol* 1977;68:21.

62. Stewart FW, Treves N. Lymphangiosarcoma in postmastectomy lymphedema. *Cancer* 1948;1:64–81.
63. Eby CS, Brennan MJ, Fine G. Lymphangiosarcoma: a lethal complication of chronic lymphedema. *Arch Surg* 1967;94:223.
64. Friederici HH, Roberts SS. The fine structure of two postmastectomy angiosarcomas. *Lab Invest* 1967;16:644.
65. Govoni E, Pileri S, Bazzocchi F, et al. Postmastectomy angiosarcoma: ultrastructural study of a case. *Tumori* 1981;67:79–86.
66. Hilfinger MF, Eberle RD. Lymphangiosarcoma in postmastectomy lymphedema. *Cancer* 1953;6: 1192.
67. Miettinen M, Lehto V, Virtanen I. Postmastectomy angiosarcoma (Stewart–Treves syndrome): light-microscopic, immunohistological, and ultrastructural characteristics of two cases. *Am J Surg Pathol* 1983;7:329–339.
68. Nemoto T, Stubbe N, Gata J, et al. Pathogenesis of lymphangiosarcoma following mastectomy and irradiation. *Surg Gynecol Obstet* 1969;128:489.
69. Schreiber H, Barry FM, Russell WL, et al. Stewart–Treves syndrome. *Arch Surg* 1979;114:82–85.
70. Silverberg SG, Kay S, Koss LG. Postmastectomy lymphangiosarcoma: ultrastructural observations. *Cancer* 1971;27:100.
71. Gray G. Angiosarcoma in lymphedema: an unusual case of Stewart–Treves Syndrome. *Bull Johns Hopkins Hosp* 1966;119:117.
72. Towsell HF, Soule EF, Coventry MB. Lymphangiosarcoma in chronic lymphedematous extremities—report of 13 cases and review of the literature. *J Bone Joint Surg Am* 1962;44:277.
73. Woodward AH, Ivans JC, Soule EH. Lymphangiosarcoma arising in chronic lymphedematous extremities. *Cancer* 1972;30:562.
74. Salm R. The nature of the so-called postmastectomy lymphangiosarcoma. *J Pathol Bacteriol* 1968; 85:445–446.
75. Capo V, Ozzello L, Fenoglio CM, et al. Angiosarcomas arising in edematous extremities: immunostaining for factor VIII-related antigen and ultrastructural features. *Hum Pathol* 1985;16:144–150.
76. Macias-Martinez V, Murrieta-Tiburcio L, Molina-Cardenas H, et al. Epithelioid angiosarcoma of the breast. Clinicopathological, immunohistochemical, and ultrastructural study of a case. *Am J Surg Pathol* 1997;21:599–604.
77. Strobbe LJ, Peterse HL, van Tinteren H, et al. Angiosarcoma of the breast after conservation therapy for invasive cancer, the incidence and outcome. An unforeseen sequela. *Breast Cancer Res Treat* 1998;47:101–109.
78. Marchal C, Weber B, de Lafontan B, et al. Nine breast angiosarcomas after conservative treatment for breast carcinoma: a survey from French comprehensive Cancer Centers. *Int J Radiat Oncol Biol Phys* 1999;44:113–119.
79. Cozen W, Bernstein L, Wang F, et al. The risk of angiosarcoma following primary breast cancer. *Br J Cancer* 1999;81:532–536.
80. Pendlebury SC, Bilous M, Langlands AO. Sarcomas following radiation therapy for breast cancer: a report of three cases and a review of the literature. *Int J Radiat Oncol Biol Phys* 1995;31:405–410.
81. Fineberg S, Rosen PP. Cutaneous angiosarcoma and atypical vascular lesions of the skin and breast after radiation therapy for breast carcinoma. *Am J Clin Pathol* 1994;102:757–763.
82. DiBonito L, Luchi M, Giarelli L, et al. Metastatic tumors to the female breast. An autopsy study of 12 cases. *Pathol Res Pract* 1991;187:432–436.
83. Laifer S, Buscema J, Parmley TH, et al. Ovarian cancer metastatic to the breast. *Gynecol Oncol* 1986;24:97–102.
84. Salyer WR, Salyer DC. Metastases of prostatic carcinoma to the breast. *J Urol* 1973;109:671–675.
85. Bobrow LG, Richards MA, Happerfield LC, et al. Breast lymphomas: a clinicopathologic review. *Hum Pathol* 1993;24:274–278.
86. Mattia A, Ferry JA, Harris NL. Breast lymphoma. A B-cell spectrum including the low grade B-cell lymphoma of mucosa associated lymphoid tissue. *Am J Surg Pathol* 1993;17:574–587.
87. Aozasa K, Ohsawa M, Saeki K, et al. Malignant lymphoma of the breast: immunologic type and association with lymphocytic mastopathy. *Am J Clin Pathol* 1992;97:699–704.
88. Jeon HJ, Akagi T, Hoshida Y. Primary malignant lymphoma of the breast. Lymphoma of the mucosa-associated lymphoid tissue. *Cancer* 1992;60:3033–3041.
89. Arber DA, Simpson JF, Weiss LM, et al. Non-Hodgkin's lymphoma involving the breast. *Am J Surg Pathol* 1994;18:288–295.
90. Cohen PL, Brooks JJ. Lymphomas of the breast—a clinicopathologic and immunohistochemical study of primary and secondary cases. *Cancer* 1991;67:1359–1369.

91. Topalovski M, Crisan D, Mattson J. Lymphoma of the breast: a clinicopathologic study of primary and secondary cases. *Arch Pathol Lab Med* 1999;123:1208–1218.
92. Windrum P, Morris T, Catherwood M, et al. Mantle cell lymphoma presenting as a breast mass. *J Clin Pathol* 2001;54:883–886.
93. Kuper-Hummel MJJ, Vrints W, Coebergh W, et al. High grade MALT-lymphoma of the breast. *Netherlands J Med* 1999;54:235–38.
94. Brogi E, Harris N. Lymphomas of the breast: pathology and clinical behavior. *Semin Oncol* 1999; 26:357–364.
95. Travis WM, Balogh K, Abraham JL. Silicone granulomas: report of three cases and review of the literature. *Hum Pathol* 1985;16:19–27.
96. Baker JL, Chandler ML, LeVier RR. Occurrence and activity of myofibroblasts in human capsular tissue surrounding mammary implants. *Plast Reconstr Surg* 1981;68:905.
97. Baker JL, LeVier RR, Spielvogel DE. Positive identification of silicone in human mammary capsular tissue. *Plast Reconstr Surg* 1982;69:56.
98. Barker DE, Retsky MI, Schultz S. "Bleeding" of silicone from bag-gel breast implants and its clinical relation to fibrous capsule reaction. *Plast Reconstr Surg* 1978;61:836.
99. Bergman RB, van der Ende AE. Exudation of silicone through the envelope of gel-filled breast prostheses: an *in vitro* study. *Br J Plast Surg* 1979;32:31.
100. Rudolph R, Abraham JL, et al. Myofibroblasts and free silicone around breast implants. *Plast Reconstr Surg* 1978;62:185.
101. Huang TT, Blackwell SJ, et al. Migration of silicone gel after the "squeeze technique" to rupture a contracted breast capsule. *Plast Reconstr Surg* 1978;61:277.
102. Winding O, Christensen L, Thomsen JL, et al. Silicone in human breast tissue surrounding silicone gel prosthesis: a scanning electron microscopy and energy dispersive x-ray investigation of normal, fibrocystic and peri-prosthetic breast tissue. *Scand J Plast Reconstr Surg* 1988;22:127–130.
103. Gayou RM. A histologic comparison of contracted and non-contracted capsules around silicone breast implants. *Plast Reconstr Surg* 1979;63:700.
104. Hardt NS, Yu L, LaTore G, et al. Complications related to retained breast implant capsules. *Plast Reconstr Surg* 1994;95:364–371.
105. Thomsen JL, Christensen L, Nielsen M. Histologic changes and silicone concentrations in human breast tissue surrounding silicone breast prostheses. *Plast Reconstr Surg* 1990;85:38–41.
106. Wickham MG, Rudolph R, Abraham JL. Silicone identification in prosthesis associated fibrous capsules. *Science* 1978;199:437.
107. Kasper CS. Histologic features of breast capsules reflect surface configuration and composition of silicone bag implants. *Am J Clin Pathol* 1994;102:655–659.
108. Emery JA, Spanier SS, Kasnic G Jr, et al. The synovial structure of breast-implant-associated bursae. *Mod Pathol* 1995;7:728–733.
109. Hameed MR, Erlandson R, Rosen PP. Capsular synovial-like hyperplasia around mammary implants similar to detritic synovitis: a morphologic and immunohistochemical study of 15 cases. *Am J Surg Pathol* 1995;19:433–438.
110. Kitchen SB, Paletta CE, Shehadi SI, et al. Epithelialization of the lining of a breast implant capsule: possible origin of squamous cell carcinoma associated with a breast implant capsule. *Cancer* 1994; 73:1449–1452.
111. Carter D. Tissue reaction to breast implants. *Am J Clin Pathol* 1994;102:565–566.
112. Corrin B. Silicone lymphadenopathy. *J Clin Pathol* 1982;35:901.
113. Hausner RJ, Schoen FJ, Mendez-Fernandez MA. Migration of silicone gel to axillary lymph nodes after prosthetic mammoplasty. *Arch Pathol Lab Med* 1981;105:371.

Appendix

The 6th Edition of the AJCC classification scheme (AJCC CANCER STAGING MANUAL, 6th Edition, Springer, New York, 2002) has some differences from the currently used 5th Edition in the definitions of the node status that are shown in the chart below. Lymph node staging can now be done with 6 lymph nodes in an axillary dissection or by sentinel lymph node(s). Cancerous nodules in axillary breast fat are classified as lymph node metastases. Additional sub-designations added to nodal sstatus include (sn) for sentinel lymph node, I+ or - for positivity or negativity by immunoperoxidase stain only, and mol+ or - for data derived by RT-PCR.

	AJCC 5th Edition	AJCC 6th Edition
PNX	Unknown	Same
pN0	No metastases	Same
	<=2 mm	<=0.2mm
		mol+/- only
pN1mi		.0.2mm<0.2cm
pN1a	<=0.2cm	>0.2cm, 1 to 3 +ALN
pN1b	>0.2cm	IMLN (sn)
pN1bi	1 to 3 +ALN, any>0.2cm, all<2cm	
pN1bii	>=4+ALN, any>0.2cm, all<2 cm	
pN1biii	Tumor beyond node capsule	
pN1biv	ALN+ and >= 2cm	
pN1c		ALN 1 to 3 + and IMLN (sn)
pN2	Matted Ipsilateral ALN	4 to 9 ALN +
		or clinically + IMLN with ALN -
pN2a		4 to 9 + ALN
pN2b		IMLN+,ALN-
pN3	+ I IMLN	ALN >=10 +
		or clinically + IMLN with >1ALN +
		or >3 ALN + with microscopically + IMLN
		or ipsilateral supraclavicular LN +
pN3a		>= 10 ALN +
		or infraclavicular LN +
pN3b		Clinically + IMLN with +ALN
		or 3 + ALN with microscopic IMLN + (sn)
pN3c		Ipsilateral Supraclavicular LN +

A, axillary; LN, lymph node; IM, internal mammary; I, Ipsilateral

In both the 5th and 6th editions, staging categories 0, I, IIA, IIB, IIIA, and IV are identical, but IIIB and IIC are slightly different (see chart below).

Stage	**AJCC 5th Edition**	**AJCC 6th Edition**
IIIB	T4 any N M0 any T N3 M0	T 4 N0 MO T4 N1 M0 T4 N2 M0
IIIC		any T N3 M0

Subject Index

Note: Page numbers followed by f indicate figures; those followed by t indicate tables.